The Lips –
45 Injection Techniques
for Esthetic Lip Treatment

The German National Library (Deutsche Nationalbibliothek, DNB) has listed this publication in its Deutsche Nationalbibliografie database; detailed bibliographic data may be found on the internet at *http://dnb.d-nb.de*

Publisher's address:
KVM – Der Medizinverlag
Dr. Kolster Verlags-GmbH
Ifenpfad 2–4
12107 Berlin

Authors' addresses:
Regine Reymond
Urs Graf-Strasse 1
4052 Basel, Switzerland
hello@regine-reymond.ch
www.regine-reymond.ch
www.easinject.ch

Dr. med. Christian Köhler
PREVENTION-CENTER AG
UTOSCHLOSS
Utoquai 31
8008 Zürich, Switzerland
c.koehler@prevention-center.ch
www.prevention-center.com

www.kvm-medizinverlag.de

1st edition, 2021

Project management: Sonia A. Piskorowska
Photos: Martin Frick (www.martinfrick-photographie.de), Lörrach-Brombach
Graphics: David Kühn, Berlin
Anatomical drawings: Karl H. Wesker, Berlin
Layout and typesetting: Petra Jentschke, Berlin
Overall production: KVM – Der Medizinverlag, Berlin
Printed by: GZH d.o.o. (www.gzh.hr), Zagreb
Printed in Croatia

ISBN: 978-1-78698-109-7

Important notes:

Like every other science, medicine is subject to constant development. Research and clinical experience widen our knowledge base. For all the treatment recommendations covered in this book, the reader can be confident that the authors, editors, and publishers have taken great care to ensure that the information provided is in line with the latest knowledge available at the time of publication.

Furthermore, the publisher cannot give guarantees for any information regarding administration methods, techniques, and frequencies. All users are requested to take great care to check the package insert leaflets of the products used and to establish, if necessary by consulting a specialist, whether the dosage recommendations or details of contraindications given therein differ in any way from the information given in this book. This type of check is particularly important with rare indications and locations as well as with rarely used or recently launched products.

Every treatment takes place at the user's own risk. The authors and publisher appeal to all users to inform them if they spot any obvious inaccuracies.

The Lips –
45 Injection Techniques for Esthetic Lip Treatment

Regine Reymond
Christian Köhler

K|V|M

About the authors

Regine Reymond, alternative practitioner, pharmaceutical representative, and co-owner of the company "easinject" is an expert in the area of esthetic lip treatment with hyaluronic acid (fillers). Based on her professional activities, she is able to demonstrate almost 20 years of expertise in the use of minimally invasive injection techniques. Having partially completed a university course in medicine, she worked as a marketing manager for international pharmaceutical companies for several years; since then, she has either organized or personally led more than 150 workshops, seminars, and symposia on the topic of filler techniques.

Dr. med. Christian Köhler is an expert in esthetic surgery, non-surgical techniques, and esthetic laser treatments. For more than 10 years, he has been heading up the Prevention Center in Zürich, Zug and Schaan, Switzerland. His specialist areas include procedures such as breast augmentation, eyelid tightening, and facelifts. Dr. Köhler has more than 18 years of hands-on experience in general, vascular, reconstructive, and plastic surgery. To date, he has also performed more than 50,000 non-surgical treatments with botulinum toxin and fillers.

Dear colleagues

The perfect, beautifully shaped mouth, with its soft fullness and healthy blush, really does exist: it is the mouth of a child. The childish mouth with its pouting lips has a direct, disarming effect on adults, triggering a protective instinct. In the adult face, this type of mouth takes on the attribute of sensuality – which is the desired effect in any lip treatment using minimally invasive procedures.

A beautiful mouth has a rather magical quality. It can have a positive effect on an individual's appearance and charisma, even where the proportions of the face are not entirely harmonious. Nevertheless, every mouth has its own natural shape, and this shape is subjected to highly individual mimic activity. With increasing age, this mimic activity influences not only the expression of the lips, but also the expression of the face as a whole, so that the emotional traces of a lifetime can supposedly be read on a person's face.

Since the lips are in constant, three-dimensional movement, which changes their shape and thereby affects overall facial expression, it is a huge challenge to shape or augment the lips with filler injections. Mistakes can be made here, and these become obvious even if they involve only the tiniest deviations or areas of asymmetry. More than one injection technique will be needed to reshape the lips. Even if we can say exactly how much of any particular material needs to be placed at a specific location on the lip, we can be certain that this will produce different results in each individual. There is no universal treatment regimen. Instead, we have multiple technical options at our disposal, and their use must always be preceded by a profound analysis and good communication with the patient. The better the interaction of these factors, the more likely a successful result will be achieved.

During my early professional days in esthetic medicine in 2001, the lips were injected using two techniques: the contours were always treated first, followed by subtle linear filling starting from the mouth corners. Plumped lips were not in fashion, and imperfections were not yet being corrected. It is incredible to see how rapidly these techniques have been evolving over the years, and how this trend is now generating an enormous demand for treatment. However, this also demonstrates the vital and changing nature of esthetic work, and shows that a dedicated and experienced therapist can never stop adopting innovations or learning and perfecting new refinements.

Injection treatment of the lips remains a challenge, even for highly experienced therapists, since the mouth does not tolerate errors. Since lips are so well-perfused, they swell quickly, which can cause complications. The patient's wishes represent an additional challenge of lip treatment, and one which must never be underestimated. Unfortunately, what a patient wants is often shaped by unrealistic expectations or extreme fashion trends. As a therapist, you may end up with a moral conflict and a dissatisfied patient, detracting from the enjoyment you derive from your work.

Some two years ago, the idea occurred to document the knowledge I had amassed over the past 20 years in workshops, international training events, conferences, and online professional development courses, with the aim of sharing this knowledge with my colleagues. Numerous conversations with eminent authorities of injection treatment, extensive research, the active support of my friends and family, and the motivation provided by the publisher, KVM, encouraged me to translate my idea into action. I have neither invented nor changed the techniques presented here. The knowledge comes from various trainers, educators, speakers, and doctors working in esthetic medicine, and shows different approaches and directions. I have collected and categorized all the techniques presented in this book for quality and feasibility, optimizing some of them, and have done so in constant dialogue and close cooperation with my co-author, Dr. Christian Köhler. The aim was to produce a practical manual about injection techniques for use in the lip region, to be applied as required or according to preference.

The various problem-solving approaches form the focus of this book, which also strives to optimize the finer points of injecting the lips with fillers; all this is presented under the aspect of realistic working practices. In this respect, we have created a matrix that can be used as a guide to match up the indications most commonly occurring at esthetic practices to the recommended techniques. However, this does not mean that therapists should reduce their skills to this matrix – on the contrary, the many different approaches shown here will allow therapists to broaden their own ranges and creatively elaborate the finer points of the treatment, perhaps even developing some of the techniques further. The recommendations on filler volumes to be injected are based on average practice-based figures in Central Europe. These values will vary according to regional beauty preferences or trends.

In the main, we have refrained from the use of before/after images, since these can easily lead to expectations that may not necessarily relate to the individual face being treated.

Dr. Christian Köhler, MD has demonstrated the techniques on models in video recordings. These are available to you as additional visual aids via the QR codes included in the book, which are a valuable add-on to the information on the various injection techniques described in the text. I would like to extend my warm thanks to Dr. Köhler and his team for their wonderful, highly positive collaboration as well as for the superb quality of the injection procedures depicted.

A further word on the 45 filler injection techniques that are presented here and form the core of this book: for each of these techniques, the images and videos of the lip treatment procedure are supplemented with details of the technique, the direction of needle insertion, skin layer, material and volume, type of injection needle, and anesthesia. All of these particulars are in line with our recommendations and experience-based values, but they should not be seen as requirements set in stone. In addition, each technique includes a "Treatment protocol" box with a key points summary of the technique as well as an "Important notes" box, which also lists the possible and undesirable side effects for each treatment technique. These may occur at varying severity in most lip injection procedures and need to be borne in mind: the principal side effects include asymmetries, inflammation, hematomas, nodules, necrosis, reddening, pain, swellings, and overcorrection. These two text boxes, which inherently contain repetitions, should provide a useful reminder of all the key aspects of the lip treatment for each individual technique.

This book is aimed at medical doctors and licensed therapists with experience of filler injection treatment. The endorsement and use of the demonstrated techniques remain the responsibility of the individual therapist conducting the treatment. It is important to remember that each lip is unique, and that no hard and fast formulae exist: the use of any of the presented techniques must be preceded by an assessment and by the therapist's decision, made in agreement with the patient, regarding when and to what extent a particular technique can be used in that patient.

Acknowledgments

Many people have provided me with their active and passive support in the form of their studies and publications. In this respect, I would like to extend particular thanks to Dr. Tom van Eijk, Dr. Daniel Brusco MD, Dr. Niklas Iblher MD, Prof. Vincenzo Penna MD, Prof. Björn G. Stark, Dr. Petra Becker-Wegerich MD, Dr. Philippe Snozzi MD, Dr. James Bouzoukis, Dr. Phillip Chang, Dr. Anil Rajani, Dr. Polsak Worakrai, and Zita Hesse. My warm thanks also go to all of those who have given their kind permission to publish their images.

Particular credit needs to be given to the graphic representations in this book. With admirable patience, David Kühn from KVM has provided outstanding depictions of every detail. This has made it possible to illustrate the various points described in the book, making them clear and easy to understand. The photographic services of Martin Frick and the filming by Andreas Grabherr also provide vivid visualizations of descriptions given in the text, closing any remaining gaps in the written material. My warmest thanks go to them for doing this!

Last but not least, my thanks go to my dear husband, Dr. Jean François Reymond MD; with his clear head and constructive criticisms, he was a valuable though strict mentor, and helped me to make the procedures comprehensible even for less experienced therapists.

I wish my readers not only professional and practical gain, but also enjoyment in reading this volume. In addition, I hope it will stimulate you to question familiar and established practices and to try new ones, and thereby to advance your continued professional development. In doing so, you might have the same experience as I did, having discovered three additional, relevant techniques after the press deadline for this book. I look forward to your feedback. Should you be aware of any techniques that have won you over but are not described herein, I would be pleased to include these, once tried and tested, in the next edition.

Basel, October 2021
Regine Reymond

Table of Contents

The following abbreviations are used in this book:

Medical abbreviations

	Sharp needle
	Blunt cannula
▲	Viscous (HA material)
●	Soft (HA material)
Ala	Attachment point of the wing of the nose
AN	Tip of the nose (apex nasi)
B′	Soft tissue B-point (the deepest point of the labiomental fold)
BDDE	Butanediol diglycidyl ether
C	Cervical point (junction of the submental and neck contours, neck–throat junction)
Cm	Columella nasi (fleshy external end of the nasal septum)
CPM	Cohesive polydense matrix
DCLT	Dynamic cross-linking technology
DN	Dorsum nasi (bridge of the nose)
Gl	Glabella (skin of the forehead between the eyebrows)
HA	Hyaluronic acid
Li	Labiale inferius (foremost edge of the lower lip)
LL	Lower lip
Ls	Labiale superius (foremost edge of the upper lip)
Me′	Soft tissue menton (the most inferior point on the soft tissue of the chin)
N′	Soft tissue nasion
NASHA	Non-animal stabilized HA
Or′	Soft tissue orbitale
Pg′	Soft tissue pogonion
Ph	Philtrum
PL	Perioral zone of the lower lip
Pn	Pronasale
Por	Porion (external auditory meatus)
PU	Perioral zone of the upper lip
RHA	Resilient hyaluronic acid
SMART	Supreme monophasic and reticulated technology
SMAS	Superficial musculoaponeurotic system
Sn	Subnasale
St	Stomion (oral fissure when the lips are closed)
Trg	Tragus
Tri	Trichion (hairline)
TWN	Thin wall needle
UL	Upper lip
UTWN	Ultrathin wall needle

Editorial abbreviations

c.	Circa (approximately)
cf.	Confer/conferatur (compare with)
e.g.	Exempli gratia (for example)
et al.	Et alteri (and others)
etc.	Et cetera (and so on)
i.e.	Id est (that is)
f.	And the following page
ff.	And the following pages
Fig.	Figure
max.	Maximum
n.d.	No date
No.	Number
p/pp	Page/pages
Syn.	Synonym
Tab.	Table

Units of measurement

%	Percent
°	Degrees
G	Gauge
g	Grams
L	HA particle size for a thick material with lifting capacity
M	HA particle size for a material of medium thickness with lifting capacity
mg	Milligrams
ml	Milliliters
S	HA particle size for a material with weak lifting capacity
XL	HA size for a very thick material with strong lifting capacity
XS	HA particle size for a thin material with no lifting capacity

1 The Lips

1 The Lips

1.1 Beauty

Regardless of era or culture, the lips always play a key role as a feature of beauty. Full, mobile, well-perfused, moist red lips are associated with youthfulness, health, sensuality, and the sexual attractiveness that goes with them. A full mouth is generally seen as an ideal of beauty and attracts attention to itself – and this has been the case since time immemorial.

This begs the question of a neutral evaluation of lip beauty that is not dependent on fashion. A pertinent investigation was reported in the "JAMA Facial Plastic Surgery" study by the surgical team headed by Natalie Popenko (University of California, Irvine), in which USA researchers showed portraits of pale-skinned women to 580 subjects. Lip shape, the ratio of upper lip to lower lip (UL : LL), and the size of the lip surface relative to the lower third of the face were altered in these portraits. The UL : LL ratio of 1 : 2 was assessed as the most attractive, with the highest mean and highest proportion of "most attractive" placings, while the UL : LL ratio of 2 : 1 was rated as the least attractive.

However, it is particularly in the current age of selfies, taken by the million and posted on Instagram with a prominent pout, that extreme lip augmentation has gained in significance – regardless of whether this lip shape fits harmoniously into the face.

In the past two years, celebrities and influencers have also effected changes in the conventional features of lip beauty, so that a disproportionately enlarged upper lip with an altered shape is now seen as attractive. This can then often lead to an unnatural result: in some circles, having thick, "bee-stung" (or "dinghy") lips is equivalent to wearing certain designer brands.

Symmetry, or the balance between the lips and rest of the face, is deliberately ignored, causing conspicuous disruption in the harmony of the facial features: the artificial lips are put on show with pride and carried on the body like a work of art.

An association between lip shape and character is another aspect that is under discussion. This subject is less well researched, although there are many disputed, popular science interpretations of this (Bunte.de Redaktion magazine website 2018), e.g.:

- Harmonious lips convey calmness and serenity.
- Thin lips stand for grimness, lack of passion, single-mindedness, perseverance.
- Large lower lips stand for impulsiveness.
- Lopsided, crooked lips stand for a loving, trustworthy nature.

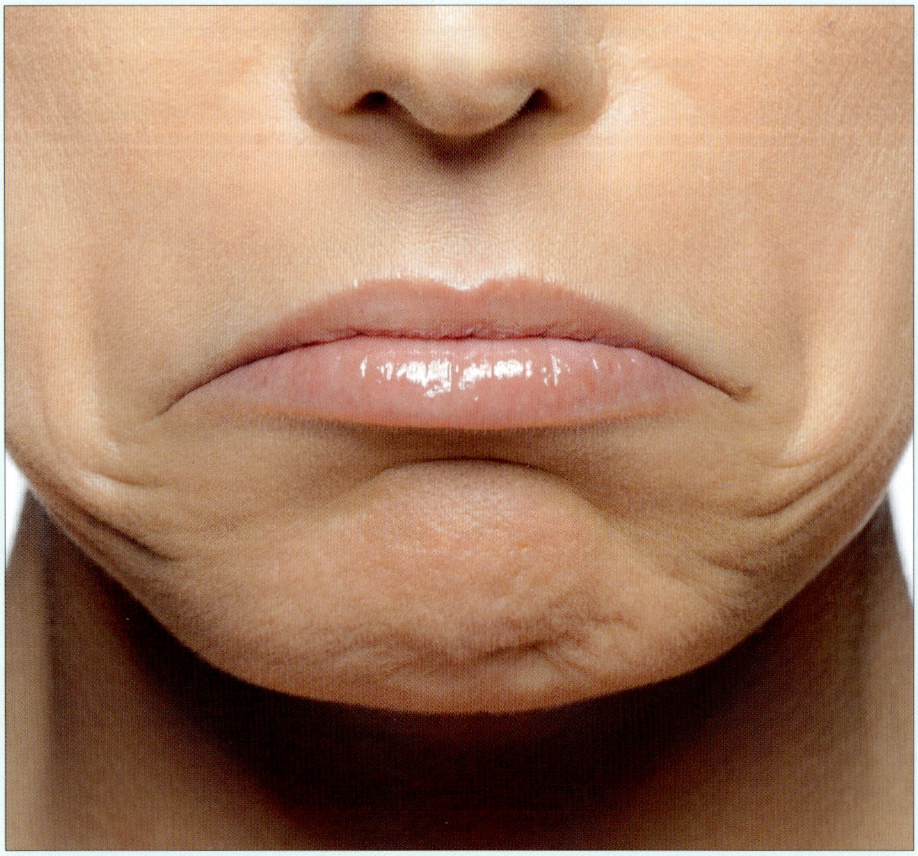

Fig. 1.1 Facial expressions show feelings that change the shape of the lips, creating visually identifiable emotions. A mouth with its corners pulled down is a display of sorrow or disgust.

However, the movements made when speaking and eating, the muscle tone of the lips, and the changes in shape caused by the facial muscles as an expression of feelings (→ Fig. 1.1), which can make a mouth beautiful or special but can also express a negative attitude, all exist independently of the anatomical structures and the genetically determined shape of the lips. These movements may be symmetric and harmonious in themselves, or asymmetric and crooked, lending a personal note to the overall appearance. Regardless of the shape of the lips when relaxed, these influences can make a pair of lips seem sensual, charismatic, erotic, pinched, disdainful, lascivious, etc. Inferences about an individual's character are made as a result of lip expression: this person has a labile mouth, an intelligent mouth, an idiotic mouth, an aggressive mouth, and so on.

1.2 Function

The lips have important functions far beyond their role as a feature of beauty. They are intended for food ingestion. Their musculature makes them very mobile so that they can hold onto food items and convey them into the mouth. Closing the lips produces an airtight seal, holding food and saliva inside the mouth and keeping out unwanted objects. This airtight seal is also important when taking in food by suction. In addition, lip closure and lip shape are of great significance when producing sounds (→ Fig. 1.2) by speaking, singing, whistling or playing wind instruments.

Since the lips contain numerous nerve endings, they comprise one of the most sensitive regions of the body. The thin skin of the lips feels pleasantly soft and reacts with enormous sensitivity to external stimuli such as temperature, touch, and pain. The lips act as an organ of touch for infants and have a highly sensitive function as an erogenous zone in sexuality, e.g. during kissing. Thus, beautiful lips can increase a person's sexual attractiveness.

1.3 Anatomy

The lips are the soft tissue folds formed in the lower, anterior part of the face, and they seal off the oral cavity against the outside world. They possess inherent mobility, and, with the cheeks (buccae), they form the vestibule of the mouth (vestibulum oris). The lips are embedded in the oral and chin region, forming its center (DocCheck Flexikon 2019). In this book, we have concentrated predominantly on this region, leaving out treatment of the nasolabial zone, as any complete treatment of that zone would also affect treatment of the upper half of the face. We had to draw a line here. We have also taken a selective approach in the anatomical depictions, and have refrained from describing regions that have no relevance to injection treatment in the lip area, such as the maxilla, even if these structures are of significance to the changes in appearance that occur during the aging process.

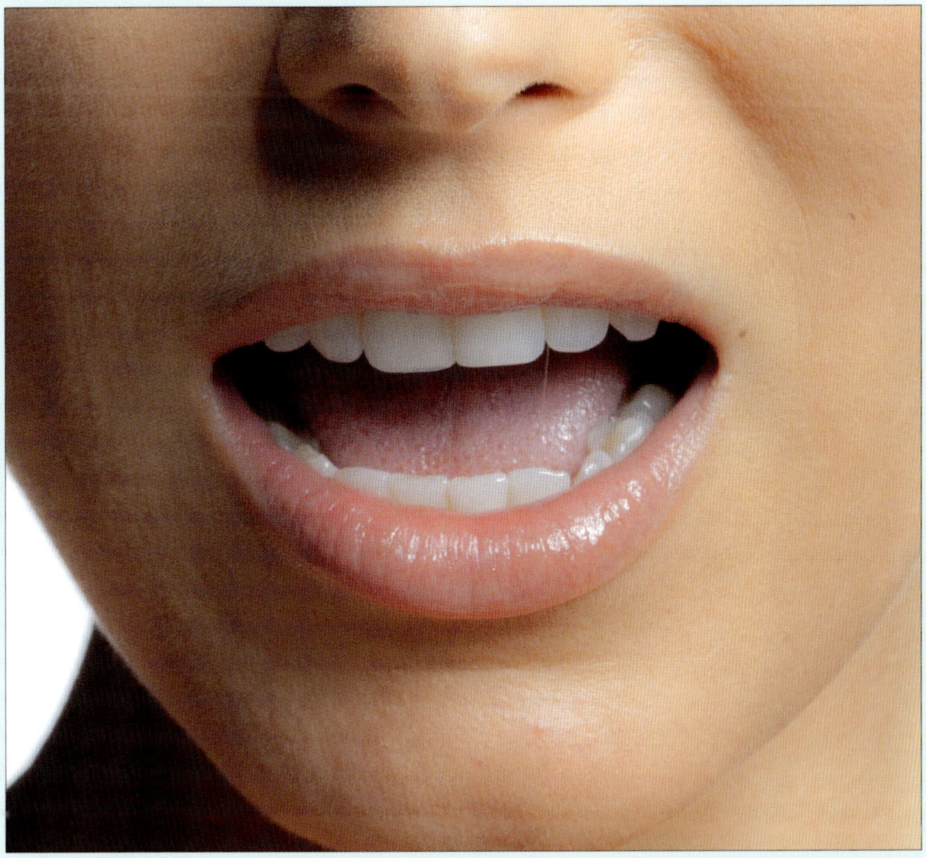

Fig. 1.2 An example of lip shape during singing.

1.3.1 Mouth region

The outer part of the mouth, i.e. the extraoral region, is distinct from the oral cavity. The section between the nose and aperture of the mouth is referred to as the upper lip, while the lower lip is the region from the aperture of the mouth to the labiomental fold. Thus, the vermillion is only one part of the lip.

Topographic Anatomy of the Mouth Region (→ Figs. 1.3–1.18)

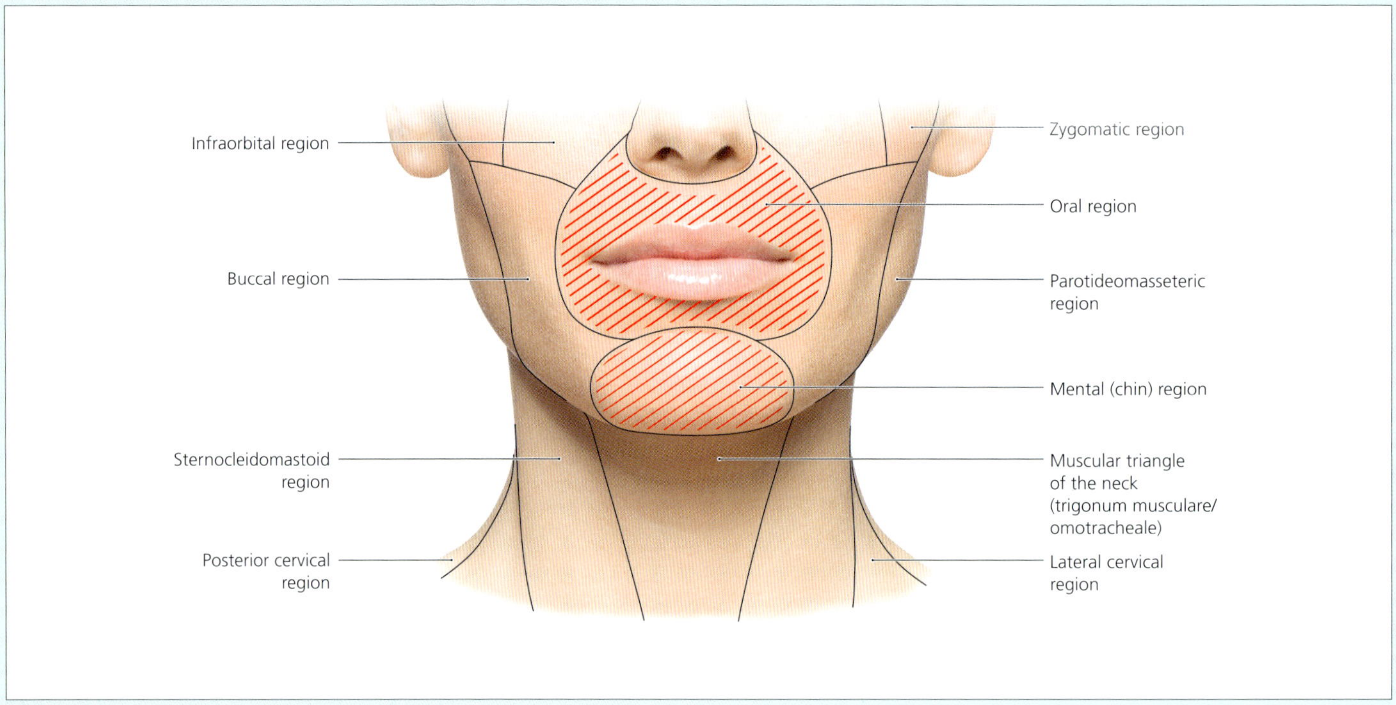

Fig. 1.3 Mouth region (oral and mental region), anterior view (hatched in red).

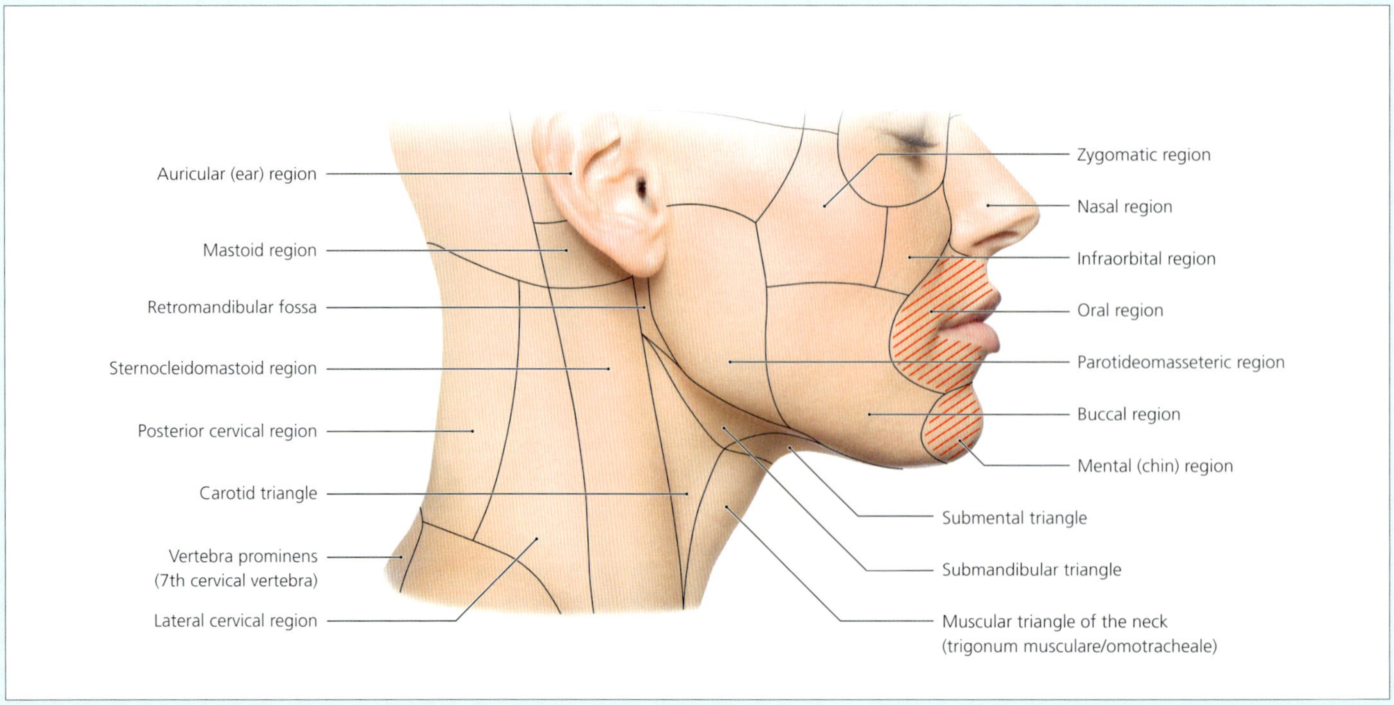

Fig. 1.4 Mouth region (oral and mental region), lateral view (hatched in red).

1

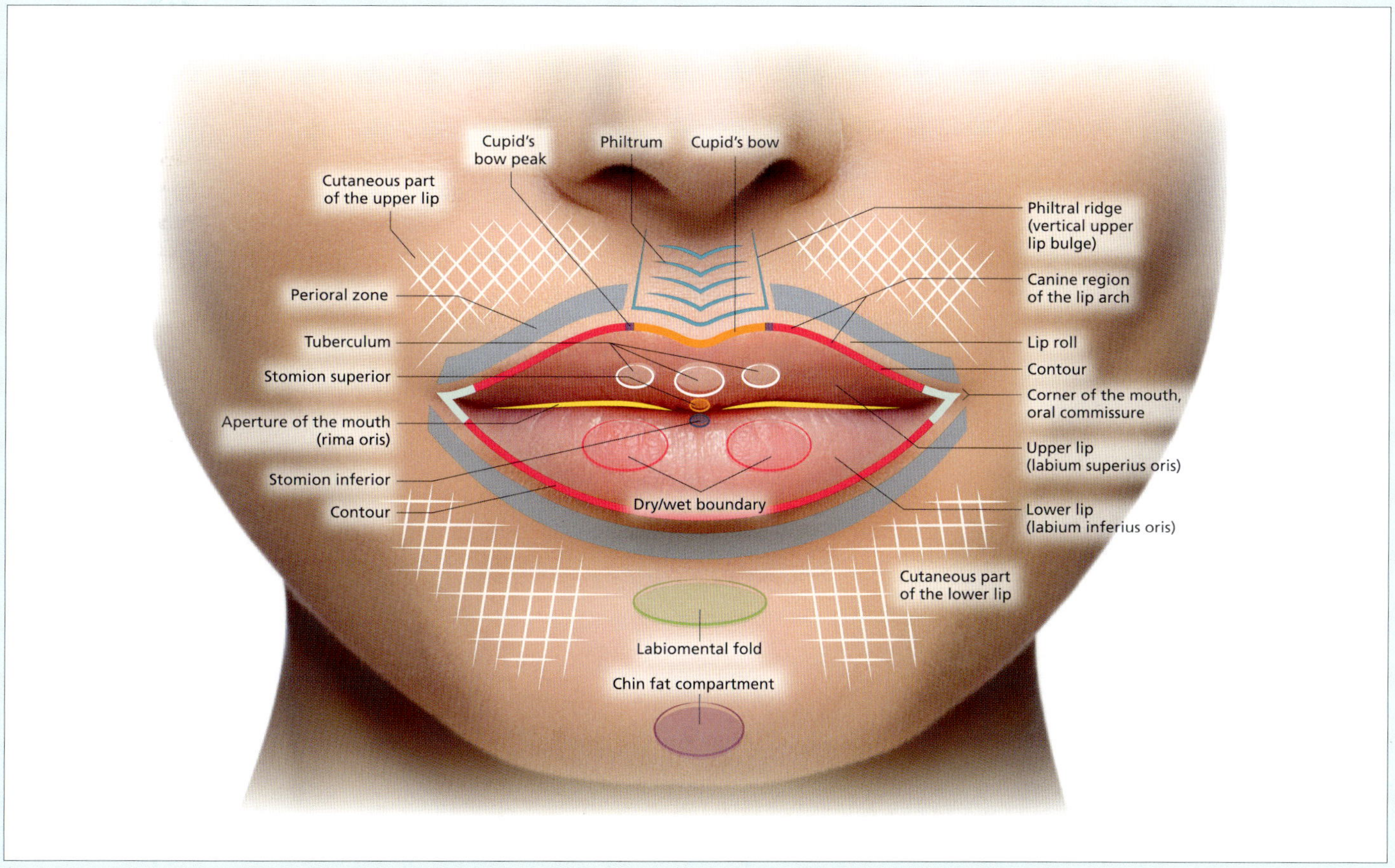

Fig. 1.5 Anatomical terms used to describe the outer lip region.

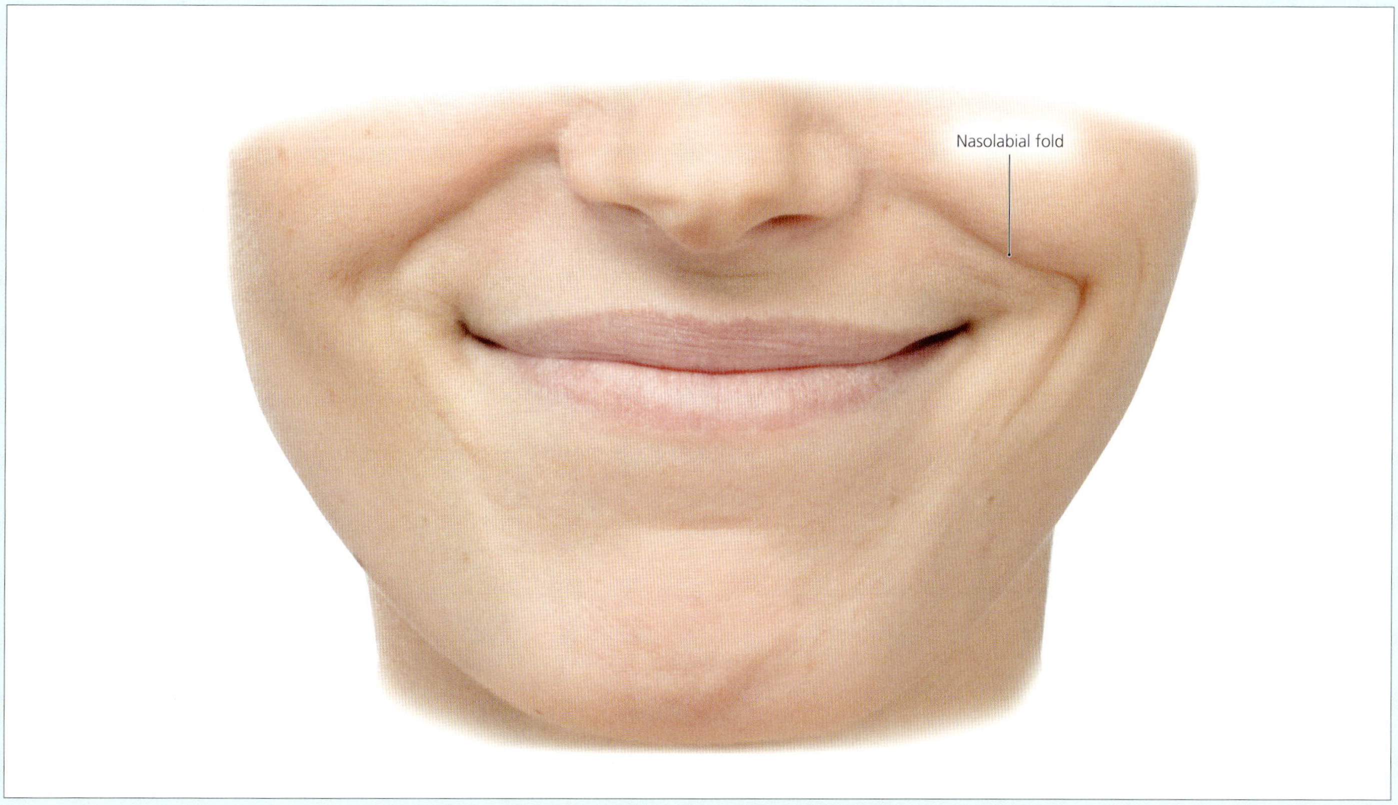

Fig. 1.6 The oral region is bounded on both sides by the nasolabial fold. In children and adolescents, this fold may be effaced when the face is at rest. However, it is always visible when a person smiles. It becomes permanent with increasing age; its prominence depends on the volume of cheek fat.

1

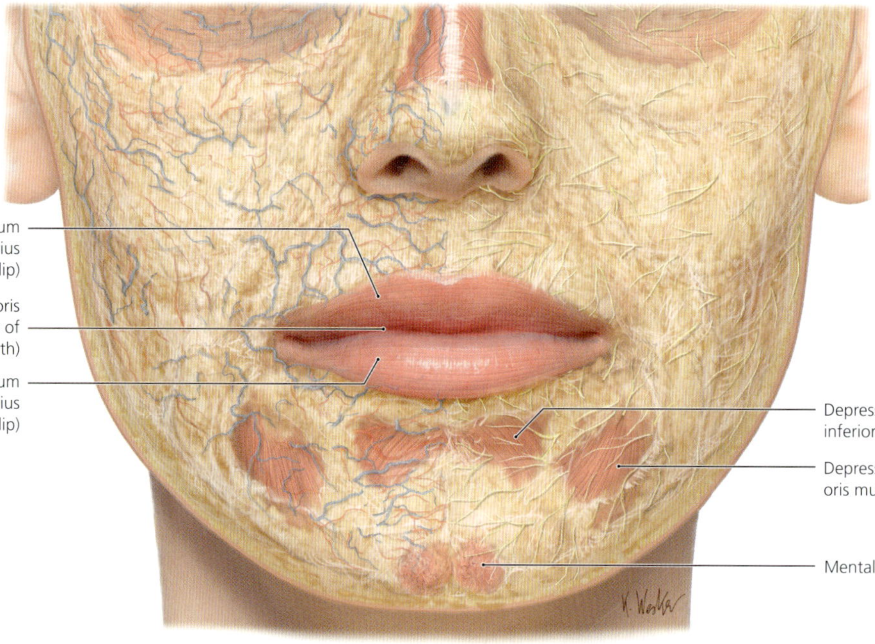

Subcutaneous fat distribution in the mouth region

Fig. 1.7 Distribution of subcutaneous fat (extensive yellowish-white structure) in the mouth region. In the lip region, the subcutaneous fat layer is comparatively thin.

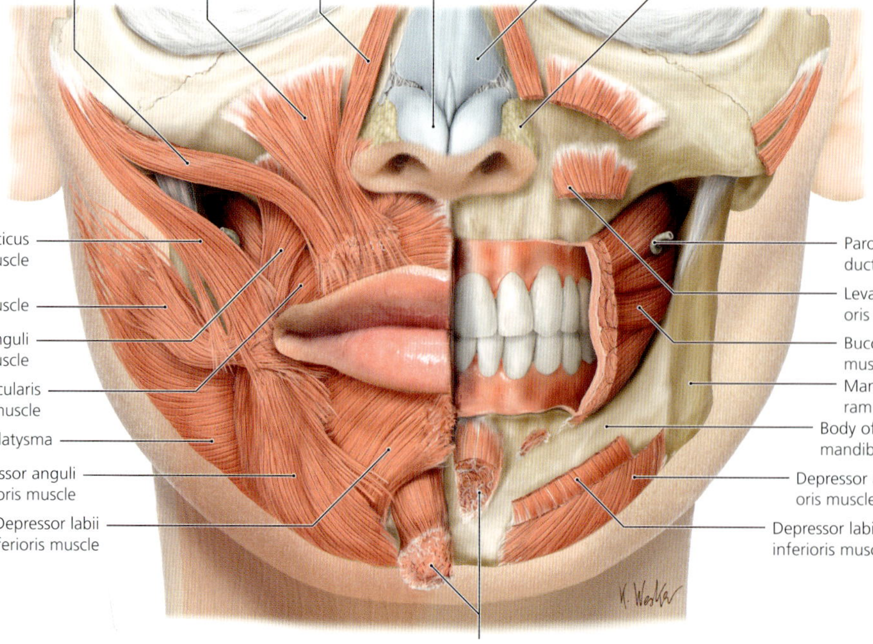

Musculature of the mouth region with the deeper sites and insertion points exposed
(in the right half of the image)

Fig. 1.8 The oral cavity is enclosed laterally by the buccinator muscle, which merges into the orbicularis oris muscle further anteriorly. Several individual muscles run toward the mouth at the side of the nose and are capable of lifting the upper lip in several directions, depending on the angle of insertion. Originating from the zygomatic arch, they show an oblique course. The risorius muscle and the platysma run horizontally. The lower lip is also reached by muscles that can pull it in all directions. This radial arrangement of the musculature is a key prerequisite for the impressive range of movements shown by the mouth. The junction of muscles at the corners of the mouth is referred to as the modiolus. Here, fibrous tissue holds the various muscle fibers together.

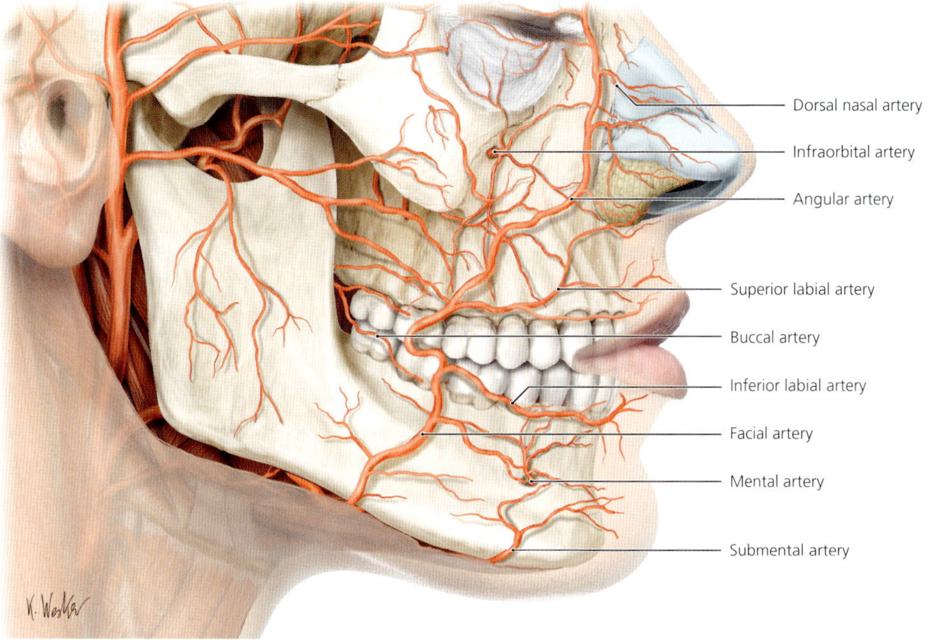

Arterial supply of the mouth region, lateral view

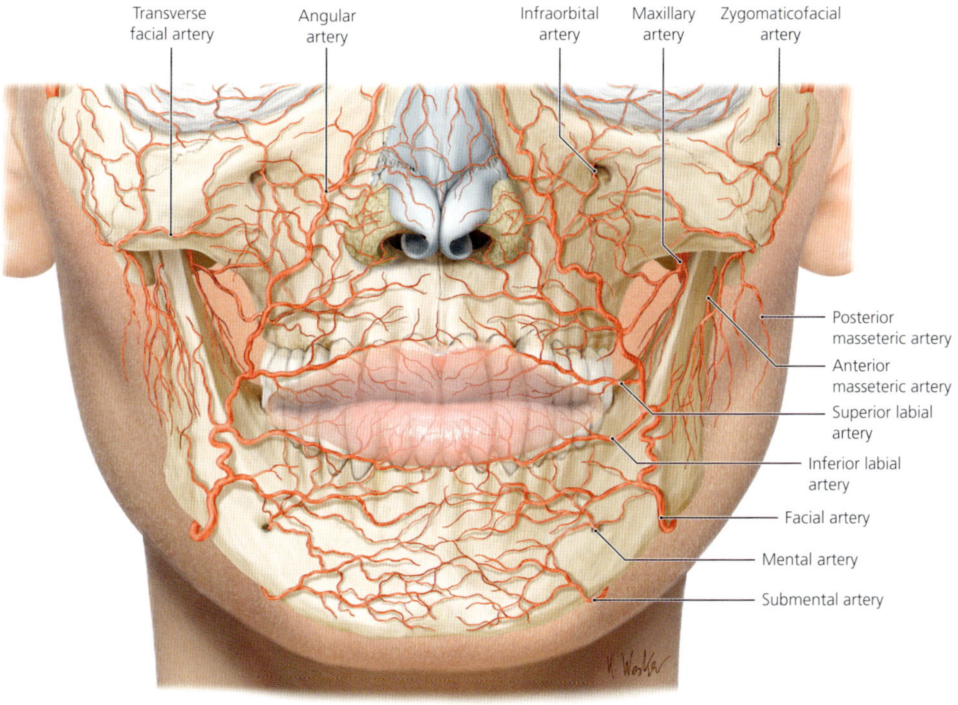

Arterial supply of the mouth region, anterior view

Fig. 1.9 The mouth region is supplied by two branches of the external carotid artery and one branch of the internal carotid artery: the facial artery originates from the external carotid artery and runs along the lower edge of the mandible to arrive at the oral commissure. Here, it sends out two branches, the inferior and superior labial arteries.

After continuing its course along the nose, it anastomoses with the dorsal nasal artery, which originates from the ophthalmic artery, that is, from the internal carotid artery. Originating from the external carotid artery, via the maxillary artery, the infraorbital artery not only exchanges anastomoses with the facial artery, but also independently supplies the cheek and lip region.

Another vessel that originates from the maxillary artery, and thus also from the external carotid artery, is the mental branch of the inferior alveolar artery, which runs below the mandible and supplies the lower lip and chin region. However, the chin region is also supplied by direct branches of the facial artery, i.e. the submental artery.

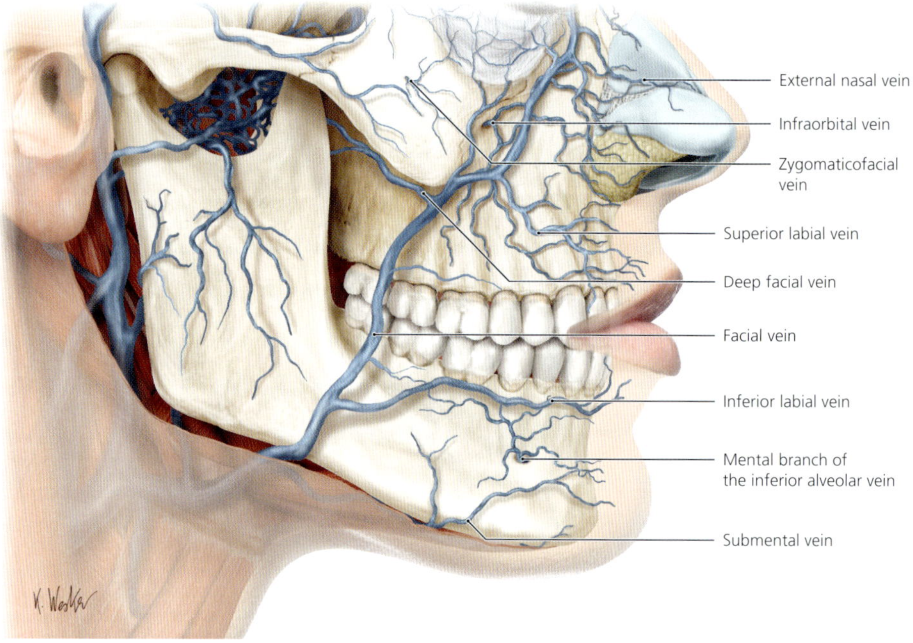

Venous drainage in the mouth region, lateral view

Fig. 1.10 The venous drainage from the cheek and lip region takes place mainly via the facial vein, and thus into the internal jugular vein.

However, venous blood also drains through the mental foramen into the inferior alveolar vein, which runs into the pterygoid plexus. The infraorbital vein also drains into the pterygoid plexus.

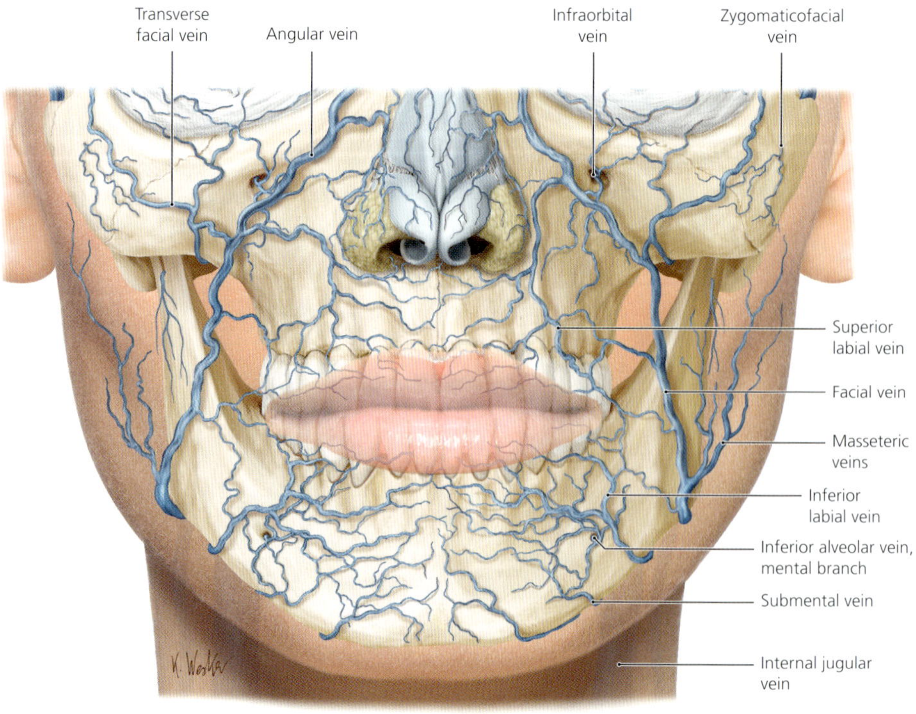

Venous drainage in the mouth region, anterior view

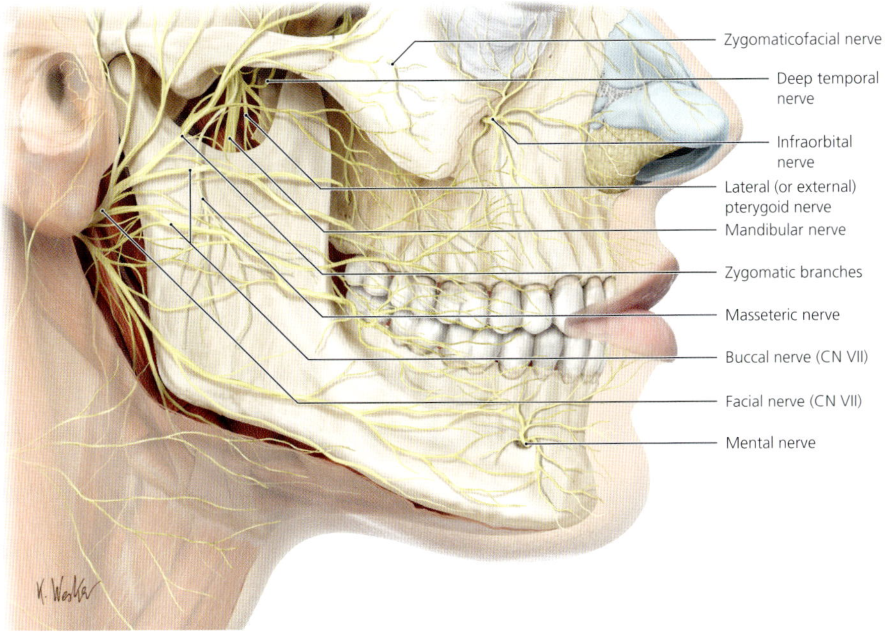

Innervation of the mouth region, lateral view

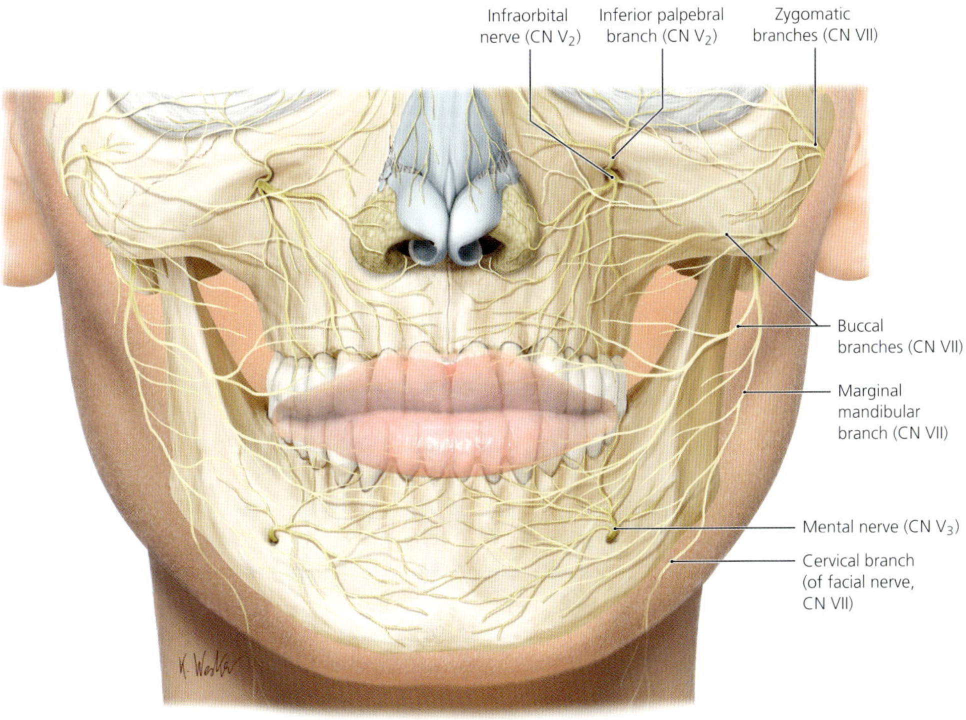

Innervation of the mouth region, anterior view

Fig. 1.11 The sensory innervation of the mouth region is provided by the infraorbital nerve and the mandibular nerve. The motor innervation of all the muscles of facial expression is provided by the facial nerve. The chewing muscles are innervated by the motor branch of the mandibular nerve.

Fig. 1.12 Images depicting the network of blood vessels and nerves that serve the mouth region clearly show how intricately this area is perfused and innervated.

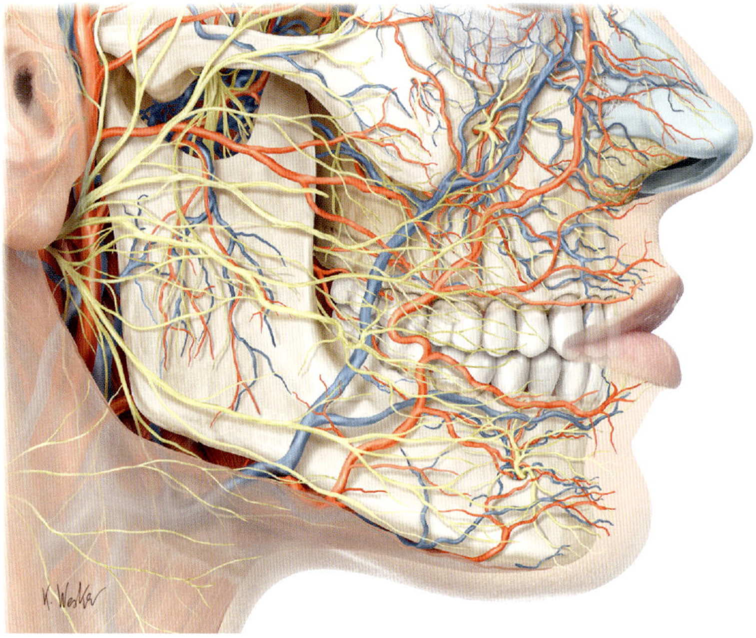

Network of blood vessels and nerves supplying the mouth region, lateral view

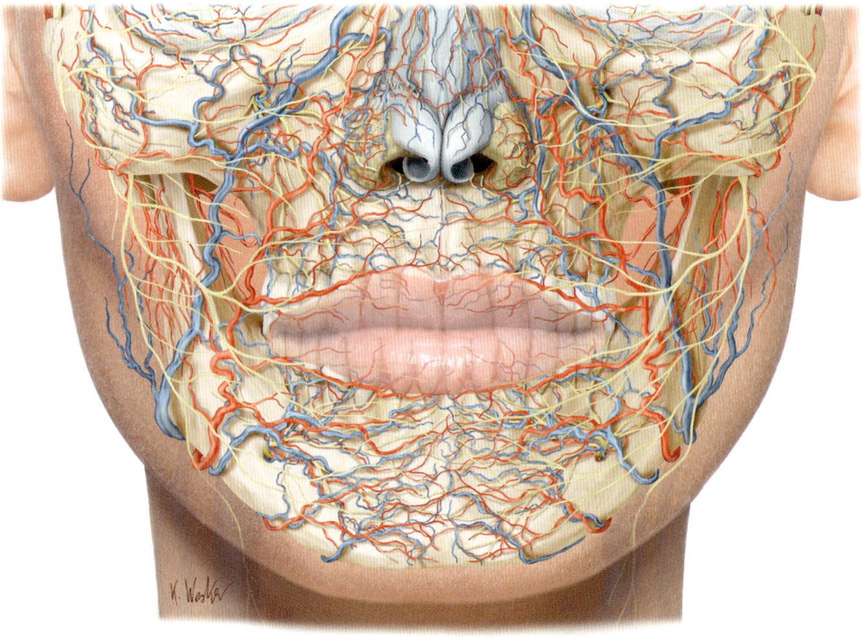

Network of blood vessels and nerves supplying the mouth region, anterior view

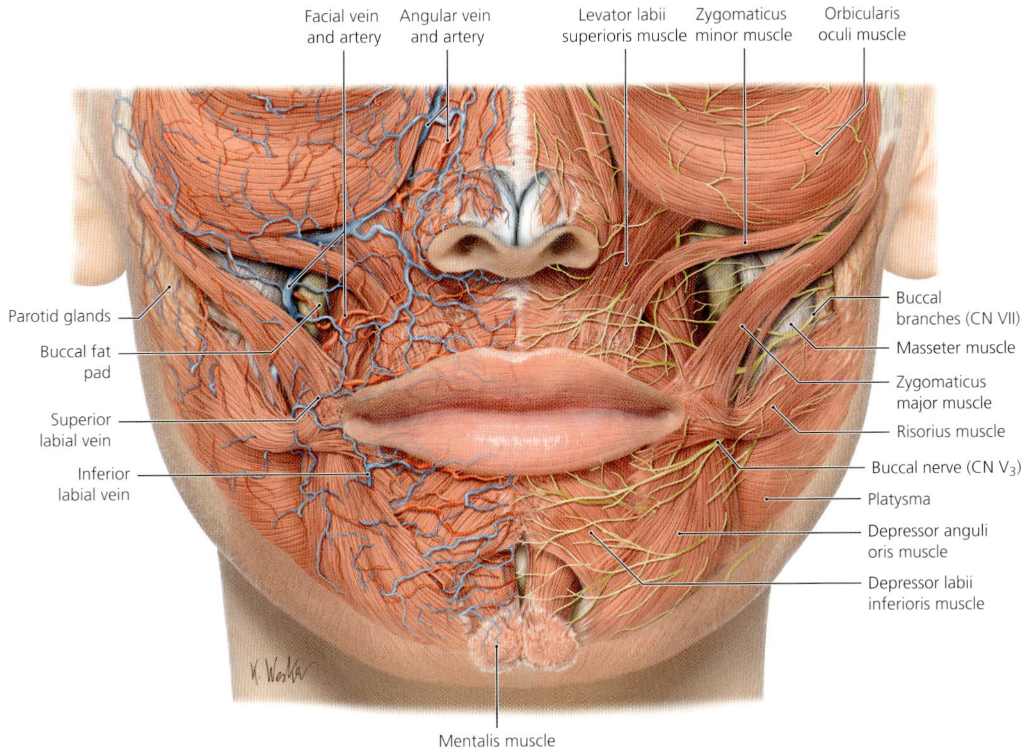

Musculature, vascular supply (left) **and innervation** (right) **in the mouth region, superficial layer**

Fig. 1.13 The mouth is surrounded by muscles of facial expression that run toward it from almost every direction. The central section of the lips is formed by the orbicularis oris muscle (see Fig. 1.15). The arteries in this superficially located muscle layer of the mouth region branch off from the facial artery, which sends out branches to the nose, the cheek, and both the upper and lower lip. The lower lip region is also supplied by the mental branch (see Fig. 1.15), which originates from the alveolar artery and emerges through the mental foramen. Venous blood from the superficial mouth region is drained via the facial vein, while all the muscles of facial expression are innervated by branches of the facial nerve. Motor innervation of the chewing muscles is provided by the motor root of the trigeminal nerve, which is distributed to the target areas via the mandibular nerve (see Fig. 1.11). Sensory innervation of the mouth region is provided by the trigeminal nerve.

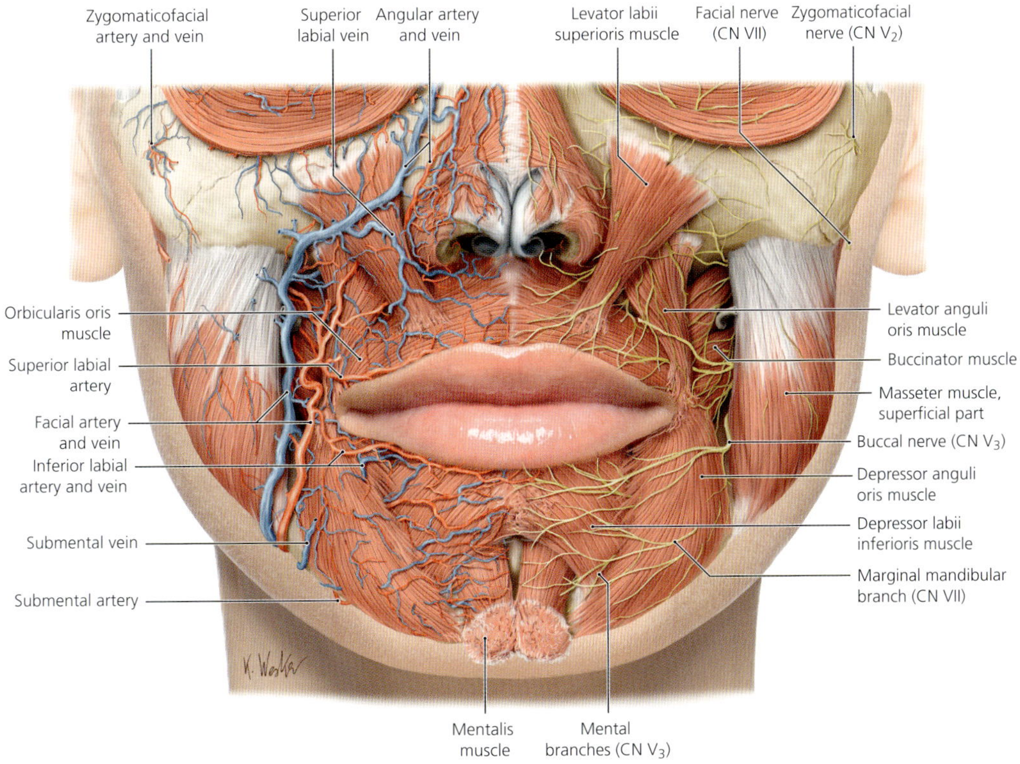

Musculature, vascular supply (left) **and innervation** (right) **in the mouth region, zygomaticus minor/major muscle, risorius muscle, and platysma removed**

Fig. 1.14 Removing the zygomaticus minor/major muscles, the risorius muscle, and the platysma exposes the entire lengths of the levator labii superioris muscle, the superficial part of the masseter muscle, and the levator anguli oris muscle, with visible origins and insertions. The buccinator muscle is partly visible.

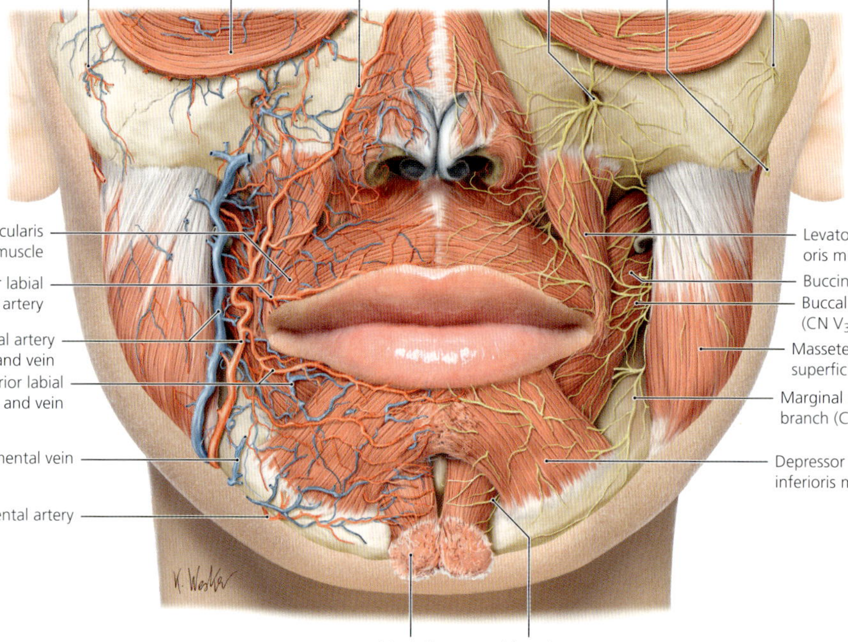

Musculature, vascular supply (left)**, and innervation** (right) **in the mouth region, superficial muscles of facial expression removed**

Fig. 1.15 The facial artery originates from the external carotid artery and reaches the facial region with its mandibular branch. After running diagonally over the cheek and along the side of the nose, where it is referred to as the angular artery, it anastomoses with the dorsal nasal artery, a terminal branch of the ophthalmic artery, which in turn originates from the internal carotid artery. The angular vein runs across and above the levator labii superioris muscle, while the angular artery runs below it. The facial artery takes a highly convoluted course in the cheek region and is stretched when the mouth opens. The facial vein shows considerably fewer twists and turns in this region. It extends accordingly when the mouth opens.

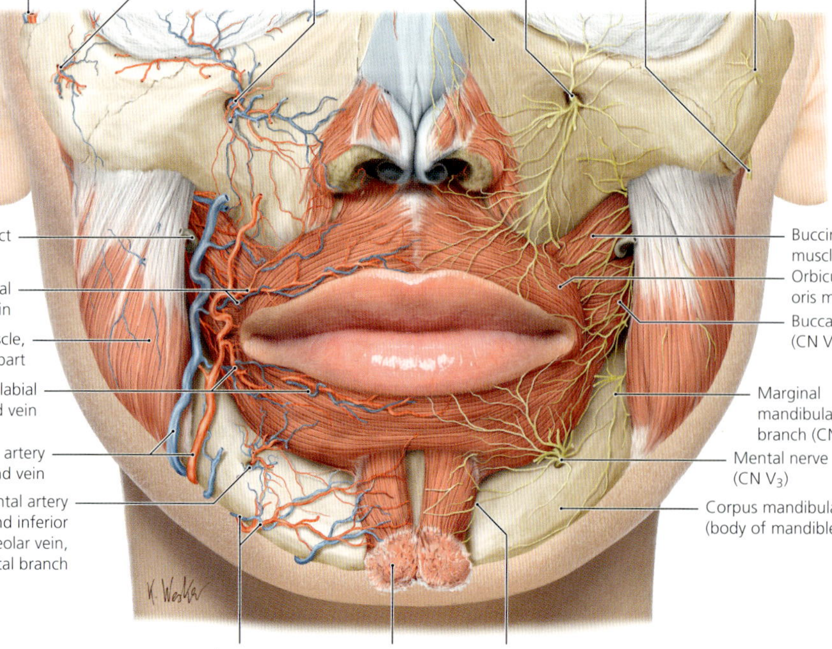

Musculature, vascular supply (left)**, and innervation** (right) **in the mouth region, orbicularis oris muscle exposed, levator labii superioris and levator anguli oris muscles removed**

Fig. 1.16 Removing the levator labii superioris and levator anguli oris muscles exposes the infraorbital foramen. After running through the infraorbital canal, the infraorbital artery and vein respectively run inward and emerge at this point, forming numerous anastomoses with the angular artery and vein. The infraorbital nerve also leaves the infraorbital canal here. The cheeks and the lip region are served by branches of the infraorbital artery and vein in the maxilla, and by the mental branches of the inferior alveolar artery and vein in the mandible. Substantial tributaries also originate from the facial artery or drain into the facial vein. Correspondingly, sensory innervation is provided by the infraorbital nerve and the mental nerve. The buccal nerve provides sensory innervation to the cheek.

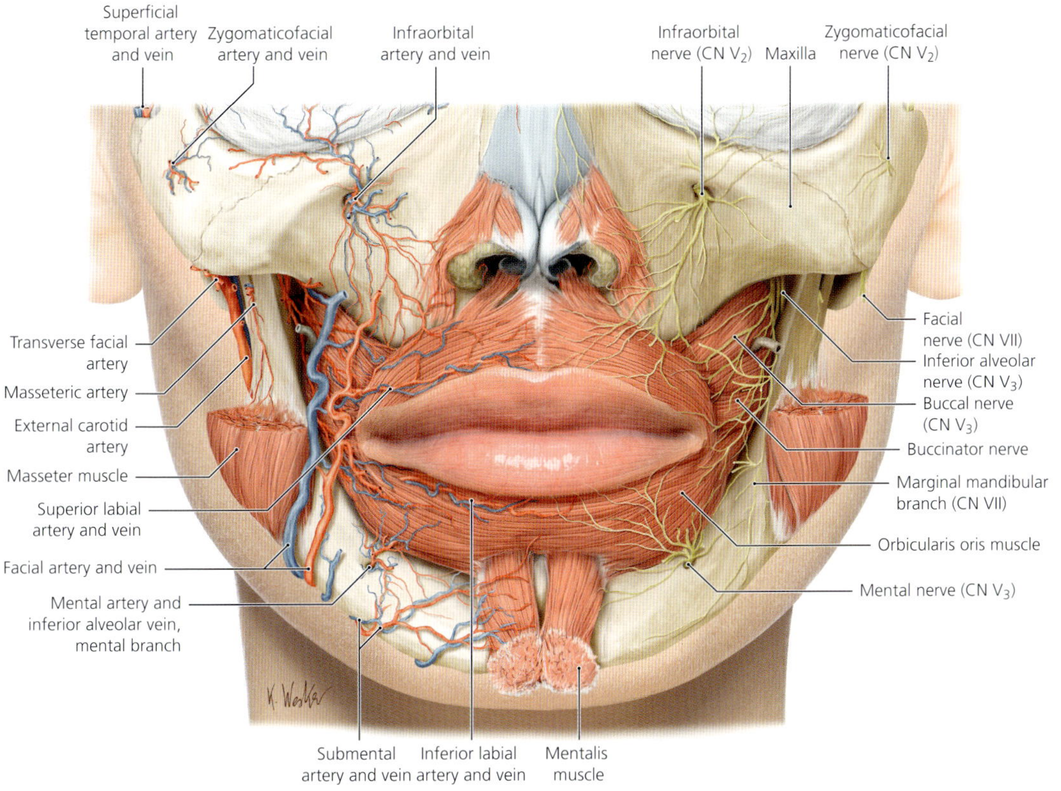

Musculature, vascular supply (left)**, and innervation** (right) **in the mouth region, orbicularis oris muscle exposed, masseter dissected**

Fig. 1.17 The outer walls of the oral cavity are formed predominantly by the orbicularis oris muscle together with the buccinator muscle. In this respect, the paired buccinator muscles and the orbicularis oris muscle, taken together, may easily be seen as a continuous muscle system, even though they are separate muscles. This muscular system is normally in balance with the tongue and determines the space for the dental arches.

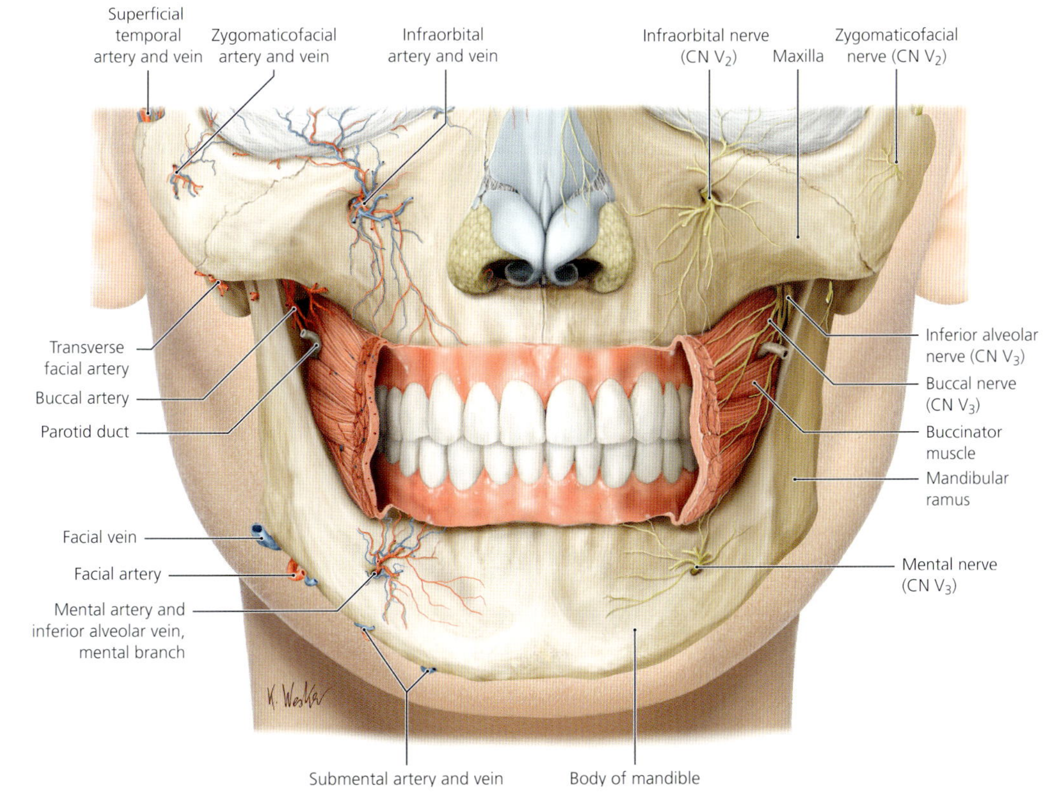

Musculature, vascular supply (left)**, and innervation** (right) **in the deepest layer of the mouth region**

Fig. 1.18 The vestibular oral mucosa of the cheeks and lip region is served by branches of the infraorbital artery and vein in the maxilla, and branches of the mental artery and vein in the mandible. Correspondingly, sensory innervation is provided by the infraorbital nerve and the mental nerve. The buccal nerve provides sensory innervation to the cheek.

1.3.2 Lips, Teeth, Periodontium, and Alveolar Processes

■ Anterior Mouth Region (→ Fig. 1.19)

The alveolar processes and the teeth are bounded by the tongue from the inside and by the lips (and then laterally by the cheeks) from the outside. Correct, natural alignment of the incisors requires the cutting edge of the maxillary incisor to overlap the cutting edge of the mandibular incisor (overbite). The biomechanical ideal is for the cutting edge of the mandibular incisor to abut onto the maxillary incisor at the point of inflection between the maxillary incisor's palatal concavity and the convexity of its tubercle. Consequently, the cutting edge of the maxillary incisor sits slightly in front of the labial surface of the mandibular incisor (overjet). The position of the dental axes is significantly influenced by the forces exerted by the tongue and the lips. In this respect, however, swallowing and speaking have less of an effect than the constant push and pressure of the tongue and lips.

■ Upper and Lower Lip (→ Fig. 1.20)

On its outer side, the lip carries the typical hairy skin of the epidermis. Below it is the connective, tissue-rich dermis that houses the sweat glands, hair follicles, and sebaceous glands.

The intermediate zone – usually known as the vermillion or red margin – is the transitional zone between the outer and inner side. It covers the lips in the area between the outer skin and the oral mucosa. This intermediate zone is coated with a thin, multilayered, translucent, squamous epithelium that is weakly cornified and unpigmented and contains isolated sebaceous glands. The epithelium is particularly thin and hairless over the papillae. The vermillion also lacks salivary glands and therefore constantly needs to be moistened with saliva. This takes place predominantly by means of the salivary film that is formed when speaking or eating. The loose connective tissue of the lamina propria (a thin, subepithelial connective tissue layer) is traversed by capillary loops, which give the lips their intense color.

The inner oral side of the lip, known as the mucosal zone (the mucous membrane side), is characterized by its lining of lip mucosa, with an uncornified, relatively thick epithelium. The lamina propria is thin and contains loose connective tissue traversed by elastic fibers. The submucosa contains fat deposits, along with numerous individual salivary glands, jointly known as the labial glands. Blood vessels and nerves run through this area as well, with branches that extend into the lamina propria. Free nerve endings also extend into the epithelium. The muscular layer (also known as the tunica muscularis) consists of striated muscle tissue (DocCheck Flexikon 2019).

Mouth Region and Lower Lip in Sagittal Sections

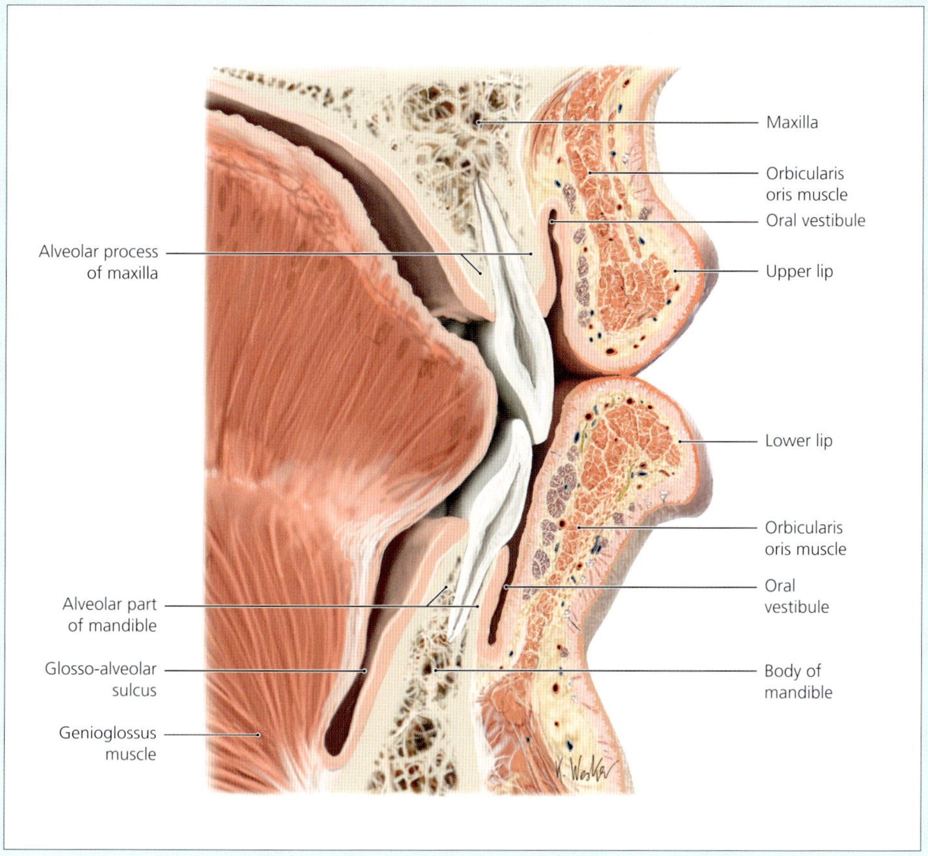

Fig. 1.19 Sagittal section through the anterior region of the mouth (taken slightly laterally of the center).

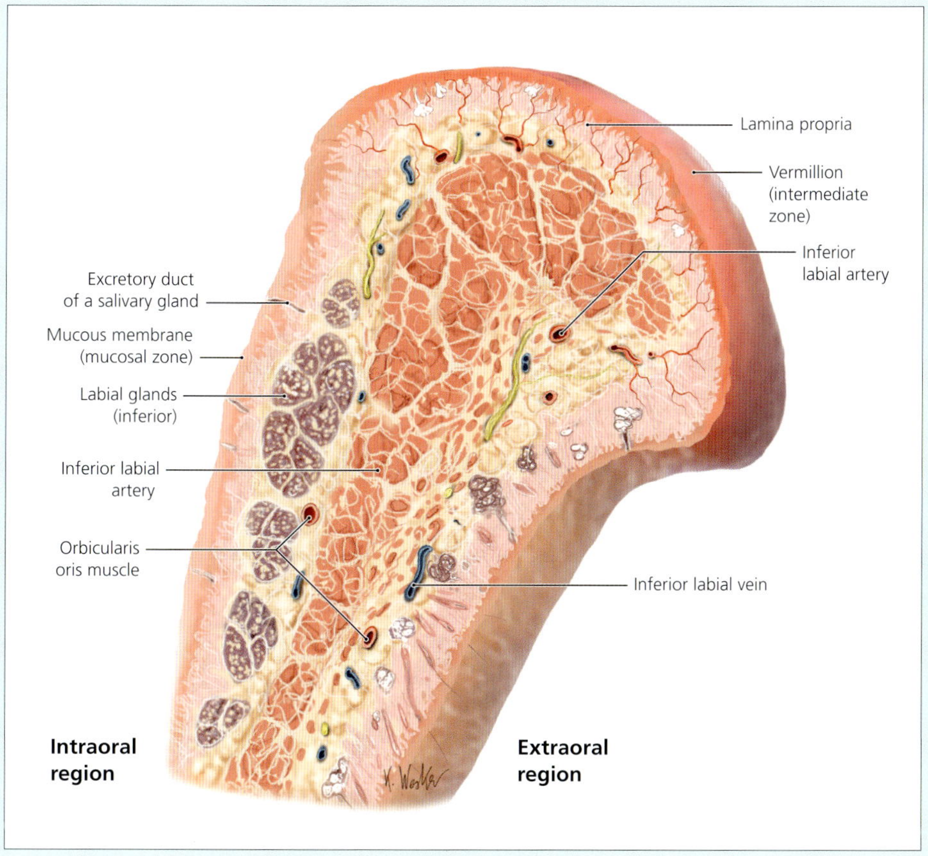

Fig. 1.20 Sagittal section through the lower lip.

1

■ Periodontium and Surrounding Area (→ Fig. 1.21)

The space between the lip and the alveolar process with teeth is referred to as the oral vestibule. At rest, it is reduced to a narrow gap, as the soft tissue of the lips nestles tightly against the teeth and gums in this region.

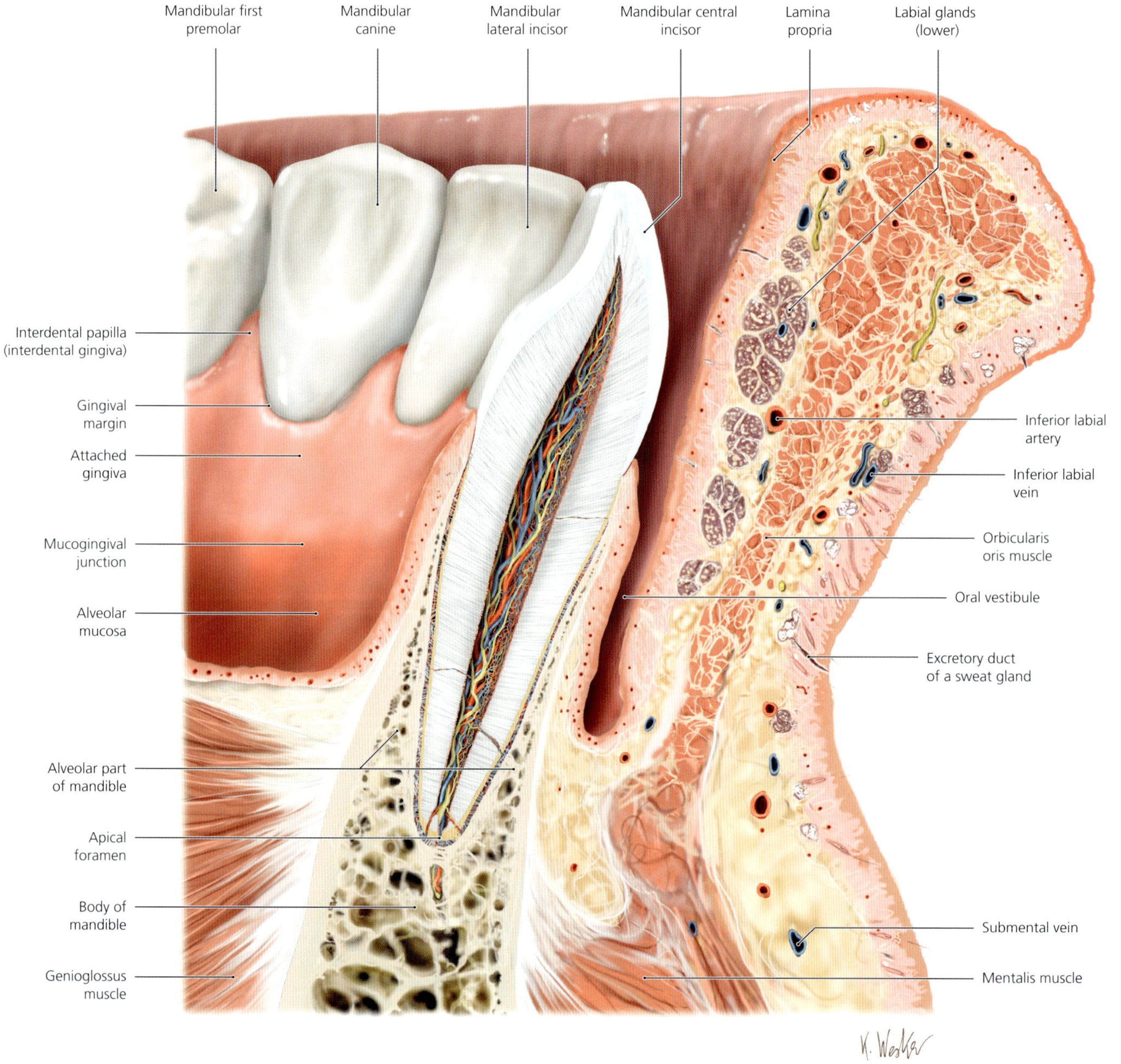

Fig. 1.21 Sagittal section through the left mandibular central incisor and its surroundings. The large vessels are located subcutaneously in the zone that adjoins the muscle.

1.3.3 Anterior Vestibule (→ Fig. 1.22 a–c)

The vestibule is lined with highly mobile mucosa. The alveolar bone is covered with the alveolar mucosa, with a network of collagenous and elastic fibers running through its lamina propria. It is highly mobile. This elastic fiber network ends so abruptly against the adjoining attached gingiva that a clear junction is visible as a morphologic feature.

The mucous membrane in the mandible does not differ from that of the maxillary vestibule. The mentalis muscle has its origin medially at the bone of the mandible on both sides and extends toward the skin of the chin. When it contracts, it produces the typical cobblestone skin pattern. The depressor labii inferioris muscle has its origin at the bone margin of the mandible, caudally of the mental foramen. In the chin region, the vestibular gingiva, the alveolar mucosa, and the mucous membrane of the oral vestibule are served by blood vessels and nerves that emerge from the mental foramen. The lip is also served by these blood vessels and nerves: it feels numb when mandibular nerve block anesthesia is administered into the mental foramen. In most cases, the mental foramen is located in the region between the root apices of the first and second premolars. If the dental arch sits further in the anterior direction on the body of the mandible, the mental foramen is located closer to the first molar. This is the case when the front teeth show pronounced anterior inclination, a feature that is frequently encountered in patients of African or Asian origin.

Vestibule

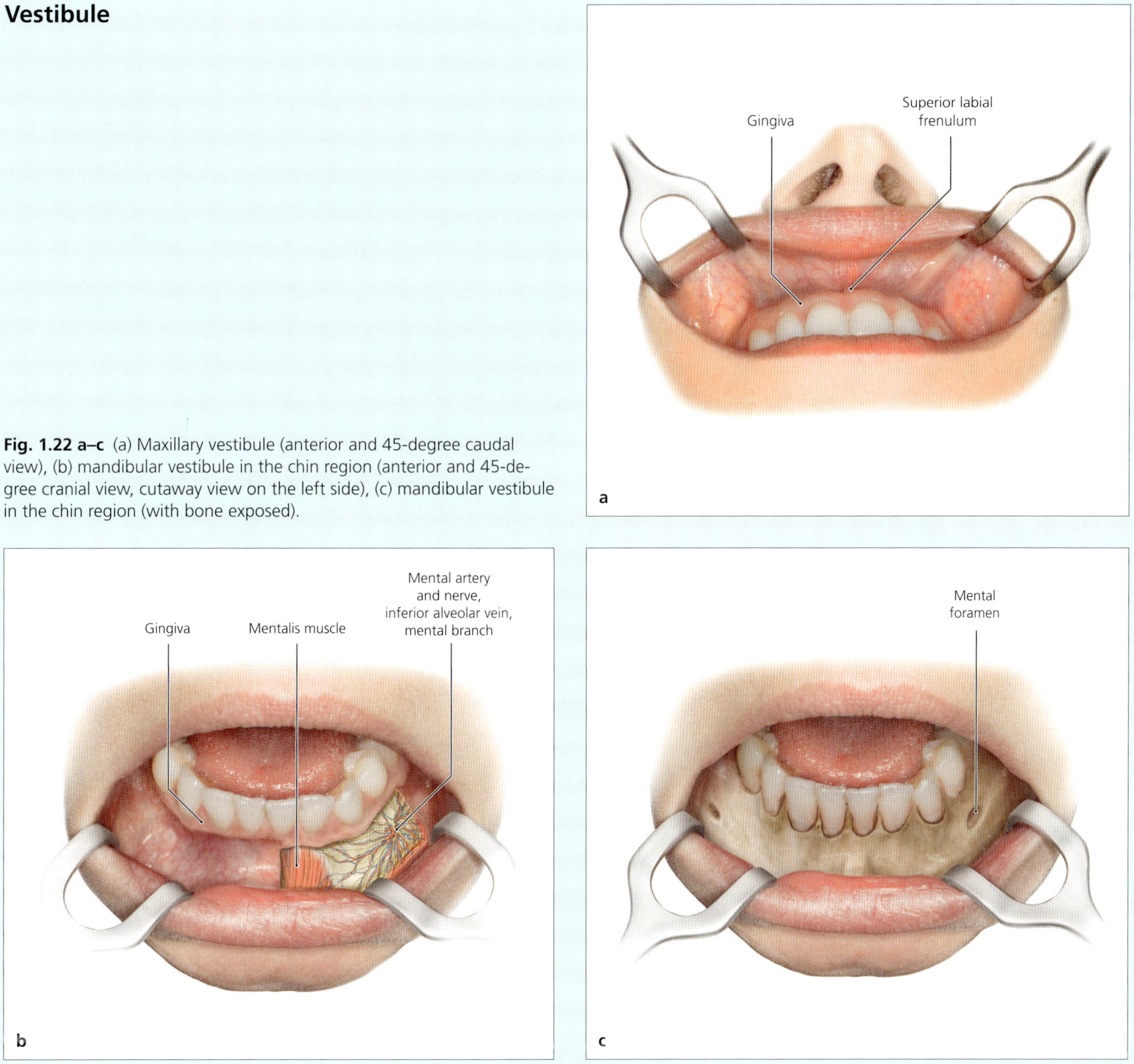

Fig. 1.22 a–c (a) Maxillary vestibule (anterior and 45-degree caudal view), (b) mandibular vestibule in the chin region (anterior and 45-degree cranial view, cutaway view on the left side), (c) mandibular vestibule in the chin region (with bone exposed).

1.3.4 Skin

■ Structure and Function

The skin is the largest organ of the human body. Its principal functions are as a barrier and for protection, by enclosing all the body's other components. It is referred to as the integument (integumentum commune), i.e. the outer skin. In addition to being a purely mechanical barrier and providing direct UV protection, the skin plays an important role in thermoregulation and body water homeostasis. On the other hand, this barrier function also requires an assured way of communicating with the outside world. For this reason, the skin takes on a variety of stimulus transmission functions, which keep us informed about the state of our environment. In addition, the skin shields us from harmful influences. It thus exercises sensory, contact, and protective functions. A differentiated architecture of cellular and acellular components also underlies this complex range of functions (→ Fig. 1.23).

The upper layer of the skin, known as the epidermis, is of ectodermal origin, whereas the dermis is of mesodermal origin. The basement membrane represents the link between these two components and is also referred to as the junction zone or interface. Located below the dermis is the subcutis, a cushioning layer made of adipose tissue.

The epidermis exerts its barrier function by means of its horny layer (stratum corneum) and is anchored by connective tissue. It is served by blood vessels and nerves. The nails, hair, sebaceous glands, and sweat glands form integral skin appendages.

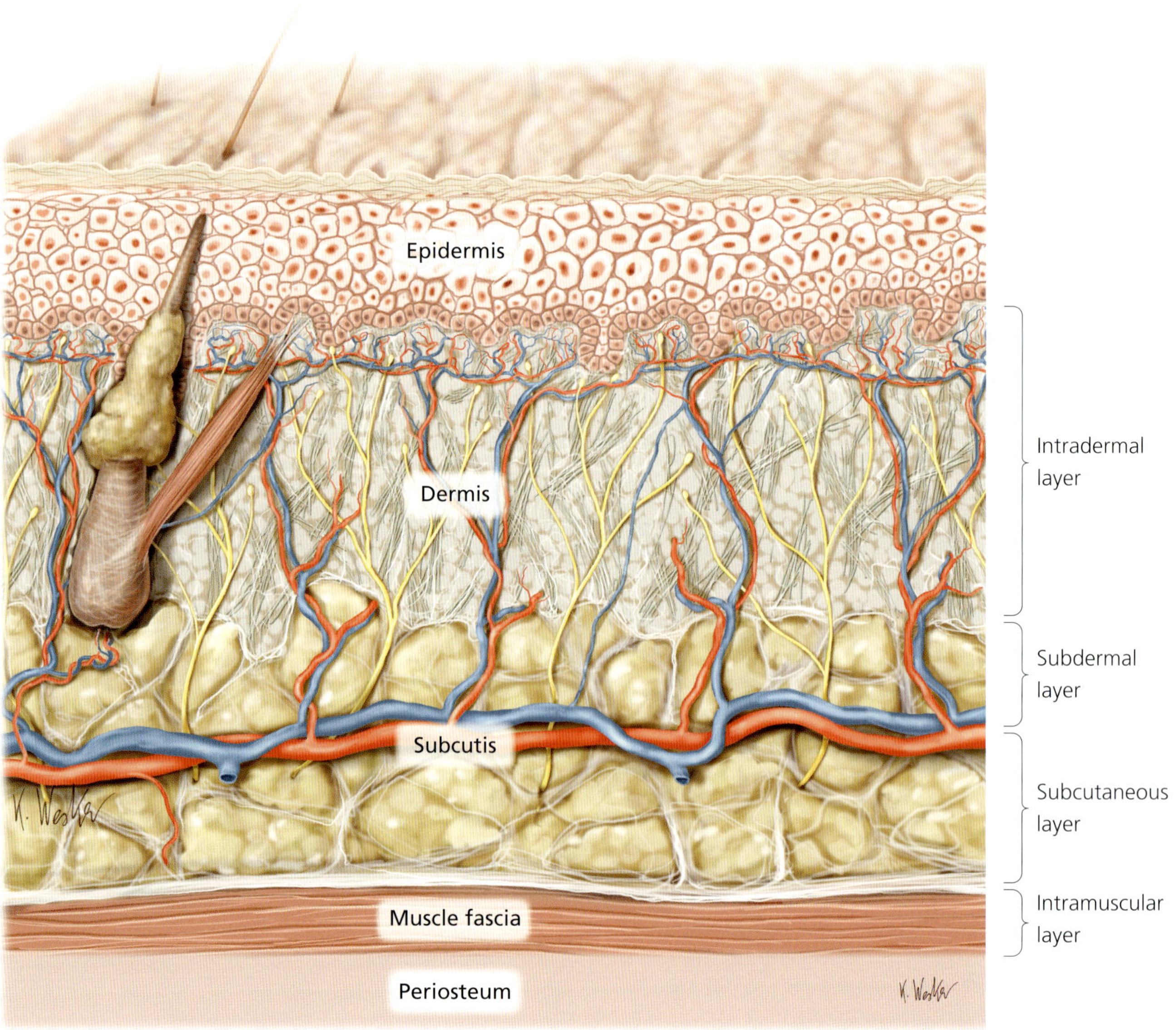

Fig. 1.23 Schematic diagram showing the skin layers.

Lip Skin

The skin of the vermillion is very thin and hairless. Cold, heat, and wind are the worst enemies of healthy lips. An inadequate fluid intake is also rapidly reflected in the lips, with the appearance of small cracks, wrinkles, and dry spots. When a lot of moisture is withdrawn from this thin layer of skin, parts of the epithelium will shed in scales, which can lead to minor sores, rhagades, and resultant inflammation.

Skin Texture

Although the principal structure of the skin is the same in all humans, there are significant differences in the epidermal architecture of facial skin between the sexes and between different ethnic groups, manifesting in the number and size of pores, water content, and elasticity.

Differences in skin texture are not caused merely by ethnic, cultural, and genetic factors. There are also extrinsic and intrinsic influences and the normal aging processes, which have an additional effect on differences in skin quality. All of this is expressed in the skin's external appearance (→ Fig. 1.24 a–c).

Skin Consistency

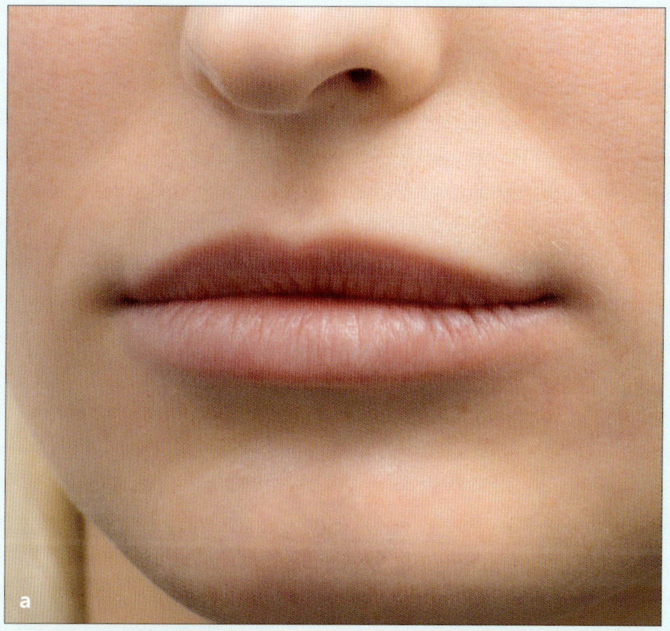

Fig. 1.24 a–c Young women with different skin textures: (a) very fine skin with small pores, (b) somewhat irregular skin with slight skin impurities and larger pores, (c) very uneven skin structure with larger pores and extremely dry lips.

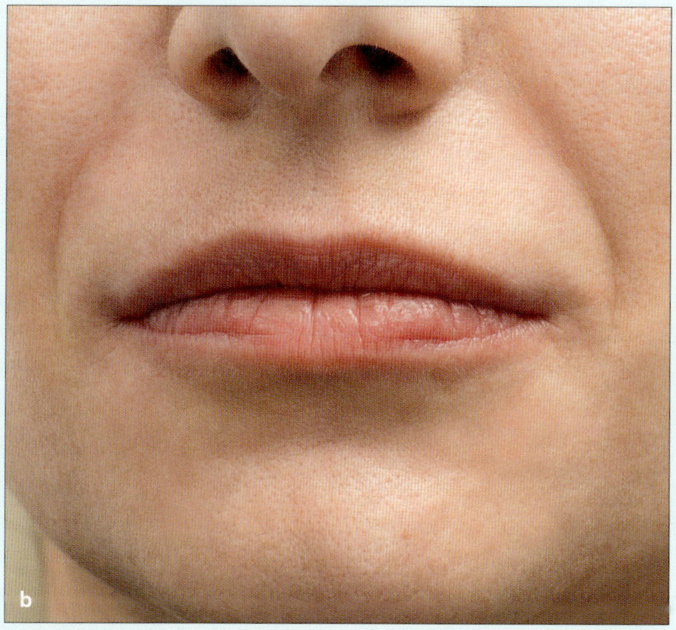

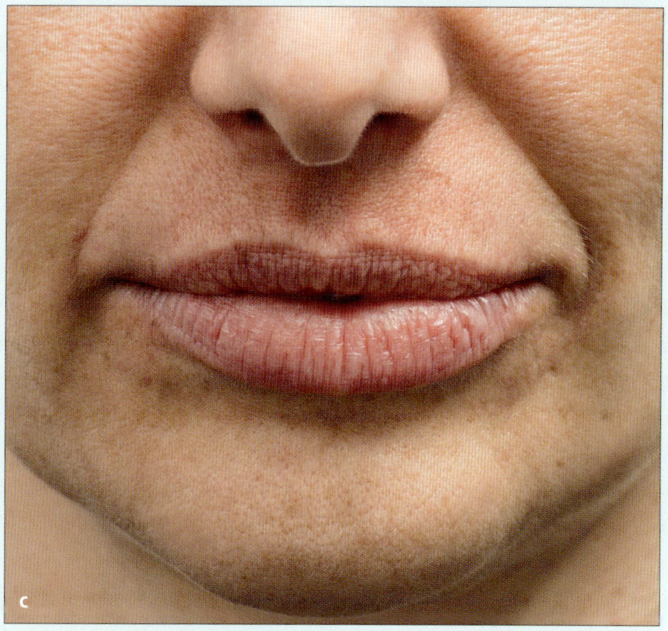

1.4 Aging Process of the Mouth Region

A lip altered by aging processes represents a challenge for the therapist. Remodeling processes and changes take place here, and these can influence the shape and surroundings of the lips. Being aware of these changes and taking them into consideration are two of the prerequisites for selecting the appropriate treatment technique, with the aim of achieving a result that is as naturally harmonious as possible.

The aging process of the mouth region is subject to the following structure-altering factors:

- Changes to the skin and its turgor
- Changes to the fat tissue
- Changes to the musculature
- Changes to the retaining ligaments
- Changes to the jaw bones and teeth

Apart from the genetic contribution to lip aging (which amounts to approximately 20% to 30%), key roles are also played by extrinsic factors such as UV radiation, smoking, and negative environmental influences (Becker-Wegerich 2011, 2016), and intrinsic factors such as hormonal changes, nutritional factors, metabolic disorders, and the side effects of other disorders.

1.4.1 Changes to the Skin and its Turgor

The skin's aging processes are subject to ethnic differences and cannot be generalized. Nevertheless, it can be said that the skin of the mouth region changes with increasing age, with the following characteristics:

- The dermis becomes atrophic, dry, and thinner, resulting in the formation of vertical aging lines. The skin also becomes susceptible to microcracks in the mouth region, which manifests in the form of deeper cracks in the oral commissures and a wrinkled vermillion.
- The dermis shows a progressive loss of elasticity. Excess tissue is formed, which then follows the force of gravity. This results in the corners of the mouth being pulled down, the cutaneous region of the lips becoming longer, and the formation of perioral and marionette lines.
- As time passes, the perioral lines sink deeper into the subcutaneous layer of the skin. In the advanced stage of wrinkling, this is associated with cornification of the epithelium in the center of the line. This makes treatment of this zone more difficult, necessitating several consecutive sessions if a satisfactory result is to be achieved.
- The loss of elasticity in the skin of the lips also causes lip shape to change, while the loss of the vermillion border blurs the contours. The consequence of this may be that the injected dermal filler can no longer expand in the desired direction.
- The commissures become thinner and elongated, the gaps become wider, and the corners droop, making the mouth look sad (in men, the loss of elasticity of the lip skin has fewer effects because the roots of the beard hairs make the skin thicker and thus more compact).
- Skin texture becomes coarser, with larger pores, and more macules and warts develop.

1.4.2 Changes to the Fat Tissue

The signs of aging as regards the subcutaneous fat and superficial musculoaponeurotic system (SMAS) are strongly associated with the distribution and thickness of the fat as well as with interindividual differences. In its function as a natural filler, a well-developed subcutaneous fat layer, as is often the case in overweight individuals, counteracts the formation of perioral lines.

Atrophy of the deep fat compartments with the corresponding loss in volume – in the mouth region, these compartments are located in the vicinity of the depressor anguli oris muscle – intensifies the appearance of aging, which is manifested by marionette wrinkles and lines.

1.4.3 Changes to the Musculature

As humans age, there is a decrease in the volume and tone of the musculature and the muscles lengthen. For the perioral region, this means that the orbicularis oris muscle becomes thinner, but longer. As a result, the lips also become thinner and the reduced tone favors the formation of perioral lines.

1.4.4 Changes to the Retaining Ligaments

True and false retaining ligaments lose their tension as a result of the progressive loss of volume; the consequence is sagging of the skin and soft tissue that is induced by gravity: in the lower part of the face, this leads to marionette lines (Sattler and Sommer 2015).

1.4.5 Changes to the Jaw Bones and Teeth

Since the soft tissue of the mouth region, especially the lips, is supported by the dentition and the structures of the jaw bones, these have a considerable effect on the esthetic features of the mouth region.

As described in the article by Daniel Brusco,* "the position of the maxilla, the mandible and the chin, relative to each other and in relation to the plane of the face and, in turn, the position and form of the dental arches and alveolar process within the maxilla or mandible, can have a definitive influence on the aforementioned soft tissues."

* Text mostly taken, with kind permission, from the as yet unpublished work by Daniel Brusco, entitled "Dentoskeletal Influences on the Esthetics of the Lips."

1.4.6 Age-related Dentoskeletal Changes*

(→ Fig. 1.25)

Once growth is complete, the facial skull is subject to constant bone remodeling, which is influenced by a variety of factors (genetics, metabolism, hormone balance), so that increasing age can also result in certain relevant changes: it is worth being aware of these changes when contemplating filler treatment of the perioral region.

Of course, the age-related dentoskeletal changes rarely become manifest in isolation, but instead mostly in combination and at varying degrees of intensity. These changes are easily hidden using skillful volume enhancement, at least to some extent, and can be offset for a while. However, if they go beyond a certain level, filler treatment reaches its limits and other causal treatment approaches should be considered if the goal of natural and harmonious facial esthetics is to be achieved.

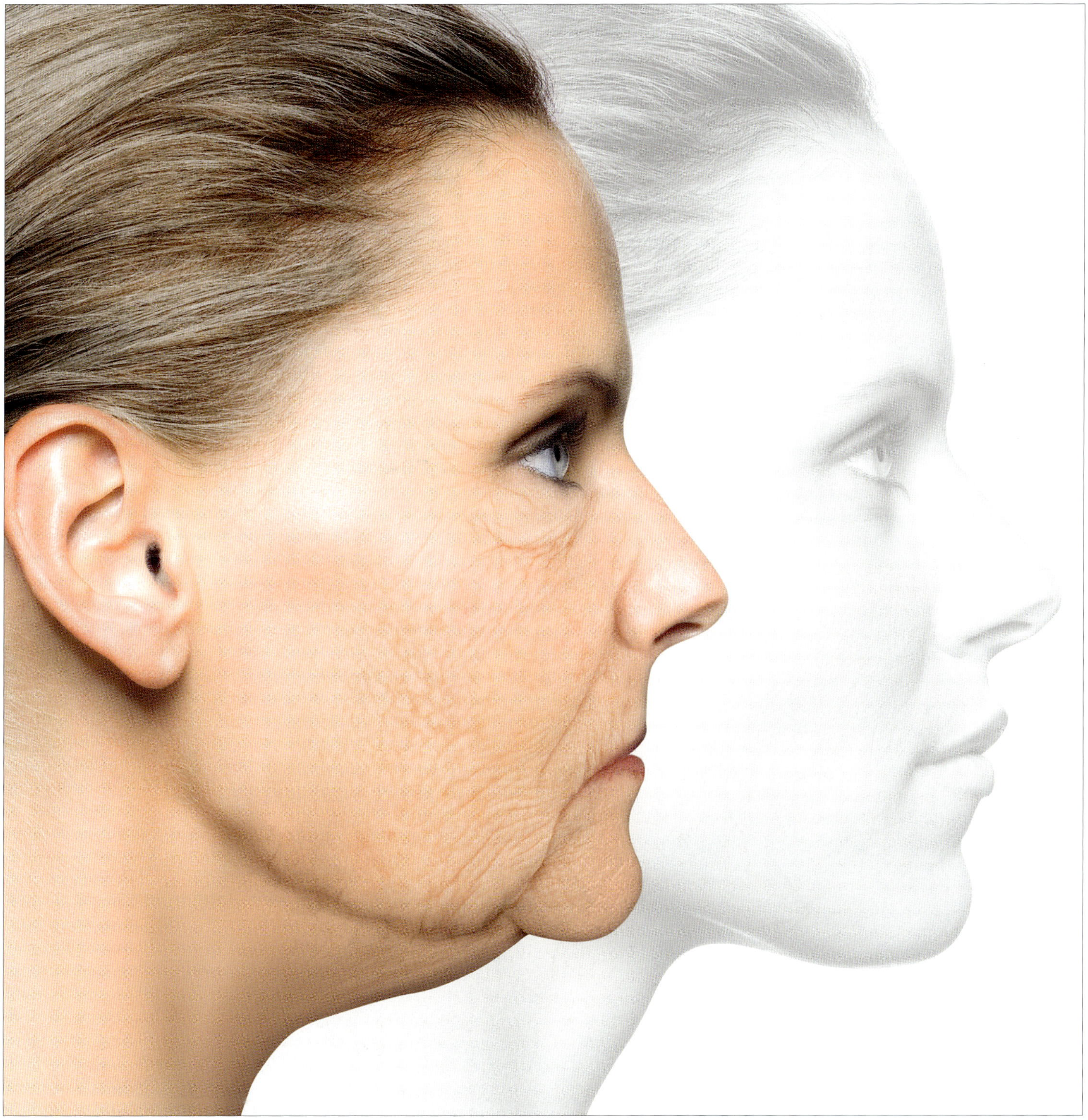

Fig. 1.25 Facial contours altered by the aging process (adapted from Daniel Brusco).

■ Maxilla

With age, even with the dentition fully preserved, the maxillary bone tends to lose its degree of projection: this is evident far into the midface and even up to the periorbital region, thus reducing the support it offers to the soft tissue. The lower margin of the orbital cavity (infraorbital margin) is displaced backward and downward, and the malar prominences of the cheekbones also become visibly reduced. We should remember that this anterior wall of the maxilla also acts as an attachment point for most of the muscles of facial expression, and provides support for the various fat compartments of the midface. Consequently, it becomes immediately apparent that skeletal aging can further intensify the sagging and loss of volume of the soft tissue. This is particularly true in the region of the upper lip if individual teeth from the anterior or premolar region are also lost, leading to additional, sometimes even complete, loss of the alveolar process, with resultant backward displacement of the entire maxilla.

■ Mandible

Increasing overlap of the anterior teeth (tertiary crowding) frequently develops in the maxilla, leading to a so-called deep bite, thus also decreasing the vertical dimension and reducing support for the lips. Taken together with the unavoidable loss of tone and elongation of the upper lip, this causes the maxillary anterior teeth to be less visible at rest and when smiling, while the mandibular teeth are increasingly revealed, representing another unmistakable stigma of old age.

■ Teeth

The same effect is produced when excessive wear, grinding of the teeth, etc. causes flattening of the cusps of the lateral teeth and a reduction in the incisal edges of the anterior teeth. When combined with tooth loss in the lateral region, this causes the additional forward tilt of the entire mandible, which also makes the chin more prominent. This can contribute toward the typical appearance of old age.

1.4.7 Classification of the Aging Lip

If all the factors of aging described above are taken into consideration, a "time lapse" event ensues, characterized by various processes that take place concomitantly. The study by Penna et al. (2015) with regard to average, symmetric lips confirms that "using the classification helps to tailor an appropriate treatment to the individual patient and aids to achieve a natural rejuvenation result." Two interdependent parameters of perioral aging are described in the study: perioral lip shape and perioral lip surface. These influence the perioral changes associated with aging lips and lead to different treatments, with the upper lip playing a more important role than the lower lip. The change in shape of the aging lip is classified into three stages, based on the front and side view with the lips slightly parted (→ Fig. 1.26).

Corresponding photos and treatment recommendations demonstrate the clinical manifestations of the three-stage model (→ Figs. 1.27–1.29).

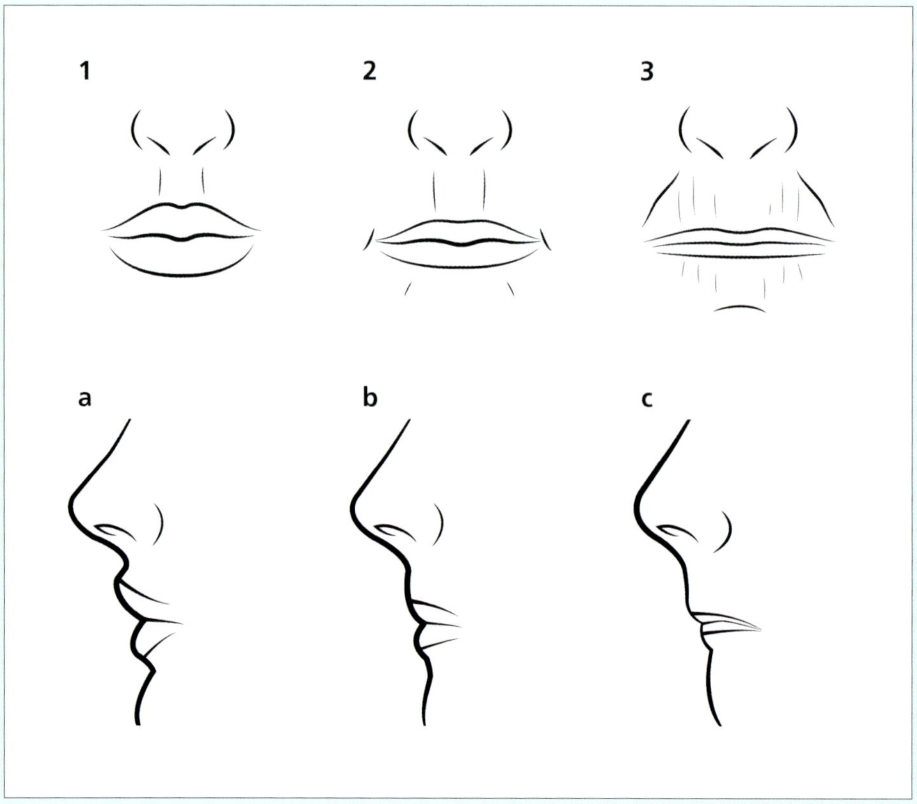

Fig. 1.26 Classification of the aging lip (modified from Penna et al. 2015).

(1–3) Perioral aging based on changes in lip shape: The cutaneous part of the upper lip lengthens increasingly in the caudal direction, producing a convex shape; the maxillary incisors are covered by the lip, and the lip vermillion inverts.

(a–c) Perioral aging based on changes in the lip surface: The philtrum, Cupid's bow, and lip roll become increasingly flattened, and static and dynamic perioral lines are formed.

Aging of the Lip Region according to the Three-Stage Model

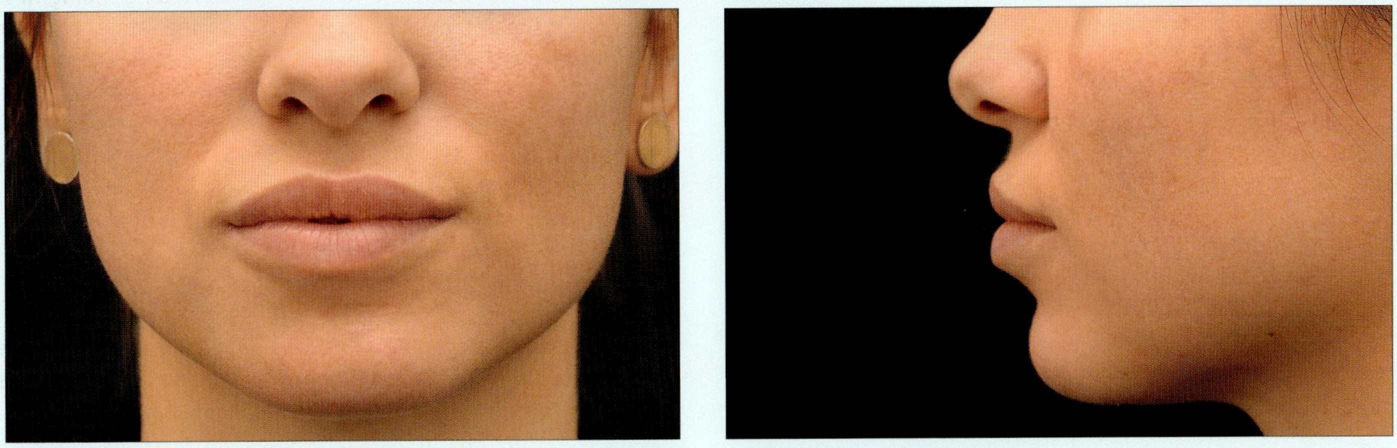

Fig. 1.27 28-year-old woman – Stage 1A: No rejuvenation necessary. Only beautification measures were undertaken, as follows: volume enhancement, evening out any asymmetries, improving contours, mouth corner lift, altering the shape, improving skin texture.

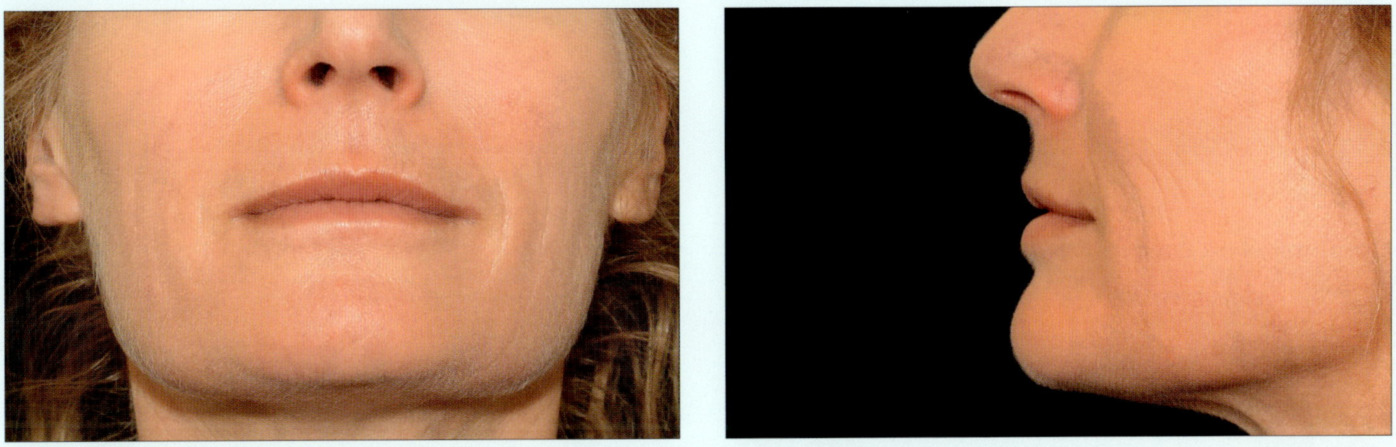

Fig. 1.28 40-year-old woman – Stage 2B: Rejuvenation and beautification required. In this case, if a natural result is to be achieved, thorough consultation and agreement is required in terms of the patient's wishes and the limits of the available treatment options. Lip augmentation should be carried out subtly, as beautification no longer looks natural if the upper lip is too long. Refreshing the contours and the philtrum with hyaluronic acid (HA) can counter the "incipient flattening of the structural elements of the lips."

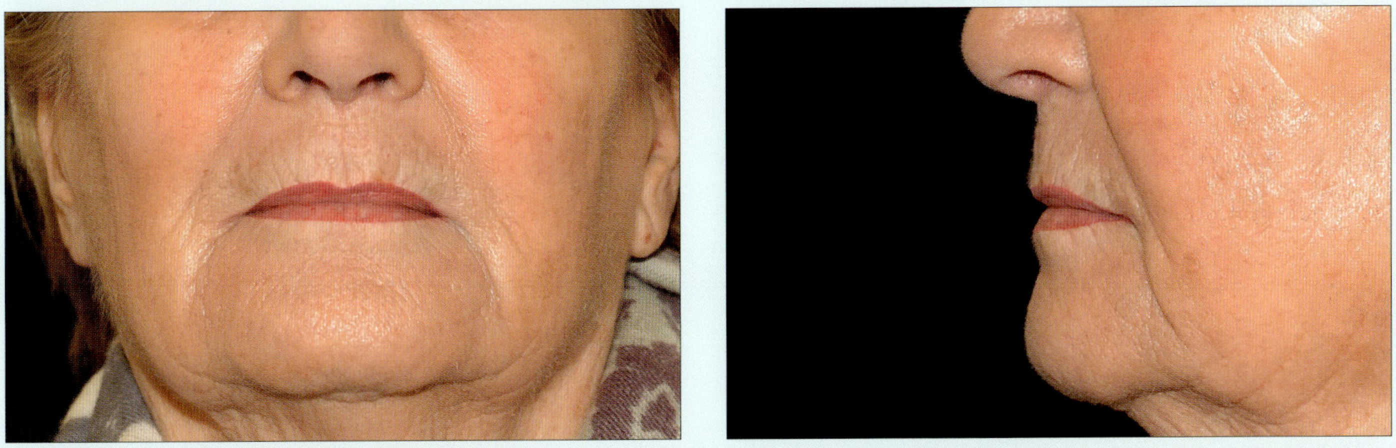

Fig. 1.29 68-year-old woman – Stage 3C: Features to be noted are the perioral lines on the upper lip; the deepening of the labiomental fold; the inversion of the vermillion; and the stretched, elongated upper lip. At this stage of the aging lip, beautification by adding volume leads to unnatural results. In this patient, it is possible to improve the structures (Cupid's bow, philtrum, contours), smooth out the perioral lines, improve skin texture using revitalizing products, and treat the corners of the mouth and the marionette lines.

1

Key Points

The various aging classifications involve different treatment concepts:

- The aim of perioral rejuvenation is to reverse the aging process of this specific esthetic unit.
- The aim of perioral beautification is to enhance the beauty of an intact young lip (Penna et al. 2015).
- The various individual deformities and anatomical circumstances affecting the lip need to be factored in and taken into account when treating aging lips (average, symmetric lips were selected for the aforementioned study).

1.5 Lip Shape and Expression

Lip shape has a pronounced, defining effect on the face. If the natural shape of the lips is inadvertently altered as a result of a treatment error or due to the unrealistic wishes of the patient, facial expression will be altered as well. The same applies if too much volume is injected into the atrophied lip of an elderly patient: the lip looks artificial and does not harmonize with the rest of the face. Improving a face harmoniously is often a balancing act between injecting as much as necessary and as little as possible.

Figures 1.30–1.41 show how changing the lips in the same face can lead to conclusions about someone's personality, mood, and general presence. These examples also illustrate what can happen if the natural shape of the face is ignored. For this reason, if a patient's wishes are based on fashion trends, they need to be evaluated by the therapist with regard to these potential effects, and the issue explored in detail with the patient.

The examples given here assume that the teeth are normally positioned. Only the mouth has been changed in each case. It is amazing how the expression of the eyes also changes when the lip shape is altered.

Lip Shape and how it Defines the Face

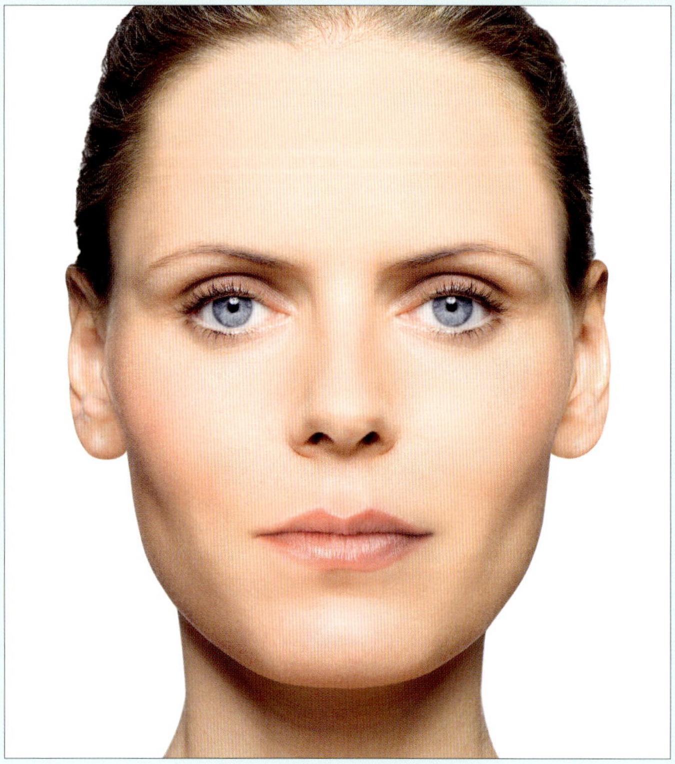

Fig. 1.30 Pronounced Cupid's bow and well-defined philtrum.

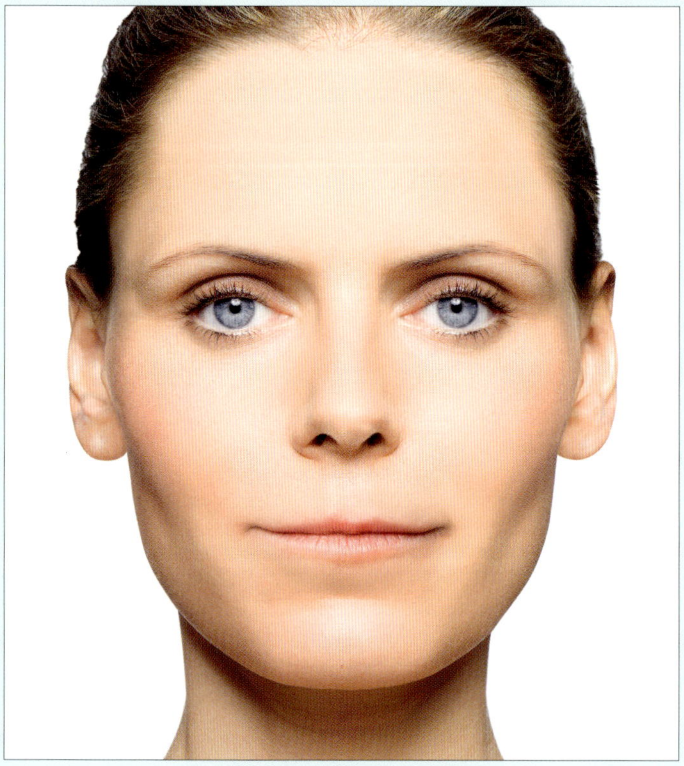

Fig. 1.31 Thin upper lip, blurred contours, and dry lips.

Lip Shape and how it Defines the Face

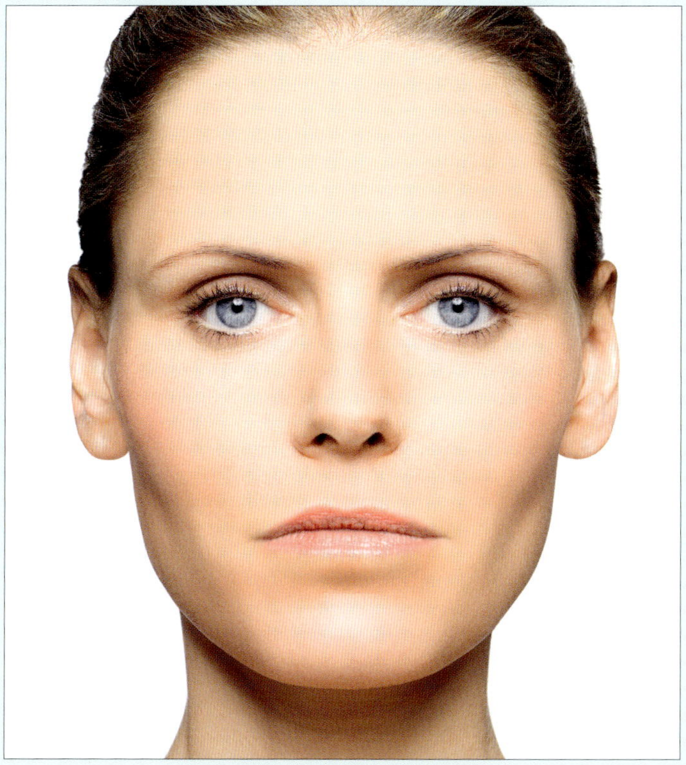

Fig. 1.32 The corners of the mouth have sagged slightly, the Cupid's bow is flat.

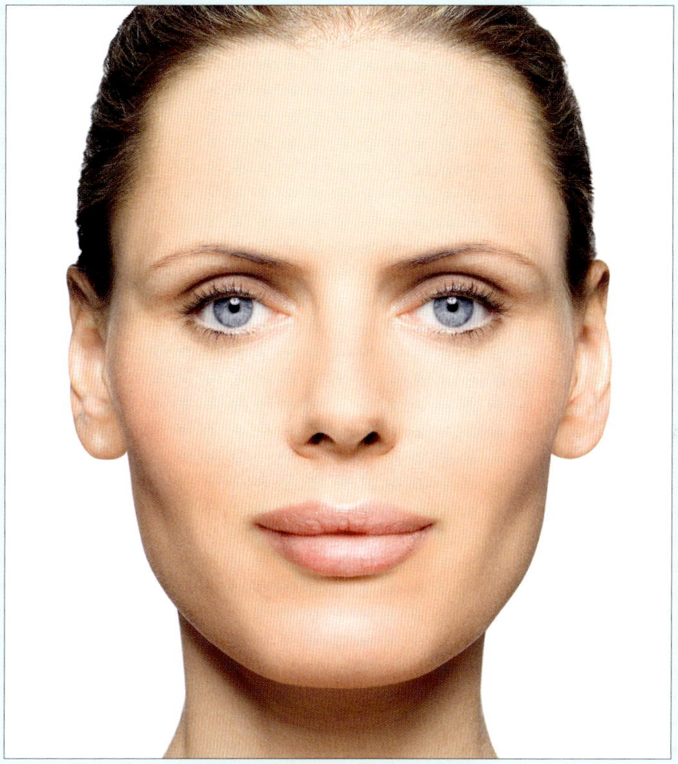

Fig. 1.33 Full lips, with the upper lip wider than the lower lip, larger lateral tubercles, and a natural central groove. The volume of the lip falls forward slightly, with a lateral deficit.

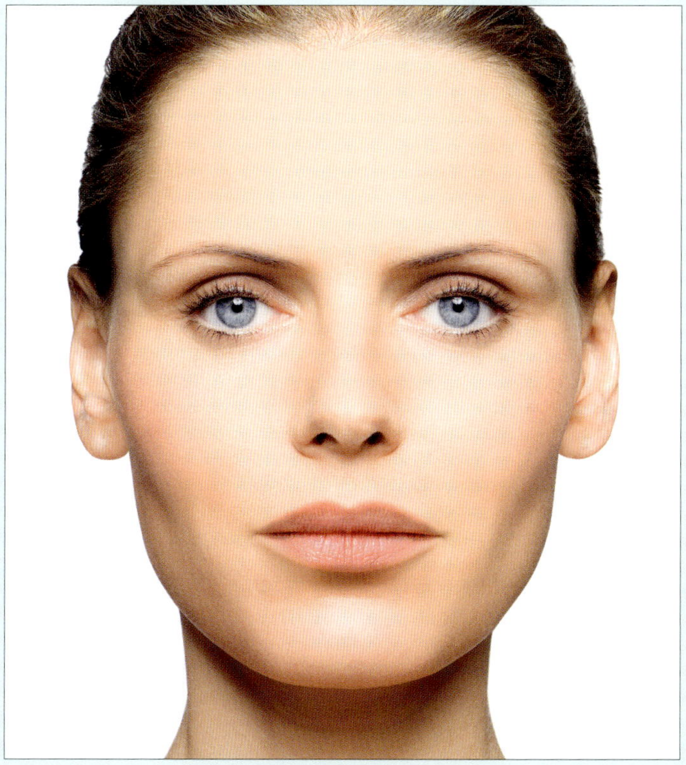

Fig. 1.34 In this image, the upper to lower lip ratio is 1 : 1, making the lower lip appear narrower.

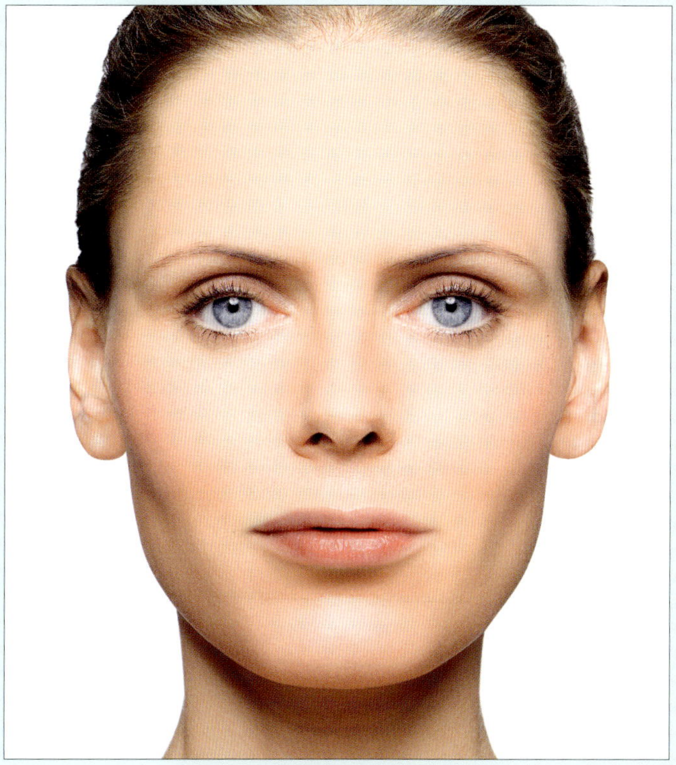

Fig. 1.35 Poorly defined Cupid's bow in a thin, stretched upper lip. The lower lip is not as wide but is more voluminous.

1

Lip Shape and how it Defines the Face

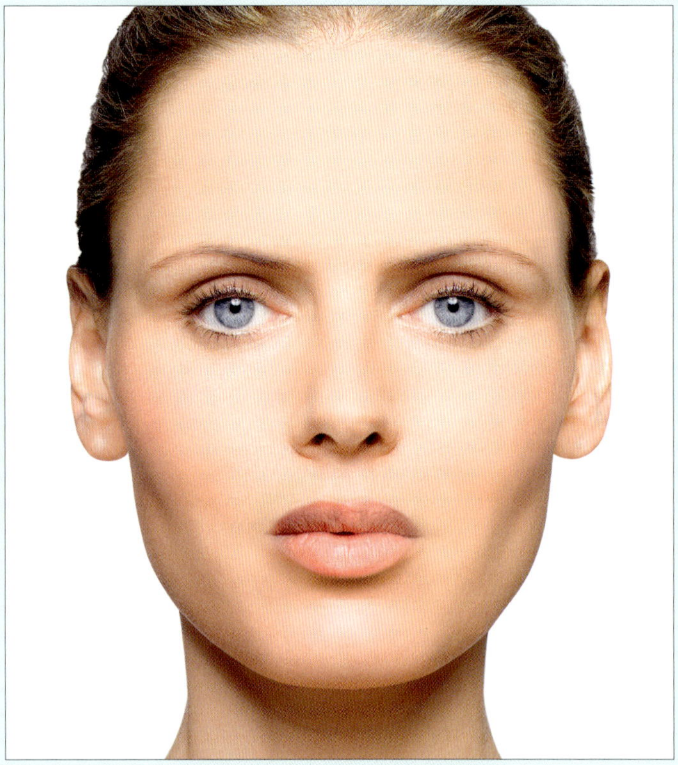

Fig. 1.36 Small, round mouth, poorly defined Cupid's bow, central groove, and dry lips.

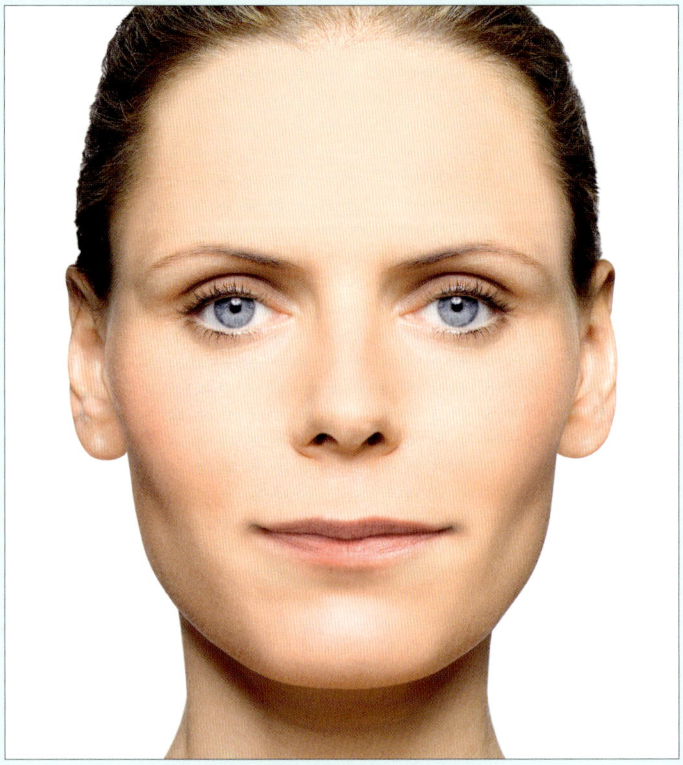

Fig. 1.37 Slightly asymmetric mouth with the central tubercle of the upper lip falling forward. The thin lower lip has a pointed anterior region and slopes gently backward. The corners of the mouth are slightly raised.

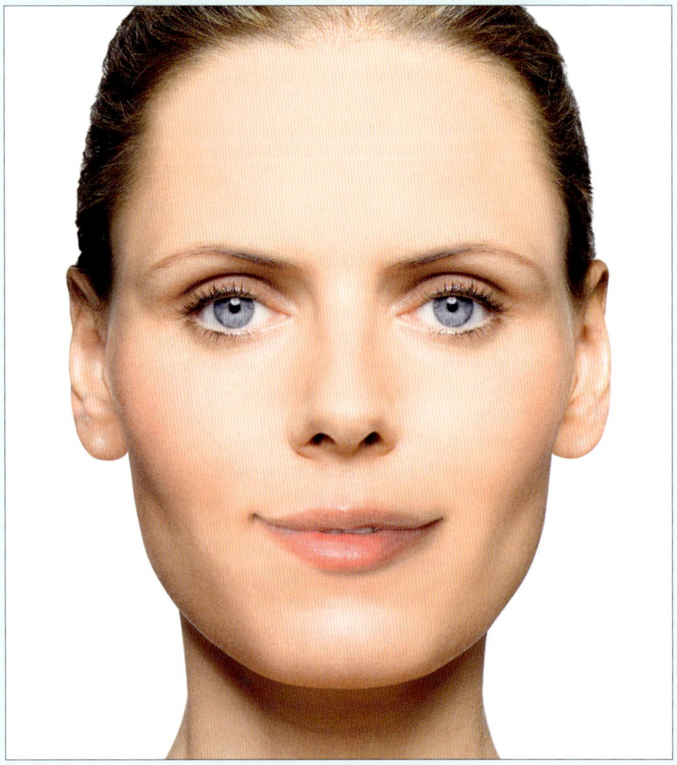

Fig. 1.38 Poorly defined, asymmetric upper lip with no contour, set against a lower lip with a central bulge, becoming thinner toward the corners of the mouth.

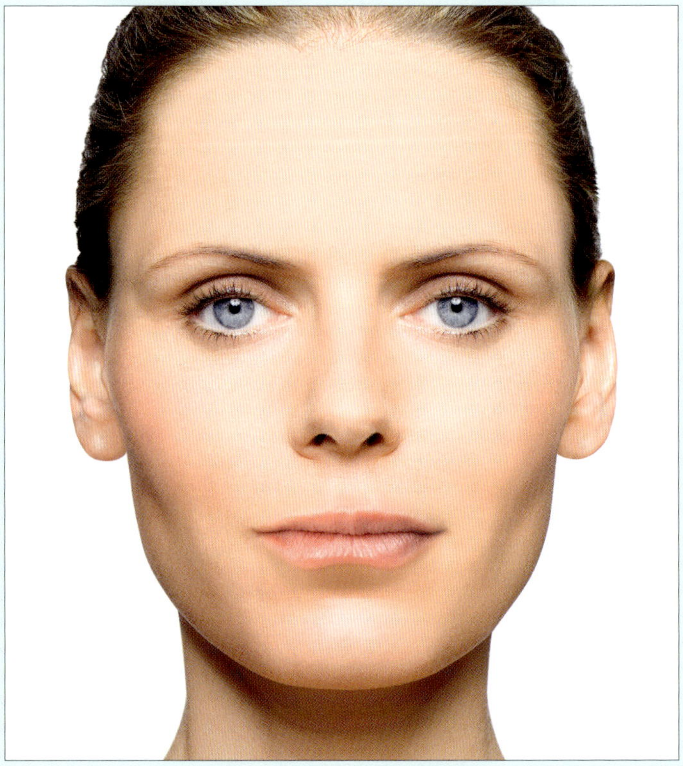

Fig. 1.39 Lower lip with a pronounced Cupid's bow.

Lip Shape and how it Defines the Face

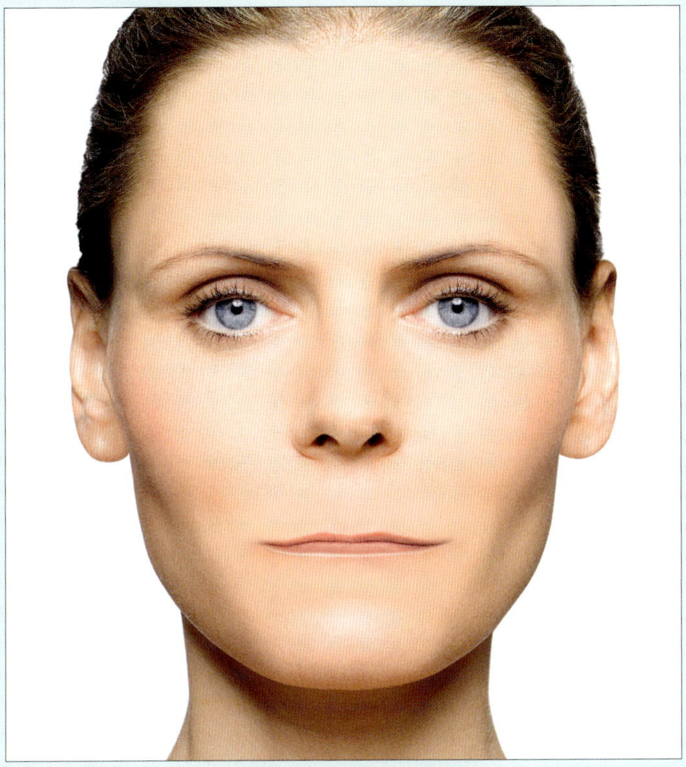

Fig. 1.40 Extremely thin lips with no visible vermillion.

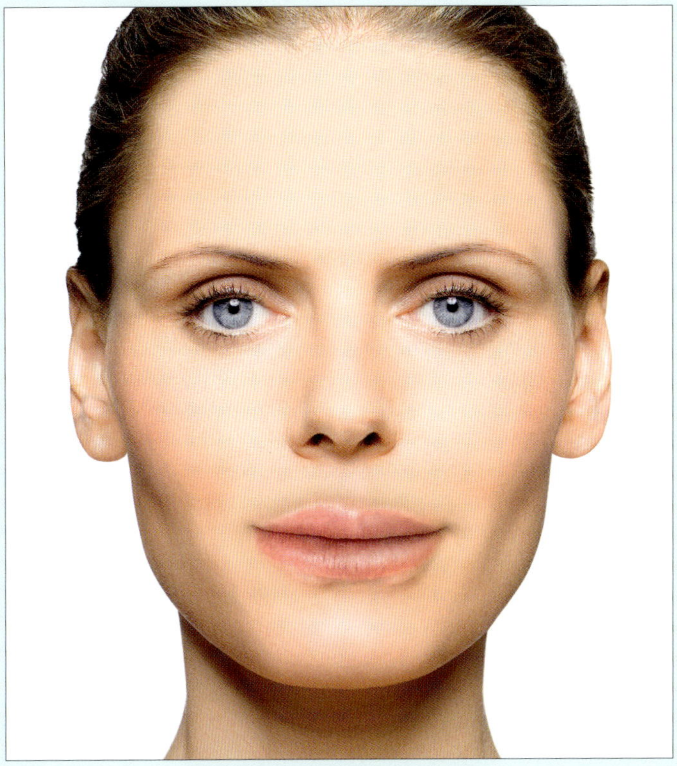

Fig. 1.41 Overcorrected lips. The material has sagged below the contours of the lower lip.

1.6 Analysis of the Lip Region

The analysis of the lip region forms the basis for a successful treatment with a realistic treatment goal, which can be implemented once all the determining factors and technical know-how have been taken into consideration. It is here that the therapist often comes up against the limits of what is possible.

After a first look at the patient, the trained eye will soon determine whether the lip is thin or full, asymmetric or symmetric; whether the corners of the mouth sag; whether perioral lines or loss of volume are present; whether there have been any incorrect previous treatments, etc.

After this first look, a fine analysis of the lips is undertaken to determine what sort of problem is involved and which treatment modalities are available. Various aspects and associated procedures are available for this fine analysis (described in detail below). An analytical guideline includes the various steps of the approach that needs to be taken.

The analysis is conducted from the morphologic perspective and always assumes an ideal profile. The therapist is free to decide how extensive the analysis will be and which analytical methods to use.

The following four major analytical procedures are presented here:
1. Inspection
2. Measurement
3. Analysis of the movements of facial expression and mobility
4. Palpation

1.6.1 Inspection

The inspection is a means of evaluating the proportions, the thickness, the curves, the size, the symmetries, the age, and the color of the lips. When conducting the inspection, factors that need to be taken into account include the relationship with the bone structures, the fat compartments, the ligaments, the SMAS, and the surrounding muscles of the whole face (Becker-Wegerich 2016). In detail, the lip inspection is carried out from the front and from the side, taking the following aspects into consideration:

- **Shape**: Size (UL/LL), width, volume (UL/LL), contours, sagging mouth corners, asymmetry, fat reduction, harmony (UL/LL), age, position of the teeth, the area surrounding the lips.
- **Skin Color** (as an index of certain underlying disorders):
  - Red discoloration: possible indication of inflammatory reactions, high blood pressure, alcohol abuse, allergies or disorders affecting the skin surface (Sattler & Sommer 2015)
  - Yellow discoloration: indication of certain metabolic or hepatic disorders
  - Red lips: indication of good blood circulation
  - Blue lips: possible indication of reduced blood oxygenation or pulmonary and cardiac disorders (Sattler & Sommer 2015)
  - Pigments and macules: indication of sun damage, metabolic abnormalities or certain disorders
- **Skin Relief**: Naevi, areas of keratosis, warts, scars, rashes, and telangiectasias are accompanying signs of certain metabolic, pathologic or aging processes. These should be investigated before the start of any treatment.
- **Texture**: Assessment of the perioral skin, the skin of the lips, and the mucous membranes. Skin texture is genetically determined and is altered by extrinsic and intrinsic factors. Lifestyle, exposure to sunlight, psychologic factors, and incorrect personal care can lead to dryness, laxity, enlarged pores, actinic damage, elastosis, wrinkling of the lips and perioral region, and the appearance of perioral shadows.
- **Lighting and Photo Documentation**: (see also p. 61 ff.): Lighting and photographic documentation of the target zone prior to the treatment are very simple tools for the accurate detection of details. When the light comes from one direction (from above, from the side or from below), the relief is illuminated, and the smallest shadows and irregularities become visible (→ Fig. 1.42).

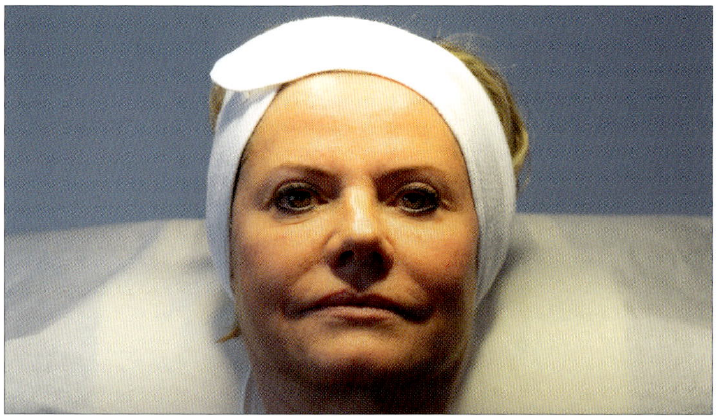

Fig. 1.42 Illuminating the skin relief: the light is being directed straight from above. The smallest irregularities, lines, and shadows become visible.

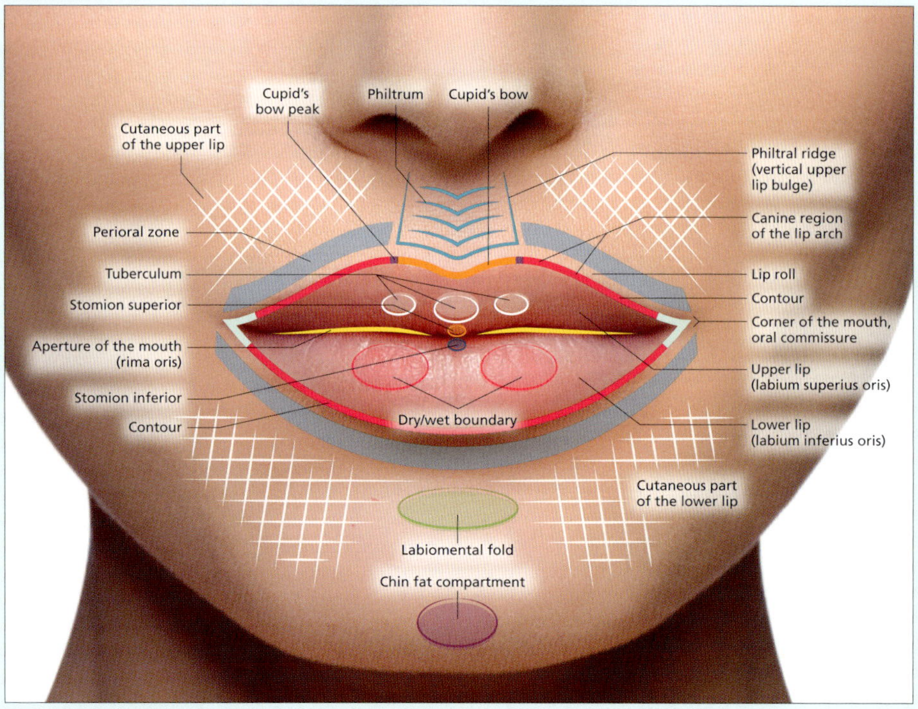

Fig. 1.43 Lip segments.

1.6.2 Measurement*

■ Anatomical and Three-dimensional Classification

(→ Figs. 1.43, 1.44)

The lip is divided into various anatomical units, which serve as a basis for a clearly defined description of the area being treated. By looking at the lips from the side, from above, and from below, the therapist gains a better understanding of the three-dimensional shape of the lips. The contours form the frame of the lips.

In its medial region, the upper lip has three tubercles that can show varying degrees of prominence. In some people, the medial tubercle is more pronounced and points slightly downward; in others, the lateral tubercles are more pronounced than the medial tubercle. Sometimes, there are either only two tubercles or they are so flattened that they are no longer apparent. There are many different variants of this feature, which give the lips their character (Rejuvent, Medical Spa & Surgery 2017).

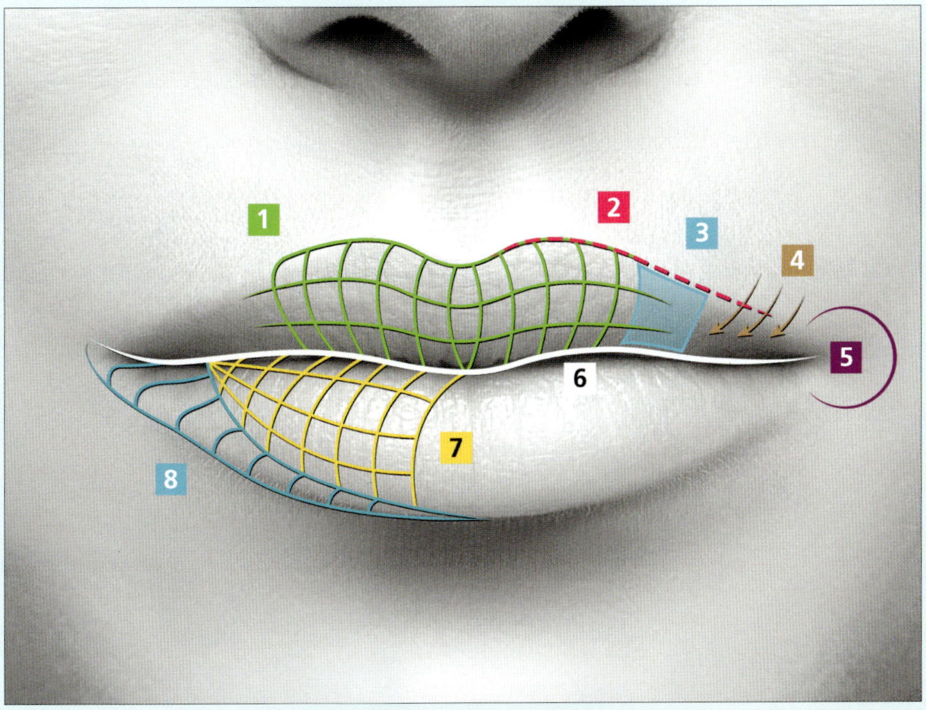

Fig. 1.44 This three-dimensional representation of the lip bumps helps to analyze lip volume (Rejuvent, Medical Spa & Surgery 2017).

1 Hump, bulge, bump
2 Sharp edge
3 Flat part
4 Rolled-in (inverted) part
5 Corner
6 Aperture of the mouth
7 Bump (bulge)
8 Ridge

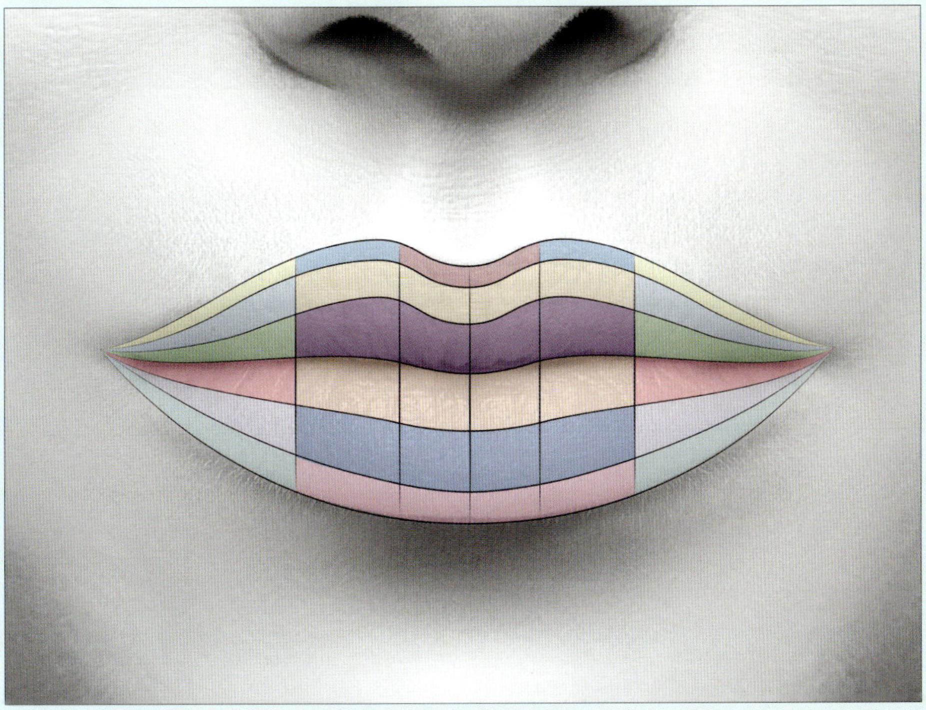

Fig. 1.45 This grid allows the distribution of lip volume to be mapped accurately and evenly on both sides, which helps the therapist, particularly one who is not yet very experienced, to inject the lip symmetrically.

* A series of passages in this section have been taken, with kind permission, from the as yet unpublished work by Daniel Brusco, entitled "Dentoskeletal Influences on the Esthetics of the Lips."

The lateral two thirds of the upper lip consist of a flat, inverted part, which shows such pronounced inward flattening in some patients that the vermillion is no longer visible. Technical know-how is required in this case if the lip shape is to be changed to achieve a harmonious result.

The lower lip has two tubercles that are generally larger than those of the upper lip. At two-thirds of its length from the center, the lower lip flattens toward the corner of the mouth. An unnatural result is produced if this flattening is not respected.

The philtrum is regarded as sexually attractive and emphasizes the contour of the upper lip. It should always be included in any treatment (Rejuvent, Medical Spa & Surgery 2017).

■ Grid

Segmental Mapping (→ see Fig. 1.45, p. 29)

Lengths and proportions can be recorded in the front view using a grid, which allows asymmetries, volume deficiencies, and proportions to be depicted. Injecting a filler changes the shape, volume, and bulge of the lips.

Quadrants (→ Fig. 1.46)

The lip is divided into four quadrants with a horizontal and a vertical line. This way of dividing the lips is a simplification of the segmental approach.

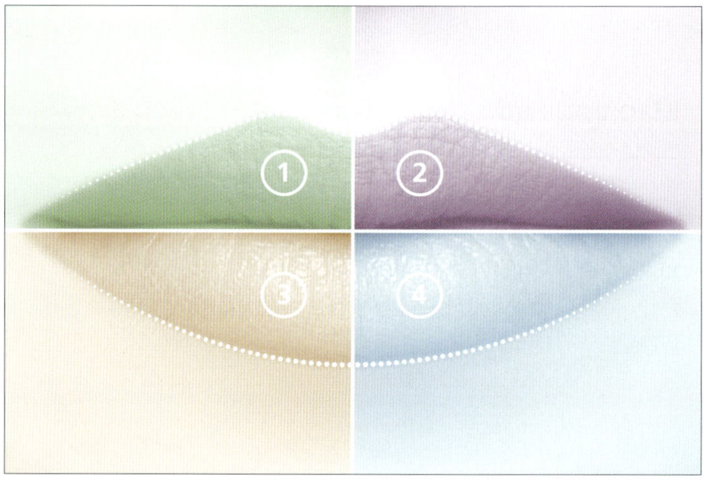

Fig. 1.46 Quadrant grid: 1 = UL, right quadrant; 2 = UL, left quadrant; 3 = LL, right quadrant; 4 = LL, left quadrant.

Mapping and Landmark Points

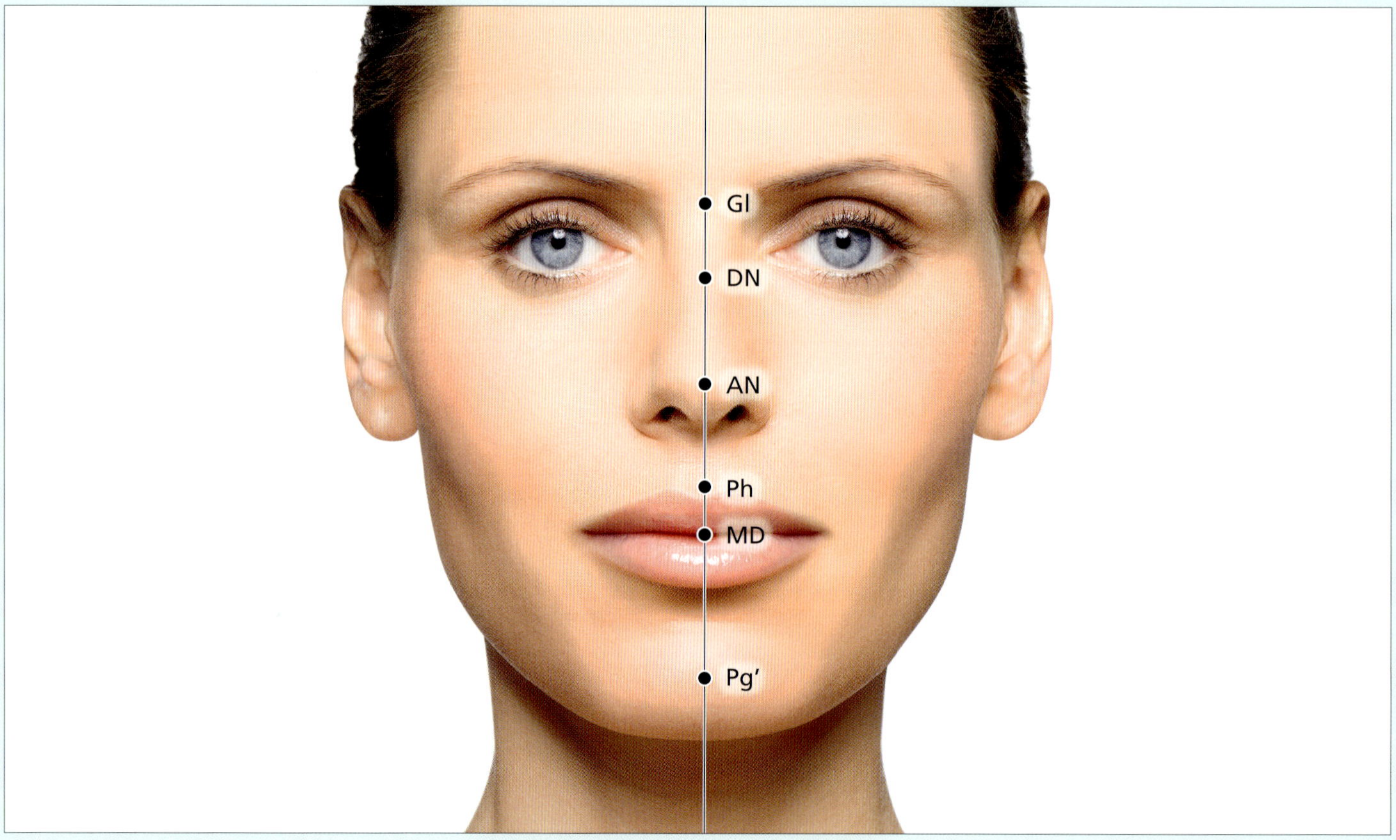

Fig. 1.47 The glabella (Gl), bridge of the nose (dorsum nasi, DN), tip of the nose (apex nasi, AN), philtrum (Ph), and soft tissue pogonion (Pg') are used to find the midline of the face. The dental midline (DM) is also included in this diagnostic measure.

■ Proportions

Mapping using Ratios (→ Figs. 1.47–1.48)

A consideration of the proportions of the face is of great significance because an understanding of the ratios and their differences relative to one another has a key influence on the implementation of a successful treatment.

There are various approaches used for measuring the face from the front and from the side. Here, for practical reasons, we have decided in favor of the most commonly used form of mapping from these two points of view. The various regions are quantified using landmarks, which are then used to determine the relationships between specific ratios and angles.

Mapping and Landmark Points

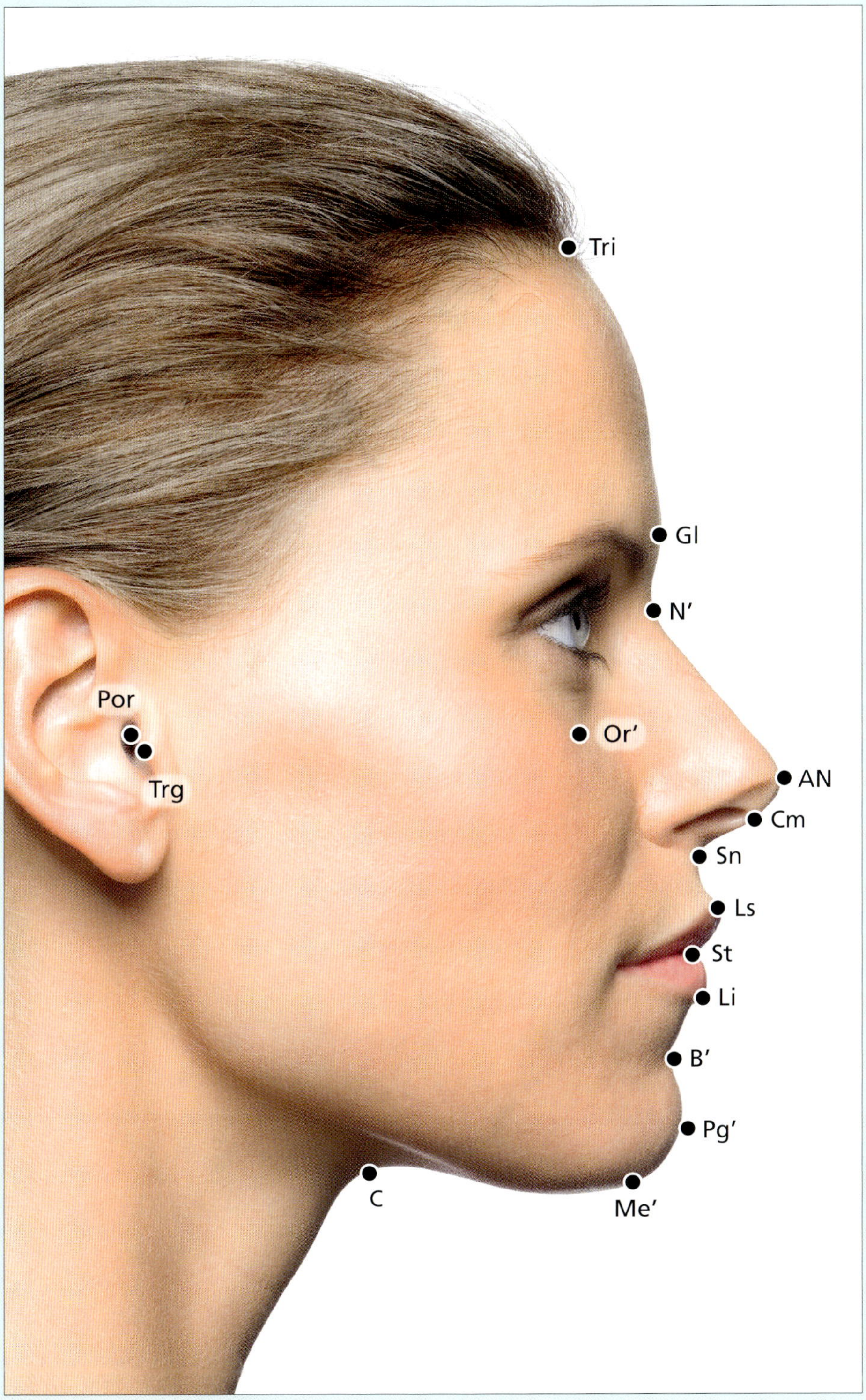

Fig. 1.48 The most commonly used facial landmarks in side view:

Tri	Trichion (hairline)
Gl	Glabella (skin of the forehead between the eyebrows)
N′	Soft tissue nasion (deepest point at the root of the nose)
Or′	Soft tissue orbitale (deepest point of the curvature of the orbital margin)
AN	Tip of the nose (apex nasi)
Cm	Columella nasi (bridge of the nose)
Sn	Subnasale
Ls	Labiale superius (foremost edge of the upper lip)
St	Stomion (oral fissure when the lips are closed)
Li	Labiale inferius (foremost edge of the lower lip)
B′	Soft tissue B-point (deepest point of the labiomental fold)
Pg′	Soft tissue pogonion
Me′	Soft tissue menton (most inferior point on the soft tissue of the chin)
C	Cervical point (junction of the submental and neck contours, neck–throat junction)
Por	Porion (external auditory meatus)
Trg	Tragus. The peaked upper edge of the tragus is referred to as the tragion and used for a few measurements

1

Golden Ratio (according to Dr. A. Swift) – Proportions according to the "Golden Mean" (→ Figs. 1.49–1.53)

Another method of facial measurement follows the proportions of the golden mean, which "describes the dividing ratio of a line segment, where the ratio of the whole to its longer part is equal to the ratio of the longer part to the shorter part" (citation from Becker Wegerich 2016).

This results in the principle of the ratio of 1 : 1.6. All objects that are consistent with this ratio are perceived as being harmonious or beautiful. The 1 : 1.6 ratio is encountered in objets d'art, in nature, and in architecture, in medieval and modern times: e.g. in works by Leonardo Da Vinci (1452–1519) and Salvador Dali (Rejuvent, Medical Spa & Surgery 2017).

In Central European esthetic medicine, this code is applied to all the proportions of the face, including the lips. Here, the "code of beauty" corresponds to the golden ratio, but this code can be quite different in other cultures: thus, for example, the code of beauty in a non-white culture defines the ideal UL : LL ratio as 1 : 1. This gives the mouth, with a pronounced lip volume, an almost round shape, which does not generally occur among pale-skinned, Caucasian individuals. Adopting a beauty ideal that is not widespread in one's own cultural circles when considering the options for esthetic treatment ("cosmetic surgery") would likely result in unharmonious proportions that would make the treatment outcome highly conspicuous – an option that some patients expressly request.

Mapping of the lips according to the golden mean is done both vertically and horizontally. The deviations in size between the two methods are very small. According to Swift and Remington (2011), for perfect lip proportions, the columns of the philtrum should line up exactly with the centers of the Cupid's bow peaks. The width of the nose should be equal to the distance between the medial corners of the eyes. From these lines, we can derive the medial segment of the lower lip, which makes up two thirds of the whole lower lip and is therefore its largest segment.

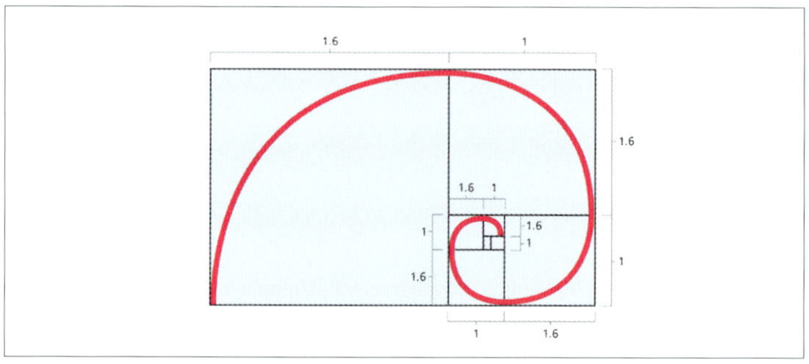

Fig. 1.49 Mapping a snail shell spiral according to the golden mean principle, producing the so-called golden or Fibonacci spiral. The ratio of the whole to its larger part is equal to the ratio of the larger part to the smaller part.

1

Golden Mean in the Lip Region

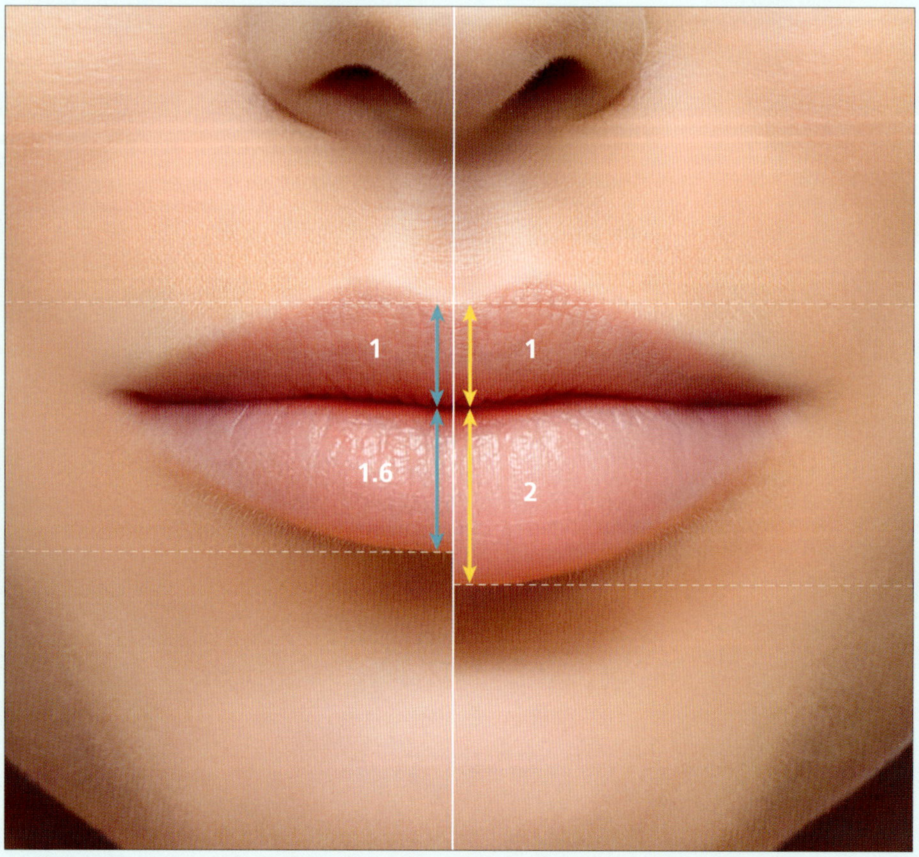

Fig. 1.50 Cupid's bow with lines drawn according to the golden mean (1 : 1.6) and using a ratio of 1 : 2.

Golden Mean in the Lip Region (continued)

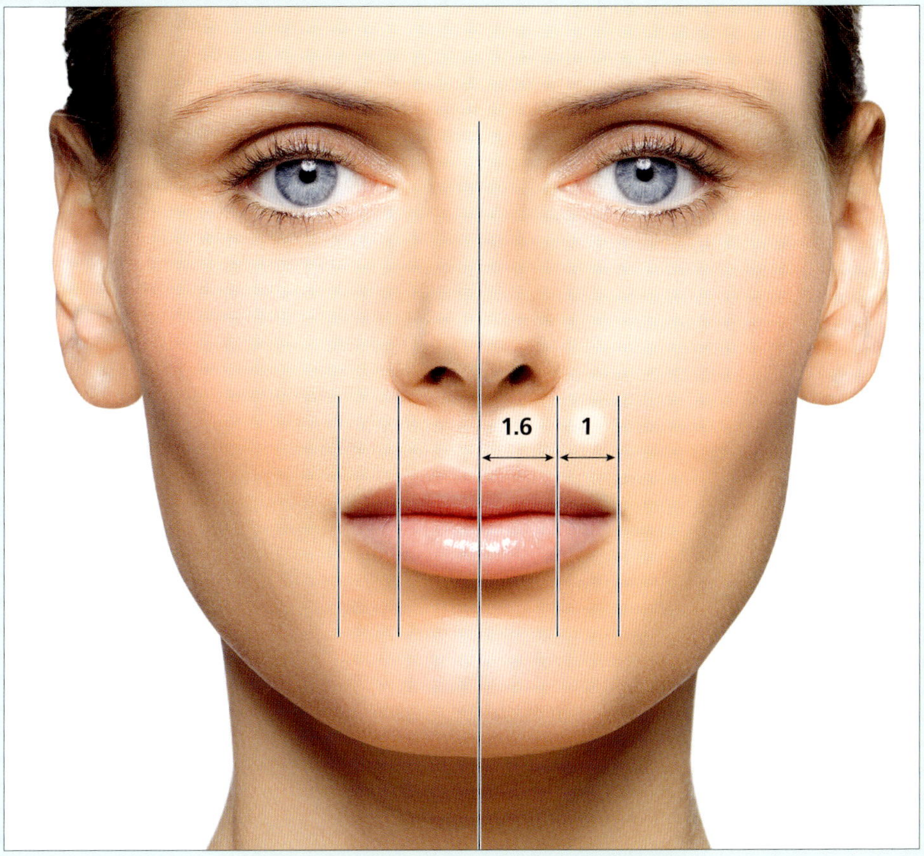

Fig. 1.51 Vertical lines mapping the lip region according to the golden mean (1 : 1.6).

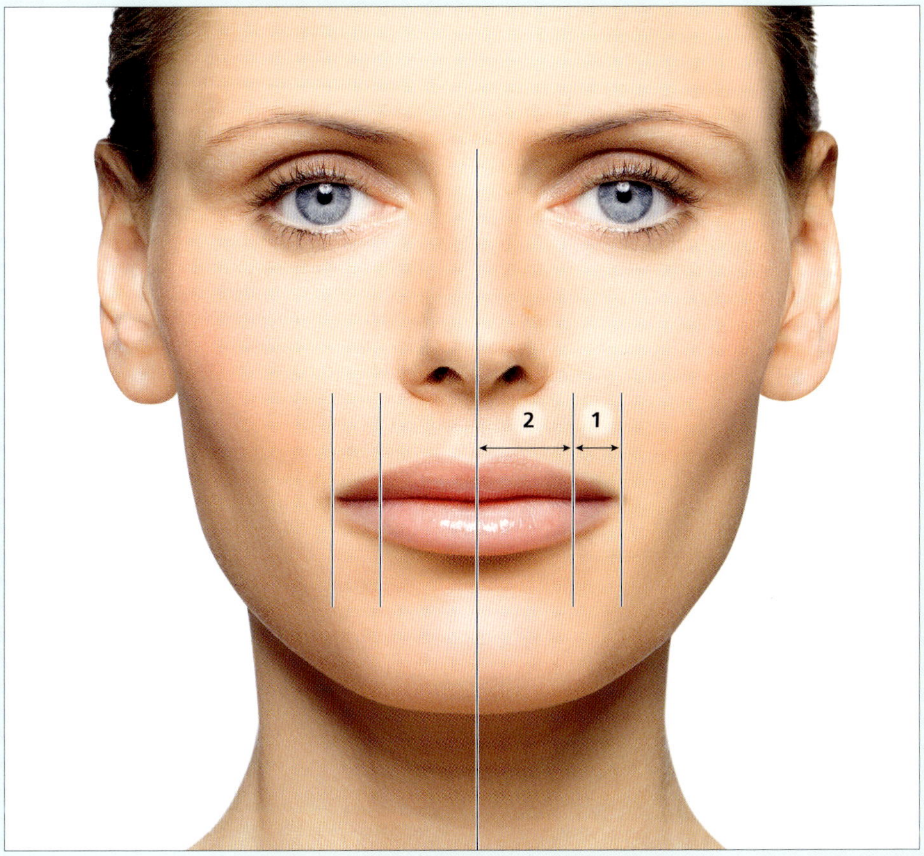

Fig. 1.52 Vertical lines mapping the lip region according to a ratio of 2 : 1.

Golden Mean in the Lip Region (continued)

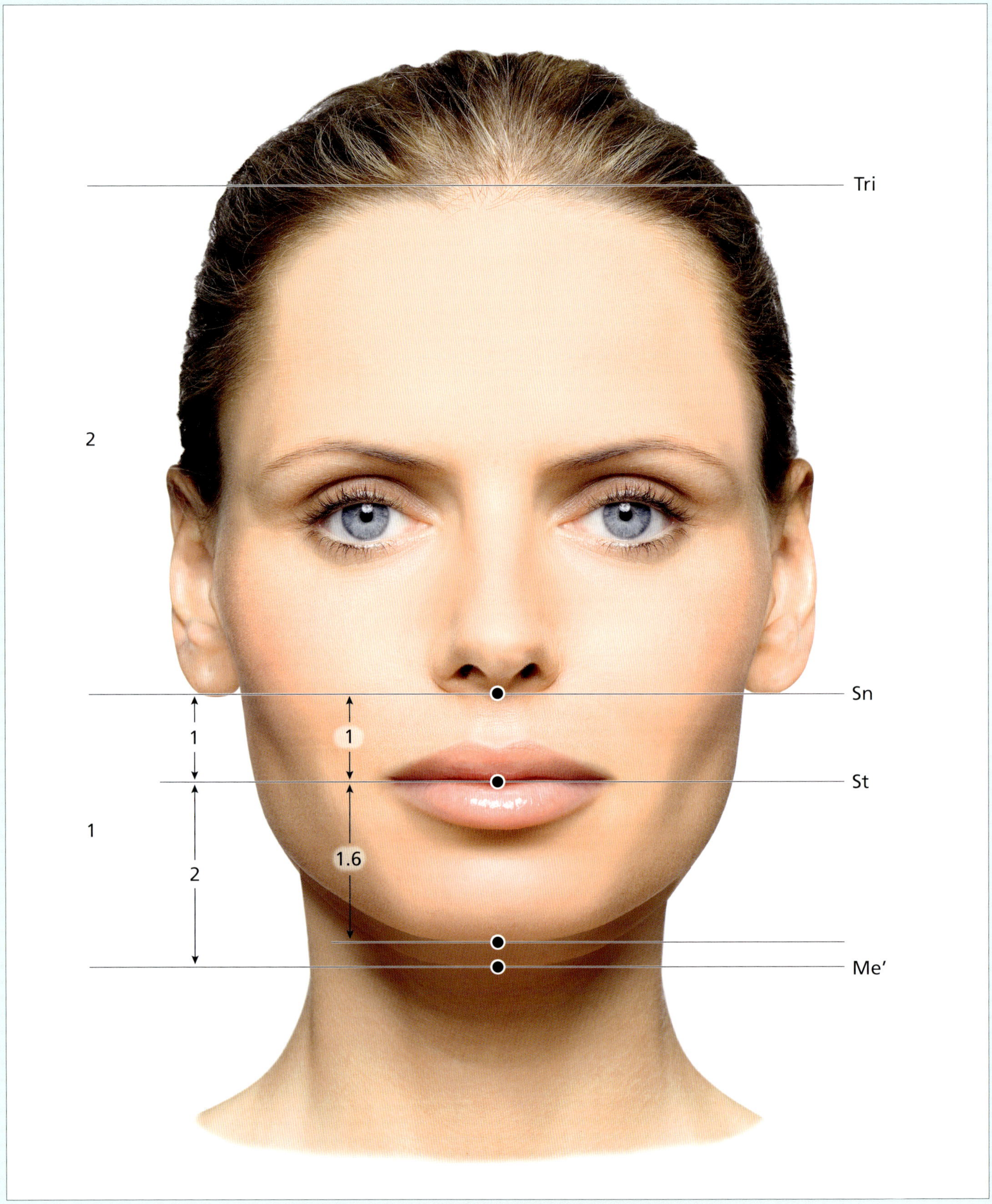

Fig. 1.53 Horizontal lines mapping the lip region according to the golden mean (1 : 1.6) and according to a ratio of 1 : 2 (Tri: trichion, Sn: subnasale, St: stomion, Me': soft tissue menton).

Tools used for Measuring the Golden Mean

The therapist can use calipers to assess lip proportions (→ Fig. 1.54). This makes it possible to determine the extent to which the proportions deviate from the ideal, and which areas can be touched up with HA to even out these proportions (→ Fig. 1.55–1.58).

This tool works in a similar way to a slide rule: the area is measured using the smaller end of the calipers (e.g. upper lip = 1); the larger end opens up accordingly, so that the ratio between the openings of the small and large ends is 1 : 1.6. This opening is then held to its counterpart (lower lip = 1.6). By doing so, one can immediately see whether the lower and upper lip are in the ideal ratio based on the golden mean. The instrument is also highly suitable for measuring all other regions of the face.

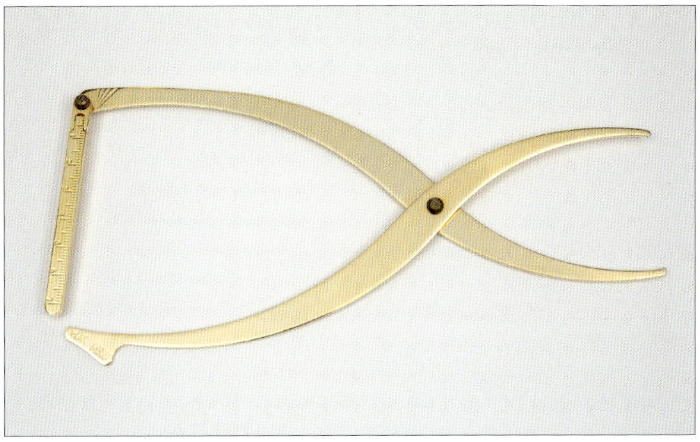

Fig. 1.54 Calipers used for measuring proportions according to A. Swift: 1 : 1.618 or 0.618 : 1.

Measuring Proportions using the Calipers

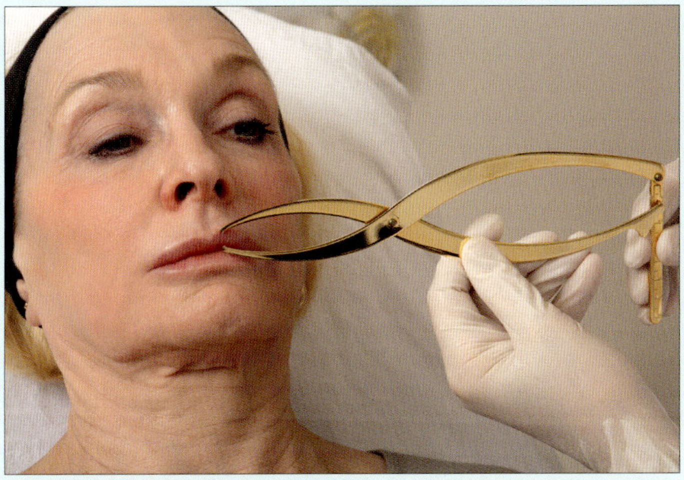

Fig. 1.55 The small end of the calipers is held with the upper half against the upper margin of the vermillion and the lower half against the aperture of the lips.

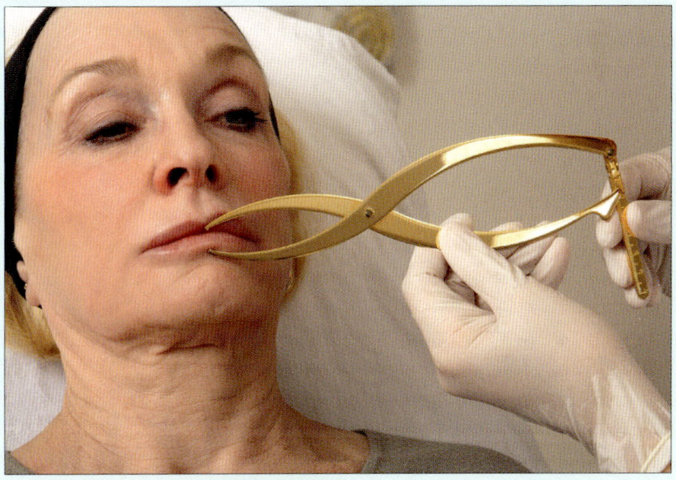

Fig. 1.56 A similar procedure is followed for the lower lip. The desired size of the lower lip according to the 1 : 1.6 ratio can be read off on the gauge at the large end of the calipers. This allows differences to be identified and evened out accurately.

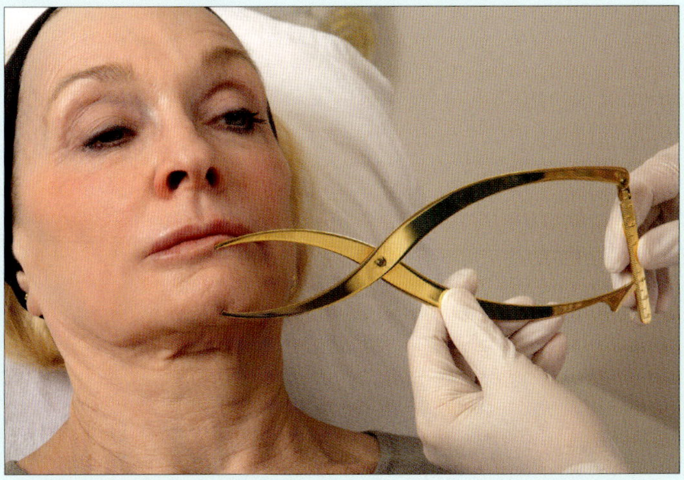

Fig. 1.57 This method can also be used to measure and evaluate the ratio of the entire mouth region. Here, the chin measures 4.8 cm.

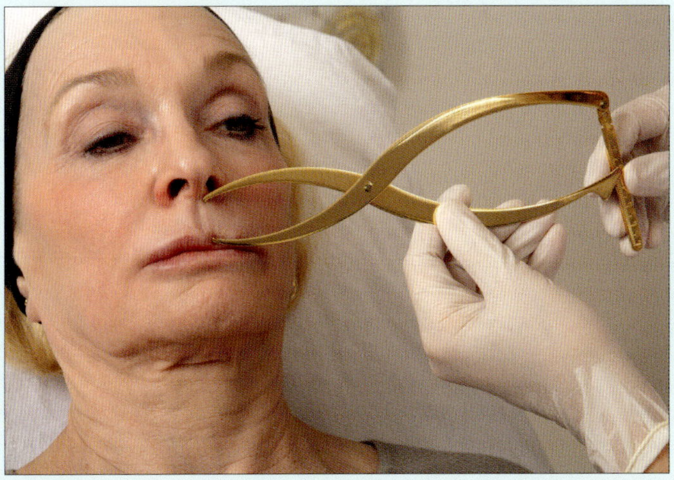

Fig. 1.58 Conclusion: this patient's proportions correspond to the golden mean as regards the ratio of the maxilla to the mandible.

1

1.6.3 Landmarks according to Daniel Brusco
(→ Fig. 1.59)

To give a more complete perspective, we have also included the approach of Daniel Brusco, maxillofacial surgeon in Zürich, Switzerland, who kindly shared his findings with us.

■ Ideal Profile

Side View

When photographed in a strictly lateral view, we perceive a profile as harmonious if the foremost points of the upper lip (labiale superius, Ls), lower lip (labiale inferius, Li), and chin (soft tissue pogonion, Pg') lie on a line that, when taken from the midpoint between the tip of the nose (pronasale, Pn) and the point of attachment of the wings of the nose (alare, Ala), forms an angle of 82 to 86 degrees (in men, this may be as high as 90 degrees) with the absolute vertical (modified Steiner line, S-line). In this context, the lips should be closed but completely relaxed, with a soft labiomental depression (no sharp line or true fold).

Front View

In the front view, the rule of thirds, if fulfilled, is regarded as esthetic for the anterior height of the face. According to this rule, the distance between the attachment point of the nasal septum (subnasale, Sn) and the oral fissure when the lips are closed (stomion, St) is half the distance from the oral fissure (with the lips closed) to the tip of the chin (soft tissue menton, Gn'). With the lips slightly parted, the incisal edges of the anterior teeth should still be clearly visible (2–4 mm), while the gum margin should be only just revealed (1–2 mm) when the lips are open in a full smile. When conducting maxillary and orthopedic surgical procedures of varying complexity, all of these points can be taken into account, and, above all, influenced almost at will to produce a natural and esthetically appropriate result.

■ Deviations from the Ideal Profile

It is essential to bear in mind that the soft tissue of the perioral region is supported by the underlying dentoskeletal structures, which differ in shape from one individual to another, with corresponding alterations to the appearance of the perioral soft tissue. Good knowledge and correct interpretation of these differences in shape are relevant when deciding which treatment strategy might be promising and which might not.

It soon becomes clear that treatment with a dermal filler will not be sufficient to achieve a harmonious result under certain anatomical conditions (→ author's treatment recommendations) (→ Figs. 1.60–1.64).

1

Ideal Profile Proportions according to Daniel Brusco

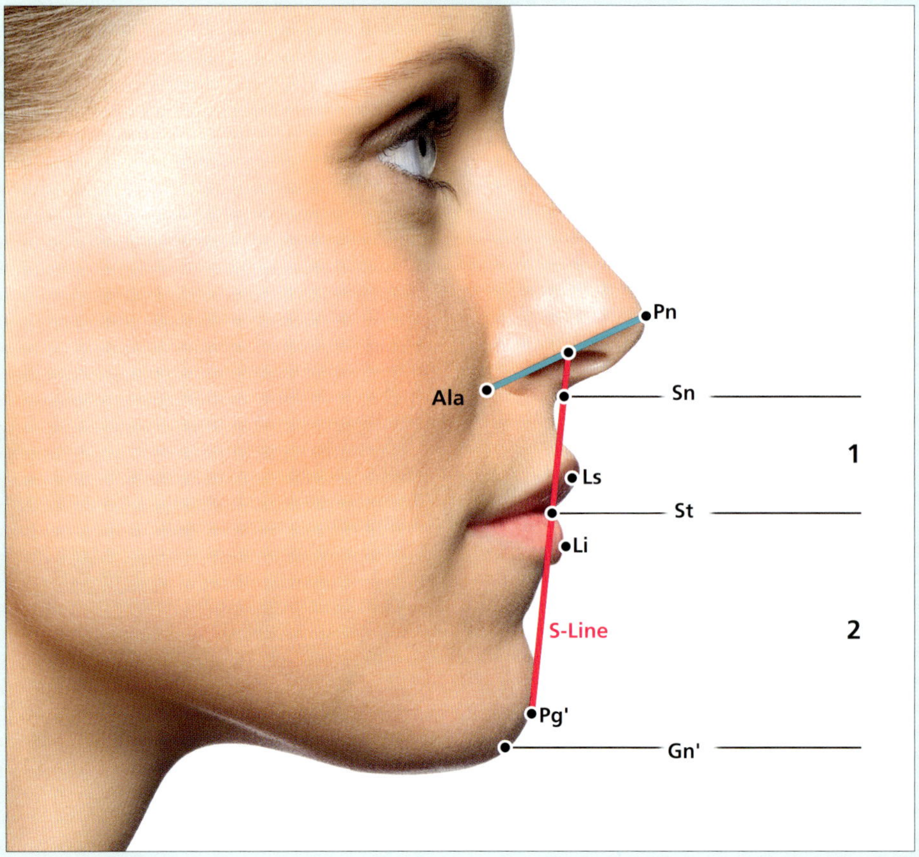

Fig. 1.59 The most commonly used landmarks and mapping lines (see Fig. 1.48, p. 31), limited to the mouth region, with two additional lines to better represent deviations from the norm of the mouth and jaws (modified from Brusco et al. 2013).

Pn	Pronasale
Ala	Attachment point of the wings of the nose
Sn	Subnasale
Ls	Labiale superius
St	Stomion
Li	Labiale inferius
Pg'	Soft tissue pogonion
Gn'	Soft tissue menton

Dentoskeletal Variants and Perioral Soft Tissue

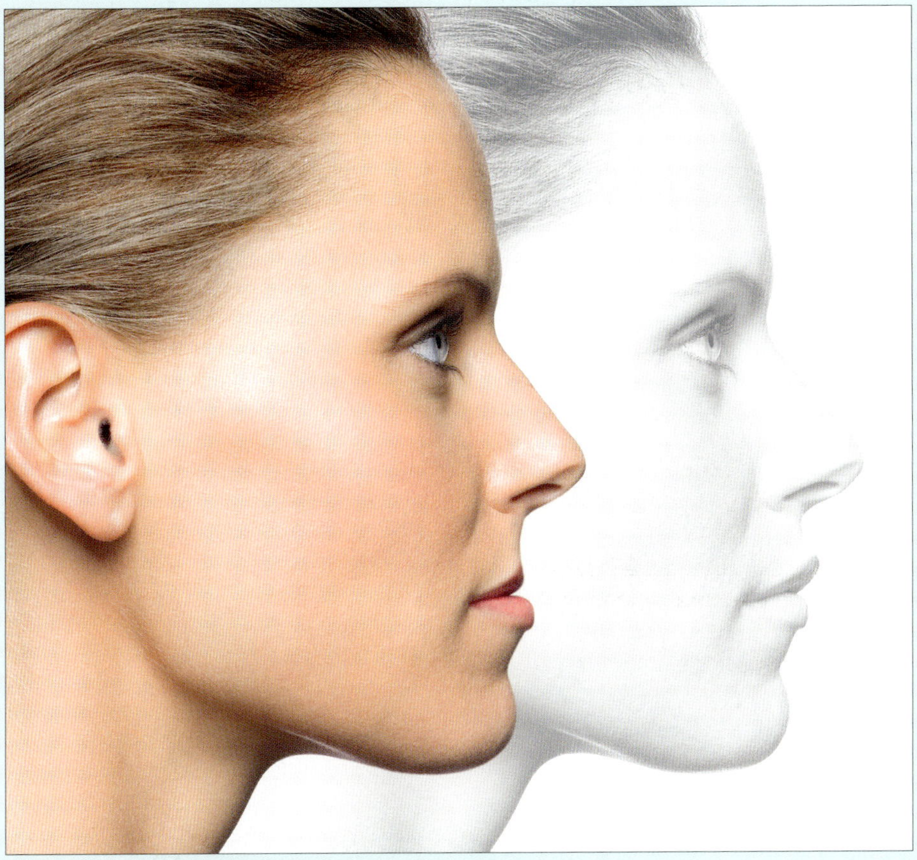

Maxilla too Far Back

Fig. 1.60 As an example, if the maxilla lies too far back relative to the mandible or the facial plane, this automatically produces a "hanging" or even inverted upper lip as a whole, with a wider nasolabial angle, a negative lip profile, and insufficient vermillion eversion. In the front view, the upper lip is thin with insufficient Cupid's bow support and a narrower or less pronounced philtrum. The paranasal region is also flattened, and nasolabial lines are almost universal, even at a young age. The same effect can also be caused by vertical (or, in extreme cases, even lingually inclined/retroclined) maxillary anterior teeth, of the kind that commonly need adjustment following an orthodontic treatment that involves the extraction of two premolars due to overcrowding.

→ **In this case, improvement can be achieved with dermal fillers in the upper lip and in the cutaneous part of the upper lip. If tooth displacement/poor alignment is the cause, the result can be considerably improved by measures to correct this displacement.**

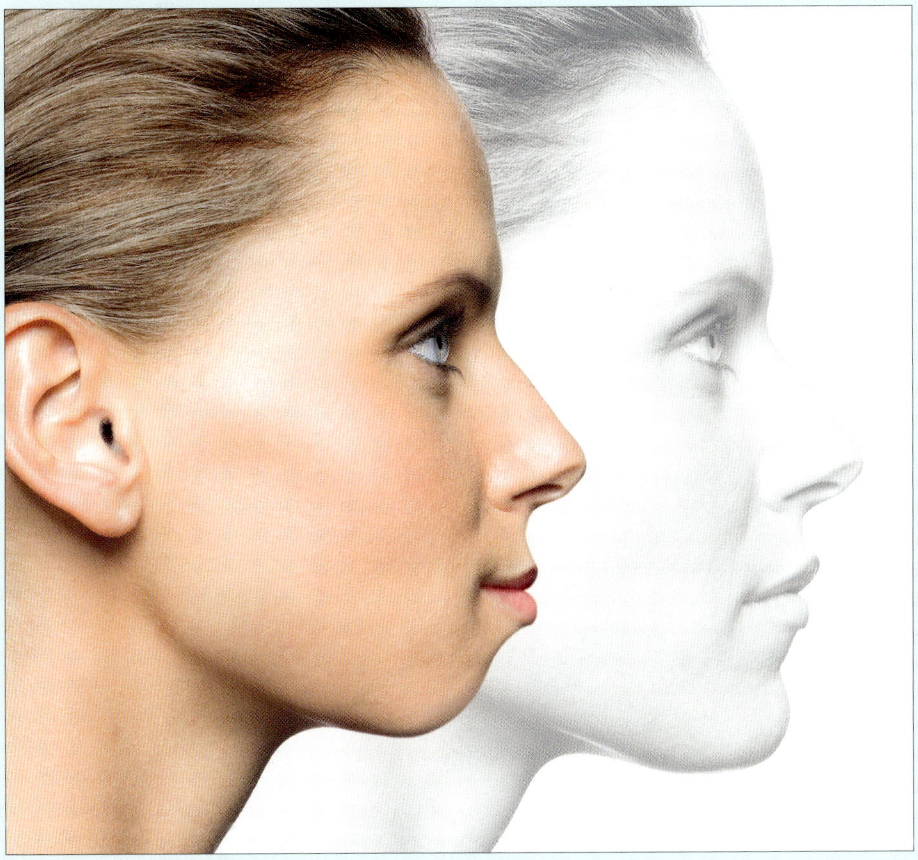

Mandible too Far Back with Everted Lower Lip

Fig. 1.61 If the mandible is too far back, the lower lip, with a receding chin, is frequently excessively everted, producing a negative lip profile, while the labiomental groove is often deeper or even takes the form of a line. This effect is also seen if the mandibular anterior teeth have no contact with the maxillary teeth or if they create a gap into which the lower lip can retract.

In the front view, relaxed closure of the lips is generally not possible but needs to be forced, with a corresponding crinkling of the lip margin (activation of the orbicularis oris muscle) and the formation of skin retractions on the chin, known as cobblestone chin (overactivity of the mentalis muscle).

→ **Slight improvement in the upper lip region is possible here. The curve between the nose and lip can be straightened slightly by augmentation of the subnasale part. The receding chin cannot be harmonized using fillers.**

Dentoskeletal Variants and Perioral Soft Tissue (continued)

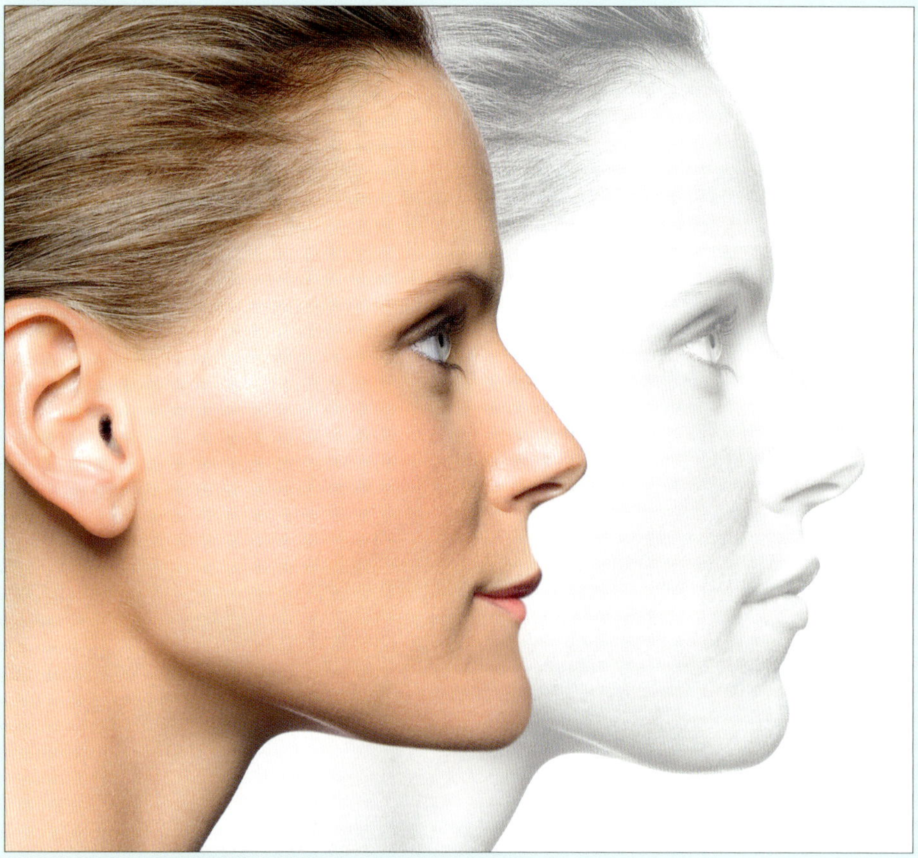

Mandible too Far Forward

Fig. 1.62 If the mandible lies too far forward, the "sturdy" (progenic) impression is often accompanied by a narrow upper lip with a flattened or even completely effaced labiomental fold and, in some cases, the formation of a plateau over the chin.

In general, the mandibular anterior teeth attempt to maintain contact with the anterior maxilla as far as possible, so that they tilt back within the alveolar process. As a result of this reclination, they offer insufficient support to the lower lip.

→ **An improvement with fillers is possible here, by proportionally evening out the upper/lower lip volumes and filling the labiomental fold slightly in order to visually reduce the prominence of the chin.**

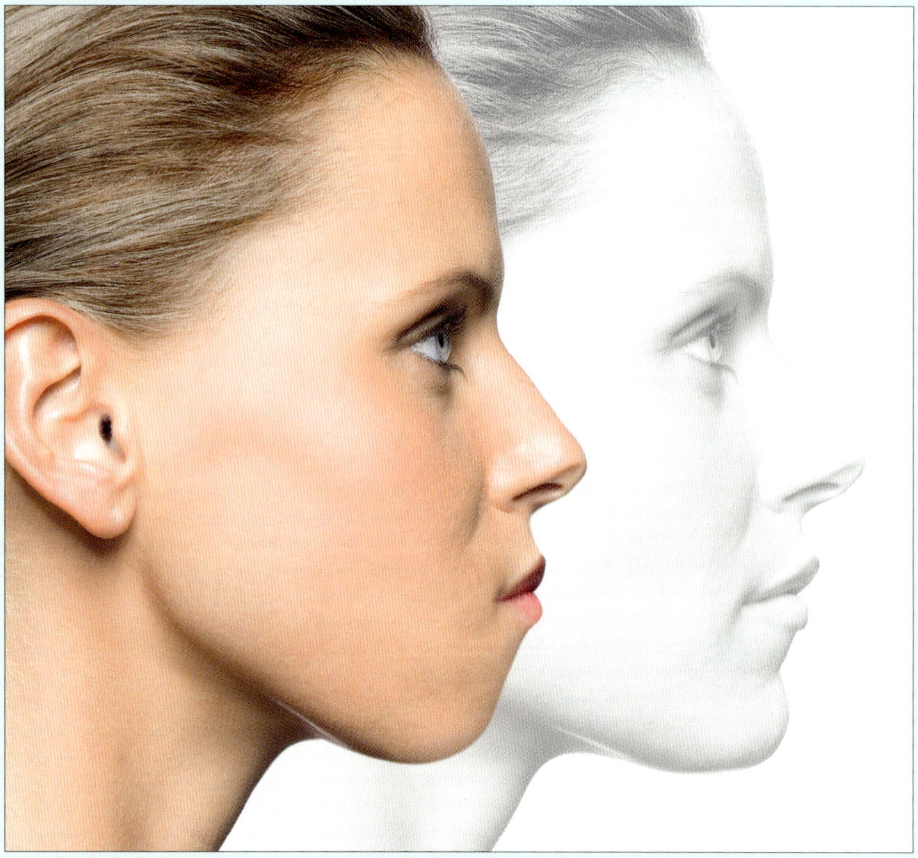

Increased Anterior Face Height

Fig. 1.63 Increased anterior face height (vertical dimension) will also lead to forced lip closure and the symptoms described further above, if the existing soft tissue volume is insufficient relative to the underlying bone. The edge of the mandible appears steep and poorly defined.

In the front view, this is often associated with a so-called gummy smile (excessive gum exposure when smiling or even with the mouth at rest).

→ **In these cases, it is difficult to achieve a satisfactory result with fillers, since the chin recedes too much. One can bring the upper lip forward slightly by injecting volume.**

1

Dentoskeletal Variants and Perioral Soft Tissue (continued)

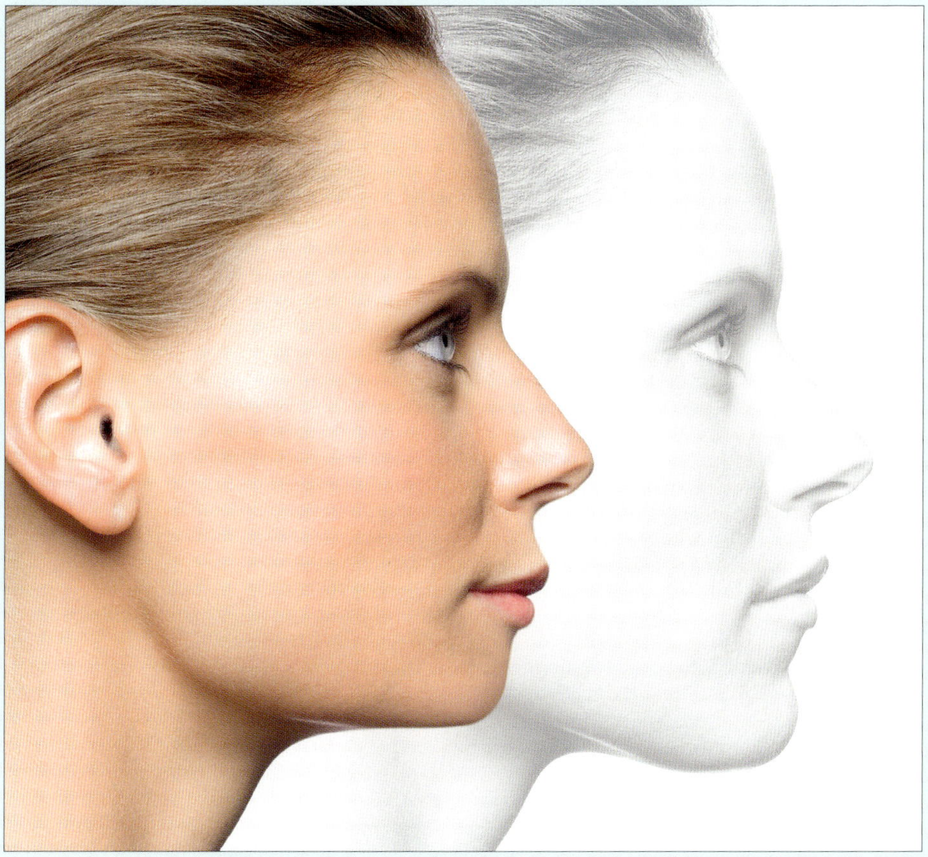

Loss of Vertical Dimension

Fig. 1.64 Conversely, a loss of vertical dimension leads to compression of the soft tissue, and the tendency toward a "duck's bill." In these cases, it is much more difficult to follow the rule of thirds. The edge of the mandible tends to be prominent, and the face appears squat.

→ Only limited improvement with dermal fillers is possible here. A satisfactory result cannot be expected even if the philtrum or the cutaneous part of the upper lip is built up.

1.6.4 Analysis of Facial Expression and Movement

The shape of the lips is altered by the muscle play involved in facial expressions. A dynamic assessment reveals how the lip behaves during movement: for instance, the movement of the lips during a smile may expose the gums (gummy smile) or obscure the teeth until they are no longer visible (toothless smile) – depending on the aging process, dental substance, and anatomical conditions. After a treatment, it is advisable to use facial expressions to check how the material behaves in the lips. In this context, we recommend keeping photographic records.

Following lip augmentation, in which irregularities often occur due to injuries to the blood vessels in the lip, it is particularly important to ask the patient to smile and say "cheese" in order to check whether the irregularity is due to a traumatic swelling or the uneven delivery of dermal filler. The latter would manifest as a small, raised bolus when the lips are stretched during facial play.

Thickness and plasticity can be analyzed by means of various expressions involving the lips (→ Figs. 1.65–1.71). Sound evidence of baseline status can be obtained using thorough photographic documentation (→ Chap. 3.2, p. 60) at the patient's first visit. Any specific lip features such as pigment disorders, herpes, scars, lip tinting or tattoos should be clearly recorded in close-up photographs. The following figures show a few examples that can be used for the analysis.

Note

The more facial play is included in the analysis, the better one can identify details that are of relevance to the analysis and the treatment. However, care must be taken to ensure that the same detailed photographs are taken in the same order at every subsequent session.

Expressive Lip Shapes

■ Smiling

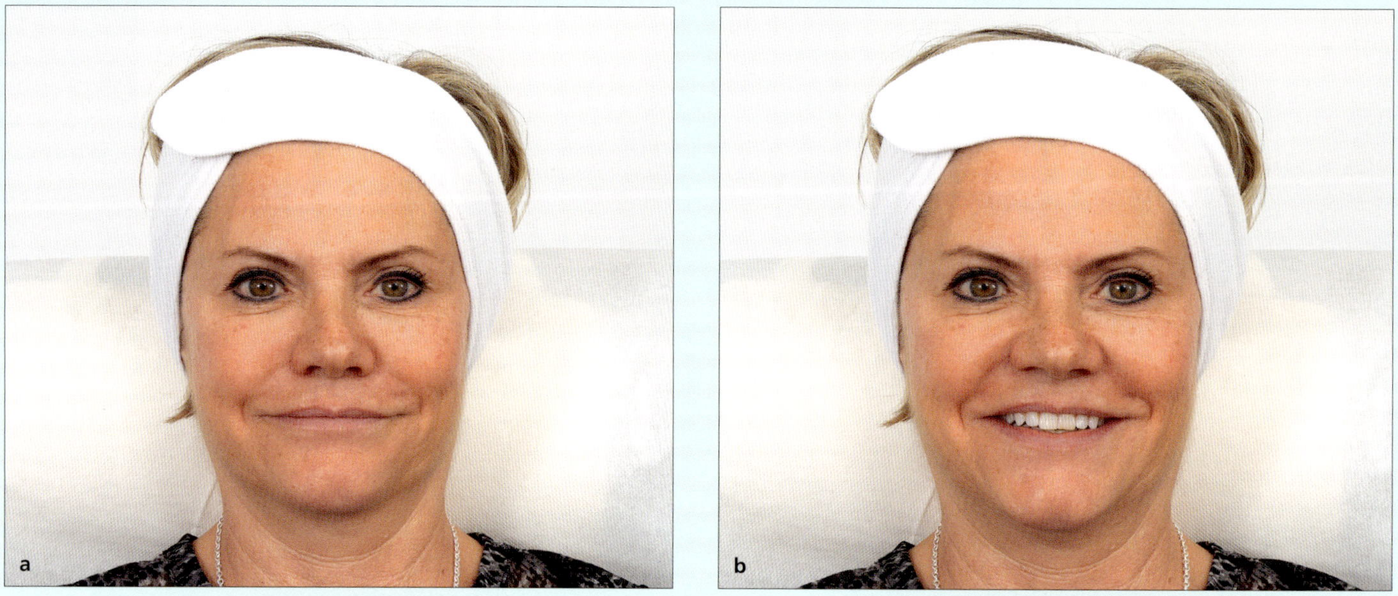

Fig. 1.65 a+b (a) Smiling with the mouth closed makes the lips thinner, while the lines at the corners of the mouth become visible. (b) Smiling with the mouth open makes the lips even thinner and clearly reveals the teeth.

When a person smiles, the mouth widens, which causes the lips to become thinner due to stretching of the orbicularis oris muscle. The corners of the mouth are lifted. The extent to which the teeth and gums are visible, the width of the lip, and the UL : LL ratio are all criteria that need to be considered with particular care before any treatment. In this respect, it is also important to respect and harmonize the various ratios that are involved. Immediately after an injection of HA into the lips, smiling would push up any asymmetrically injected boluses, whereas any minor internal bleeds caused by damaged blood vessels are flattened. By asking the patient to smile, the therapist can check whether any asymmetry is due to unevenly placed material or to a swelling caused by hematoma.

■ Pulling Down the Corners of the Mouth

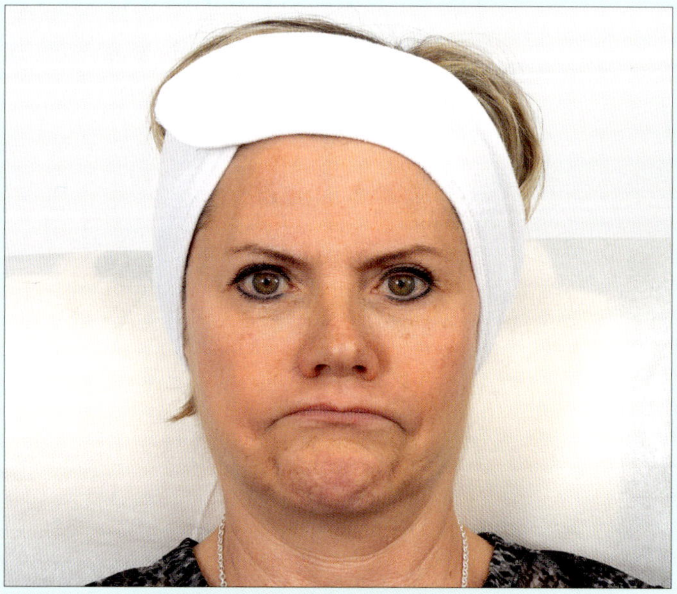

Fig. 1.66 Asking the patient to pull down the corners of the mouth allows the activity of the depressor anguli oris muscle to be evaluated. In older patients, this reveals perioral shadows, drooping oral commissures, and lines on the chin.

■ Cobblestone Chin

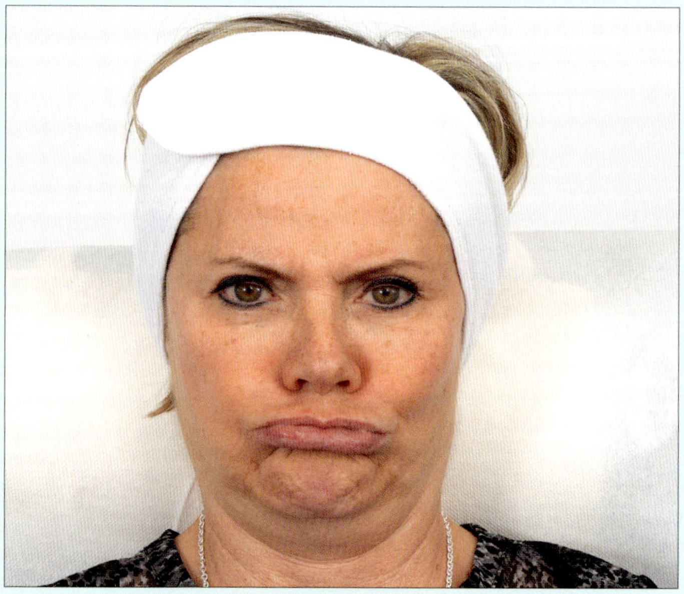

Fig. 1.67 Pulling the lips into a pout and tensing the chin activates the mentalis muscle, making the mental crease (chin crease) more visible. A cobblestone chin is more commonly found in Asian patients. Treatment with botulinum toxin is preferable to HA in this case, as it relaxes and thus "elongates" the chin.

Expressive Lip Shapes (continued)

■ Relaxed Mouth

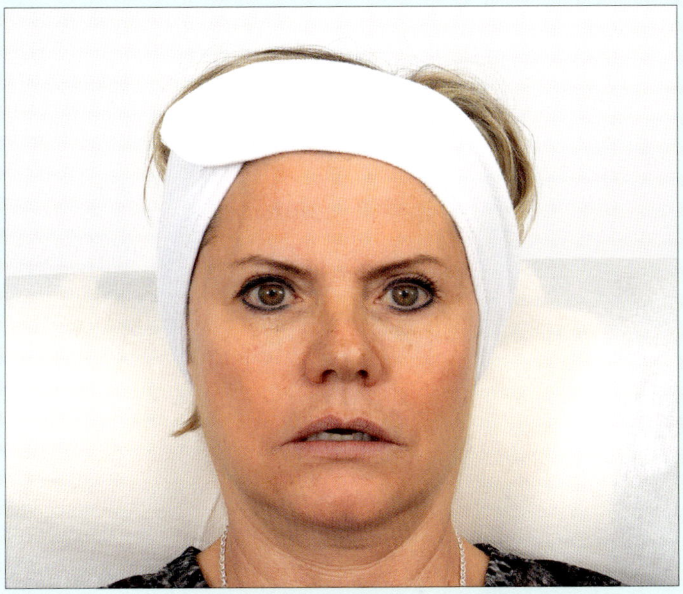

Fig. 1.68 A front view of the patient with the mouth open but relaxed clearly reveals special features of the lips, such as pigment disorders, herpes, scars, tinting, and tattoos; these can then be documented using close-up photographs. The drooping of the corners of the mouth when the mouth is open and relaxed may be, but need not always be, an expression of negative emotions. Drooping mouth corners develop in elderly patients in particular, as a result of excess fat in the cheeks or loss of elasticity in the skin.

■ Speaking

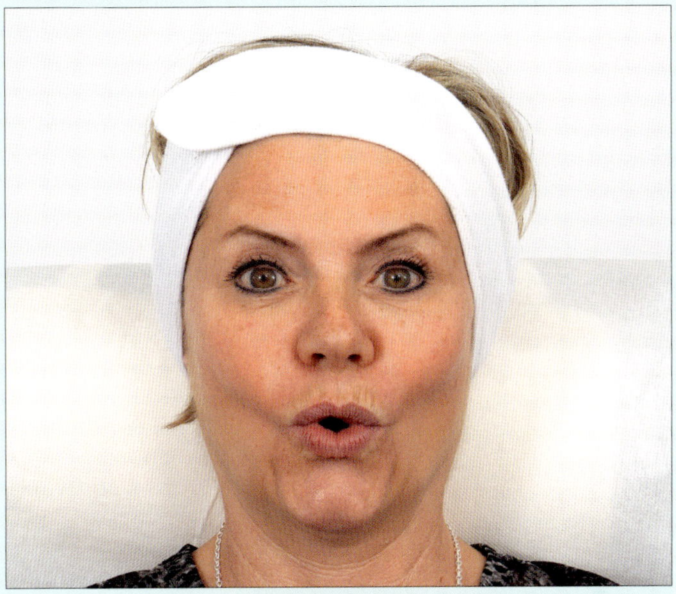

Fig. 1.69 When a person speaks, sings or yawns, the lips are open and more relaxed in shape than they are in a smile. The shaping of the lips during speaking shows up perioral lines and shadows. The way the lips move after a treatment can also be assessed by asking the patient to speak.

■ Saying "Cheese"

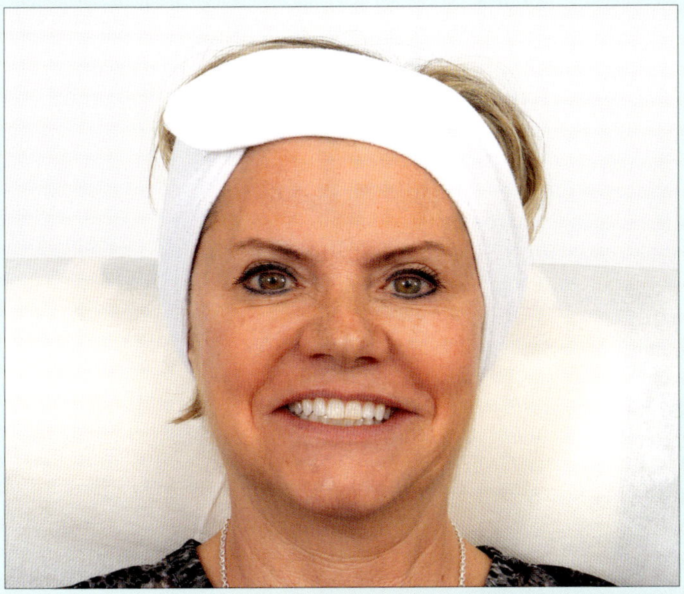

Fig. 1.70 The lips are tightened and become thinner when the patient is asked to say "cheese." This is a very good method of checking whether the material has distributed evenly after the treatment, or whether any asymmetries or nodules have been produced.

■ Puckered Lips

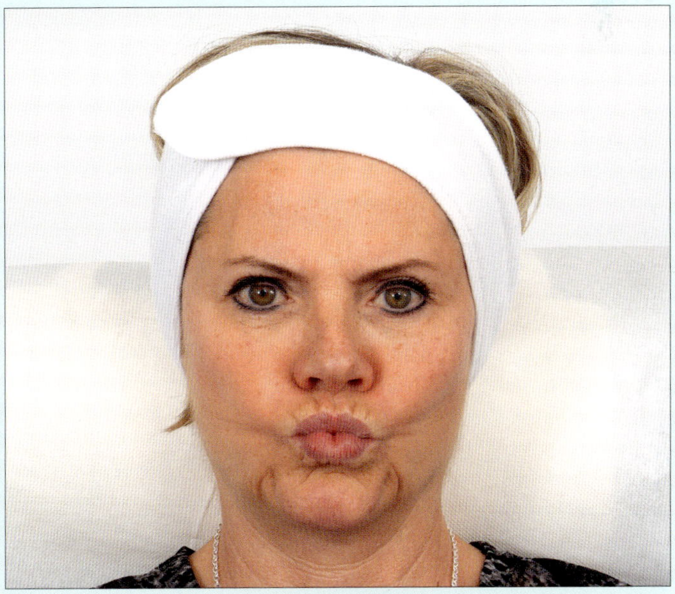

Fig. 1.71 When the lips are puckered, the orbicularis oris muscle contracts, pulling the lips together. The visibility of the resultant perioral lines and wrinkles clearly reveals the extent to which the aging process has advanced. There are numerous possible intermediate stages between fine perioral "ripples" and large shadows surrounding the lower lip.

1.6.5 Palpation

By palpating the lips (→ Figs. 1.72, 1.73), the therapist can feel their condition and assess the following features:

- Temperature
- Moisture
- Surface consistency
- Turgor
- Scars
- Pain
- Volume
- Nodes, indurations

1

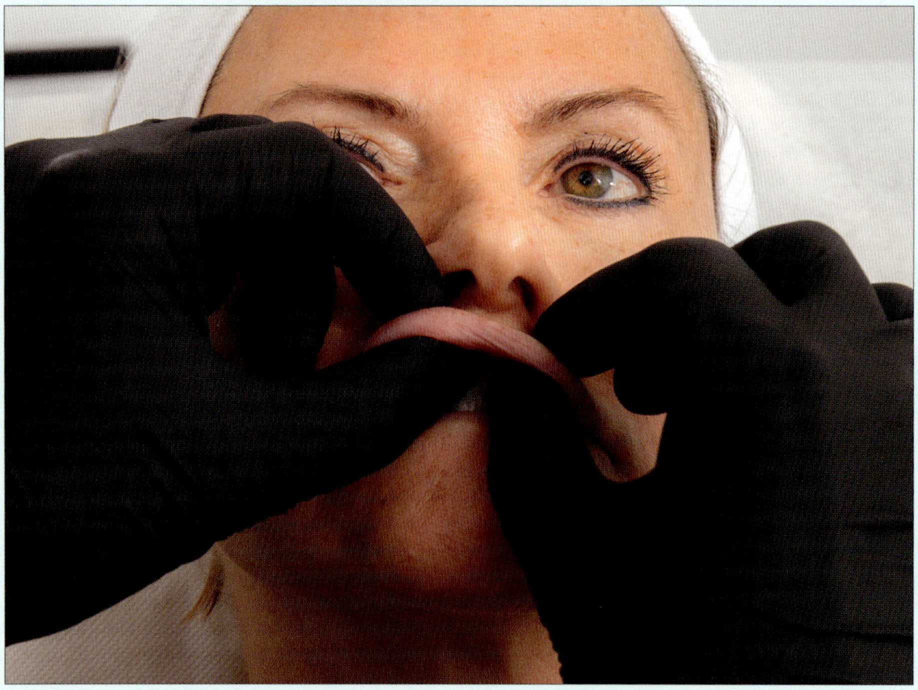

Fig. 1.72 An analysis by palpation of the upper and lower lip is important when planning the optimal lip treatment. For example, any nodes and scars are indicators of previous treatments and injuries, which could complicate a treatment.

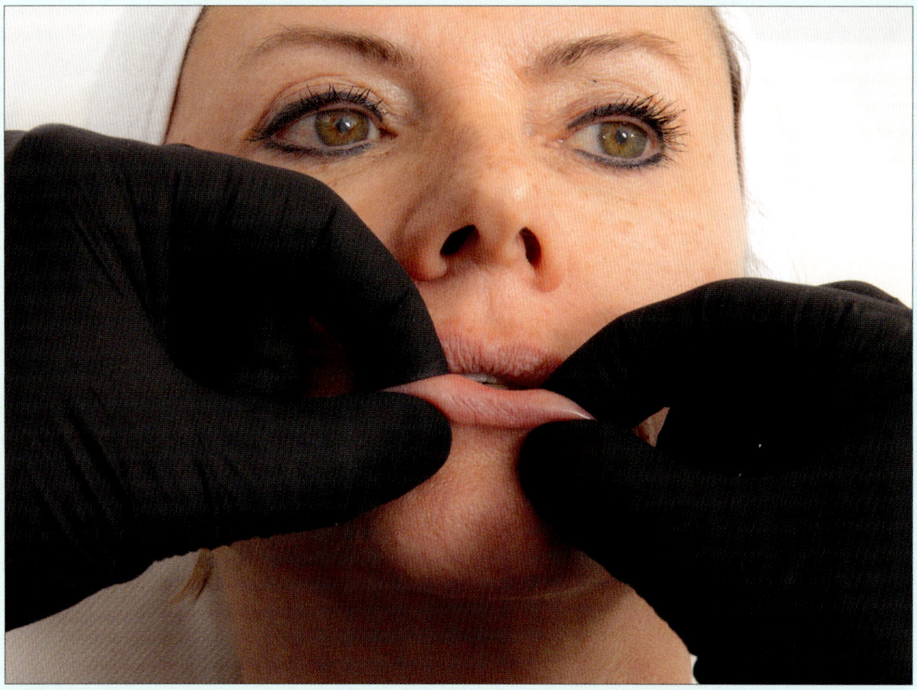

Fig. 1.73 A young, firm, smooth lip is also easier to augment than a lip that shows lax skin turgor or a lip with skin that is very brittle, cracked or wrinkled.

1.7 Merz Scales

These images (reproduced with the kind permission of Merz Pharmaceuticals GmbH, Frankfurt) demonstrate various aspects of the lips. Each five-point scale shows five degrees of change. The scales help the therapist to assess the baseline status, from which a variety of potential treatment options may result. A score of 1 represents the intact lip, which can generally only be treated preventively. The scale then moves incrementally from scores 2 to 5, with a score of 5 representing the most pronounced form of the change involved.

1.7.1 Puckered Lips

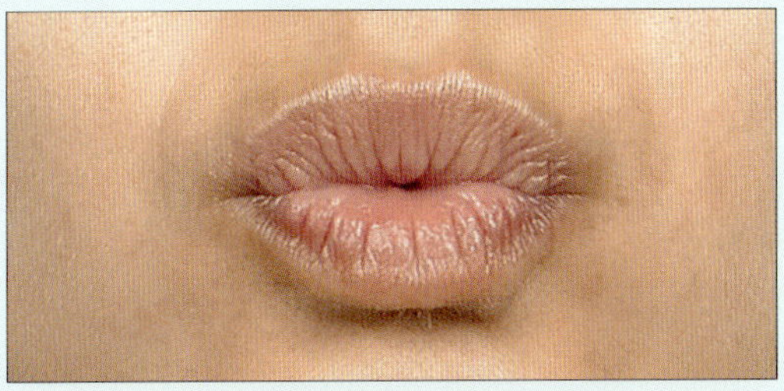
1

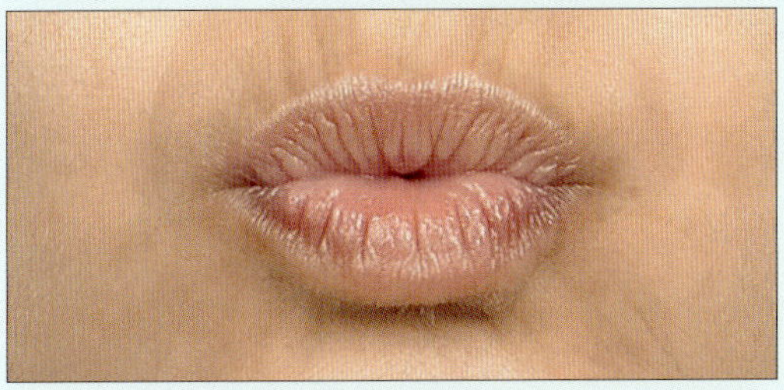
2

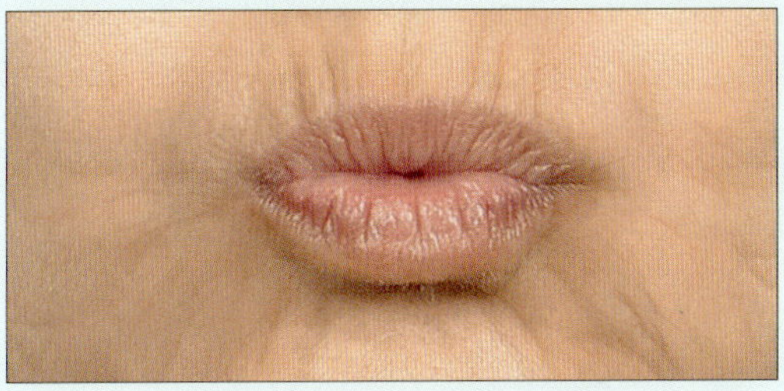
3

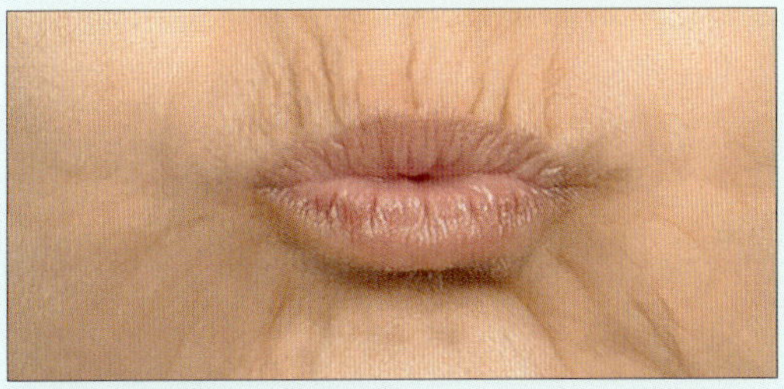
4

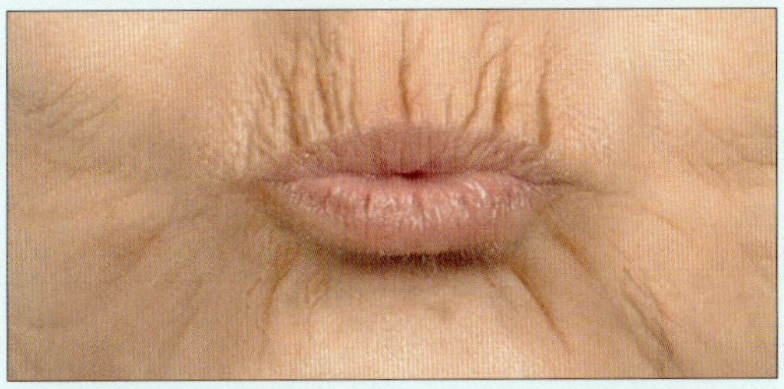
5

If the score is 1, the perioral region should be enhanced preventively. If the score is 2 or 3, a good treatment result may be expected; here, the perioral shadows below the lip should be treated by adding volume. If the score is 4 or 5, several consecutive treatments will often be needed, although a 100% successful outcome is not likely.

1.7.2 Perioral Lines

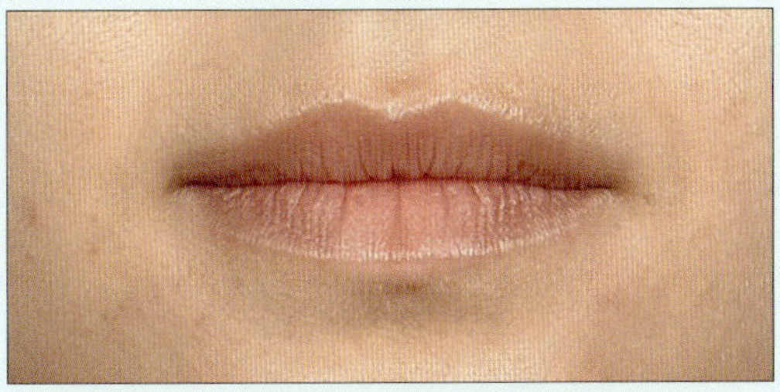
1

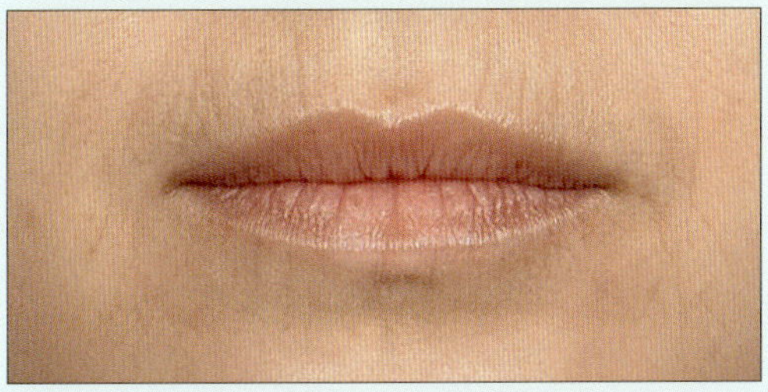
2

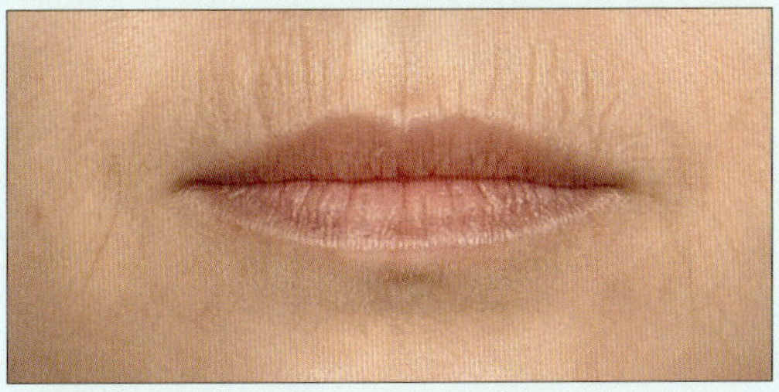
3

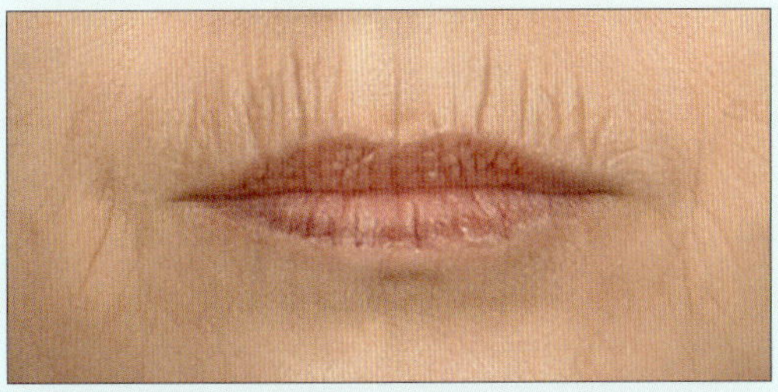
4

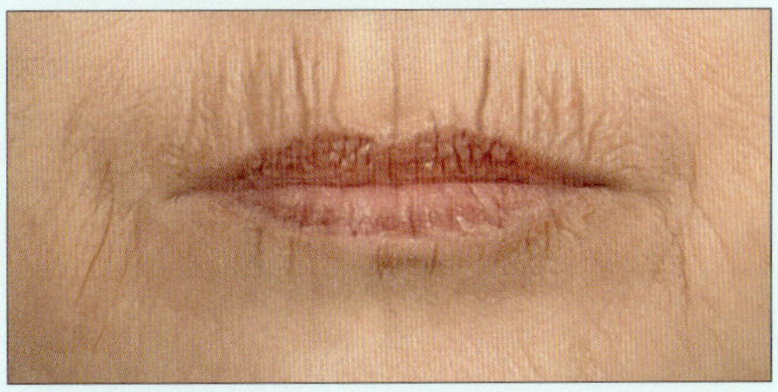
5

If the score is 1, the perioral region and the contours should be enhanced preventively. If the score is 2 or 3, a good treatment result may be expected. However, if the score is 4 or 5, several consecutive treatments will often be needed, although a 100% successful outcome is not likely.

1.7.3 Corners of the Mouth/Oral Commissures

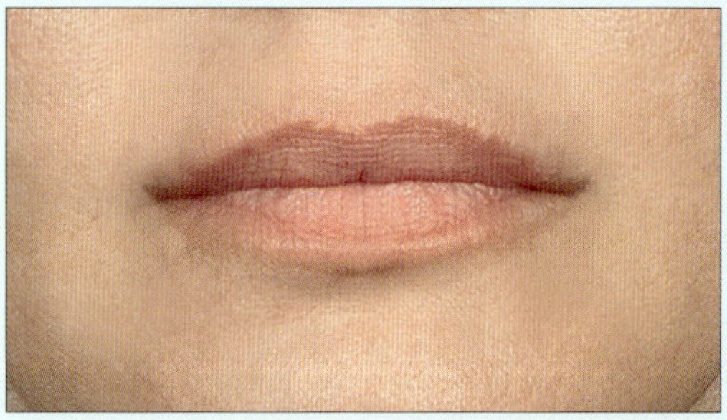
1

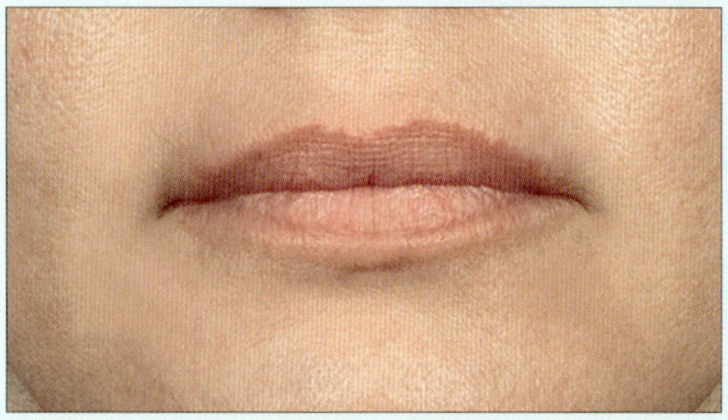
2

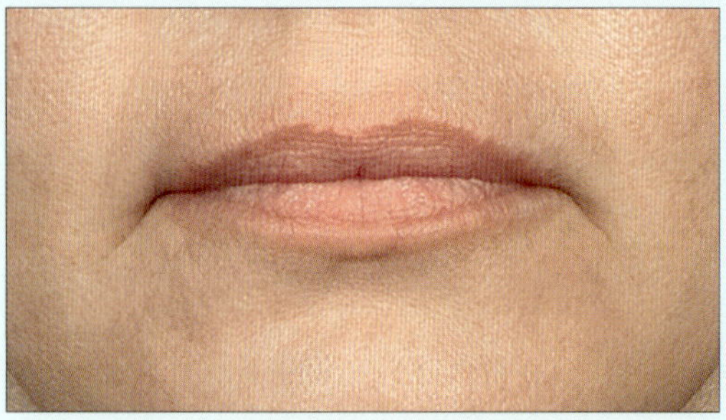
3

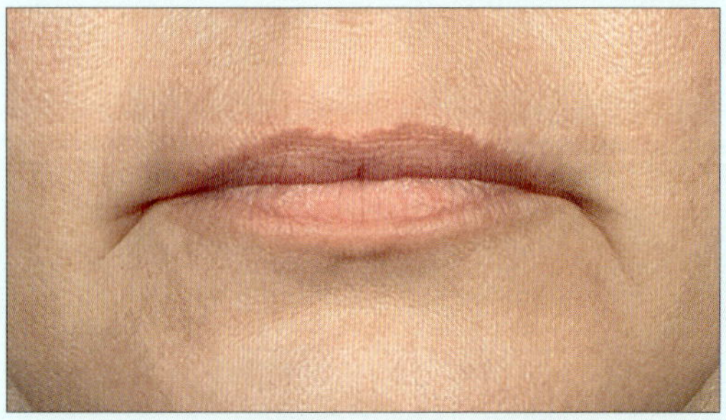
4

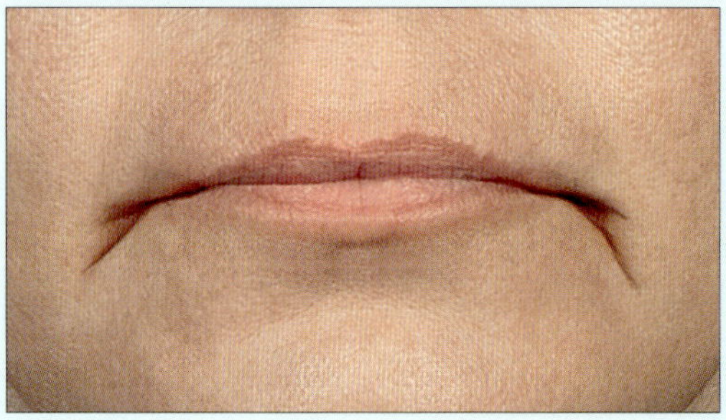
5

Whereas a good degree of improvement is possible if the score is 2 to 3, more challenging treatment techniques will be needed if the score is 5. At this stage, it not always possible to correct drooping oral commissures fully.

1.7.4 Nasolabial Lines

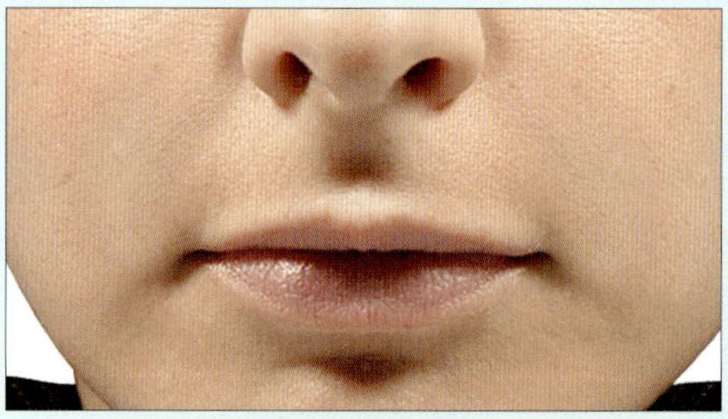
1

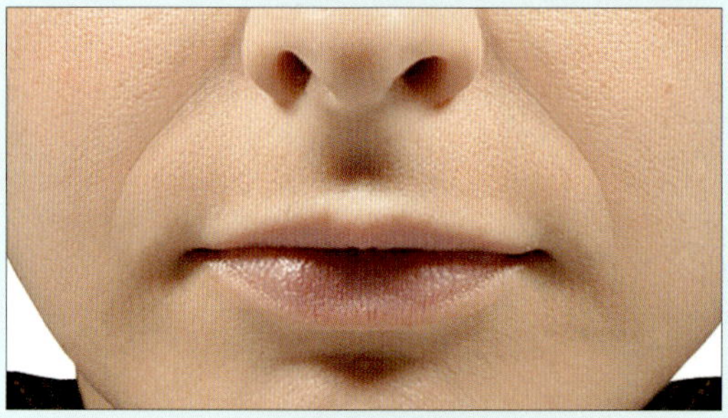
2

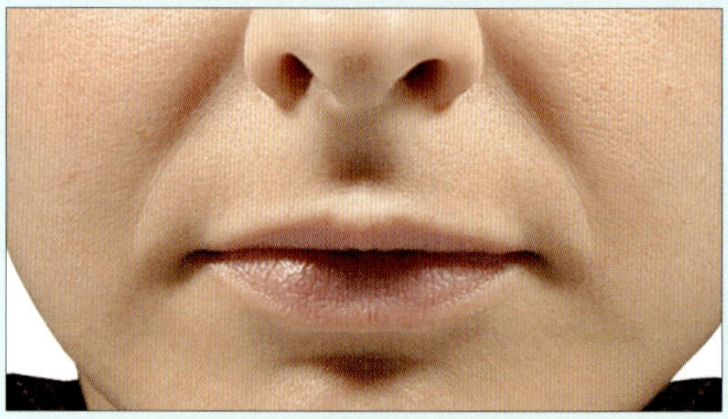
3

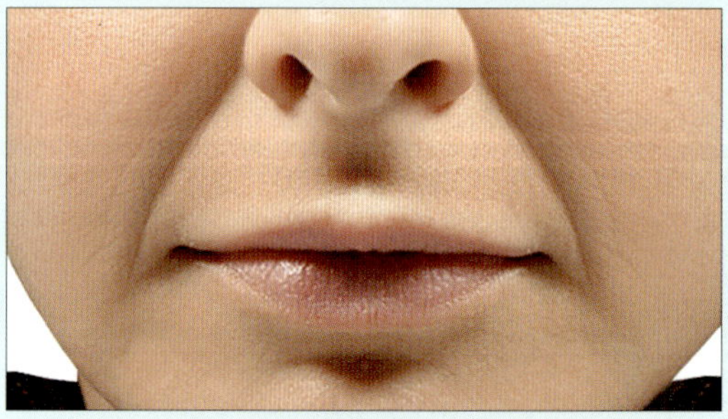
4

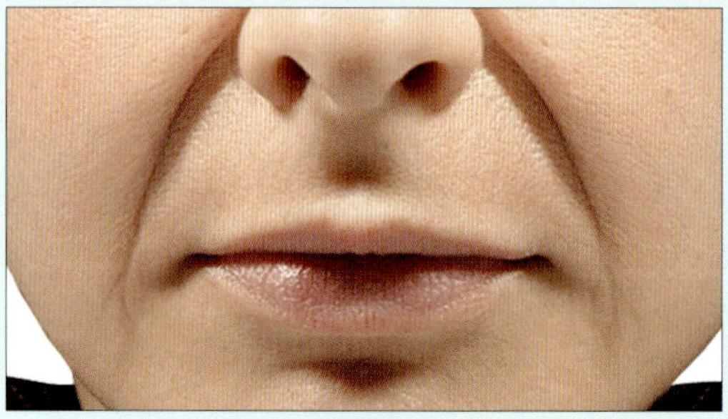
5

Since nasolabial lines are always part of the overall picture of the oral region, it is important to include them in any lip treatment. If the score is 2 to 4, very good treatment results can be achieved with the cannula technique or with a sharp needle. However, if the score is 5, several techniques should be used in combination. Furthermore, complete correction of the nasolabial lines is not likely with a baseline score of 4 or 5.

1.7.5 Marionette Lines

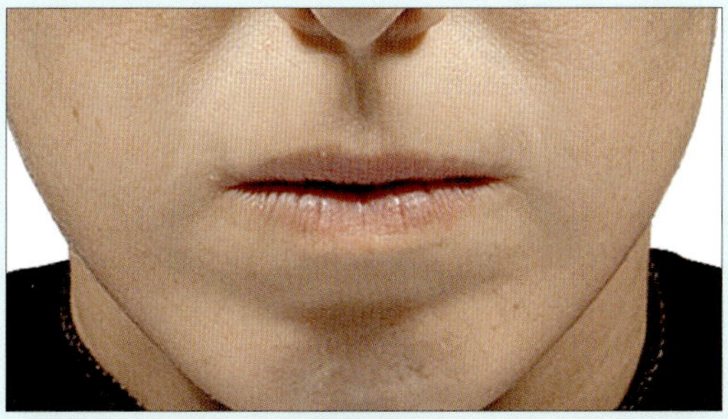

1

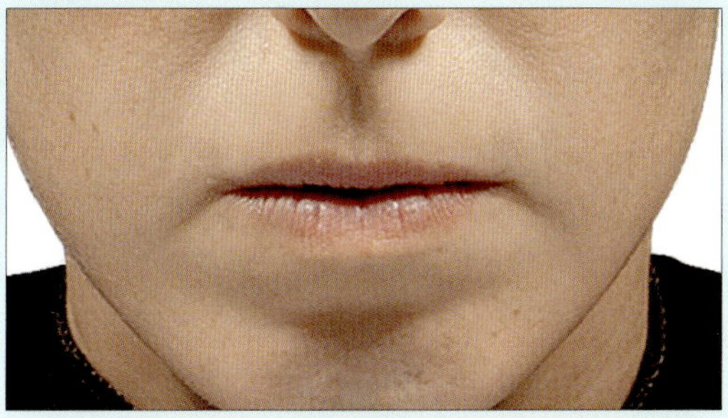

2

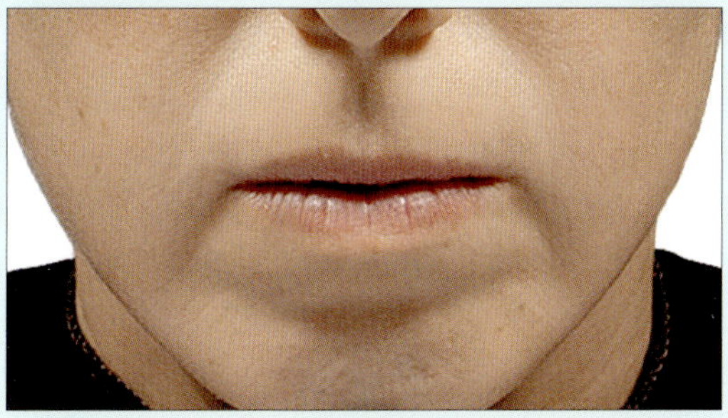

3

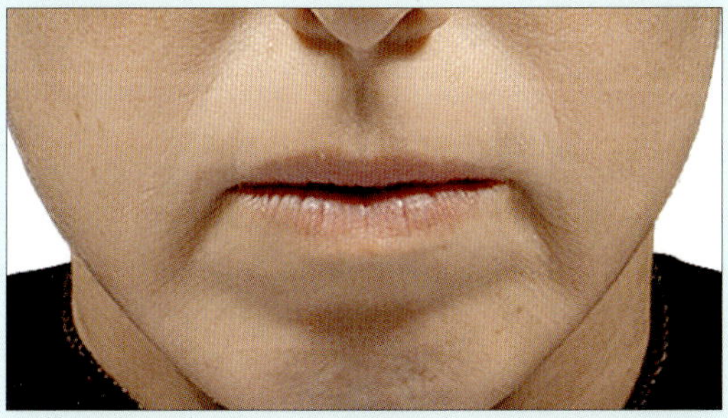

4

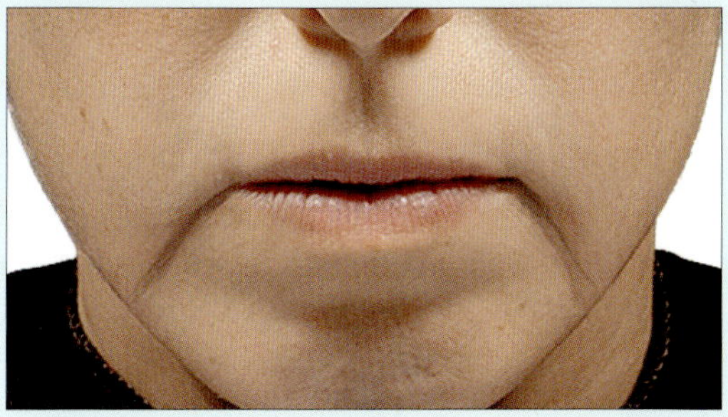

5

While a good degree of improvement is possible if the score is 2 to 3, more challenging treatment techniques will be needed if the score is 5. At this stage, it not always possible to correct marionette lines fully.

1.7.6 Lip Volume

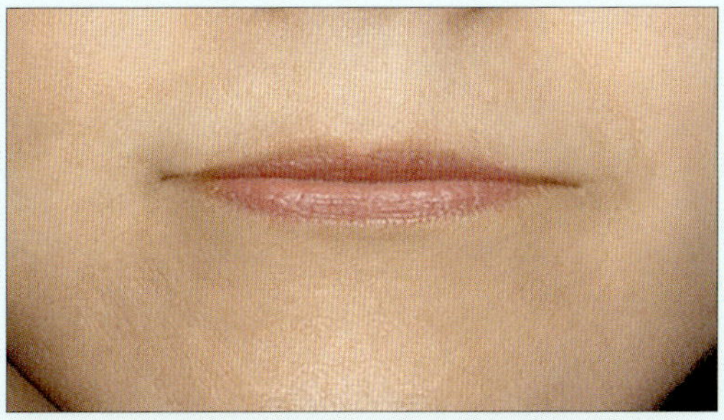

1

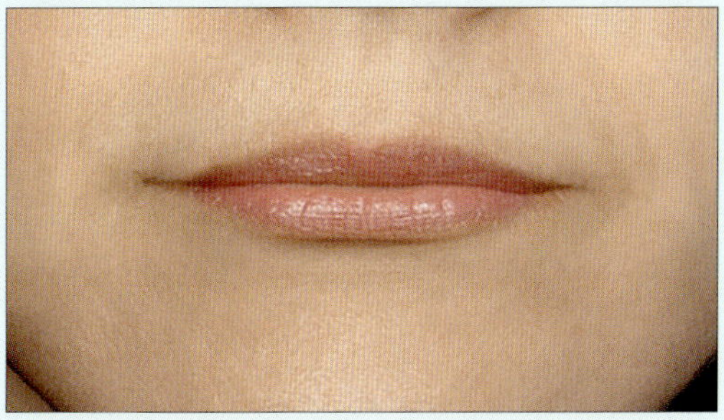

2

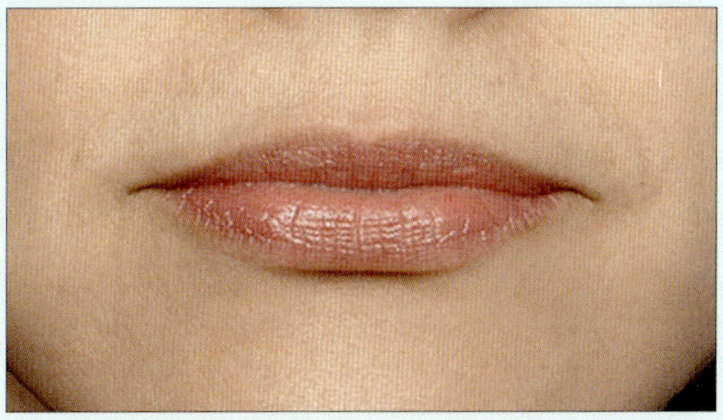

3

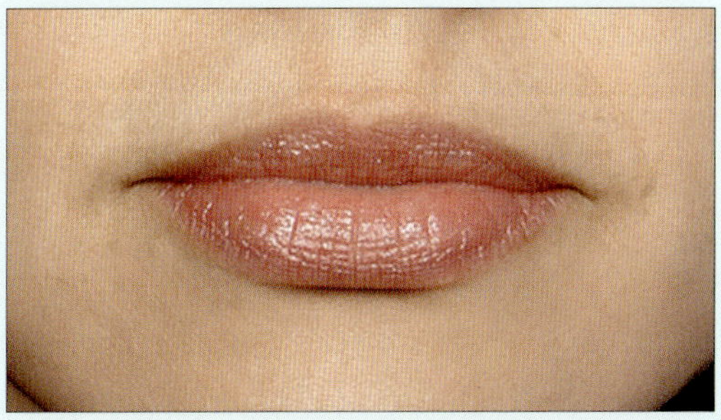

4

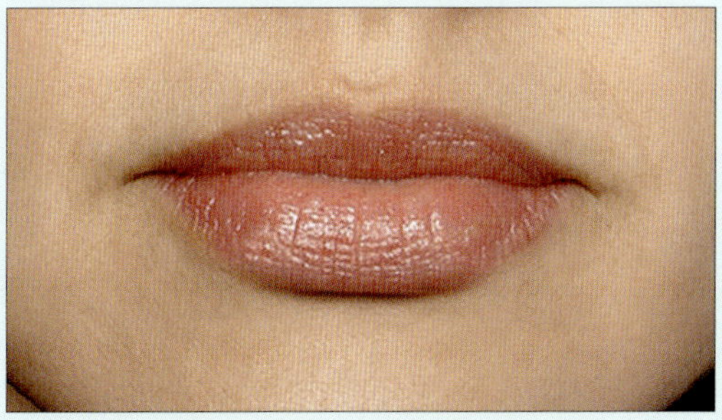

5

If the lip is young, the treatment goal will be much easier to achieve than with an atrophied, older lip. Here, the main aim is beautification by changing the shape and increasing the volume of the lip. By respecting the original shapes, the treatment outcome should always blend into the face harmoniously.

2 Consultation

2 Consultation

A consultation has a starting point and a goal. "Natural beauty is a destination" (Swift 2017). This long road requires a systematic approach. The various steps involved in a consultation are presented in this chapter, though slight variations are always possible.

As with all medical consultations, the medical history takes center stage in any filler treatment. However, unlike standard medical treatments, the patient's motivation for requesting the treatment is not subject to a true therapeutic goal. In an esthetic treatment, therefore, there is less demand for therapeutic competence and more for the therapist's counseling, technical, and artistic skills. The aim is to align the patient's wishes with the feasibilities and limitations of a treatment, and to communicate this properly and transparently.

We recommend that the following aspects be included in a consultation:

1. The patient's wishes
2. The patient's medical history and emotional make-up
3. Contraindications
4. Analysis
5. Examination findings
6. Documentation
7. Counseling and information session
8. Budgeting
9. Treatment planning

2.1 The Patient's Wishes

2.1.1 Motivation

A person's desire for a change in external appearance is often associated with an internal emotional event. All patients who embark on the journey toward a beauty treatment have one thing in common: they want to alter an aspect of themselves that bothers them. However, there is a broad range between minor wishes for improvement or slight dissatisfaction and extreme changes driven by an obsession with constant beautification of one's appearance due to the desire to "become a different person," and the transition between the various stages is fluid.

When clarifying patients' expectations, it is important to understand what they wish for and what motivates them to change something about themselves. Although images from social networks can help to identify a general direction in which to go, they should never be used as a model to be copied. It is also essential to ask patients about their ethnic or cultural ideals. Thus, for example, the desired upper to lower lip (UL : LL) proportions in Russia tend to be a ratio of 1 : 1, while in South America the prevailing ratio is 2/3 : 1/3, and in Europe the inverse ratio of 1/3 : 2/3 applies.

It is very difficult to satisfy a patient's wishes if the desire for a beauty treatment is a replacement for some other shortcoming. A tendency toward treatment addiction (beauty neurosis) may also develop.

People's most common motivation is a general dissatisfaction with their own appearance. This dissatisfaction could be with something they have always disliked about their appearance or it could be due to aging or to the influence of fashion trends. These days, patients are much clearer about what they want changed than was the case only a few years ago. Patients presenting to the esthetic medicine practice for a rejuvenating and beatifying lip treatment expect a natural result. However, this desire for change often goes hand in hand with unrealistic expectations, which sometimes cannot be realized due to reasons such as the patient's age or lip shape (see Chap. 1.6.3, p. 36).

Note

The term **body dysmorphic disorder** or **body dysmorphia** (also known as body dysmorphophobia) describes a state of impaired self-perception, which has a variety of psychologic causes. People with body dysmorphia have a constant compulsion to compare themselves with others, which is fed by the media and social networks. "The fear and delusion of being ugly, combined with a heightened sense for esthetics and the accompanying expectations" (Thess 2010) lead to chronic dissatisfaction with the treatment outcome and a constant need to switch therapists. The more accurately the therapist collects information about the patient, the clearer the patient's motivation for the treatment will become.

Furthermore, it is important to keep a detailed record, including photographic documentation, in order to demonstrate the change that has been produced after the treatment (Thess 2010).

Caution

Changes in anatomical structures due to fillers: Baseline anatomical parameters limit the room for maneuver (Rejuvent, Medical Spa & Surgery 2017). It is not always possible to create full lips from thin ones without producing an unnatural result (→ Fig. 2.1). Since there is often insufficient space for the injected volume, the lips project outward, producing a "duck's bill" effect.

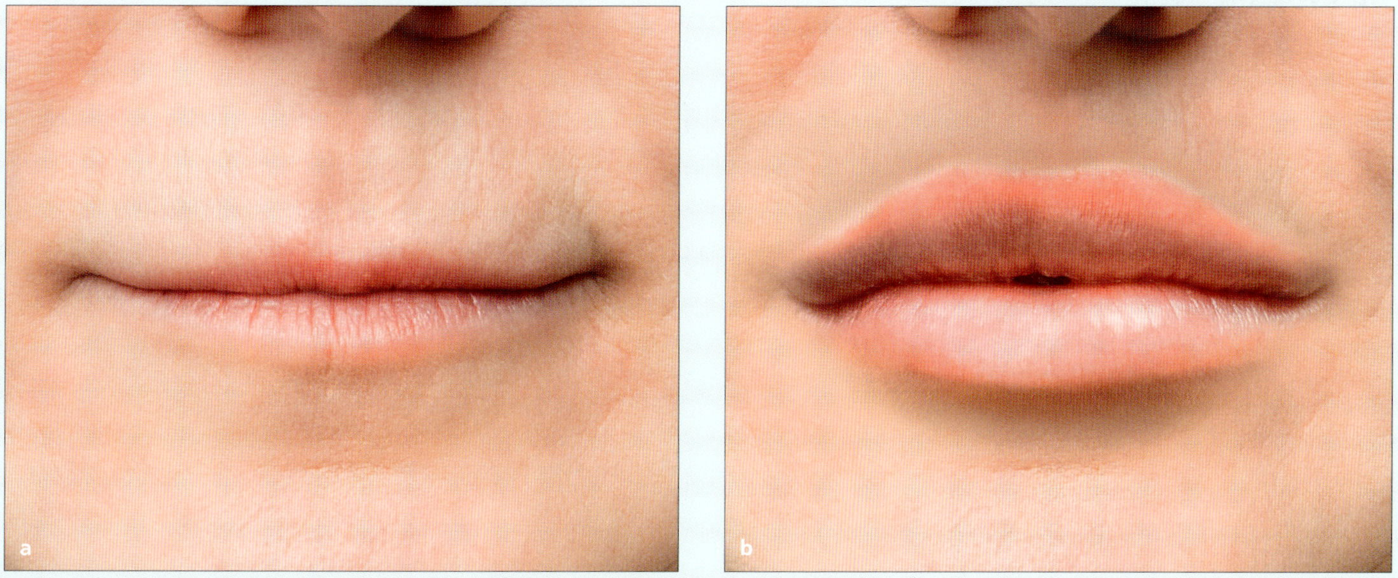

Fig. 2.1 a+b Thin (a) versus full (b) lips in the same female patient.

2.1.2 Fashion and Trends

We are writing in 2020, when we are constantly being bombarded by opportunities for beautification or self-optimization in the form of social media images, advertising or celebrities such as models. Many people are influenced by fashion trends and wish to alter the appearance of their mouths. For example, extremely full, "bee-stung" lips, sometimes also known as "dinghy lips" (→ Fig. 2.2), are in vogue among young women in Europe. Patients in Asia, on the other hand, tend to have their mouths altered to a heart shape, using a combination of surgery and filler augmentation (→ Fig. 2.3 with the kind permission of Dr. Apple, Thailand, © www.doctorappleclinic.com).

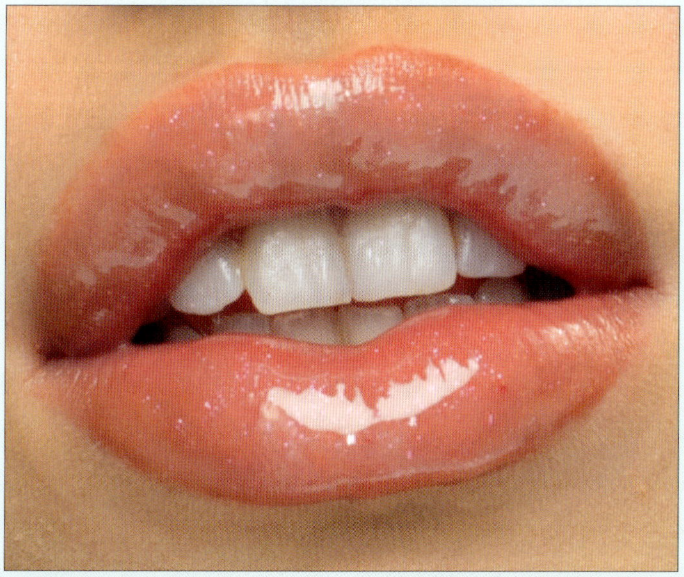

Fig. 2.2 Fashion trend: "bee-stung" lips (sometimes also known as "dinghy lips").

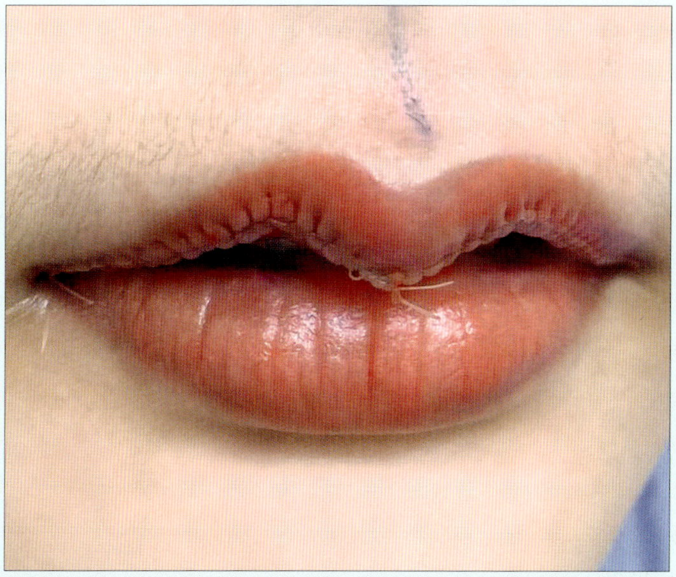

Fig. 2.3 Fashion trend: heart-shaped lips (© www.doctorappleclinic.com).

2.1.3 The Desire for Rejuvenation

In older patients, it is often the case that expectations cannot be realistically implemented. Here, it is important to give the patient a mirror and to discuss the possibilities and limitations of the treatment in detail, demonstrating the discrepancy between the feasibility of a treatment and what the patient wants to get from it.

2.1.4 Volume versus Budget

Some previously untreated patients will require several treatments and bigger volumes. In most cases, treating the lips alone is not enough to optimize overall appearance. For example, targeted lip volume augmentation is often combined with treatment of the perioral region.

Financial limitations frequently stand in the way of the optimal treatment result. If the patient's budget is not sufficient to achieve the optimal treatment, therapists should restrict themselves to one region on the wish list that can be treated with the available amount of hyaluronic acid (HA). Thus, the patient will see a clear result after the treatment, which would not have been the case had the HA been distributed over several areas of the face.

2.2 Medical History and Examination

Taking the patient's history and performing the examination before a lip augmentation should include an evaluation of skin consistency as well as the patient's esthetic and medical baseline status and lifestyle habits. Features specific to ethnic origin, culture, and gender should also be included. The medical history is essential when determining the indications and contraindications for HA treatment. The following points should be investigated and documented in a questionnaire:

- Age-related changes
- Skin structure
- Previous esthetic treatments
- Surgical procedures
- Use of medication
- Infections
- Delayed wound healing
- Keloid formation
- Intolerances and allergies
- Autoimmune disorders
- Metabolic disorders
- Thyroid disorders
- Bleeding diathesis (tendency to bleed)
- Pregnancy
- Lifestyle habits

2.3 Contraindications

2.3.1 Complicating Baseline Situations

The following circumstances represent complication factors in the baseline status:

- Old lips
- Asymmetric lips
- Dryness
- Pretreated lips
- Scarred lips (following permanent makeup, herpes)

2.3.2 Relative Contraindications

If the following diagnoses or conditions apply, any injection treatment should be performed at the therapist's discretion:

- Immunosuppressed patients
- Children and adolescents under 18 years of age (only in exceptional cases)
- Disposition towards keloids
- Use of nonsteroidal anti-inflammatory drugs
- Connective tissue disorders
- Thin, atrophic skin
- Sarcoidosis
- Anticoagulant medication (ensure correctly timed discontinuation before the treatment) and/or coagulation disorders
- Existing autoimmune disorder (decision should be made on a case-by-case basis, see 2.3.4 below, special monitoring necessary)
- Granulomatous inflammation
- Recent dermabrasion, laser treatment or chemical peels
- Patients with a disease caused by streptococci (e.g. recurrent tonsillitis)

2.3.3 General Contraindications

The product leaflet of the dermal filler should be read carefully in order for the therapist to become well acquainted with the contraindications that apply with a particular product. Generally speaking, treatment with any HA dermal filler is contraindicated in the following situations:

- Previous treatment with a non-absorbing material or material of unknown origin
- Complications occurring in a past filler treatment
- Rhagades, cracks, wounds or inflammations of the oral commissures
- Pregnancy
- Facial surgery in the past 6 months
- Excess scarring
- Acute infection
- Inflamed and cracked lips
- Perioral acne
- Acute herpes infection
- Bleeds

2.3.4 Case-related Contraindications

The following autoimmune disorders require a case-by-case decision regarding lip treatment, and will necessitate medical investigation and monitoring if such a treatment is performed:

- Bullous pemphigoid
- Churg-Strauss syndrome
- Ulcerative colitis
- Dermatitis herpetiformis (Duhring's disease)
- Dermatomyositis
- Epidermolysis bullosa acquisita
- Idiopathic thrombocytopenic purpura
- Lupus erythematosus
- Crohn's disease
- Multiple sclerosis

- Pemphigus erythematosus
- Pemphigus foliaceus
- Pemphigus vulgaris
- Polychondritis
- Psoriasis
- Henoch-Schönlein purpura
- Rheumatic fever
- Rheumatoid arthritis
- Giant cell arteritis

Good to Know

- Hypothyroidism is associated with a longer product life in the body.
- Hyperthyroidism is associated with a shorter product life in the body.
- The effect of exogenous hormones on the breakdown of HA is not clear.

2.4 Analysis and Findings

Various analytical techniques are used (see Chap. 1.6, p. 27) to accurately document the status of the lip being treated and to produce precise findings. The better the analysis, the more reliable and conclusive the examination findings and expected treatment outcome. On this basis, and considering the data collected in the history taking, the therapist can decide whether anything stands in the way of HA treatment. These data then form part of a comprehensive patient documentation record.

2.5 Documentation

The comprehensive patient documentation record consists of the documented history, photographic documentation, patient information sheet, informed consent form, and treatment form (see Chap. 3.1, QR code, p. 60). Once proper and fully comprehensive information has been provided, which states the indication, risks and side effects, treatment alternatives, and any preliminary and follow-up treatment, this information needs to be checked and signed by the patient. Failure to do so would constitute bodily harm.

2.6 Counseling, Information Session

The therapist is not only requested to provide counseling and information but has a duty to do so. To ensure that good medical advice is provided, as many of the aforementioned factors as possible need to be considered, the baseline parameters need to be defined, and everything needs to be communicated to the patient in as much detail as possible during the information session.

If a lip-altering treatment is requested, it is advisable to ask the patient for a photograph taken in earlier years. Once the patient's requirements and the treatment goal have been assessed for feasibility, the baseline findings have been recorded objectively, and the status of the lip has been technically recorded and documented, including all parameters, the treatment goal should be agreed upon and put into writing.

In so doing, the subjective factors should be explored with the patient during the discussion, and then summarized into a treatment goal on an advisory basis. The exact demarcation line between the patient's requirements and the treatment goal should then be set out.

Especially if a patient's esthetic preconceptions are extreme and fashion-driven, it is often a balancing act for the therapist to bring the patient's wishes down to a realistic level. A gradual, gentle approach is required to achieve consensus about a treatment outcome that looks as natural as possible.

The initial treatment session is always more time consuming because the preliminary analysis, documentation, counseling, and treatment planning take more time than the preparations involved in any follow-up appointments. In addition, patients are more anxious during the first session, and this requires an empathetic, soothing mode of communication.

2.7 Budgeting

Clear budgeting of the treatment costs is a key prerequisite for obtaining an optimal treatment result. For example, if the patient cannot meet the cost requirements for a complete treatment in the first stage, the therapist will inspire trust by presenting a staged treatment plan that gives the patient time and confidence to split the required financial output into several sessions. Another positive side effect of this is that it boosts patient loyalty. In addition, if large volumes of filler are required, a better result will be achieved by gradual augmentation.

A variety of factors need to be taken into consideration when calculating the cost of treatment. One set of determining parameters arises from the country's economic situation: it makes a big difference if one lives and works in a country such as Switzerland, with its high cost of locally produced goods and locally supplied services, as opposed to a country with a relatively low cost of living. Other factors include regional circumstances (population, accessibility, per capita income of the region where the practice is located), purchase prices, and competing offers, along with factors specific to the therapist (skills and experience/status, motivation, "company philosophy," unique selling point, business goals). These factors all directly influence the budgeting of a treatment and should be thoroughly analyzed before a price is set.

Another key point is the therapist's motivation: Is it a passion for esthetics and for making the patient happy that motivate and allow the therapist to meet any demand without stress, or does the focus lie more on economic aspects such as "making a quick buck"? Bear in mind that one does not necessarily rule out the other. All the aforementioned factors should be taken into consideration, and once a business plan has been drawn up, it should be used in combination with those factors to guide the therapist toward achieving the specific goal.

One simple method is to do an internet search of the prices of various competitors with whom one can identify, and then to factor in one's own costs in order to set a basic price that assures profit and allows for a bit of experimental upward leeway.

It is advisable to prepare a price list in advance, which conveys transparency to the patient and can be used as a basis for decision making. A certain amount of leeway should be factored into the pricing, for example, offering an inclusive price for treatments that use more than 2.0 ml of HA.

2.8 Treatment Planning

The planning should include precise details of the technique and product as well as how much volume will be used.

Treatment planning should comprise more than just a one-off treatment, since treatment with HA fillers should be repeated regularly to achieve a good long-term result. For patients with several treatment zones, it causes less discomfort if these zones are not all treated in one session, but over the course of several consecutive appointments.

A treatment plan defines how long term the augmentation should be in order to prevent age-related changes for a prolonged period or to make gradual improvements to the mouth region in several stages. An action plan, a schedule, and a costing plan with the expected results should be drawn up for this purpose. The time window may extend over 1 to 2 years.

For patients, the advantage of a treatment plan is that they are kept in the picture accurately about the treatment goal, the exact financial outlay involved, and the time required for the treatment. This lets patients know that they are being cared for in a controlled manner and are being guided toward a more long-term treatment goal.

The following points should be clarified during the treatment planning process (Sattler & Sommer 2015):

- What is the expected result?
- How quickly should the result become visible?
- What financial means are available?
- How long should the effect persist?
- How much discomfort and inconvenience is the patient prepared to take on?

2.8.1 Treatment Planning for the Lip Region using a Case Example

In the case example (→ Figs. 2.4–2.13), we demonstrate an optimal treatment that is built up over a number of consecutive stages. Bear in mind that this is an example tailored specifically to this female patient, and not a formula that can be applied to any patient. The prerequisites are an adequate budget and the patient's willingness to cooperate with the treatment.

In this case, we have concentrated only on the mouth region, though this would not normally be the case.

The procedure used in the sample treatment for the lip region may be summarized as follows:

- Medical history and findings
- Whether or not this is a first-time treatment
- Treatment wishes, e.g. rejuvenation and beautification
- Limited/unlimited budget
- Treatment plan:
  - Gradual familiarization during the first session
  - Revitalization takes priority initially
  - Gradual buildup of the lip region
  - Setting up a treatment rhythm

Color scheme of the marked treatment zones in the case example:

- **HYDRATION, REVITALIZATION**
- **ACCENTS**
- **PERIORAL LINES**
- **LIP VOLUME**
- **PERIORAL VOLUME**
- **SHAPING, BEAUTIFICATION**

Treatment Planning for a 9-Month Period

An extensive, protracted treatment requires a precise analysis and detailed photographic documentation.

Analysis

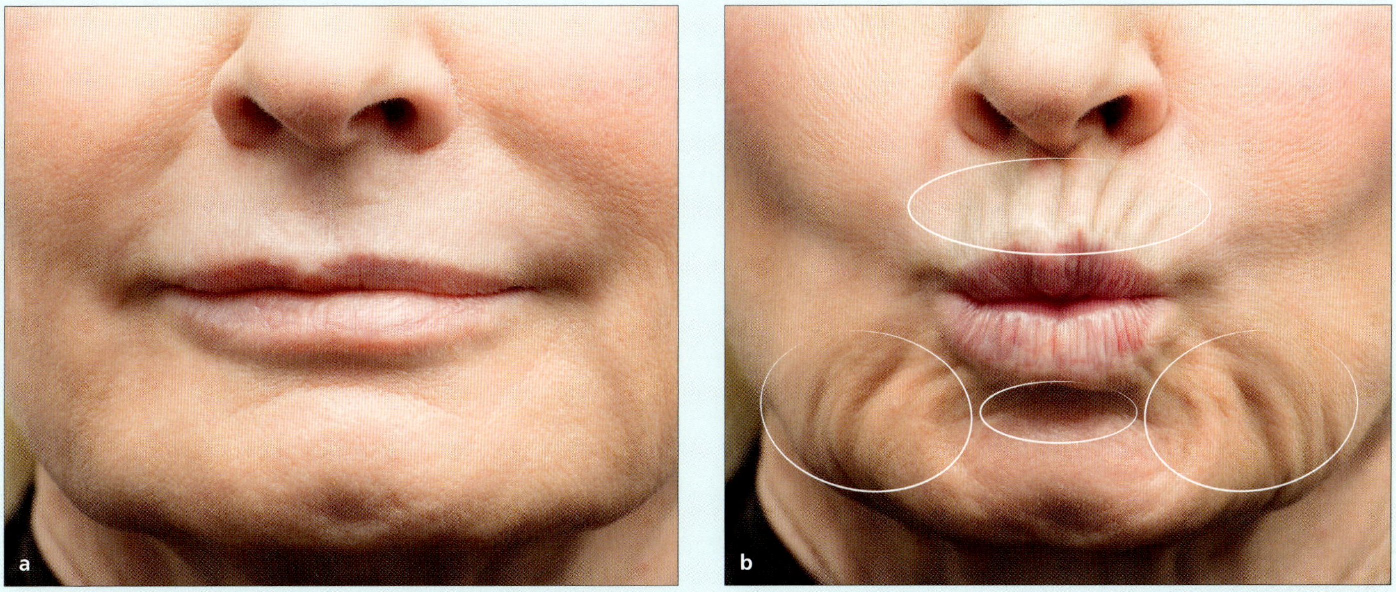

Fig. 2.4 a+b The baseline situation, with the mouth relaxed, of a 60-year-old female patient who has already had several injection treatments (a). Tensing the muscles around the mouth to pucker the lips reveals the perioral shadows caused by volume deficit (b).

- Slightly atrophied, older lip
- Asymmetries in the lips
- Irregular lip contours
- Pronounced chin crease
- Flattened philtrum
- Skin dryness (lips and perioral zone)
- Sagging of the perioral zone
- Slightly drooping mouth corners

Analysis by Segmental Lip Mapping

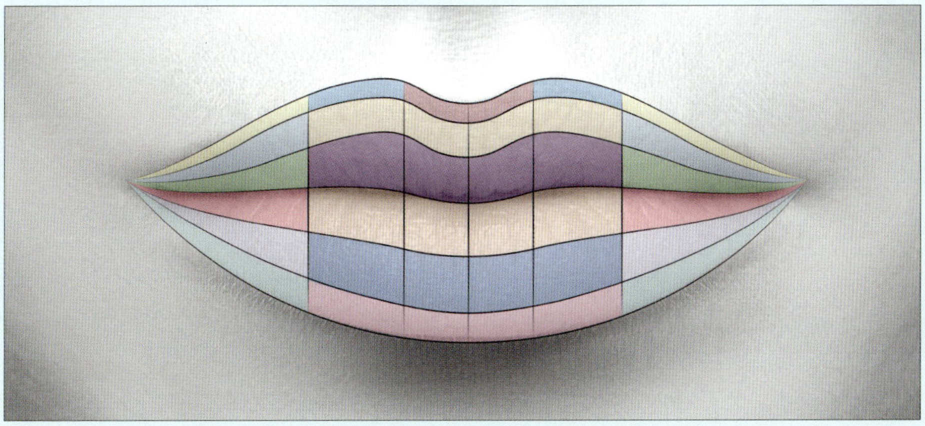

Fig. 2.5 The segmental mapping of the lip using various gridlines helps determine irregularities, asymmetries or deficits. The grid can be placed over the lips on the patient photograph like a template: deviations from the template reveal problem zones and the potential need for treatment. The reference points provided by the grid can also be used as the baseline, allowing any beautification or alteration of the lips to be defined in agreement with the patient.

Analysis using a Quadrant Template

Fig. 2.6 The quadrant template allows the therapist to determine the ratios of the four parts of the lips in relation to each another, i.e. to ascertain whether these ratios are "correct."

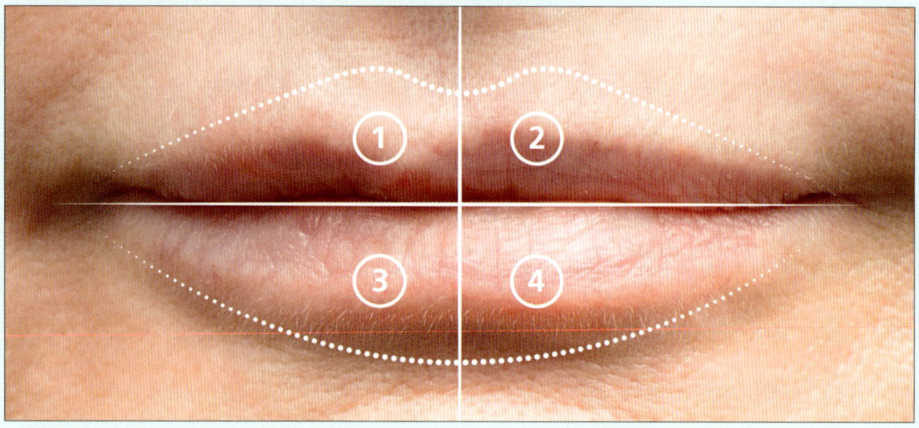

Fig. 2.7 Use of this analytical template clearly shows up the asymmetry of the lips.

The Cupid's bow shows a shift to the right (from the patient's point of view). The right upper lip is smaller, thinner, and more inverted in the center. The tubercle is not located in the center but more toward the right. The two philtral columns are flattened, more so on the right side than on the left. There is also a small scar on the right philtrum near the contour. The right lower lip is less pronounced than the left one: it is flatter, thinner, and shorter. The center of the lower lip is parallel to the center of the Cupid's bow.

Treatment Plan

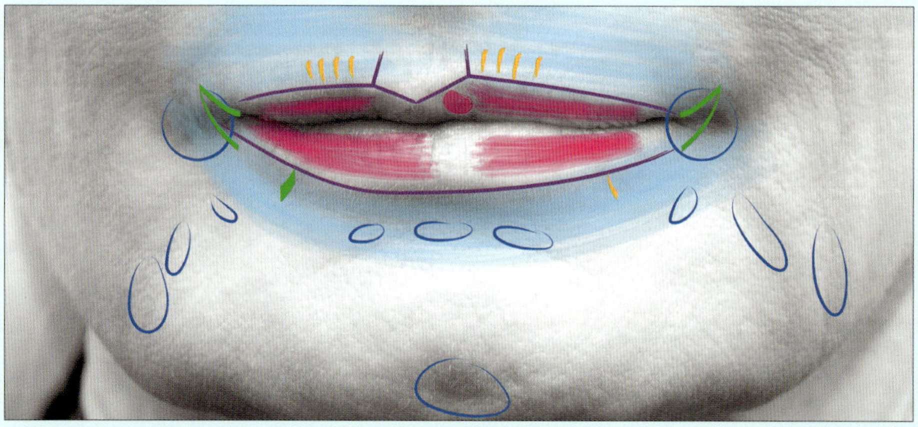

Fig. 2.8 The lips and perioral areas have been marked to indicate treatment sites for the following indications:

- Rehydration and revitalization of the perioral zone
- Contouring and accentuation of the lost shapes
- Balancing out asymmetries
- Volume replacement
- Removal of the shadows and lines on the chin
- Lip corner lift
- Lip moistening
- Reduction or removal of the perioral lines

When it comes to balancing the upper lip asymmetry, an improvement can be made by sharp contouring of the philtrum. To do this, 1.0 mm will be added to the medial side of the right philtrum, close to the natural philtral peak, to achieve visual centering of the philtrum. The tubercle should be accentuated slightly on the left side (with 0.02 ml HA). The right upper lip can be matched up with the left by balancing out the deficit. The right lower lip can be augmented laterally, using technique 42 (see Chap. 9.6.6, p. 294) with 0.5 ml HA. The volume deficit of the right lower lip will be remedied by matching it to the left lower lip. Once the symmetry has been improved, the lips as a whole can be treated over several sessions. The revitalization needs to be carried out over three consecutive sessions, to allow neocollagenesis to take place. The first session provides the basis for all subsequent treatments.

First Session: Early January

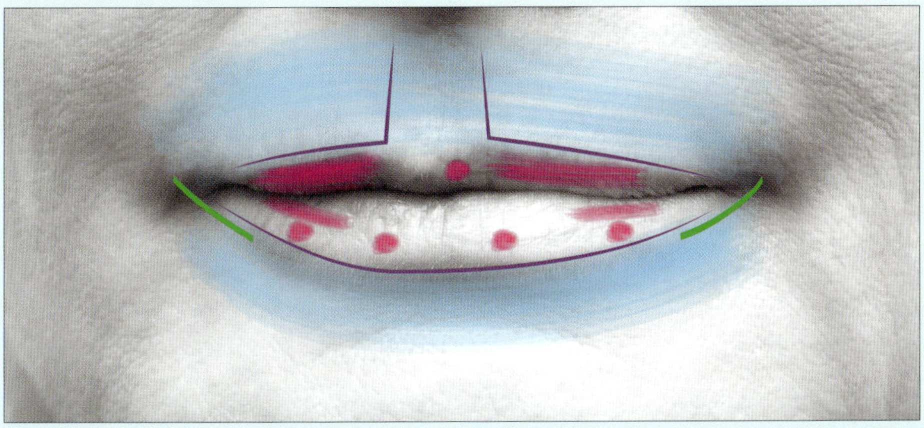

Fig. 2.9

- Revitalization, hydration in the perioral region
- Stabilization of the contours
- Balancing and shaping of the philtrum
- Volume replacement
- Gentle lip corner lift
- Widening the lips

Treatment*	Technique no.	HA product	UL	LL	PU	PL
Contour	6	M	0.3	0.35	–	–
Philtrum	9	M	0.2	–	–	–
Mouth corners	39	M	–	0.4	–	–
Volume	18	M	0.3	0.3	–	–
Tubercles	27		0.05	–	–	–
Revitalization	1	XS	–	–	0.5	0.5
HA filler in ml			2.9			

Table 2.1 *The HA volumes are given in ml. The technical details may be looked up in this book under the respective technique number. The name and batch number of the product being used would always be entered into a real treatment plan. UL = upper lip, LL = lower lip, PU = perioral zone of the upper lip, PL = perioral zone of the lower lip.

Second Session: Early February

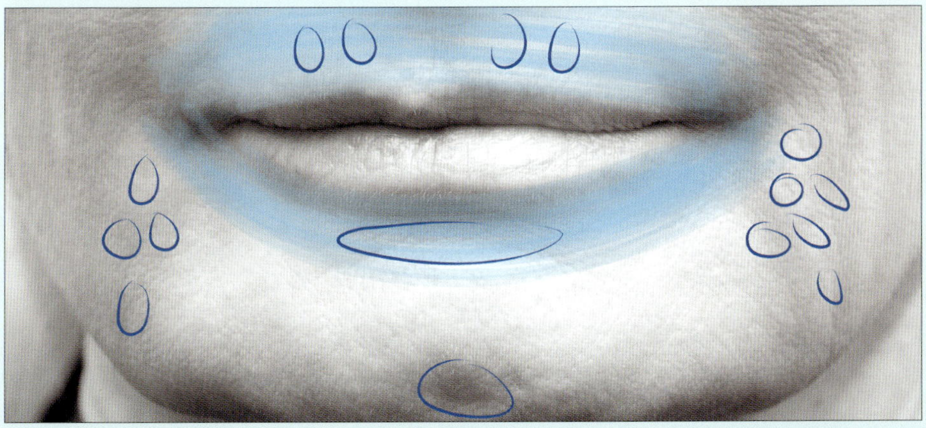

Fig. 2.10

- Second revitalization, hydration of the perioral zone
- Inject filler into the perioral shadows (vertical injection technique)
- Filling of the chin groove
- Filling of the labiomental fold

→ The second revitalization and the perioral volumization are scheduled for the 2nd session.

Treatment*	Technique no.	HA product	UL	LL	PU	PL
Revitalization	2	XS	–	–	0.5	0.5
Perioral shadows	31	M	–	–	0.4	–
Labiomental fold	29	M	–	–	0.4	–
Chin augmentation	30	M	–	–	0.2	–
HA filler in ml			2.0			

Table 2.2 *The HA volumes are given in ml. The technical details may be looked up in this book under the respective technique number. The name and batch number of the product being used would always be entered into a real treatment plan. UL = upper lip, LL = lower lip, PU = perioral zone of the upper lip, PL = perioral zone of the lower lip.

Third Session: Mid-March (6 Weeks Later)

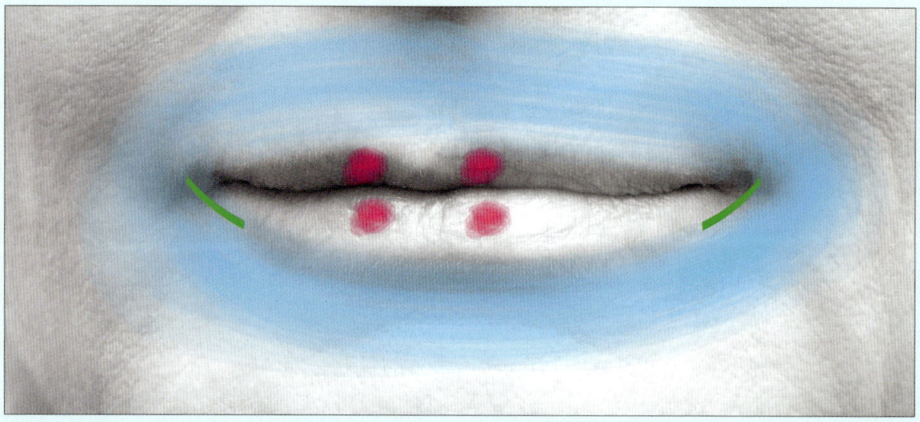

Fig. 2.11

- Third revitalization, hydration of the perioral zone
- Refresh treatment, volumization of the red part of the lip
- Gentle lip corner lift

→ In the 3rd session, the revitalization is to be completed and accents put in.

Treatment*	Technique no.	HA product	UL	LL	PU	PL
Revitalization	1	XS	–	–	0.5	0.5
Volume	5	M	0.2	0.2	–	–
Mouth corners	37		–	0.2	–	–
HA filler in ml			1.6			

Table 2.3 *The HA volumes are given in ml. The technical details may be looked up in this book under the respective technique number. The name and batch number of the product being used would always be entered into a real treatment plan. UL = upper lip, LL = lower lip, PU = perioral zone of the upper lip, PL = perioral zone of the lower lip.

Fourth Session: End June

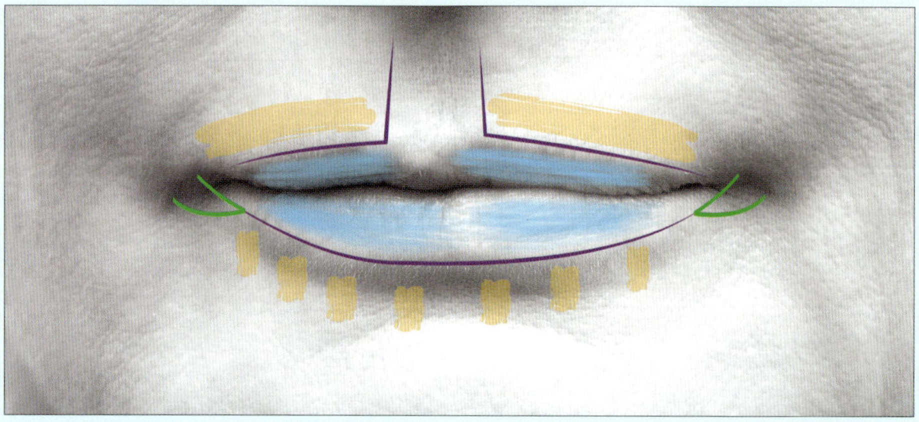

Fig. 2.12

- Reworking of the contours and philtrum
- Inject filler into the perioral lines
- Revitalization of the entire vermillion area
- Lip corner lift

→ In the 4th session, the contours are to be reinforced, with targeted filler injections into the perioral lines. The dry lips can also be rehydrated.

Treatment*	Technique no.	HA product	UL	LL	PU	PL
Perioral lines	11	XS	0.1	0.1	–	–
Philtrum	9	M	0.2	–	–	–
Contour	7	M	0.4	0.4	–	–
Oral commissures	38	M	–	0.4	–	–
Revitalization	3	XS	0.2	0.2	–	–
HA filler in ml			2.0			

Table 2.4 *The HA volumes are given in ml. The technical details may be looked up in this book under the respective technique number. The name and batch number of the product being used would always be entered into a real treatment plan. UL = upper lip, LL = lower lip, PU = perioral zone of the upper lip, PL = perioral zone of the lower lip.

Fifth and Last Session: End September/Early October

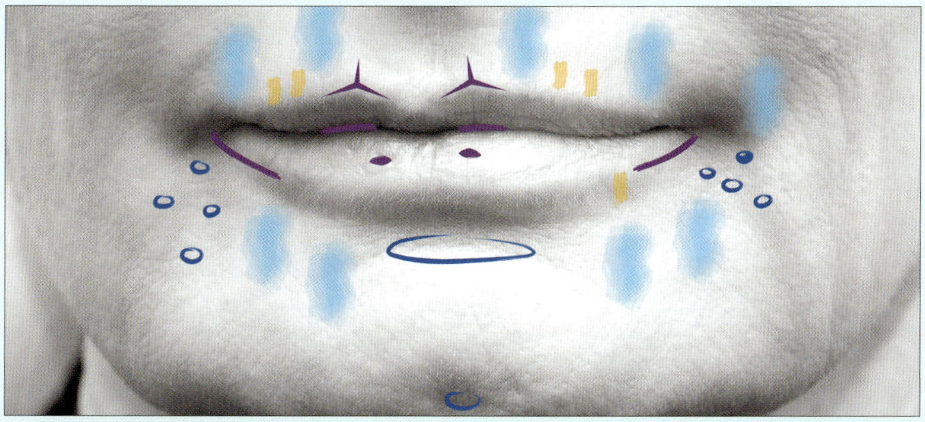

Fig. 2.13

- Accents, contour, philtrum tip, wet-dry border
- Improvement of the radial wrinkles
- Refresh labiomental fold
- Refresh chin region
- Reinjection of the perioral shadows
- Revitalization of specific points, hydration of the perioral zone

→ **In the 5th session, tiny corrective and refresher injections are to be given as required, and the treatment concluded.**

Treatment*	Technique no.	HA product	UL	LL	PU	PL
Perioral hydration	1	XS	–	–	0.3	0.3
Perioral lines	13	XS	–	–	0.2	0.2
Contour and philtrum tip	10	M	0.05	0.15	–	–
Wet-dry border (lips)	22	M	–	–	–	0.2
Perioral shadows	31	M	–	–	–	0.4
Chin groove	30	M	–	–	–	0.1
Labiomental fold	29	M	–	–	–	0.1
HA filler in ml			2.0			

Table 2.5 *The HA volumes are given in ml. The technical details may be looked up in this book under the respective technique number. The name and batch number of the product being used would always be entered into a real treatment plan. UL = upper lip, LL = lower lip, PU = perioral zone of the upper lip, PL = perioral zone of the lower lip.

2

3 Documentation

3 Documentation

3.1 Patient Documentation

Before every treatment, the therapist should conduct an information session during which the parameters that describe the baseline situation are recorded. Risks and side effects are pointed out, and the possibilities and limitations of the treatment are discussed. Once a detailed medical history has been taken, the examination findings are noted, and the medical procedure is explained and discussed. All this information is collected and recorded with the aid of questionnaires, information sheets, and the patient documentation record, taken down in writing and signed by the patient in an informed consent form (→ QR code).

The treatment itself is logged and documented by the therapist before and after each session, with a record of the product, batch number, indication, points of note, and any follow-up treatment. If side effects occur, the product's batch number provides important evidence for the indemnity insurance, to show that the therapist did not make any product-related errors. The documentation also has a precautionary role, providing proof in the event of a patient complaint. These complaints are generally based on misapprehension regarding the treatment success, once patients have become accustomed to their altered appearance.

Photographic documentation with good before-and-after photos provides a record of the baseline status and the changes resulting from several treatments. Moreover, photographic documentation provides a safeguard in the event of a dispute, for instance, patients frequently claim that the injections have not worked or that the HA has been absorbed too quickly. This kind of claim can be cleared up and, if necessary, refuted with a good photographic documentation record.

Note

The documentation records are an important aid in demonstrating the course of a treatment, thus providing the therapist with a legal safeguard.

Templates of the relevant documentation forms have been kindly provided to us by the company Teoxane and can be accessed by means of this QR code. They can also be ordered from other material manufacturers.

3.2 Photographic Documentation

Clear and informative photos are an important method of documenting the outcome of a treatment. Firstly, the images can be used as a way of communicating the further course of the treatment to the patient. Secondly, they can be used as a safeguard in the event of a dispute. Certain factors need to be taken into account when making a photographic record of the lips:

- The lips should be free of makeup
- The patient's skin should be dry and clean
- The face should be relaxed and the facial expression neutral

The first photo acts as a reference image for all the subsequent shots that are taken. It therefore requires great care and precision because it documents the baseline situation. This reference photo should always be used for any subsequent documentation of the treatment course. The photos should be comparable with respect to lighting, cutout, perspective, and quality, which requires a standardized procedure. The photo details need to be cleanly reproduced by the camera settings and must not be improved using image processing software. To achieve this, the following factors should always be set in the same way:

- Settings on the camera (focal length and lighting), smartphone or tablet
- Lighting and light source
- Sitting position and positioning
- Camera angle and distance

3.2.1 Camera and Equipment

Either a compact camera or a reflex camera may be used to take the photos. We have not given any recommendations here, as the technology is constantly changing and developing at a very rapid rate.

A tripod is required to ensure that all the photos are taken from the same perspective. Ideally, the camera should be in parallel alignment with the subject: if the subject is photographed from above or below, the proportions will be distorted. If a tripod cannot be used, the camera must be held still, either supported against the photographer's body or on a table. The basic equipment includes the following:

- Tripod
- Gray or blue image background
- Lights, flash or dedicated flash unit
- Camera
- Chair or stool with adjustable height

These objects should always be in the same place. Marks on the floor or wall may be used to fix these locations.

The optimal settings for the aforementioned parameters are best found by trial and error: camera settings, exposure time, angle, and distance from the face should be tried and tested to achieve the best possible settings for the individual circumstances. The parameters should be recorded in a checklist and adjusted accordingly, where required. Many cameras allow a specific group of settings to be saved as "custom settings" (user settings, C1, C2, C3, ...). If the same camera is used again for photographic documentation, it is then simply a case of selecting the appropriate user settings.

3.2.2 Photos taken with Smartphones and Tablets

Very good photos can be taken with a smartphone that has a good camera function, or with a tablet that has similar features. The advantages of taking photos with these devices is that the task is easier to delegate to practice assistants, since they are likely to be familiar with such devices through daily use. However, when using this technique, it is still necessary to ensure that the standards described above are followed. At present, the use of a camera is still a safer and more reliable method of producing a standard photographic documentation series over a prolonged period of time.

3.2.3 Lighting and Light Source (→ Figs. 3.1–3.4)

A room that does not admit direct sunlight is recommended for standardized lighting. A room that faces north or, even better, a room that can be blacked out is best. The light settings should be identical for each photo and each photoshoot. An artificial light source is recommended for this purpose.

The main light source should be directed at a 45-degree angle from above left or above right (→ Fig. 3.1a). Illuminating the subject from above in this way reveals the relief of skin irregularities, lines or shadows. If the face is lit directly from the front with a flash or an artificial light, the image will look less sculptural, and the skin structures will no longer be identifiable.

In addition, different light settings can reveal different shadows; this is not possible if a strong light is directed at the face only from the front. For example, allowing the light source to circle around the face after a filler injection treatment for wrinkles will make it possible for the therapist to check whether irregularities, lines or shadows have been corrected. Dedicated flash units or permanent light-emitting diode (LED) light sources should be used in professional photographic documentation records.

Lighting Effects

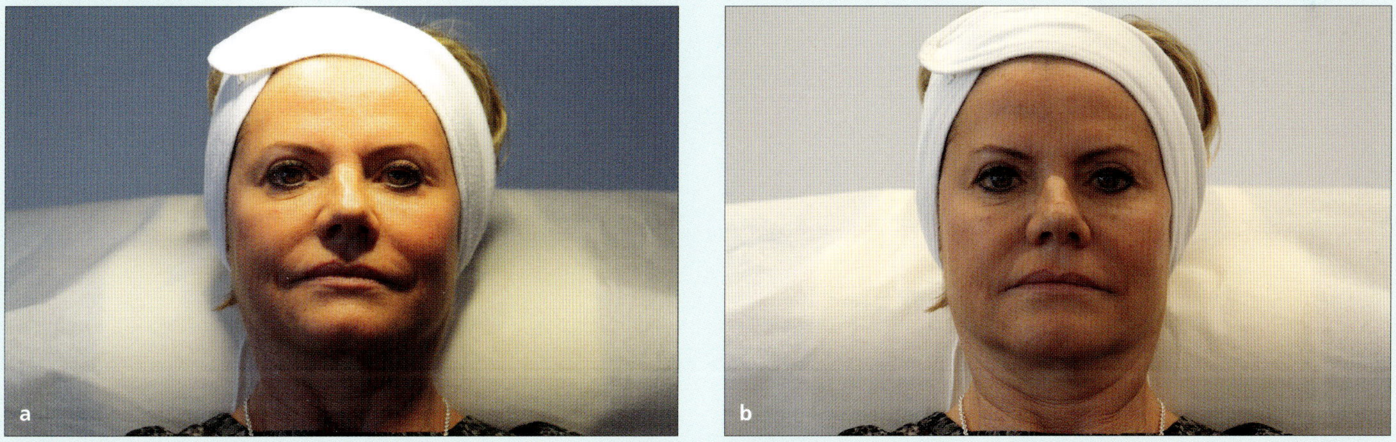

Fig. 3.1 a+b Angle of light incidence: 45 degrees from above (a), and light incidence from a diffuse ceiling light (b). The angle of incidence of the light plays an important role in identifying shadows and reliefs. The light is directed from above in both situations. In image (a), the face is lit directly with a mobile light from above, so that the major shadows are sharply illuminated. In image (b), diffuse light is being directed at the face from a fixed ceiling light, so that the shadows and skin relief are not as clearly identifiable and have become blurred.

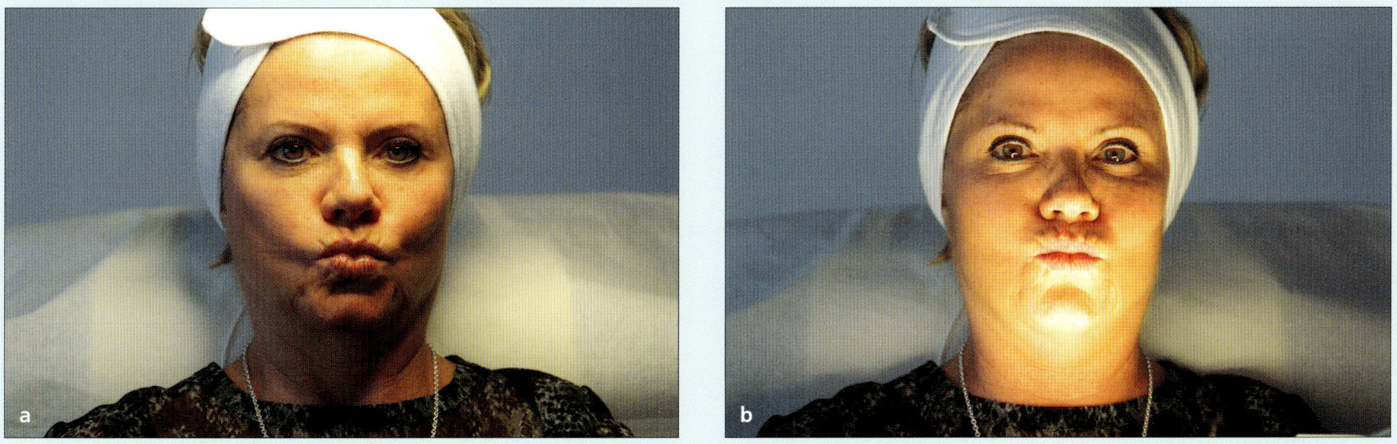

Fig. 3.2 a+b Direct light from above (a) and below (b). Different lighting setups reveal a variety of shadows; this is not possible with a strong light that illuminates the face directly from the front.

Lighting Effects

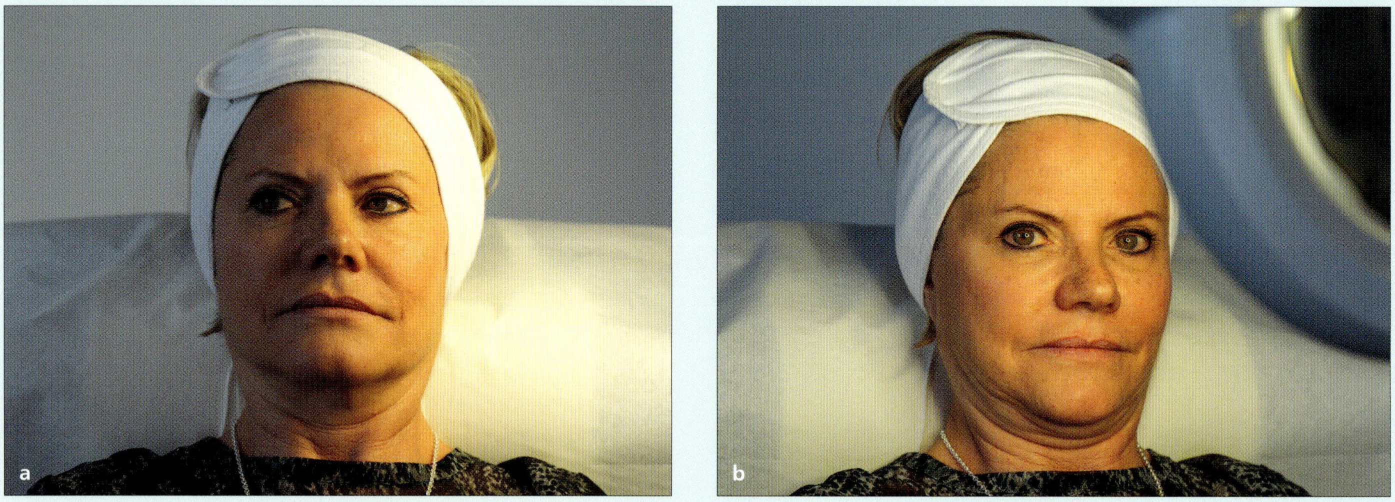

Fig. 3.3 a+b When the face is lit from the right or left side, the shadows fall sideways, revealing any prominences that run vertically (a). When the light incidence is directly from the front, it is difficult to identify the course of any lines, shadows, and irregularities (b).

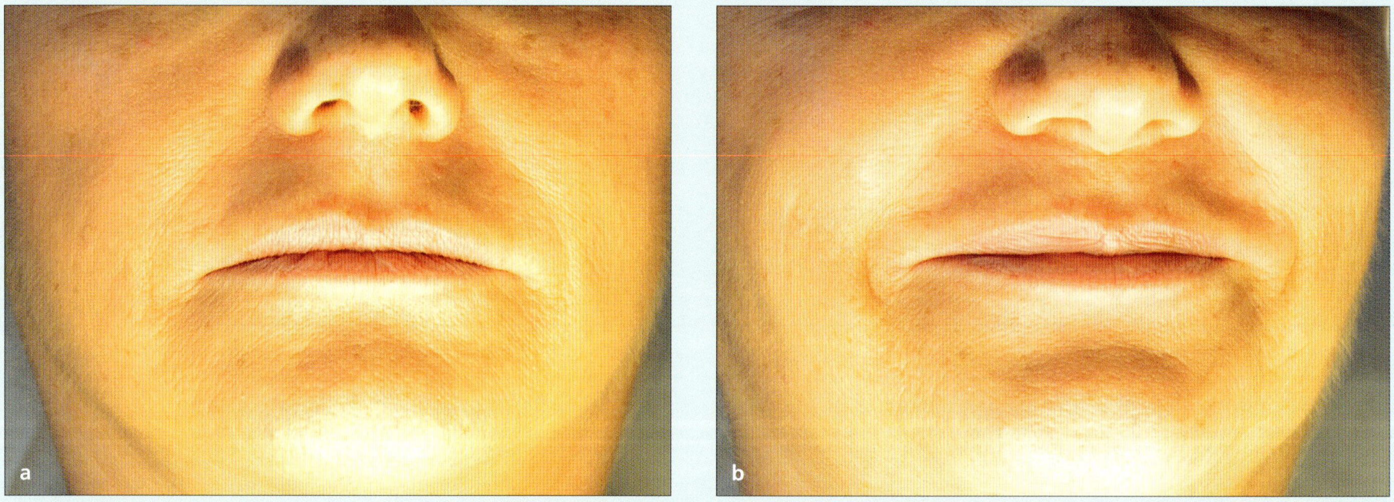

Fig. 3.4 a+b If the relaxed lips are lit from above, it clearly reveals whether the cutaneous part of the lip has been uniformly injected with filler, without any bulges or prominences (a). Facial expressions can help the therapist to check how the shadows behave and whether any irregularities occur (b).

3.2.4 Sitting Position and Positioning

The patient should sit upright on the chair, with the head held upright but without overextending the chin. The seat height should be adjusted according to a mark on the wall, to ensure that the head shot is always taken at the same height. If a camera is used, this should be on a tripod placed in a fixed position, with the lens height at the patient's eye level. The distance between the lens and the patient's face should be between 15–20 cm if a smartphone camera is being used (→ Fig. 3.5); once this distance has been checked carefully, it should always be kept the same. The camera should be at a distance of 1–1.5 m. Images of the whole head should always be taken for a photo documentation of the lips, as follows:

- With the head held upright
- With a relaxed facial expression
- With the lips closed

3.2.5 Photographs of the Lips

The first photos of the patient (→ Figs. 3.6–3.16), taken at the start of a documentation series, are the reference images that are used as a parameter for comparison with the treatment results documented with subsequent shots. For this reason, it is important to take these photographs conscientiously and with care.

Lip shapes resulting from various facial and emotional expressions should also be recorded in order to obtain comprehensive material that can be used for the analysis (see Chap. 1.6.4, p. 39). Of course, this series of images can be continued indefinitely: the more facial play is included, the better one can record details that are relevant to the pre-and post-treatment analysis, However, it is important to ensure that the same close-up shots are taken in the same order at each subsequent session if a meaningful comparison is to be made.

Reference Images for Treatment Documentation – Various Views of the Face

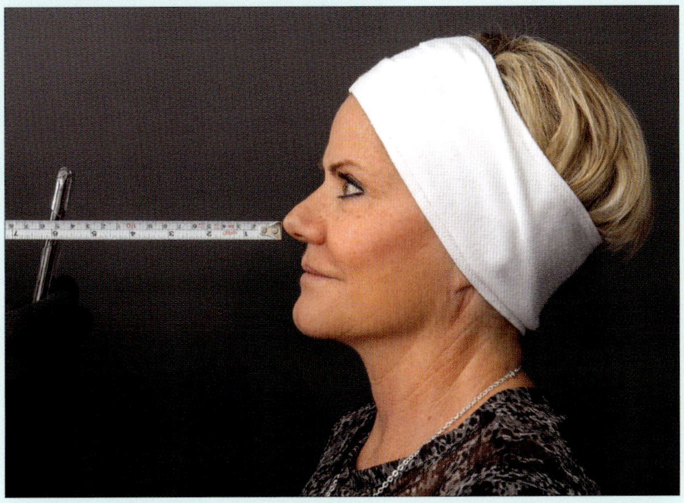

Fig. 3.5 Patient sitting upright and in profile view: the lens is at the correct distance and is at eye level (image taken using a smartphone).

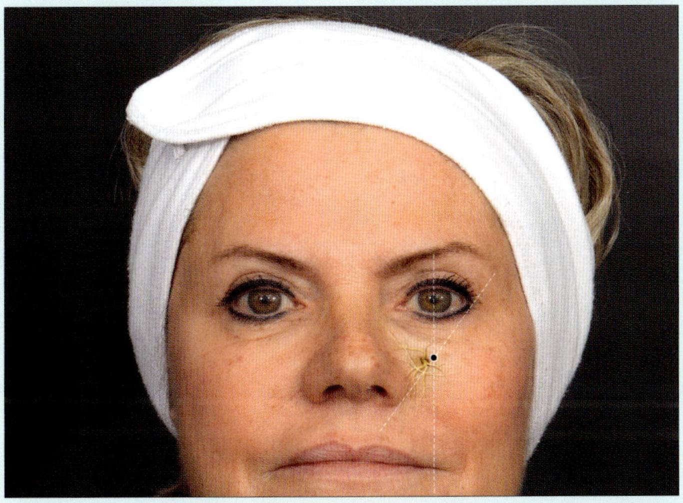

Fig. 3.6 Front view.

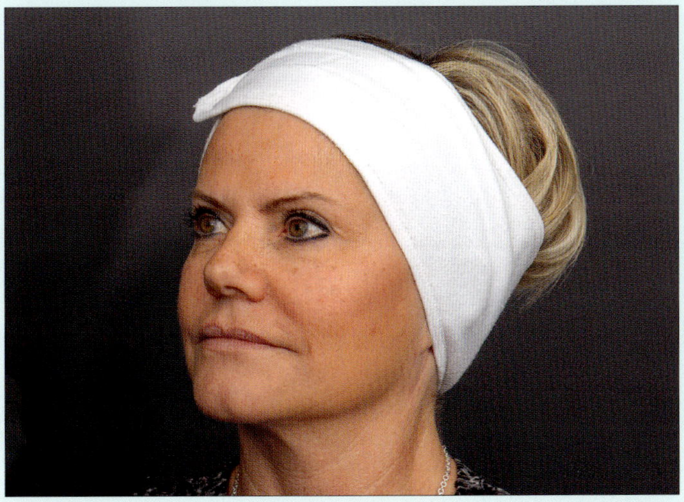

Fig. 3.7 Image taken in semi-profile, also known as three-quarter view (this type of image needs to be taken from both sides).

Reference Images for Treatment Documentation – The Lips during Facial Play and Movement

(→ see Chap. 1.6.4, p. 39)

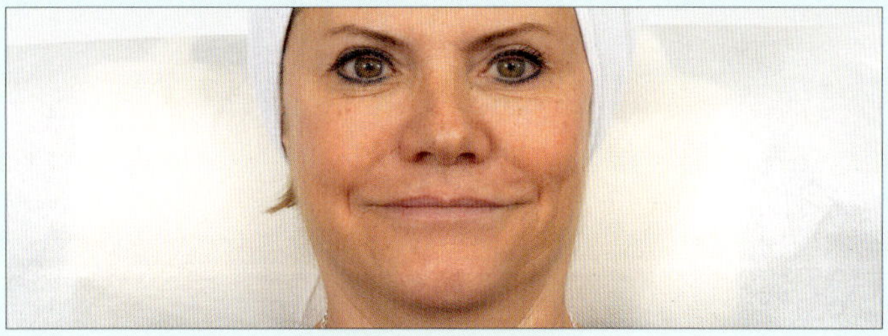

Fig. 3.8 Patient smiling with the mouth closed.

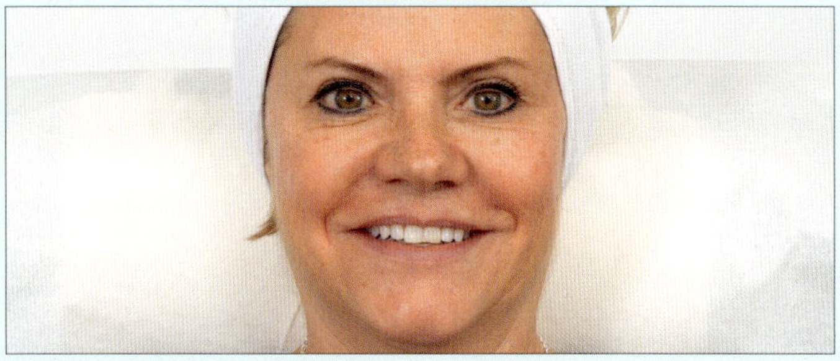

Fig. 3.9 Patient smiling with the mouth open.

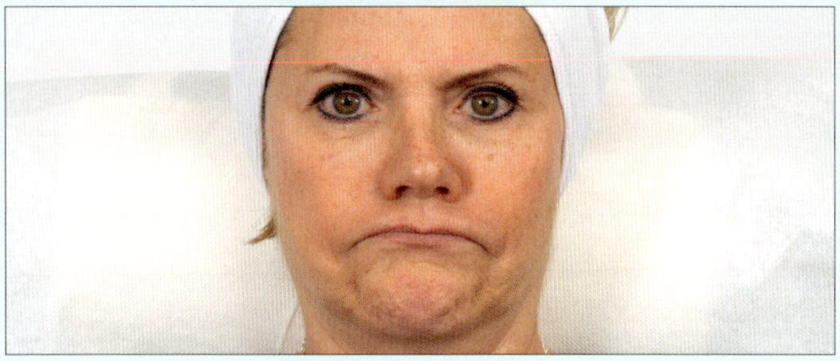

Fig. 3.10 Mouth corners pulled down.

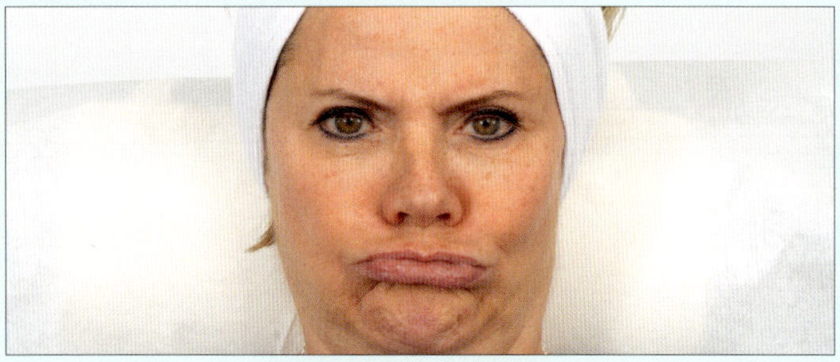

Fig. 3.11 Activity of the mentalis muscle (cobblestone chin).

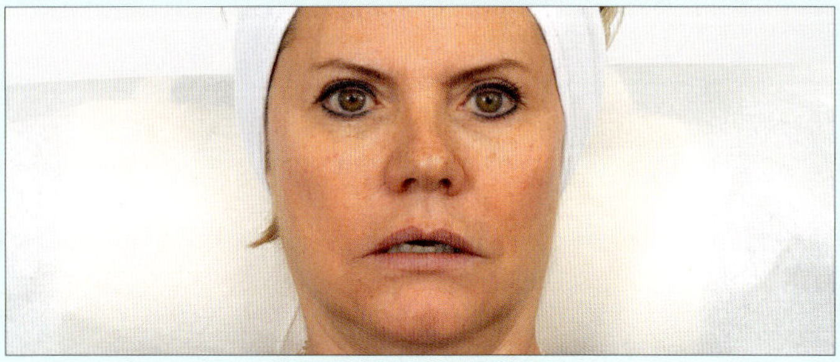

Fig. 3.12 Relaxed, open mouth.

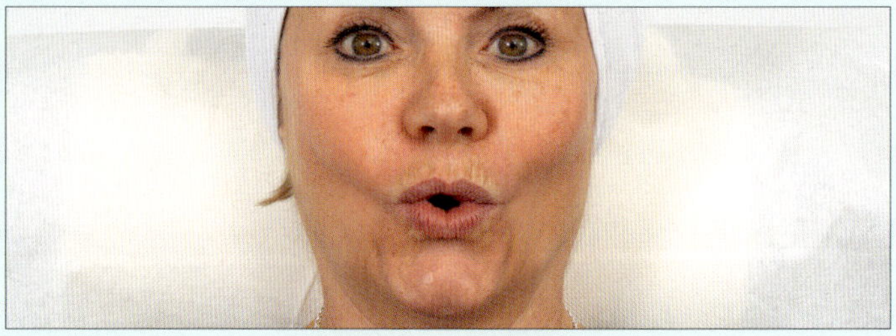

Fig. 3.13 Shaping of the lips during speech.

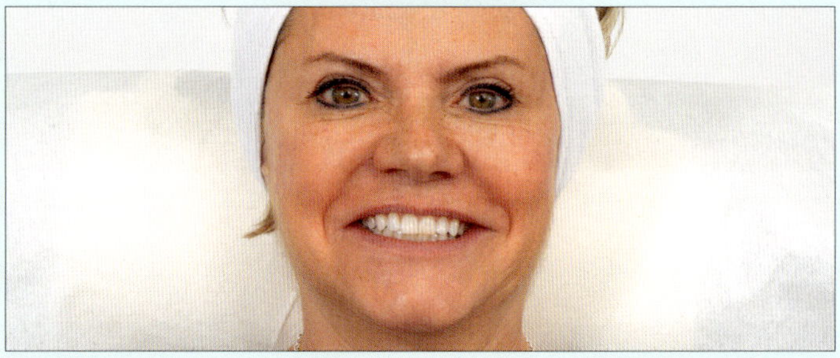

Fig. 3.14 Tightening the lips while saying "cheese."

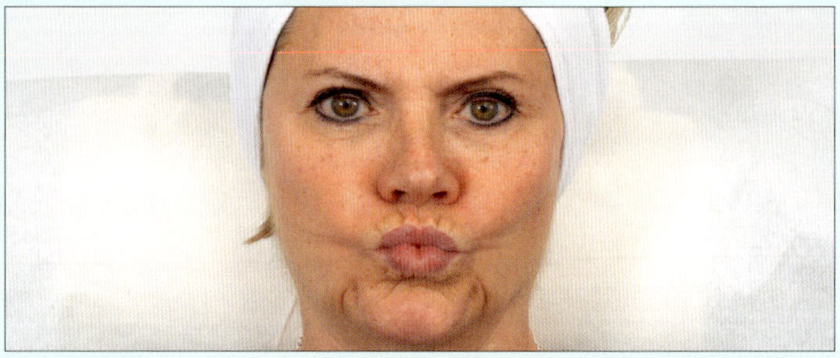

Fig. 3.15 Puckered lips.

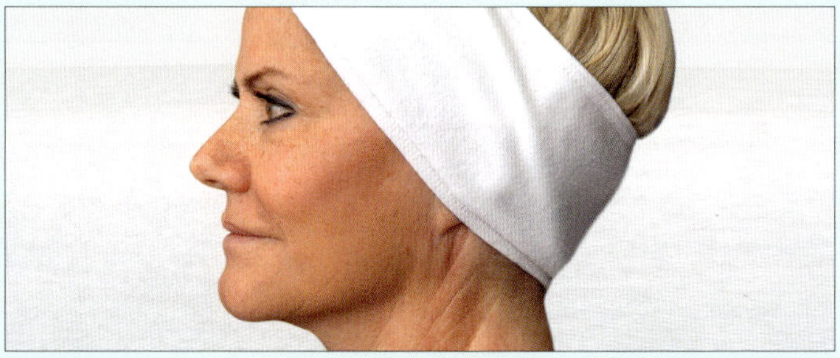

Fig. 3.16 Profile view for analysis of the UL : LL ratio and the anatomy of the jaw.

4 The Dermal Filler Hyaluronic Acid

4 The Dermal Filler Hyaluronic Acid

Hyaluronic acid (HA), first used in esthetics in 1996 (as Restylane), is an absorbable, natural gel that consists of long polysaccharide chains, which occur naturally in the human body. It is manufactured synthetically on a non-animal basis and causes virtually no immunologic reactions. Due to its properties as a filler, in combination with its water-binding capacity, HA is eminently suitable as a dermal filler for esthetic, rejuvenating facial treatments: HA revitalizes the skin by hydration and rejuvenates the appearance by treating lines and through facial augmentation. A large number of different variants of HA are now available: there are more than 200 HA products on this constantly growing market, making it difficult for the therapist to choose the right filler for the indication being treated. As far as fillers are concerned, here we will refer only to lip augmentation. In a bid to provide therapists with an overview, we have restricted ourselves to a small number of products currently on the market and, with the aid of the tables in Sattler & Sommer (2015, p. 62), have developed a lip-specific table of fillers (see Chap. 4.9, p. 75).

4.1 Requirements for Hyaluronic Acid in Lip Treatment

The most important gel property of HA for a lip augmentation treatment is its viscoelasticity, i.e. a change in consistency between soft and solid. As a result, it can adjust dynamically to the movement of the lips and also exhibits a lifting capacity. Moreover, HA should not cause any swellings.

Solid gels with a good lifting capacity are used for contours, the philtrum or marionette lines. Solid, small-particle HA products are used for injections into perioral lines, while fluid, easy-flow HA products are used for hydration of the perioral zone (Becker-Wegerich 2016).

Generally speaking, an optimal filler has the following properties (Sattler & Sommer 2015):

- Degradable
- Adjusts to the consistency of the tissue
- Low complication rate
- Non-allergenic
- Sterile
- Good value
- Easy to inject
- Biocompatible
- Compatible with other fillers
- Pain-free administration
- Does not form nodules
- As natural as possible to ensure integration into the tissue
- Long in vivo persistence
- Good lifting capacity in the appropriate indication
- Good elasticity in the appropriate indication

4.2 Filler Properties

The HA fillers differ with regard to their rheological properties, which consist of the following factors and determine their gel characteristics:

- **Particle size**: The smaller the particle size, the more superficially the product is injected and the more rapidly it degrades. The larger the particles, the deeper the product is injected and the slower it degrades.
- **Concentration per ml**: The amount of HA that a product contains determines the key properties of the filler during and after the injection.
- **Type of crosslinking**: The viscosity increases with the degree of crosslinking (Sattler & Sommer 2015); for example, a low degree of crosslinking and a small particle size result in a softer, rapidly degradable filler. A high degree of crosslinking results in a harder gel. The harder the gel, the better its lifting capacity.
- **Modification**: The modification of an HA product, which results from the type and degree of crosslinking, plays a major part in determining biocompatibility. The less modification a product has undergone, the better it is tolerated.

A product's elasticity and viscosity – and thus also its lifting capacity and tissue life – depend on the above-listed four properties. Taken together, the degree of crosslinking, the HA concentration, and the particle size determine the water content, the degradability, the elasticity, and the viscosity of an HA filler.

Viscosity describes the flow properties and thickness of a gel (Galderma, n.d.). It is crucial to be informed about the viscosity of a product: if a lip treatment is to be successful, it is important that the correct product for the appropriate treatment goal is used in the correct layer:

- The low-viscosity products are used predominantly for subdermal, horizontal HA distribution (Sattler & Sommer 2015).
- The medium-viscosity products are all-rounders that can be used for numerous indications. While still showing good plasticity, they also possess lifting capacity.
- The high-viscosity products have the best lifting capacity and show high resistance to deformation. In the lip region, they are used predominantly to strengthen and lift the tissues. They show no plasticity.

Elasticity in this context is the ability of a gel to "spring back" into its original form after being deformed (Galderma, n.d.).

Innovative Cross-Linking Technologies for Dermal Fillers

Examples of innovative crosslinking technologies that have resulted in biphasic gels include the Optimal Balance technology from Q-Med Galderma and the Vycross technology from Allergan, which allow fillers with a particularly long life to be manufactured. However, based on clinical experience to the contrary, the authors cannot agree with the manufacturers' claims that the low water-binding capacity of these fillers can prevent swellings.

On the other hand, the CPM (Cohesive Polydense Matrix) technology from Merz and the RHA (Resilient Hyaluronic Acid) technology from Teoxane have allowed for the manufacture of monophasic fillers without particles. When injected, these are distributed into the tissue interstices unaided, producing a smooth transition between the treated tissue and the adjoining areas.

There is also a likelihood of side effects due to the varying toxicity of the crosslinking agents used.

(Cited from: Sattler & Sommer 2015, p. 58)

4.3 Dermal Filler Products

A selection of filler products with their properties are presented in this chapter (see p. 68). The descriptions of these fillers and the recommendations regarding needles are taken from the relevant product information texts provided by the manufacturers.

Since the filler market has experienced huge growth, with the launch of increasing numbers of products from Asia as well as generics, it would be beyond the scope of this book to mention them all. The brand-name products presented here offer a choice of different rheological properties, viscosities, and degrees of crosslinking. The tables offer a clearly arranged palette of fillers for a variety of indications, since not only the perioral region but also the entire face needs to be treated in routine practice. For the lip techniques, we have used the tables by Sattler & Sommer (2015) as a basis (see p. 62 in that book). To simplify the entire procedure, our "Filler Navigator" table (p. 75) classifies the products with regard to their clinical properties, regardless of brand names, and also lists them according to manufacturer.

The products for lip treatment have wide-ranging uses, from the treatment of perioral lines of varying depths to lip contouring and all the way to filling of the lips and perioral parts of the face.

Three factors are of key importance for a successful lip augmentation:

- A profound knowledge of the products
- The technical and anatomical knowledge of the therapist
- The skin and aging status of the patient

Classifications and Symbols used in the Filler Tables and the Filler Navigator

Fillers are available in a variety of particle sizes and degrees of crosslinking. Fillers are classified into different particles sizes using the symbols XS to XL. However, some fillers defy precise classification and are therefore supplied by the manufacturers using different categories.

Particle size

XS stands for a thin material with no lifting capacity, suitable only for revitalization and hydration of the skin

S stands for a small-particle material with low lifting capacity, suitable for the finest lines and wrinkles

M stands for a medium-thickness material with lifting capacity, suitable for lines of medium depth

L stands for a thicker material with lifting capacity, suitable for lines of medium depth

XL stands for a very thick material with lifting capacity, suitable for deep lines and augmentation treatments

Degree of crosslinking

● **Soft –** stands for a soft, weakly crosslinked gel, which is used to replace lost tissue and fat

▲ **Strong –** stands for a strongly crosslinked gel with good lifting capacity, for contouring, the lifting of lines, and supraperiosteal augmentation

Added analgesic: Virtually all the products are available with added lidocaine.

In all cases, you can find the most up-to-date, detailed information about the products from the manufacturers themselves (see manufacturers' internet links, p. 339). The fillers best suited for treating the lips are listed in a separate table. We recommend the harder, more crosslinked gels with good lifting capacity, marked "▲" for contouring and shaping of the lips, and the softer, less crosslinked gels, marked "●" for lip augmentation and filling.

4

4.4 Filler Products for Treatment of the Lips and Perioral Region

HA Fillers for Treatment of the Lips and Perioral Zone (Authors' Recommendation)						
Product name	**Supplier**	**Indication**	**Depth of administration**	**HA concentration Viscosity Crosslinking**	**Needle/ cannula gauge**	**Special material properties**
BELOTERO Soft ●	Merz Aesthetics	• Correction of superficial lines	Upper dermis	20 mg/ml Dynamically multi-crosslinked (CPM and DCLT technology)	30G 1/2	• Polydensified, cohesive gel • Very good tissue integration • Weak water-binding capacity • Persistence of 6–9 months • Very well tolerated • Available with lidocaine (0.3%)
BELOTERO Lips Contour ▲	Merz Aesthetics	• Lip contours • Fine, perioral lines and wrinkles • Moderate lines at the corners of the mouth	Upper and middle dermis	22.5 mg/ml Multi-dynamically crosslinked (CPM technology)	27G 1/2 30G 1/2	• Medium-viscosity, polydensified cohesive gel • Very good tissue integration • Virtually no water-binding capacity • Persistence of 12 months • Very well tolerated • With lidocaine (0.3%) • Blanching possible
BELOTERO Lips Shape ●	Merz Aesthetics	• Lip volume • Highly pronounced lines at mouth corners	Middle and deep dermis	25.5 mg/ml Multi-dynamically crosslinked (CPM technology)	27G 1/2	• High-viscosity, polydensified elastic gel • Very good lifting capacity and tissue integration • Very well tolerated • Persistence of 12 months • Available with lidocaine (0.3%)
Juvéderm HYDRATE ●	Allergan	• Improvement of skin moisture and elasticity	Upper dermis	13.5 mg/ml Non-crosslinked HA with 0.9% mannitol	30G 1/6 32G	• Good water-binding capacity • Short persistence
Juvéderm ULTRA 3 ▲	Allergan	• Medium-depth and deep skin lines • Lip contours • Lip volume	Middle and deep dermis	24 mg/ml Crosslinked (HYLACROSS technology)	27G 1/2	• Smooth, supple gel • Long persistence • With lidocaine (0.3%)
Juvéderm ULTRA 4 ▲	Allergan	• Deep skin lines • Volume build-up of lips and cheeks	Deep dermis	24 mg/ml Crosslinked (HYLACROSS technology)	27G 1/2	• Smooth gel • Long persistence • With lidocaine (0.3%)
Juvéderm ULTRA SMILE ●	Allergan	• Medium-depth and deep skin lines • Lip contours • Lip volume	Middle and deep dermis	24 mg/ml Crosslinked (HYLACROSS technology)	30G 1/2	• Smooth gel • Long persistence • With lidocaine (0.3%)
Juvéderm VOLBELLA ●	Allergan	• Superficial and medium-depth lines • Volume build-up and definition of lip contours	Upper and middle dermis	15 mg/ml Cross-linked (VYCROSS technology)	30G 1/2	• Good persistence • Good distribution (reason: minimal cohesiveness) • Very good tissue integration and neocollagenesis • With lidocaine (0.3%)
Juvéderm VOLIFT ●	Allergan	• Deep skin lines • Contour deficits • Volume build-up of cheeks, chin, and lips	Deep dermis (recommendation: not for intradermal use)	17.5 mg/ml Crosslinked (VYCROSS technology)	30G 1/2	• Very long persistence (up to 18 months) • Good distribution • Very easy to inject • Very good tissue integration and neocollagenesis • With lidocaine (0.3%))
Restylane ▲	Galderma	• Lip contours • Philtrum • Perioral region	Middle dermis	20 mg/ml stabilized (NASHA technology)	29G 1/2 27G Pixl 28G Pixl +	• Solid gel with moderate lifting capacity • Available with or without lidocaine
Restylane Defyne ●	Galderma	• Deep lines • Soft to moderate facial contouring • (Oral commissures, chin crease, chin)	Deep dermis Superficial subcutis	20 mg/ml Very high degree of crosslinking and calibration (Balance technology)	27G 1/2 (UTWN)	• Moderately solid gel with high lifting capacity • With lidocaine

4

HA Fillers for Treatment of the Lips and Perioral Zone (Authors' Recommendation)						
Product name	**Supplier**	**Indication**	**Depth of adminis-tration**	**HA concentration Viscosity Crosslinking**	**Needle/ cannula gauge**	**Special material properties**
Restylane Lyft Lidocain ▲	Galderma	• Powerful lifting capacity • Deep lines • Soft to moderate facial contouring • (Oral commissures, chin crease, chin)	Deep dermis Superficial subcutis	20 mg/ml Stabilized (NASHA technology)	29G 1/2; 23–25G Pixl, 25G Pixl +	• Solid gel with high lifting capacity • Available with and without lidocaine
Restylane Skinbooster Vital ▲	Galderma	• Improvement of skin moisture, skin structure, skin elasticity • Requires more tissue coverage (thicker skin)	Intra-dermally	20 mg/ml Stabilized (NASHA technology)	System; 30G Pixl 29G TWN	• SmartClick system • Strong water-binding capacity • Well tolerated
Restylane Skinbooster Vital Light ●	Galderma	• Improvement of skin moisture, skin structure, skin elasticity • Requires more tissue coverage (thinner skin)	Subcutane-ously	12 mg/ml Stabilized (NASHA technology) Low crosslinking	29G TWN 30G Pixl	• SmartClick system • Strong water-binding capacity • Well tolerated
Restylane Kysse ●	Galderma	• Lip volume • Lip contours	Vermillion Submucosa	20 mg/ml With moderate degree of crosslink-ing and low calibration rate (Balance technology)	30G 1/2 (UTWN)	• Moderately soft gel with moderate lifting capacity • With lidocaine
saypha FILLER Lidocain ▲	Croma Pharma	• Lip volume • Correction of moderate to pronounced facial lines and wrinkles	Middle to deep dermis	2.3 % HA (23 mg/ml)	2 x 27G Terumo 1/2", thin-walled	• Sterile • Viscoelastic • Clear, colorless, isotonic, homogenized gel implant • With 0.3% lidocaine
TEOSYAL Kiss ▲	TEOXANE	• Harmonization of lip volume and lip contours • Hydration of the lips	Subdermally Intramuscu-larly	25 mg/g Crosslinked (RHA technology)	27G 1/2	• Moderately viscous gel • Persistence approximately 9 months
TEOSYAL RHA 2 ●	TEOXANE	• Moderate lines • Also universally for all indications	Middle dermis	23 mg/g Crosslinked (RHA technology) BDDE Crosslinking agent only 3.1%	30G 1/2	• Specially for the mobile regions (forehead, glabella) • With lidocaine
TEOSYAL RHA 3 ●	TEOXANE	• Deep, pronounced lines	Deep dermis	23 mg/g Crosslinked (RHA technology) BDDE Crosslinking agent only 3.6%	27G 1/2	• Specially for dynamic regions (nasolabial folds, marionette lines) • With lidocaine
TEOSYAL Global Action ▲	TEOXANE	• Medium-depth lines • Also universally for all indications except tear trough	Middle dermis Subdermally	25 mg/g Crosslinked (RHA technology)	30G 1/2	• Moderately viscous gel • Also available with lidocaine

4

HA Fillers for Treatment of the Lips and Perioral Zone (Authors' Recommendation)						
Product name	**Supplier**	**Indication**	**Depth of adminis-tration**	**HA concentration Viscosity Crosslinking**	**Needle/ cannula gauge**	**Special material properties**
TEOSYAL Redensity 2 ●	TEOXANE	• Skin booster for redensification of the skin (face, decolletage, and backs of the hands)	Into the epidermis and dermis	15 mg/g non-cross-linked HA combined with 8 amino acids, 3 antioxidants, zinc, copper, and vitamin B6 (patented "Dermo-Restructuring Complex")	30G 1/2	• Well tolerated, with lidocaine
TEOSYAL RHA Kiss ●	TEOXANE	• Harmonization of lip contours and lip volume	Subdermally, intramuscularly	23 mg/g HA 0.3% lidocaine 3.1% DoM (degree of modification)	27G x 1/2 25G x 25 mm	• Less BDDE • RHA (resilient HA technology) • Preserves the natural viscoelastic properties of the lips

4.5 Filler Products for Revitalization and Hydration

XS Fillers – Superficial Augmentation: Revitalization and Hydration						
Product name	**Supplier**	**Indication**	**Depth of adminis-tration**	**HA concentration Viscosity Crosslinking**	**Needle/ cannula gauge**	**Special material properties**
BELOTERO Soft ●	Merz Aesthetics	• Correction of superficial lines	Upper dermis	20 mg/ml Dynamically multi-cross-linked (CPM and DCLT technology)	30G 1/2	• Polydensified, cohesive gel • Very good tissue integration • Weak water-binding capacity • Persistence of 6–9 months • Very well tolerated • Available with lidocaine (0.3%)
Juvéderm HYDRATE ●	Allergan	• Improvement of skin moisture and elasticity	Upper dermis	13.5 mg/ml Non-crosslinked With 0.9% mannitol	30G 1/6; 32G	• Good water-binding capacity • Low persistence
Juvéderm VOLITE – Skin Juvénizer ●	Allergan	• Hydration and elasticity treatment (skin, fine lines and wrinkles, face, decolletage, hands)	Intra-dermally	12 mg/ml VYCROSS technology	32G 1/2	• Only one treatment • Significant hydration and patient satisfaction • Very good tissue integration • With lidocaine (0.3%)
Restylane Skinbooster Vital ▲	Galderma	• Improvement of skin moisture, structure, and elasticity • Requires more tissue coverage (thicker skin)	Intra-dermally	20 mg/ml Stabilized (NASHA technology)	30G Pixl 29G TWN	• SmartClick system • Strong water-binding capacity • Well tolerated
Restylane Skinbooster Vital Light ●	Galderma	• Improvement of skin moisture, structure, and elasticity • Requires less tissue coverage (thinner skin)	Subcutane-ously	12 mg/ml Stabilized (NASHA technology) Low degree of crosslinking	29G TWN 30G Pixl	• SmartClick system • Strong water-binding capacity • Well tolerated
saypha RICH ▲	Croma Pharma	• Improvement of tone and elasticity • Filling of fine lines (crow's feet, laughter lines)	Superficial skin tissue	18 mg/ml Not crosslinked	2 x 30G Terumo 1/2", thin-walled	• Viscoelastic, isotonic, and biodegradable gel • SMART technology • Not crosslinked • Stabilization with glycerin • High hyaluronate concentration • High molecular weight (3.0 million daltons)
TEOSYAL Meso ●	TEOXANE	• Revitalization • Rehydration	Into the epidermis and dermis	15 mg/g Non-crosslinked	30G 1/2 32G	• Soft gel • With recommended treatment protocol

XS Fillers – Superficial Augmentation: Revitalization and Hydration						
TEOSYAL Redensity 1 ●	TEOXANE	• Skin booster for redensification (face, decolletage, backs of the hands)	Into the epidermis and dermis	15 mg/g Not crosslinked Combined with 8 amino acids, 3 antioxidants, zinc, copper, and vitamin B6 (patented "Dermo-Restructuring Complex")	30G 1/2	• Well tolerated • With lidocaine

S Fillers – Superficial Augmentation						
Product name	**Supplier**	**Indication**	**Depth of administration**	**HA concentration Viscosity Crosslinking**	**Needle/ cannula gauge**	**Special material properties**
BELOTERO Soft ●	Merz Aesthetics	• Correction of fine superficial lines	Upper dermis	20 mg/ml Dynamically multi-crosslinked (CPM and DCLT technology)	30G 1/2	• Polydensified, cohesive gel • Very good tissue integration • Weak water-binding capacity • Persistence of 6–9 months • Very well tolerated • Available with lidocaine (0.3%)
Juvéderm ULTRA 2 ▲	Allergan	• Filling of medium-depth skin lines • Definition of the lips	Middle dermis	24 mg/ml Crosslinked (HYLACROSS technology)	30G 1/2	• Smooth gel • Very well tolerated • Good persistence of up to 12 months • With lidocaine (0.3%)
Juvéderm VOLBELLA ●	Allergan	• Superficial and medium-depth skin lines • Volume build-up • Definition of the lip contours	Upper and middle dermis	15 mg/ml Crosslinked (VYCROSS technology)	30G 1/2	• Good distribution (reason: minimal cohesiveness) • With lidocaine (0.3%)
Restylane Skinbooster Vital ▲	Galderma	• Improvement of skin moisture, structure, and elasticity • Requires more tissue coverage (thicker skin)	Intra-dermally	20 mg/ml Stabilized (NASHA technology)	30G Pixl 29G TWN	• SmartClick system • Strong water-binding capacity • Well tolerated
Restylane Fynesse ●	Galderma	• Superficial lines (especially in the perioral and periorbital areas)	Superficial dermis	20 mg/ml Low degree of crosslinking and low calibration rate (Balance technology)	30G 1/2 (UTWN)	• Very soft gel • Moderate lifting capacity
TEOSYAL Redensity 2 ●	TEOXANE	• Skin booster for redensification (face, decolletages, backs of the hands)	Into the epidermis and dermis	15 mg/g Not crosslinked Combined with 8 amino acids, 3 antioxidants, zinc, copper, and vitamin B6 (patented "Dermo-Restructuring Complex")	30G 1/2	• Well tolerated • With lidocaine
TEOSYAL RHA 1 ●	TEOXANE	• Very fine and superficial wrinkles and lines • Perioral lines	Middle dermis	15 mg/g Mixture of cross-linked/non-cross-linked HA (RHA technology) BDDE cross-linking agent only 1.9%	30G 1/2	• Specially for the dynamic regions (face, neck, decolletage) • With lidocaine

S Fillers – Superficial Augmentation						
Juvéderm VOLITE ●	Allergan	• Improvement of the skin quality factors of moisture and elasticity • Smoothing of fine wrinkles on the face, decolletage, and hands	Intra-dermally	12 mg/ml cross-linked HA, unique, patented VYCROSS technology, with long- and short-chained HAs for particularly rapid tissue integration, long persistence, minimal swelling of the gel	32G 1/2	• Only one treatment • Results visible for up to 9 months • Significant hydration and patient satisfaction • With lidocaine (0.3%)

4.6 Filler Products for Medium Augmentation

M Fillers – Medium Augmentation						
Product name	**Supplier**	**Indication**	**Depth of administration**	**HA concentration Viscosity Crosslinking**	**Needle/ cannula gauge**	**Special material properties**
BELOTERO Balance ●	Merz Aesthetics	• Medium-depth lines • Lip augmentation • Lip contours	Middle dermis	22.5 mg/ml Multi-dynamically crosslinked (CPM technology)	27G 1/2 30G 1/2	• Medium-viscosity, polydensified cohesive gel • Very good tissue integration • Virtually no water-binding capacity • Persistence of 12 months • Very well tolerated • Available with lidocaine (0.3%)
BELOTERO Intense ●	Merz Aesthetics	• Deep lines • Lip augmentation	Middle and deep dermis	25.5 mg/ml Multi-dynamically crosslinked (CPM technology)	27G 1/2	• High-viscosity, polydensified elastic gel • Very good lifting capacity and tissue integration • Very well tolerated • Persistence of 12 months • Available with lidocaine (0.3%)
Juvéderm ULTRA 3 ▲	Allergan	• Medium-depth and deep lines • Lip contours • Lip volume	Middle and deep dermis	24 mg/ml Crosslinked (HYLACROSS technology)	27G 1/2	• Smooth gel • Long persistence • With lidocaine (0.3%)
Juvéderm VOLIFT ●	Allergan	• Deep skin lines • Contour deficits • Volume build-up (cheeks, chin, lips)	Deep dermis (Recommendation: not for intradermal use)	17.5 mg/ml Crosslinked (VYCROSS technology)	30G 1/2	• Very long persistence of up to 18 months • Good distribution • Very easy to inject • Very good tissue integration and neocollagenesis • With lidocaine (0.3%)
Juvéderm VOLBELLA ●	Allergan	• Superficial and medium-depth lines • Lip volume • Lip contours	Upper and middle dermis	15 mg/ml Crosslinked (VYCROSS technology)	30G 1/2	• Good persistence • Good distribution (reason: minimal cohesiveness) • Very good tissue integration and neocollagenesis • With lidocaine (0.3%)
Restylane Refyne ●	Galderma	• Medium-depth lines (especially nasolabial folds and marionette lines, tear trough, and lid-cheek junction)	Middle dermis	20 mg/ml Moderate degree of crosslinking and low calibration rate (Balance technology)	30G 1/2 (UTWN)	• Soft gel with moderate lifting capacity • With lidocaine
Restylane ▲	Galderma	• Medium-depth lines (especially nasolabial folds and marionette lines, oral commissures)	Middle dermis	20 mg/ml Stabilized (NASHA technology)	29G 1/2 27G Pixl 28G Pixl +	• Solid gel with moderate lifting capacity • Available with or without lidocaine

M Fillers – Medium Augmentation						
saypha FILLER Lidocain ▲	Croma Pharma	• Lip volume enhancement • Correction of moderate to pronounced facial lines and wrinkles	Middle to deep dermis	2.3% (23 mg/ml)	2 x 27G	• Terumo 1/2", thin-walled • Sterile • Viscoelastic • Completely clear, colorless, isotonic, homogenized gel implant • With lidocaine (0.3%)
TEOSYAL Global Action ▲	TEOXANE	• Medium-depth lines • Also universally for all indications except tear trough	Middle dermis Subdermally	25 mg/g Crosslinked (RHA technology)	30G 1/2	• Moderately viscous del • Also available with lidocaine
TEOSYAL RHA 2 ●	TEOXANE	• Moderate lines • Also universally for all indications	Middle dermis	23 mg/g Crosslinked (RHA technology) BDDE cross-linking agent only 3.1%	30G 1/2	• Specially for the mobile regions (forehead, glabella) • With lidocaine

4.7 Filler Products for Deep Augmentation

L Fillers – Deep Augmentation						
Product name	**Supplier**	**Indication**	**Depth of adminis-tration**	**HA concentration Viscosity Crosslinking**	**Needle/ cannula gauge**	**Special material properties**
BELOTERO Intense ●	Merz Aesthetics	• Deep lines • Lip augmentation	Middle and deep dermis	25.5 mg/ml Multi-dynamically crosslinked (CPM technology)	27G 1/2	• High-viscosity, polydensified cohesive gel • Very good lifting capacity and tissue integration • Very well tolerated • Persistence of 12 months • Available with lidocaine (0.3%)
Juvéderm ULTRA 4 ▲	Allergan	• Deep skin lines • Volume build-up of lips and cheeks	Deep dermis	24 mg/ml Crosslinked (HYLACROSS technology)	27G 1/2	• Smooth gel • Long persistence • With lidocaine (0.3%)
Juvéderm VOLIFT ●	Allergan	• Deep skin lines • Contour deficits • Volume build-up of cheeks, chin, and lips	Deep dermis (Rec-ommenda-tion: not for intradermal use)	17.5 mg/ml Crosslinked (VYCROSS technology)	30G 1/2	• Very long persistence of up to 18 months • Good distribution • Very easy to inject • Very good tissue integration and neocollagenesis • With lidocaine (0.3%)
Restylane Defyne ●	Galderma	• Deep lines • Soft to moderate facial contouring (especially cheekbone region, chin, lower jaw contours)	Deep dermis Superficial subcutis	20 mg/ml Very high degree of crosslinking and calibration rate (Balance technology)	27G 1/2 (UTWN)	• Moderately solid gel • High lifting capacity • With lidocaine
Restylane Lyft Lidocain ▲	Galderma	• Deep lines • Soft to moderate facial contouring (especially cheekbone region, chin, lower jaw contours)	Deep dermis Superficial subcutis	20 mg/ml Stabilized (NASHA technology)	29G 1/2 23–25G Pixl 25G Pixl +	• Solid gel • High lifting capacity • Available with or without lidocaine
TEOSYAL Deep Lines ▲	TEOXANE	• Deep lines	Deep dermis Subdermally	25 mg/g Crosslinked (RHA technology)	27G 1/2	• Moderately viscous gel • With lidocaine
TEOSYAL RHA 3 ●	TEOXANE	• Deep, pronounced lines	Deep dermis	23 mg/g Crosslinked (RHA technology), BDDE crosslinking agent only 3.6%	27G 1/2	• Specially for the dynamic regions (nasolabial folds, marionette lines) • With lidocaine

4

4.8 Filler Products for Very Deep Augmentation

XL Fillers – Very Deep Augmentation

Product name	Supplier	Indication	Depth of administration	HA content Viscosity Crosslinking	Needle/ cannula gauge	Special material properties
BELOTERO Volume ▲	Merz Aesthetics	• Volume build-up	Deep into the dermis Subcutaneously Supraperiosteally	26 mg/ml Dynamically crosslinked (CPM technology)	30G 1/2 27G 1/2 27G/37 mm	• High-viscosity, polydensified malleable gel • Good for modeling • Can be injected with a very fine needle • Persistence of up to 18 months • Very well tolerated • Available with lidocaine (0.3%)
Juvéderm ULTRA 4 ▲	Allergan	• Deep skin lines • Volume build-up of lips and cheeks	Deep dermis	24 mg/ml Crosslinked (HYLACROSS technology)	27G 1/2	• Smooth gel • Long persistence • With lidocaine (0.3%)
Juvéderm VOLUMA ●	Allergan	• Volume build-up in the mid-face	Subcutaneously Supraperiosteally	20 mg/ml Crosslinked (VYCROSS technology)	27G 1/2	• Very long persistence of up to 24 months • Very easy to inject • Initially highly malleable but rapidly reaches its final solidity • Good tissue integration • Long-term lifting effect • Low material distribution • High cohesiveness • With lidocaine
Restylane Volyme ●	Galderma	• Volume build-up (temples, cheekbone region, lower jaw contours)	Subcutaneously to supraperiosteally	20 mg/ml High degree of crosslinking and very high calibration rate (Balance technology)	27G 1/2 (UTWN)	• Moderately soft gel • High lifting capacity • With lidocaine
Restylane SubQ ▲	Galderma	• Volume build-up • Strong facial contouring (chin and cheeks)	Subcutaneously to supraperiosteally	20 mg/ml Stabilized (NASHA technology)	21G 21G Pixl	• Powerful lifting effect • Available with or without lidocaine
saypha VOLUME PLUS ▲	Croma Pharma	• Correction of volume deficits in the mid-face region • Facial volume restoration • Shaping of the natural contours of the face	Deep dermis Subcutaneously Supraperiosteally	2.5% (25mg/ml)	2 x 27G Terumo 1/2", thin-walled	• Also for medically indicated build-up purposes, e.g. for the treatment of facial lipoatrophy • With lidocaine (0.3%)
saypha VOLUME ▲	Croma Pharma	• Correction of deep lines and grooves • Build-up of lost facial volume • Modeling of the facial contours	Deep dermis Subcutis	2.3% (23mg/ml)	2 x 27G Terumo 1/2", thin-walled	• Also for reconstructive treatments, e.g. in facial lipoatrophy, disfiguring scars or morphologic asymmetry • Also available with lidocaine (0.3%)
TEOSYAL Ultimate ▲	TEOXANE	• Ideal volumizer for full-face treatments	Superficial and deep fat compartments	22 mg/g Crosslinked (RHA technology)	22G 27G 1/2	• Moderately viscous gel • Soft volumizer • Good material distribution • Also available with lidocaine
TEOSYAL RHA 4 ●	TEOXANE	• Very pronounced lines • Volume addition	Subcutaneously	23 mg/g Crosslinked (RHA technology) BDDE cross-linking agent only 4%	27G 1/2	• Specially for volume in the larger dynamic regions (cheeks, facial contours) • With lidocaine
TEOSYAL Ultra Deep ▲	TEOXANE	• Targeted volume build-up • Deep fat compartments	Supraperiosteally	25 mg/g Crosslinked (RHA technology)	25G 1	• More solid gel • Extra-long persistence • Outstanding lifting effect • Also available with lidocaine

4

XL Fillers – Very Deep Augmentation						
Juvéderm Volux ▲	Allergan	• Designed for the chin and chin line; contours and defines, builds up volume, balances out volume deficits	Deep dermis Subcutis Supraperi-osteally	25 mg/ml cross-linked HA, unique, patented VYCROSS technology, with long- and short-chained HAs for particularly rapid tissue integration, long persistence, minimal swelling of the gel	25–27G	• The highest cohesiveness, lifting power, and elasticity of all the Juvéderm fillers • Very long efficacy of 18 to 24 months • Easy to inject (low plunger pressure) • With lidocaine (0.3%)

4.9 Filler Navigator

The filler navigator provides a representative choice of the products available on the market, based on our treatment experiences. It provides an at-a-glance guide to the recommended fillers according to indication group. It is self-evident that soft, fluid fillers with a low degree of crosslinking are used for the hydration and augmentation of soft tissue, while the harder fillers with a higher degree of cross-linking are used for line augmentation and lifting. Depending on the treatment goal, it will be up to the therapist to choose the correct filler (detailed descriptions and recommendations are provided in Chap. 9, p. 127 ff.).

Filler Navigator – Dermal Fillers* for Lip Treatment at a Glance

Indications Groups	Particle size	Viscosity	Teoxane	Galderma	Allergan	Croma	Merz
Hydration, Revitalization	XS	●	Teosyal Redensity 1 Teosyal Meso	Restylane Vital Light	Juvéderm Hydrate		Belotero Hydro
		▲				Saypha Rich	
Accents	S/M	●		Restylane Refyne			Belotero Lips Contour
		▲	Teosyal Global Action	Restylane	Juvéderm Ultra 3	Saypha Filler	Belotero Balance
Perioral Lines	S	●	Teosyal Redensity 1 Teosyal Redensity 2		Juvéderm Volite		Belotero Soft
		▲		Restylane Vital	Juvéderm Ultra 2	Saypha Filler	
Lip Volume	M/L	●	Teosyal RHA 2 Teosyal RHA 3 Teosyal RHA Kiss	Restylane Kysse	Juvéderm Volift Juvéderm Volbella Juvéderm Voluma		Belotero Lips Shape Belotero Intense
		▲	Teosyal Kiss		Juvéderm Ultra Smile Juvéderm Ultra 4	Saypha Filler	Belotero Lips Contour
Perioral Volume	M/L	●		Restylane Refyne Restylane Defyne	Juvéderm Volift Juvéderm Volbell		Belotero Balance Belotero Intense
		▲	Teosyal Deep Lines	Restylane	Juvéderm Ultra 3 Juvéderm Ultra 4	Saypha Filler Saypha Volume	Belotero Volume
Shaping Beautifica-tion	M/L	●	Teosyal RHA 2 Teosyal RHA 3	Restylane Defyne Restylane Volyme	Juvéderm Volift		Belotero Balance Belotero Intense
		▲	Teosyal Global Action Teosyal Deep Lines	Restylane Lyft	Juvéderm Ultra 3	Saypha Volume	

● = Soft filler (low viscosity), ▲ = Hard filler with good lifting capacity (higher viscosity)
* The products are available with or without lidocaine.

5 Anesthetic Methods

5 Anesthetic Methods

Most dermal fillers are supplied with lidocaine, making a hyaluronic acid (HA) treatment less painful. However, this still does not stop the pain caused by the insertion of the needle into the tissue. Sensitivity to pain is particularly high in the lip region. The form of anesthesia used depends on the patient's level of sensitivity and the therapist's preferences. The issue of pain relief will need to be clarified with each patient before the treatment. If pain relief is required, the following measures should be considered:

- Maximum compression of the lip
- Application of cold stimuli
- A topical anesthetic cream
- Direct lidocaine application
- Anesthetic skin wheals at the injection site
- Nerve block using the mucosal block or micro-nerve block technique
- Conduction (regional) anesthesia (infraorbital block, extraoral or intraoral approach)

5

5.1 Maximum Compression of the Lip (→ Fig. 5.1)

To minimize injection pain during lip augmentation, especially when treating the contours, it is helpful for the therapist to compress the lip when first injecting into it. To do this, the area being treated should be grasped with the thumb and index finger of the opposite hand and squeezed. The needle is then inserted into the highly compressed tissue, HA containing lidocaine is deposited by antegrade injection, and the lidocaine is left to act for a few seconds.

5.2 Application of Cold Stimuli

A cold spray or ice packs applied to the target tissue before the treatment serves to slightly reduce the sensitivity to pain. To avoid the risk of cold burn, the ice packs should not be placed directly onto the skin or left there for more than two minutes (Criollo-Lamilla et al. 2013).

5.3 Topical Anesthetic Cream

(→ Fig. 5.2)

Anesthetic creams containing lidocaine are often used to minimize injection pain during lip augmentation. Various strengths of these creams are available from different manufacturers. Pharmacies also supply their own formulations, which contain up to 30% lidocaine and tetracaine and thus have a powerful and rapid effect. To enhance the effect of these creams, the skin should first be cleansed with a disinfectant and the cream then applied and covered with a clear plastic film so that the active substances can infiltrate the skin. Unfortunately, the action of these creams is often associated with swelling, rendering the radial lines and wrinkles less visible and making the treatment more difficult.

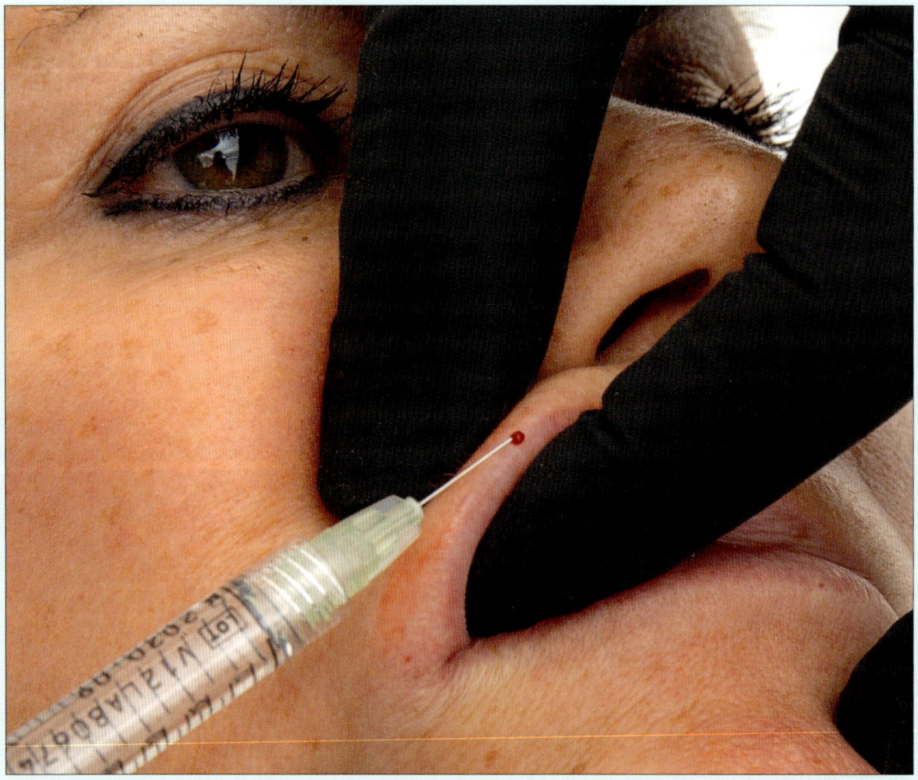

Fig. 5.1 The lip is squeezed so hard that it pales slightly.

5.4 Direct Lidocaine Application

(→ Fig. 5.3)

If the delicate skin of the perioral region is rolled once with a needle roller (0.5 mm gauge) once degreasing has taken place after the skin disinfectant, this will perforate the tissue very slightly. The area can then be anesthetized by dabbing the gently perforated skin with a local anesthetic. However, this produces only partial anesthesia of the lip, as its central region, which is also the most sensitive to pain, still remains sensitive.

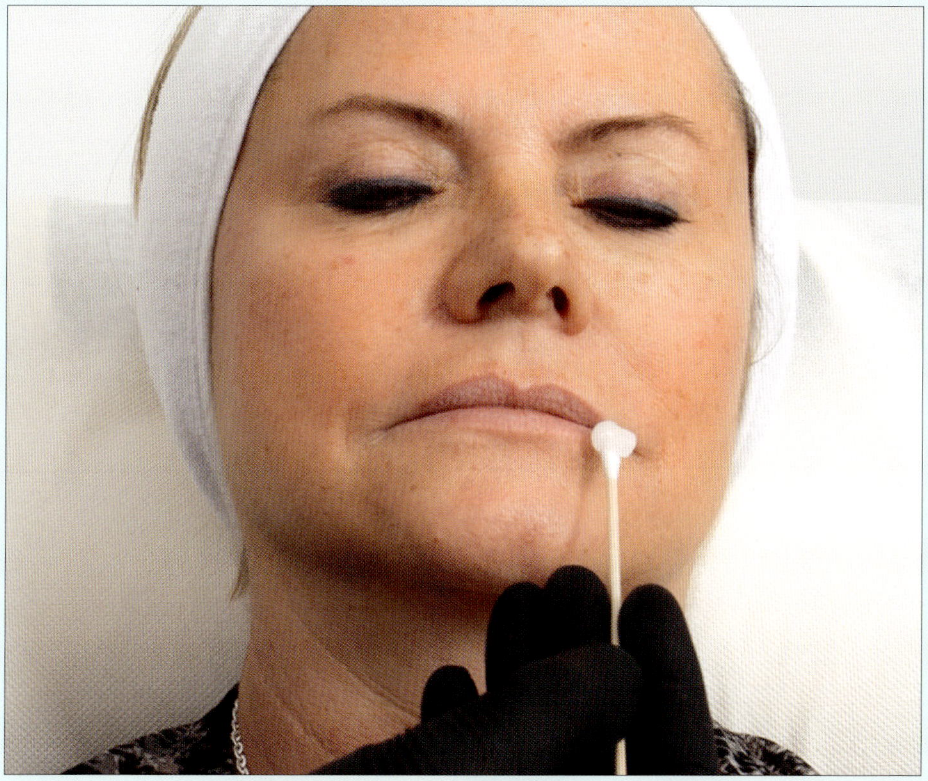

Fig. 5.2 Anesthetic creams should be applied before the treatment with a cotton bud (Q-tip) and left to act for at least 20 minutes.

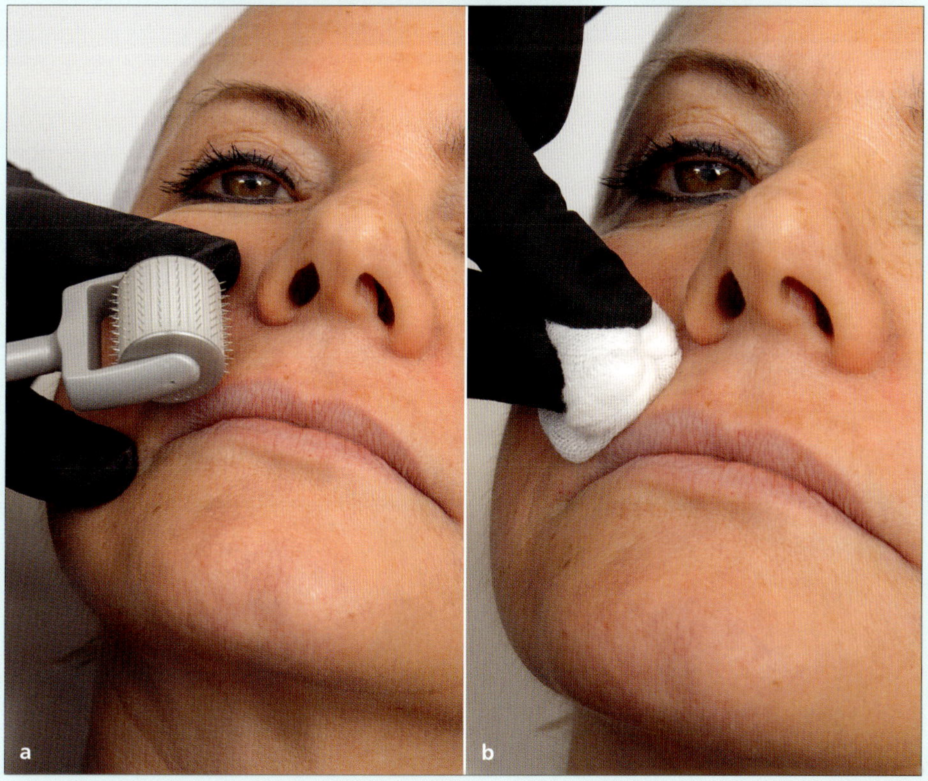

Fig. 5.3 a+b (a) Gentle rolling of the cutaneous part of the lip with a needle roller (0.5 mm). (b) Dabbing with a pad or cotton bud (Q-tip) soaked in lidocaine (2%).

5.5 Anesthetic Skin Wheals at the Injection Site (→ Fig. 5.4)

When performing lip augmentation with a blunt cannula, it is much less uncomfortable for the patient if lidocaine is injected to form a skin wheal at the injection site before the insertion of the Nokor needle. The lidocaine spreads radially for a short distance, considerably minimizing pain in the lip region.

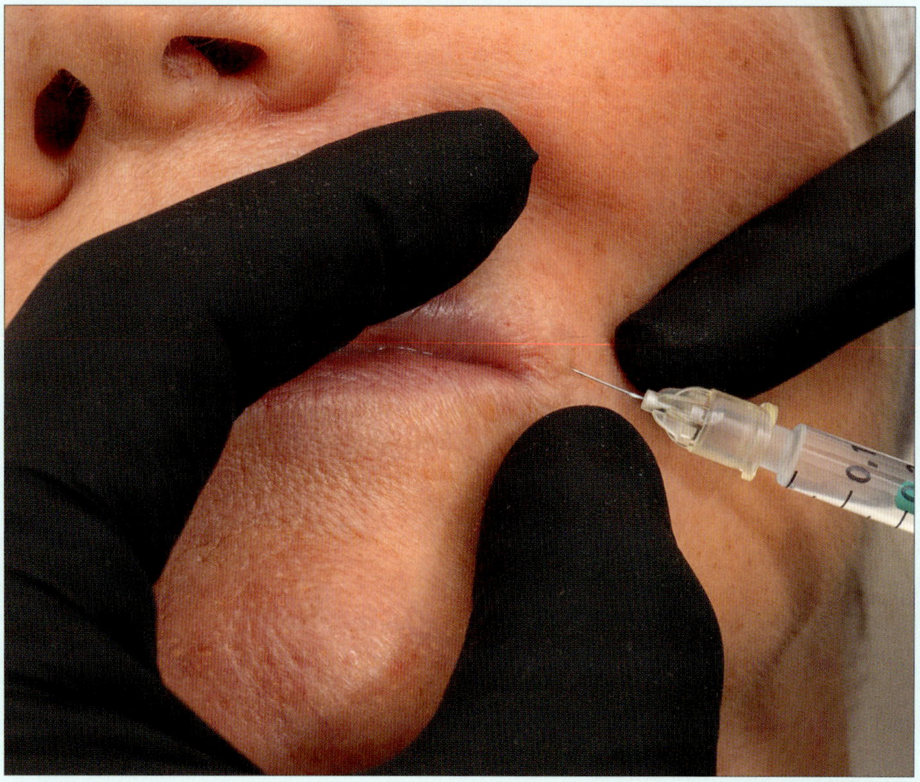

Fig. 5.4 A skin wheal containing 0.2 ml lidocaine (2%) anesthetizes the first third of the lip quadrant.

Wheal

5.6 Nerve Block using the Mucosal Block or Micro-Nerve Block Technique (→ Figs. 5.5, 5.6)

The "annular mucosal block" described by Sattler & Sommer (2015) causes infraorbital nerve block: To achieve this, lidocaine wheals are placed into the mucosa at 2-cm intervals along a line that runs I cm away from the lip line, but parallel to it. The advantages of this are that the effect sets in rapidly, does not last long, and causes no distortion of the mouth during the effective period.

Another variant of the mucosal block method consists of placing several lidocaine wheals at 1-cm intervals along the vestibule (the mucosal fold).

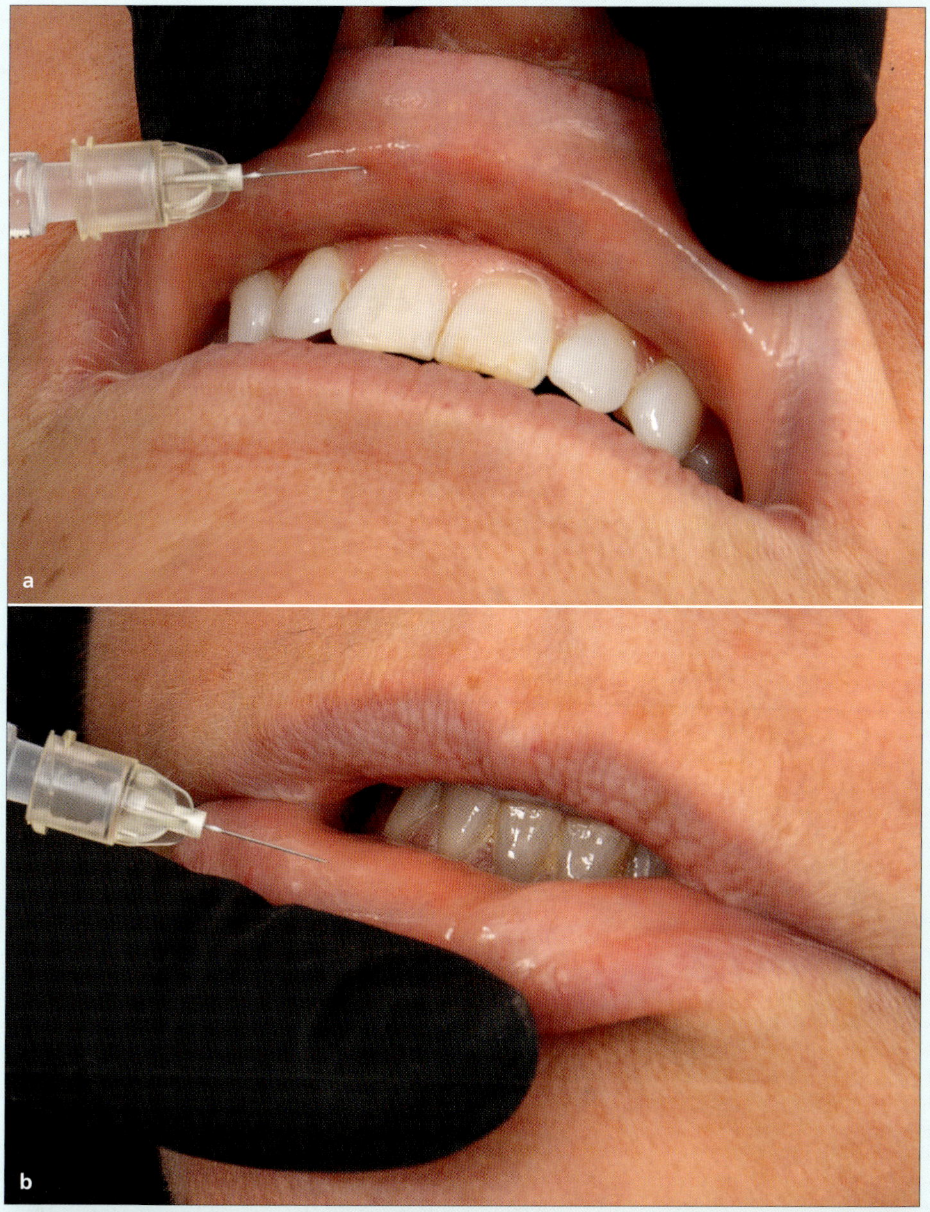

Fig. 5.5 a+b For the mucosal block technique, wheals (0.5 ml per wheal) are placed at 1-cm intervals into the mucosa of the upper lip (a) ...

... and the lower lip (b).

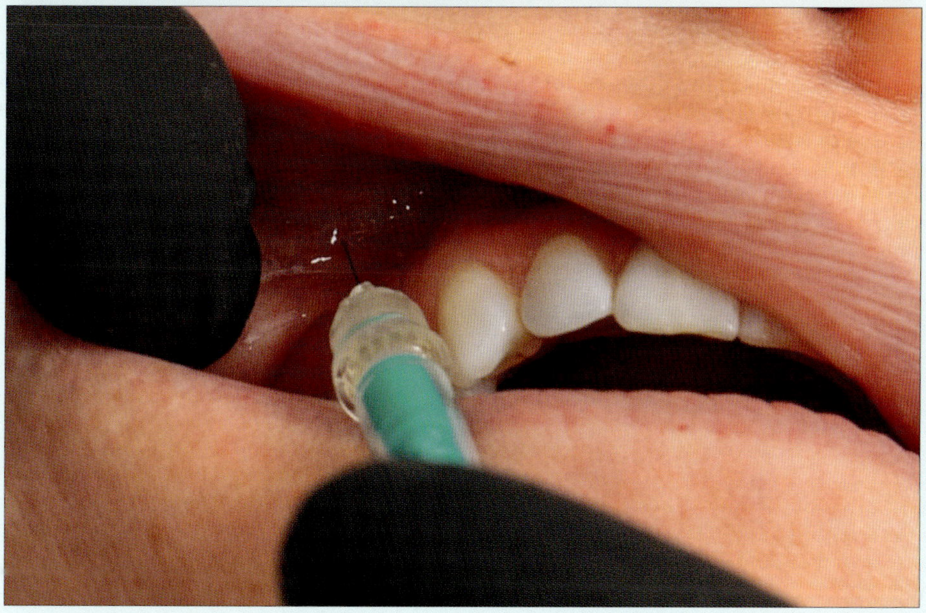

Fig. 5.6 As an alternative, lidocaine wheals may be placed along the vestibule.

5.7 Conduction Anesthesia (→ Fig. 5.7)

This form of anesthesia causes the maximum possible targeted numbing of a specific area and is familiar to the patient from dental procedures. Pain conduction is inhibited by injecting the anesthetic into the immediate vicinity of the nerve.

We do not recommend infraorbital anesthesia due to its prolonged effect; the alternative is an HA injection in combination with lidocaine. Infraorbital block is also associated with the risk of a serious side effect in the form of anaphylactic shock (see 5.8, p. 84) or of intravascular injection of the anesthetic. Another disadvantage is that the perioral lines will no longer be quite as visible, as the tissue swells up slightly after lidocaine is injected.

Since the anesthetic effect can last for up to two hours after the injection, patients may find the persistent numbness unpleasant. The more accurately the calculated minimum dose is placed at the nerve ending, the less discomfort the procedure will cause to the patient (Criollo-Lamilla et al. 2013). Since the introduction of less traumatizing injection methods with a blunt needle and with dermal filler containing lidocaine, conduction anesthesia is now generally used only in patients who are anxious and highly sensitive to pain. For this reason, it is still considered to be one of the classic anesthetic methods for lip treatment and is described here. It requires the treatment chair to be positioned at a 45-degree angle, with good lighting, a clean mucosa, and sterile gloves.

Caution

Due to the risk of injury to the infraorbital nerve, the anesthetic must not be injected directly into the infraorbital foramen and onto the nerve. It is also important to aspirate before the injection, to prevent intravascular injection (Azib 2013, p. 92).

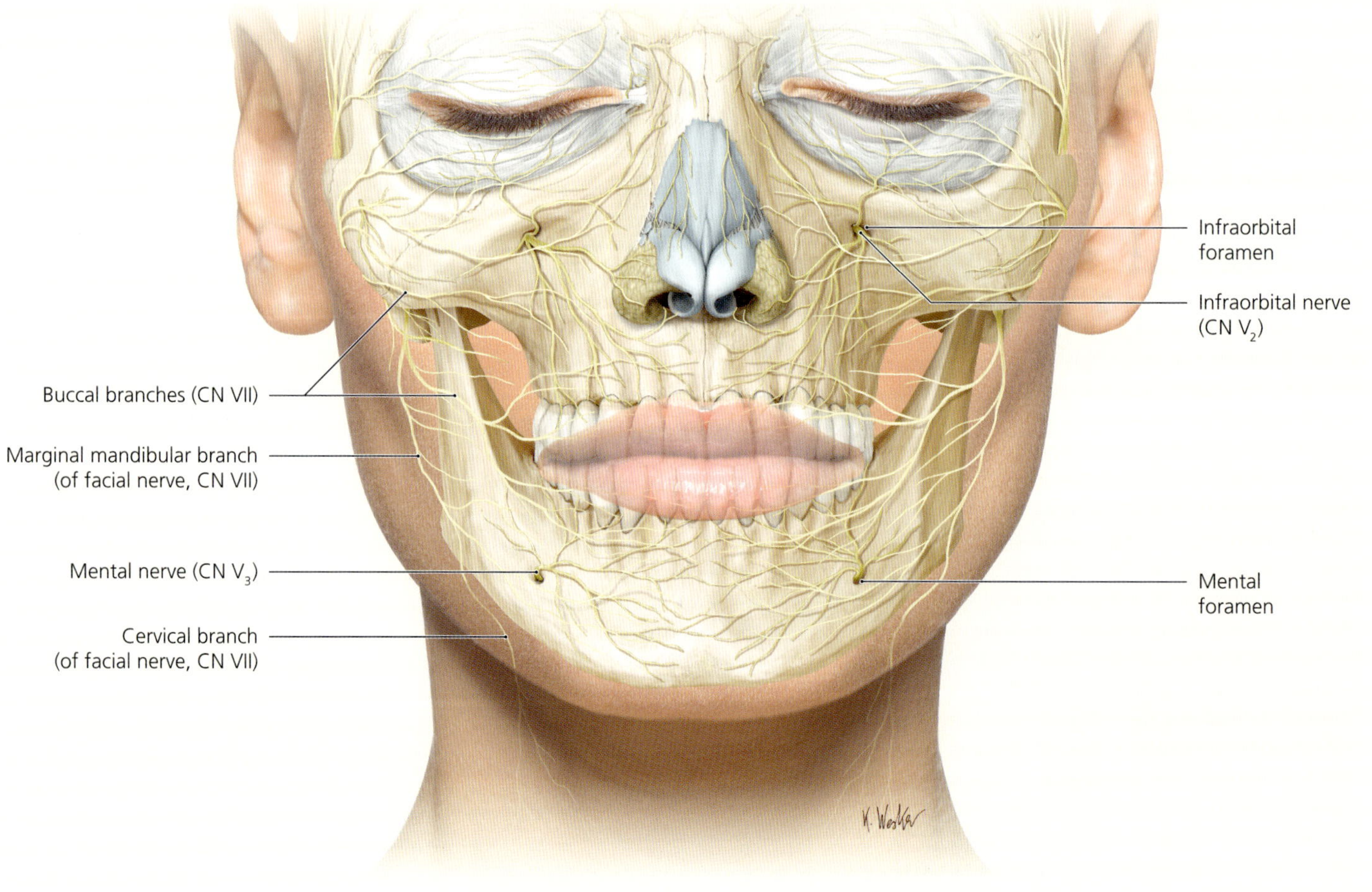

Fig. 5.7 The infraorbital nerve emerges from the infraorbital foramen and innervates the upper lip via its superior labial branches. The mental nerve emerges from the mental foramen and innervates the lower lip.

5.7.1 Infraorbital Block, Extraoral Approach

(→ Fig. 5.8)

The injection site for infraorbital block using the extraoral approach is at the intersection of the line running from the wing of the nose to the outer eyelid and the line running vertically downward from the pupil, slightly above the infraorbital foramen, which is located 1 cm below the infraorbital margin. The lidocaine depot should be injected close to the infraorbital nerve.

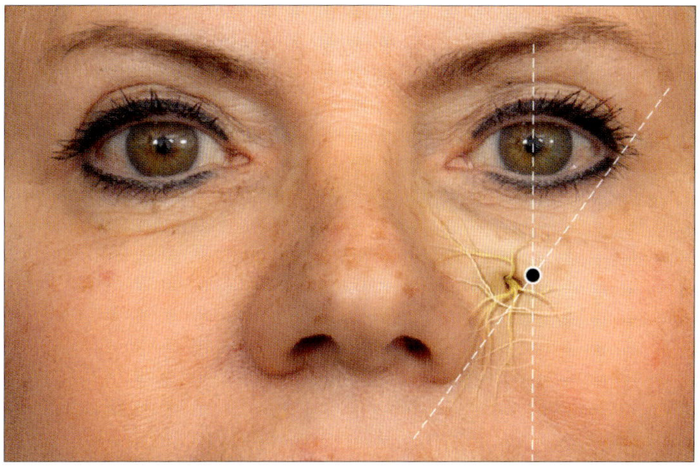

Fig. 5.8 Injection site for the infraorbital block using the extraoral approach.

5.7.2 Nerve Block, Intraoral Technique

In this form of conduction anesthesia, the infraorbital nerve should be blocked when injecting the upper lip, while the mental nerve is blocked when injecting the lower lip.

■ Upper Lip Block (→ Fig. 5.9 a–c)

Fig. 5.9 a–c (a) To determine exactly where the anesthetic should be placed in conduction anesthesia by upper lip block, the therapist should imagine a line running from the canine toward the pupil.

(b) The mucosa needs to be disinfected first. The vestibule may be anesthetized slightly in advance with a cotton bud (Q-tip) soaked in lidocaine. Pull the upper lip upward to evert it, raise the mucosa, and insert the needle into the vestibule between the first premolar and the canine, parallel to the canine's longitudinal axis. Direct the needle toward the center of the pupil.

(c) Inject the lidocaine depot in the direction of the infraorbital foramen. While doing so, protect the nerve's exit point by compressing with the free hand from outside. Gently massaging the area after the injection ensures more effective distribution of the lidocaine.

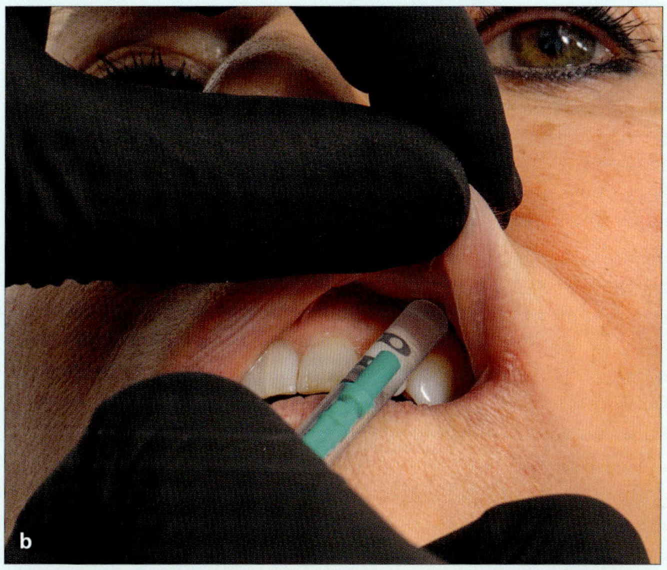

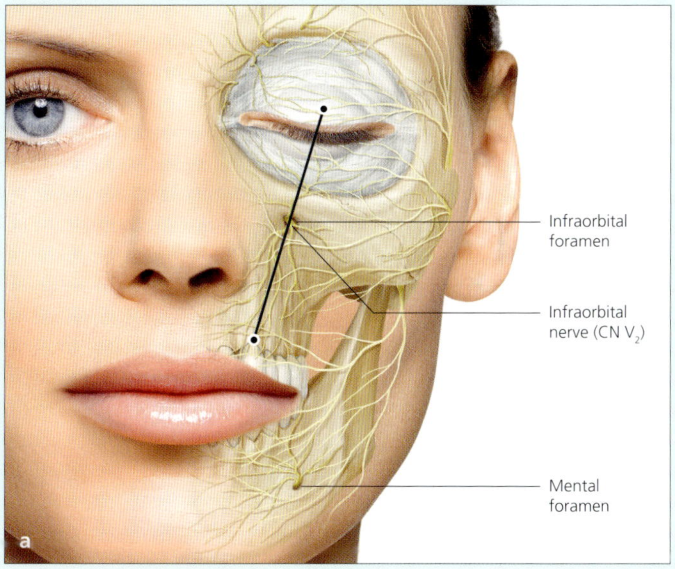

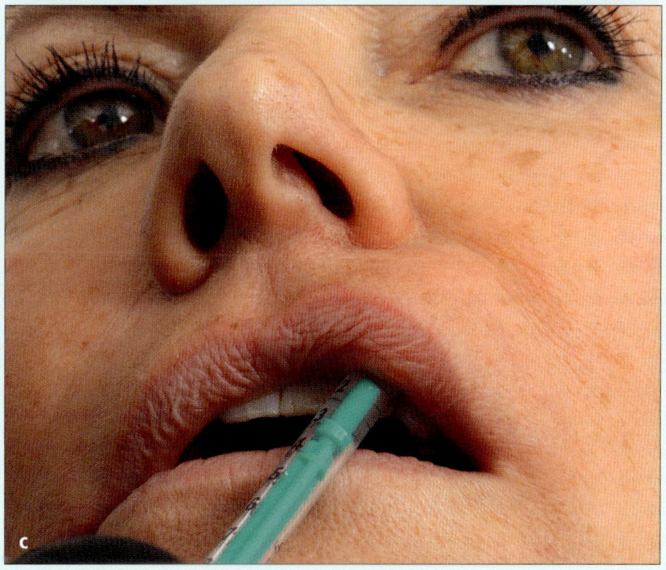

■ **Lower Lip Block** (→ Fig. 5.10 a–c)

Fig. 5.10 a–c (a) In conduction anesthesia by lower lip block, the therapist should imagine a line running from the center of the pupil to the corner of the mouth. The mental foramen, with its emerging mental nerve, lies along an extension of this line, laterally of the canine below the first premolar.

(b) The anesthetic should be injected intraorally into the periodontal pocket of the mandible in the direction of the mental foramen.

(c) The mucosa may be anesthetized slightly in advance with a cotton bud (Q-tip) soaked in lidocaine. Pull the lip downward to evert it, insert a 30G needle 5 mm below the first premolar, and advance slowly in the direction of the mental foramen. Immediately after making contact with the bone, withdraw the needle slightly, aspirate, and deliver the lidocaine depot in the direction of the mental foramen.

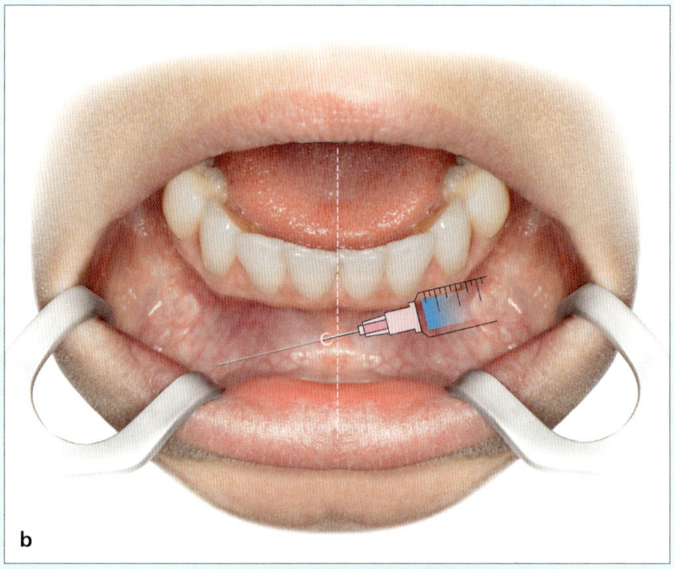

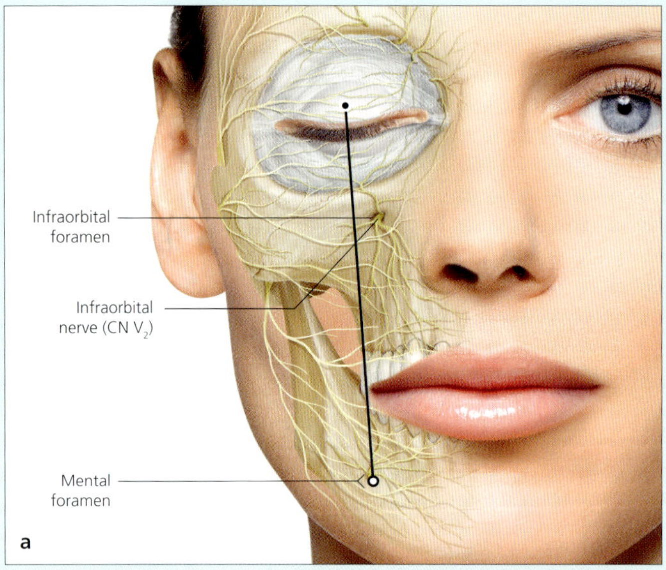

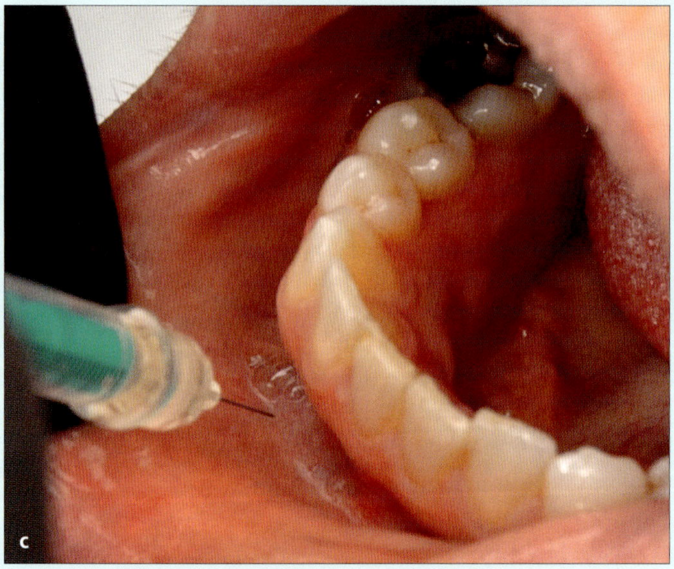

5

5.8 Complications of Local Anesthesia

Local anesthetics can diffuse into the bloodstream and may thus cause side effects in the brain and heart. For example, if administered at sufficiently high concentration, they can flood the brain and produce a toxic effect.

A toxic blood concentration of a local anesthetic can have a negative effect on the heart's conduction system. This may lead to cardiac arrhythmia, a reduction in the heart's pumping power, a fall in blood pressure, and even to cardiac arrest in some circumstances.

Anaphylactoid reactions to local anesthetics are also possible. These may manifest in the form of urticaria, an asthma attack or a fall in blood pressure, ranging in severity up to anaphylactic shock.

Important Notes

If the needle touches the nerve, it should be withdrawn slightly, the area aspirated, and the lidocaine depot then delivered. Intravascular injection must be avoided at all costs! If the numbness does not extend to the middle of the lip, an additional wheal should be placed into the superior labial frenulum. The therapist is responsible for administering anesthesia. It is therefore essential for the therapist to have the appropriate knowledge, skills, and experience. It is essential to rule out any intolerances or allergic reactions to anesthetics when taking the patient's history.

6 Complications, Side Effects, Follow-Up Assessment

6 Complications, Side Effects, Follow-Up Assessment

In rare cases, lip injection and augmentation treatments are accompanied by complications or side effects. Snozzi & Van Loghem (2018) published an overview of the main side effects of a filler treatment, with extensive therapeutic recommendations. Therefore, we would like to refer to this publication here and summarize only the key findings that apply to lip treatment. The reader is referred to the study by Snozzi & Van Loghem for their therapeutic recommendations.

Apart from the reactions that commonly accompany the treatment such as reddening, swelling, and pain, the side effects are classified into five groups: discoloration, edema, infection, the formation of nodules, and vascular complications.

6.1 Discoloration

6.1.1 Hematomas

Discoloration after an injection is common, especially in the perioral and oral regions, and usually occurs as a result of the perforation of small or medium-sized blood vessels with a sharp needle. This mainly involves hematomas, which can develop within "minutes to hours" (Snozzi & Van Loghem 2018) following the vessel trauma, but as a general rule subside after one to five days.

Compression immediately after a blood vessel injury can prevent a more major hematoma. In rare cases, a hematoma may undergo fibrous encapsulation and persist in the form of a palpable nodule (Snozzi & Van Loghem 2018). "When there is evidence of a hematoma, compression for a few minutes is advised. The recommended treatment comprises vitamin K ointment BID for 7 days, or intense pulsed light therapy. If there is persistent hemosiderin staining, pulsed-dye or potassium titanyl phosphate (KTP) laser treatment is recommended." (Becker-Wegerich 2011, 2016)

6.1.2 Tyndall Effect

The Tyndall effect is a bluish coloration in the tissue following the superficial injection of highly cross-linked hyaluronic acid (HA). This occurs most commonly when injecting the contours and perioral lines. In the opinion of experts, the Tyndall effect is caused by the partial absorption of red light and the reflection of shorter wavelength light (e.g. blue) due to the optic chamber that is formed by the deposition of HA (Snozzi & Van Loghem 2018). The effect can persist for months. If the blue discoloration is unsightly and too intense, the recommendation is to dissolve it with hyaluronidase.

6.1.3 Blanching

The superficial injection of highly cross-linked HA into thin skin can produce a blanching effect. This is most commonly seen when injecting the contours and perioral lines. In most cases, the blanching can be remedied by vigorous massaging immediately after its onset. If the blanching is perceived as unsightly, it is advisable to treat it by dissolution with hyaluronidase (see p. 96).

6.2 Edema

As a general rule, lip augmentation is always associated with mild to severe swelling. The degree of swelling depends on the injection technique and needle used, but there may also be other factors that influence it.

6.2.1 Short-term, Immediate, Post-Interventional Edema

This category of edema is common and depends on the injection technique and needle/cannula used, the extent of tissue trauma, and the volume of product injected. Generally, no specific treatment is needed. Cooling packs and medication to reduce the swelling may be recommended in isolated cases. If the swellings are severe or persistent, continued treatment should be provided by a specialist.

6.2.2 Histamine-Mediated Edema

This edema occurs as a result of the direct release of histamine following the treatment. It needs to be investigated and treated by a medical specialist. The therapist can identify histamine-mediated edema by the presence of a Quincke's edema-type swelling and/or urticaria (Snozzi & Van Loghem 2018).

6.2.3 Non-Antibody–Mediated (Delayed, Type IV) Allergic Reactions

The presence of indurations, erythema, and edema may indicate a non-antibody–mediated allergic reaction. While it may present only a day after the injection, it can also appear several weeks afterwards and persist for several weeks. This complication needs to be investigated and treated by a medical specialist (for treatment recommendations, see Snozzi & Van Loghem 2018).

6.3 Infection

6.3.1 Bacterial Infection

All invasive and minimally invasive procedures are associated with a risk of infection, although this is very rare (Sattler & Sommer 2015). The infection risk can be minimized by good antisepsis. According to Snozzi & Van Loghem (2018), erysipelas and streptococcal cellulitis are among the more common forms of bacterial inflammation, whereas abscesses tend to be rare. Antibiotic treatment depends on the severity of the infection and the pathogen and should always be prescribed by a specialist.

6.3.2 Viral Infection

The reactivation of herpes simplex is the most common viral infection to occur after an injection of HA into the lips. The antiviral agent aciclovir is recommended as prophylaxis in patients who are known carriers of herpesviruses and who frequently suffer from these infections. This medication is recommended if such an infection does break out.

6.4 Nodules

A distinction is made between non-inflammatory and inflammatory nodules.

6.4.1 Non-Inflammatory Nodules

Small, readily palpable nodules may develop immediately after the injection, linked to the non-uniform injection of crosslinked HA fillers. This phenomenon is less common with softer gels.

Smaller or larger, palpable or visible nodules are commonly found in previously treated lips. They may have occurred due to following possible reasons:

- Placement of an incorrect material
- Injection of an excessive volume of material
- Wrongly selected material
- A pre-existing material becomes visible

At first, these nodules can generally be reduced and redistributed by massage during the treatment. This becomes more difficult if the nodules have become encapsulated in connective tissue. As a second step, these nodules may be crushed mechanically or punctured, and the HA filler expressed (Sattler & Sommer 2015). If these interventions are unsuccessful, an attempt may be made to dissolve the nodules by enzyme treatment with hyaluronidase.

6.4.2 Inflammatory Nodules

In rare cases, the HA implant may lead to an inflammatory, granulomatous, and fibrotic process with inflamed, swollen nodules, erythema, and even occasional purulence.

A typical feature of inflammatory granulomatous processes is that they can set in later, i.e. weeks to months after the treatment. The causes of such an event are complex and often difficult to explain. They may be trivial infections or biofilms formed by common skin-colonizing bacteria that self-encapsulate with a complex protective adhesive matrix. This allows them to adhere irreversibly to living structures or inert surfaces. If a filler is injected, it can become coated with bacteria and form a biofilm, which induces a permanent immune response that may eventually lead to a chronic granulomatous reaction. Other possible causes are immune reactions and the excipients of the filler used (Sattler & Sommer 2015; for treatment recommendations, see Snozzi & Van Loghem 2018).

Investigation by a specialist and precise knowledge of the patient's medical history are very important.

6.5 Vascular Complications

Vascular complications are rare and highly dependent on the injection technique used. The use of sharp needles and the deposition of large boluses are both associated with a higher risk of a vascular complications.

Intravascular injection into an artery may lead to ischemia and, in the worst-case scenario, to necrosis. The course of such a complication may be described as follows (DeLorenzi 2017):

- Skin blanching immediately after the injection
- Marbling of the skin (livedo reticularis) within hours
- Slow capillary refill, and dusky blue-red discoloration a few days later
- Blister formation with subsequent tissue sloughing (necrosis)

6.6 Follow-Up Assessment

The patient should be scheduled for a follow-up appointment one to two weeks after a lip treatment. This follow-up is particularly important with a lip treatment since, more than other parts of the body, the lips need correction following hematomas, nodules or other minor irregularities.

After about one to two weeks, the therapist will be able to see what the treatment result looks like. The following points should be checked:

- Symmetry at rest
- Unwanted visible asymmetries or nodules during mobilization of the lips when smiling or speaking
- Inflammations or other unwanted side effects
- Subsidence of hematomas and bruises
- Patient satisfaction

To do this, the lips are photographed again from all sides and during movement, as in the initial analysis (see Chap. 3.2.5, p. 62). The before-and-after image documentation helps objectify the result. A corrective follow-up treatment might then take place, if required.

Caution

Actions in the event of vascular complications

A vascular event needs to be identified quickly, followed by aggressive treatment to prevent serious and possible irreversible complications such as tissue necrosis (DeLorenzi 2014).

Five steps to counter a vascular complication:

1. Immediate identification of the complication.
2. Immediate local administration of hyaluronidase (maximum dose) into the area served by the vessel. The increased vascular permeability will allow the hyaluronidase to reach the intravascular implant without the therapist having to inject into the vessel (DeLorenzi 2014).
3. Heat the area with warm compresses, a heating unit or a hair dryer to stimulate the circulation. Never cool the area.
4. Gently massage without applying pressure.
5. Refer the patient urgently to a unit where the vascular occlusion can be remedied, surgically if need be (Sattler & Sommer 2015; Snozzi & Van Loghem 2018).

Note

The use of a blunt cannula offers no protection from intravascular injections. Slow injection and working with the patient, who needs to give a sign if any unusual pain occurs, are prerequisites for reducing the risk of complications. Interdisciplinary collaboration with experienced colleagues is advisable, where necessary.

7 Practice Fittings and Facilities, Materials, Patient Management

7 Practice Fittings and Facilities, Materials, Patient Management

7.1 The Practice Ambience

At an esthetic practice, first impressions are of the utmost importance. The treatment room should be inviting in design, with a medically hygienic, professional look, bright and freshly ventilated, peaceful, set to a comfortable temperature, and also pleasantly fragranced. An esthetic practice should safeguard the patient's privacy. The documentation should be placed accessibly on a desk, ballpoint pen at the ready, with somewhere convenient for the patient to place a bag and glasses. A drink should be offered, and no rush or pressure should be apparent.

All the equipment needed for the hyaluronic acid (HA) treatment should be prepared, ready for use. The treatment chair should stand in the room unobstructed and be covered with a clean, fresh cloth. Single-use treatment couch rolls, fabric sheets or terrycloth covers are available for this purpose. The cover must be changed after every patient. The chair should be positioned so that the patient cannot be seen from neighboring buildings; if necessary, this can be ensured through the use of obscuring drapes or a window blind. The light from the treatment lamp should not shine directly into the patient's eyes. A cushion to support the neck or knees will allow the patient to sit in a more relaxed position.

7.2 Furnishings

Since basic knowledge about how to equip the room may be assumed in view of the therapist's medical training, only a few selected aspects are explored here.

7.2.1 Chair (→ Fig. 7.1)

There is a wide range of chairs on the market, from simple cosmetic treatment couches to sophisticated designer chairs. These chairs differ mainly in terms of adjustability and functionality, comfort for the patient, and quality of the materials, and thus, of course, also in terms of price.

The ergonomic features of the chair are of prime importance – both therapist and patient need to be in a comfortable position during the treatment. The chair should stand in the room unobstructed to allow the therapist comfortable access to the patient from all sides. Ideally, the area being treated should be at the therapist's chest height.

Positioning of the chair is a key point that strongly influences the quality of the therapist's work. While performing the treatment, the therapist needs to be able to approach the treatment area comfortably with a straight upper body. This avoids back strain and means that the chair can be used for firm, relaxed support if the therapist needs to twist and turn while injecting the patient. It is up to the therapist to decide whether to administer the injections sitting down or standing up.

The angle of the treatment chair should be adjustable, since some areas need to be injected with the patient upright, while for others a semi-supine position is needed. This requires a backrest that can be smoothly adjusted from a vertical sitting position to a horizontal supine one. The analysis is always conducted with the patient sitting upright (see Chap. 3.2.4, p. 62), since the lines and shadows on the face are more clearly visible when the patient is seated rather than in a supine position, in which the whole face tends to relax.

The footrest needs to be adjustable and should be adjusted to the horizontal position to allow the patient to sit or lie comfortably.

From our point of view, the basic features of a treatment chair are as follows:

- Adjustable height (3)
- A low minimum height of 55.5 cm
- A backrest angle that can be adjusted between 90–180 degrees (1)
- A footrest that can be adjusted between an upright position of 90 degrees and a horizontal position of 0 degrees (2)
- Headrest with adjustable height (5)
- A high degree of stability to prevent tilting even under maximum strain in the horizontal position
- Comfortable padding
- Armrests that are padded on both sides, that can be folded backwards up to 180 degrees and removed if necessary (4)
- Ideally (though this is not essential), the chair should be electrically operated

7.2.2 Lighting

Lighting from all angles plays a significant role in the pre-treatment analysis and the subsequent evaluation of the treatment result (see Chap. 3.2.3, p. 61 f.). Its function is to illuminate the face in such a way as to make the relief of the skin clearly visible. It is important for the light source to be movable, allowing the light to be directed at the face from all sides.

Using a magnifier light allows the therapist to perform the finest superficial injection treatments in a controlled way. Ideally, the light source should be attached to the ceiling to prevent the risk of tripping over cables. Of course, there are many simple variants, such as table lamps or tripod lights, which also do the job well.

7.2.3 Tray and Table (→ Fig. 7.2)

A flexible, adjustable table or tray, which can be wheeled into the required position during the treatment, is recommended to ensure that the necessary materials are within easy reach. A wide range of suitable trays and tables are available.

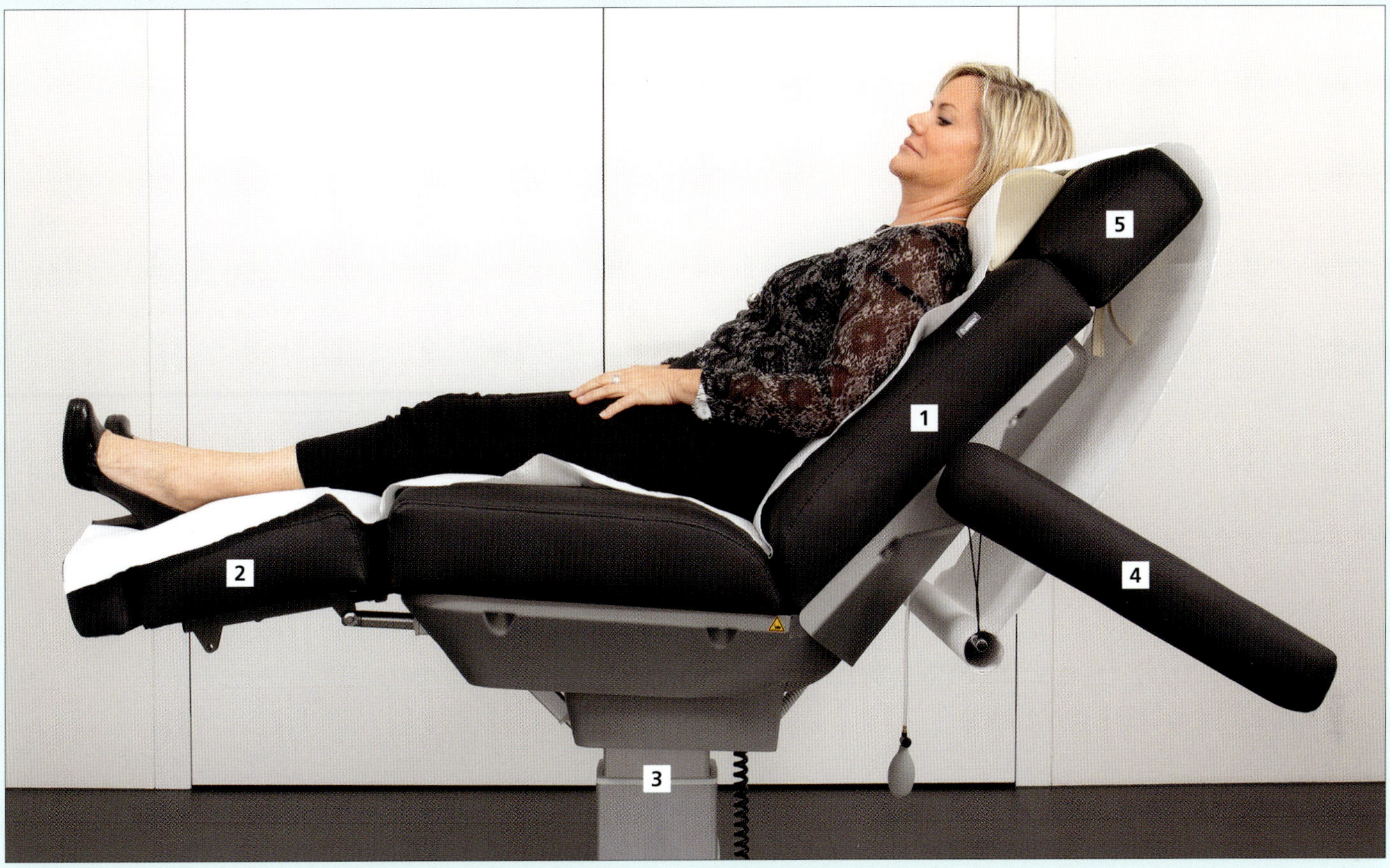

Fig. 7.1 Treatment chair with the basic features labeled: adjustable backrest (1), adjustable footrest (2), adjustable height (3), armrests that can be folded back and removed (4), adjustable headrest (5).

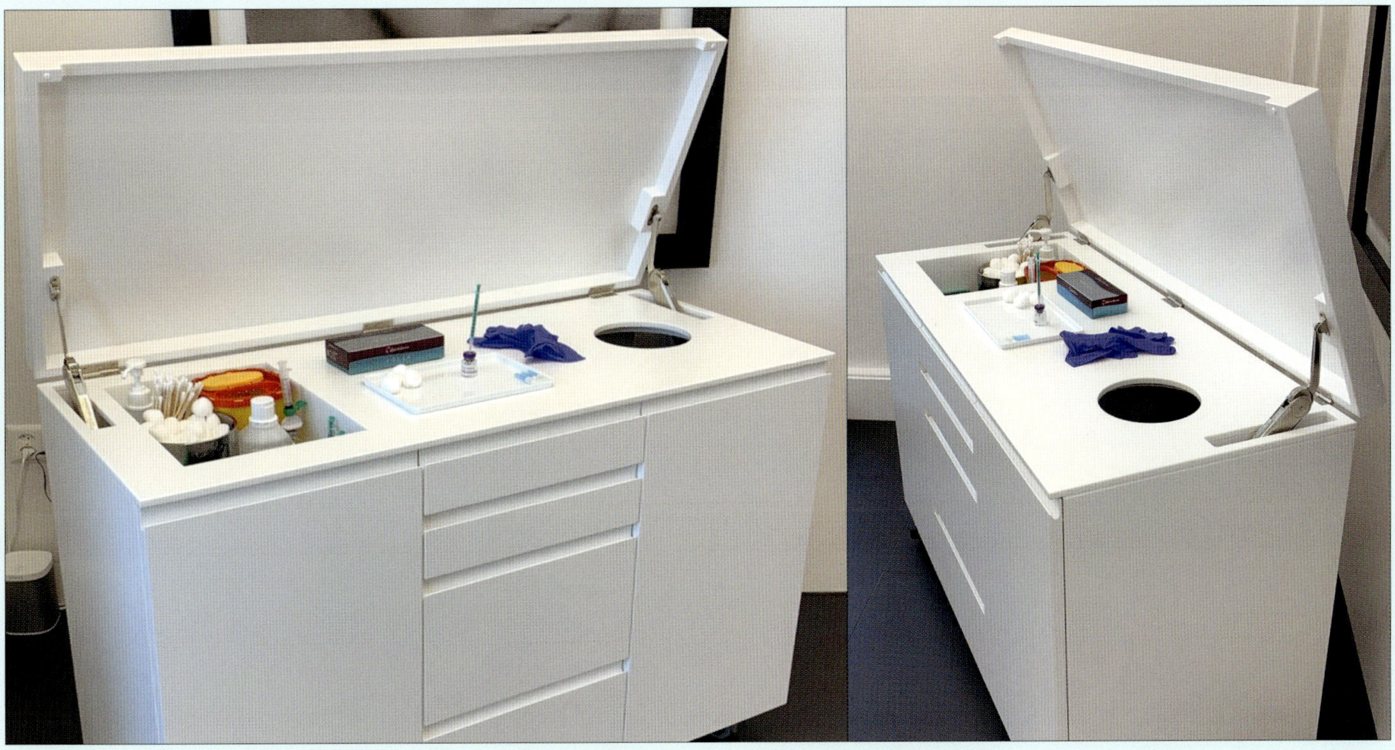

Fig. 7.2 This tray/table was developed for use in esthetic dermal filler treatments, based on practical experience. It can be wheeled into place where required, while the equipment is stored hygienically and can be firmly covered with the lid.

7.3 Hygiene

The hygienic measures during a filler injection treatment for facial lines are no different from the standard measures at any medical practice:

- Well-ventilated room
- Freshly covered treatment chair (fabric sheet/paper roll)
- Disinfected trays and other surfaces for tools and materials, with sterile coverings
- Sterilized practice tools and equipment (kidney dishes, etc.)
- Disposal of needles and cannulas in a dedicated sharps disposal box
- Disposal of waste materials after every treatment
- Cannulas and injection needles must not be touched with the fingers and must not come into contact with hair or skin
- Single-use gloves to be worn; sterile gloves should be worn when administering injections
- Use of medical masks to cover the nose and mouth
- Cleaning and disinfection of the skin area being treated

Caution

Cleaning and disinfection of the skin area being treated

Before each treatment, thoroughly remove all makeup, and disinfect the skin area being treated by wiping it with a sterile swab soaked in a product such as Octenisept or Kodan. Repeat this procedure three times in a row, using a new, freshly soaked swab each time. During the treatment, a swab soaked in an alcohol-free disinfectant should be held ready in the therapist's free hand, so that any blood can be removed and the skin cleaned. This swab should be changed immediately after use. After the treatment, clean the wound once again with disinfectant. It is advisable to apply a wound-healing cream.

7.4 Equipment used in Pre- and Post-Treatment Care

The following procedures and products are needed for pre- and post-treatment care in a lip treatment with HA (→ Figs. 7.3–7.18):

Equipment used in Pre- and Post-Treatment Care

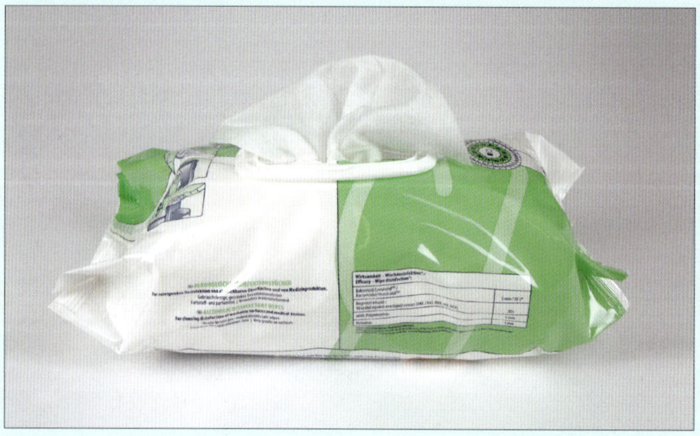

Fig. 7.3 Makeup removal – Use makeup remover wipes or swabs soaked in a facial cleansing product.

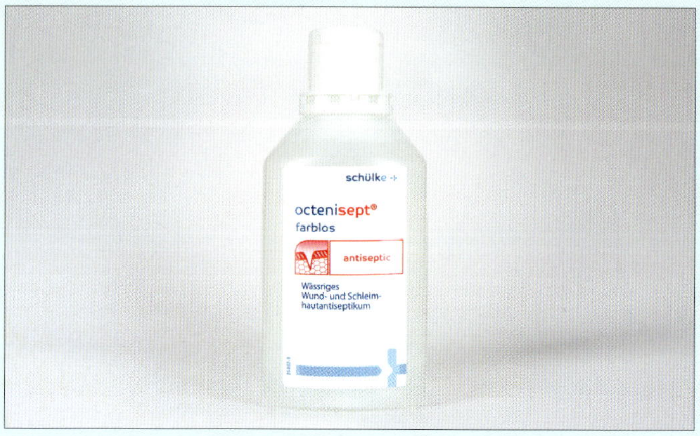

Fig. 7.4 Disinfection – Before the treatment, thoroughly disinfect the area being treated with Kodan or Octenisept (also suitable for the mucosa) or similar skin disinfectants.

Equipment used in Pre- and Post-Treatment Care (continued)

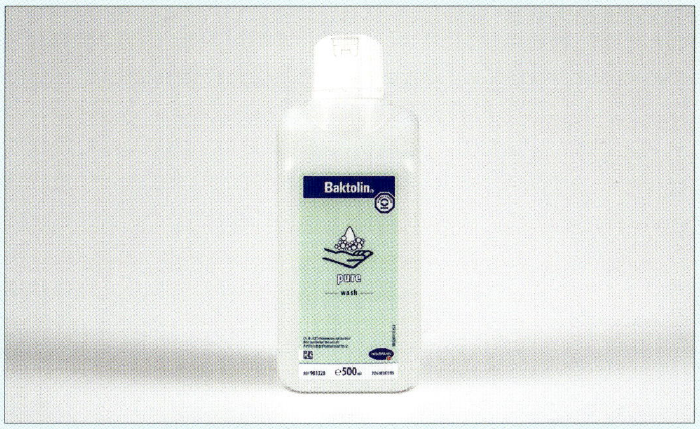

Fig. 7.5 Cleaning the hands – Before each treatment and before putting on single-use gloves, clean the hands thoroughly with medicated soap, then disinfect them.

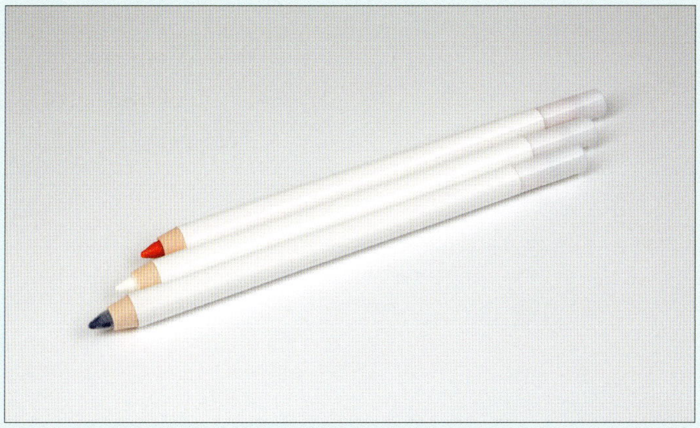

Fig. 7.6 Marking – Mark the area being treated with a white or colored skin-marker pencil.

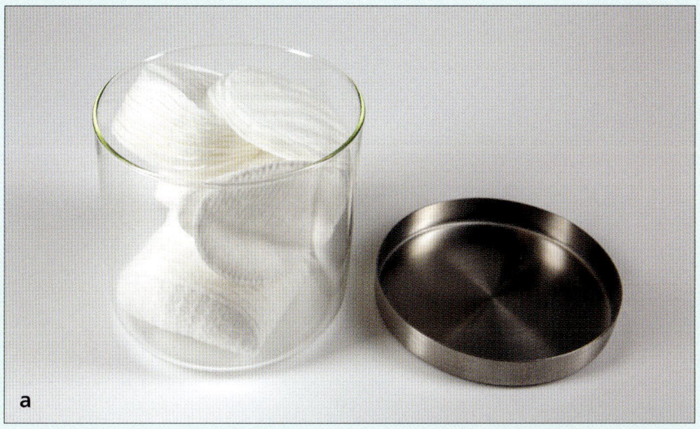

Fig. 7.7 a–c Swabs – Apart from classic medical swabs (a) and sterile swabs or compresses (b), one can also use cotton pads (c) because they are pleasant for the patient and also highly absorbent.

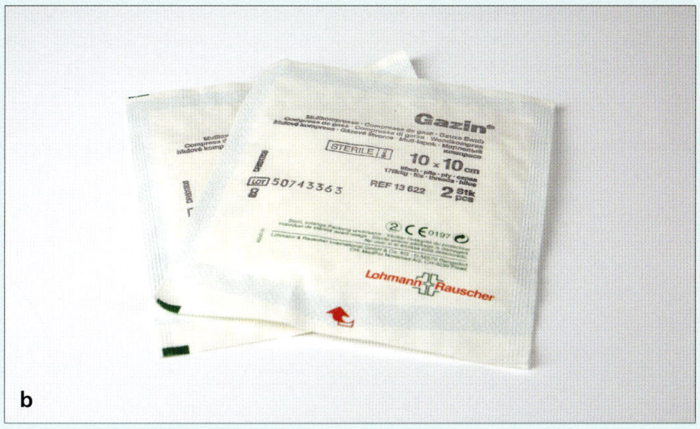

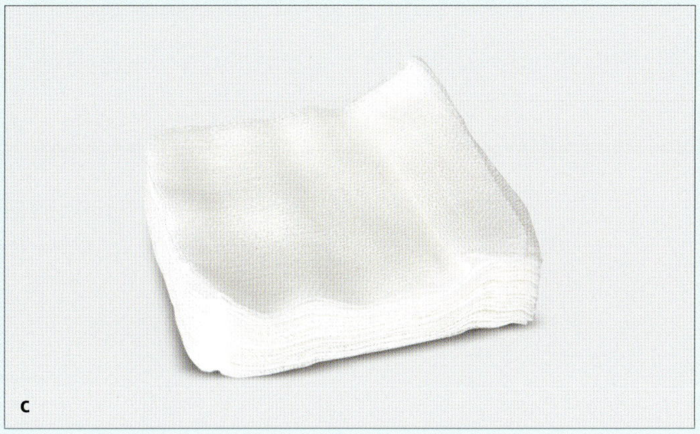

Equipment used in Pre- and Post-Treatment Care (continued)

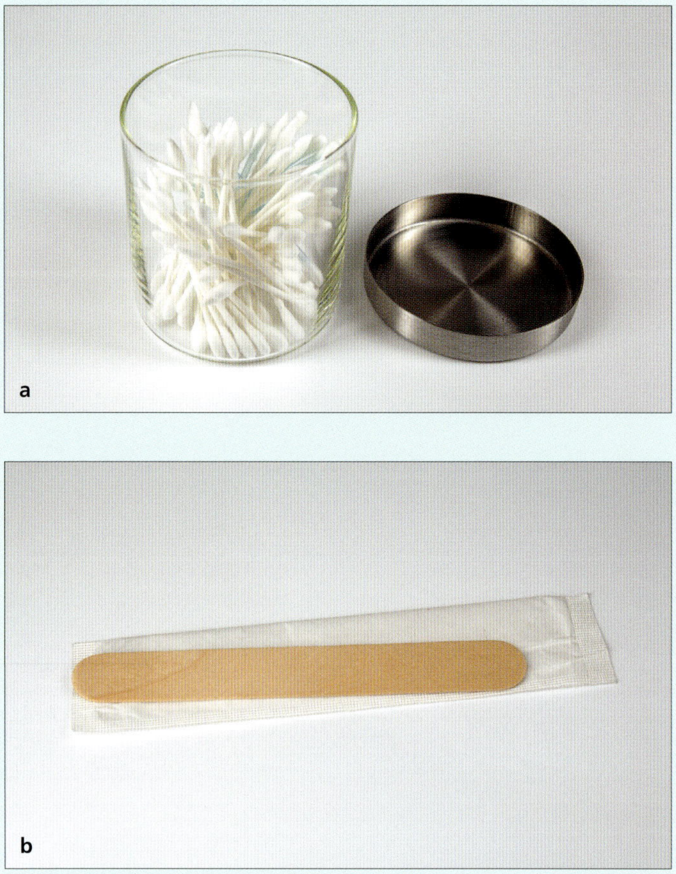

Fig. 7.8 a+b Cotton buds (Q-tips) or spatulas – Creams can be applied using a cotton bud (a) or a spatula (b).

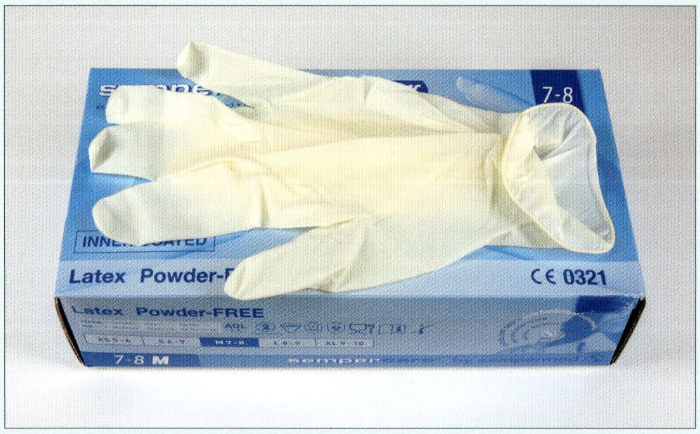

Fig. 7.9 Single-use gloves – Gloves should fit snugly with no wrinkling and must be powder-free; sterile gloves should be used for certain indications. These gloves are available in various colors (e.g. blue, black). The use of sterile gloves is recommended when injecting with a cannula. If the patient has a latex allergy, work with latex-free gloves.

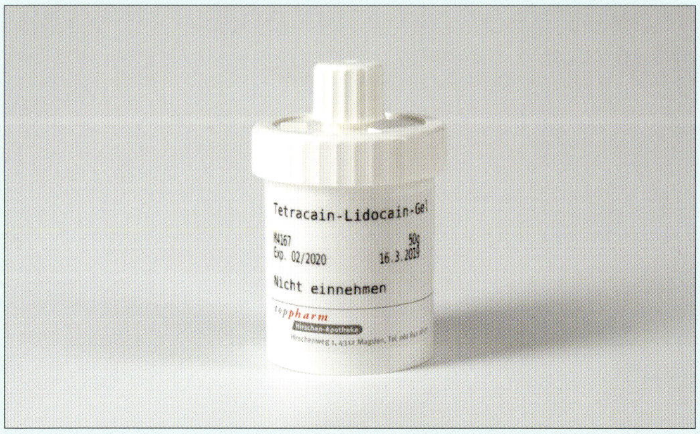

Fig. 7.10 Local anesthetic (cream, ointment) – e.g. Emla, pharmacy's own formulation containing more than 25% tetracaine and lidocaine (shown here in the photo), Pliaglis, Xylocaine Spray, etc.

7

Equipment used in Pre- and Post-Treatment Care (continued)

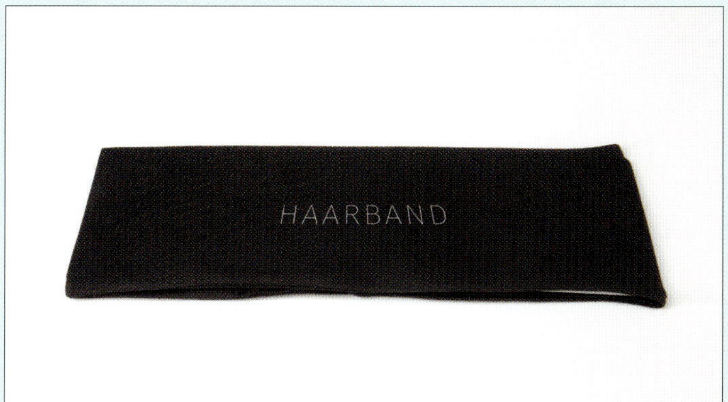

a

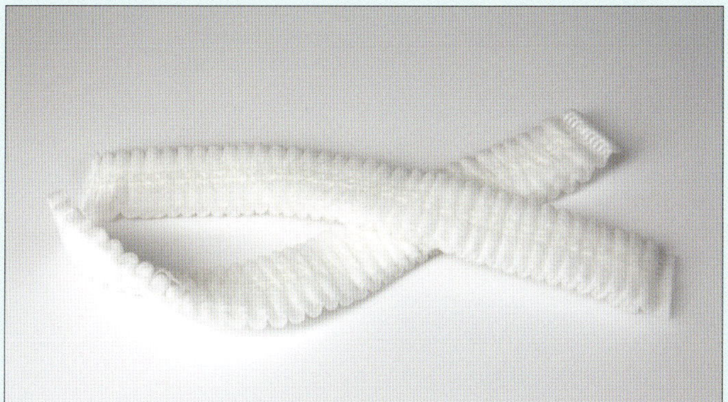

b

Fig. 7.11 a+b Hairband – It is important to keep the patient's hair off the face. A surgical cap, a hairband (a), a hairnet (b) or hairclips may be used for this purpose.

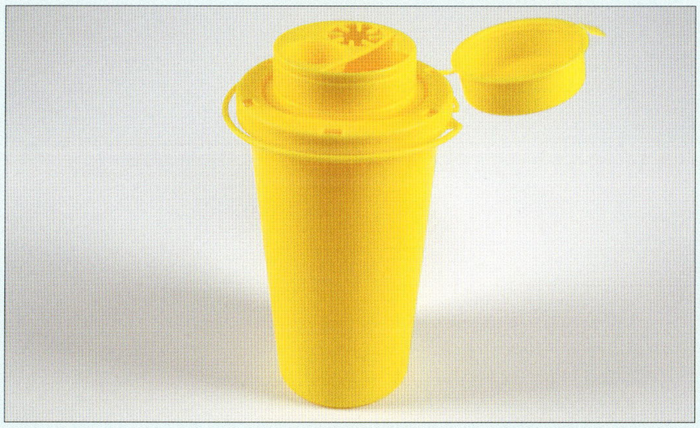

Fig. 7.12 Sharps disposal boxes and kidney dishes – must be available at every practice.

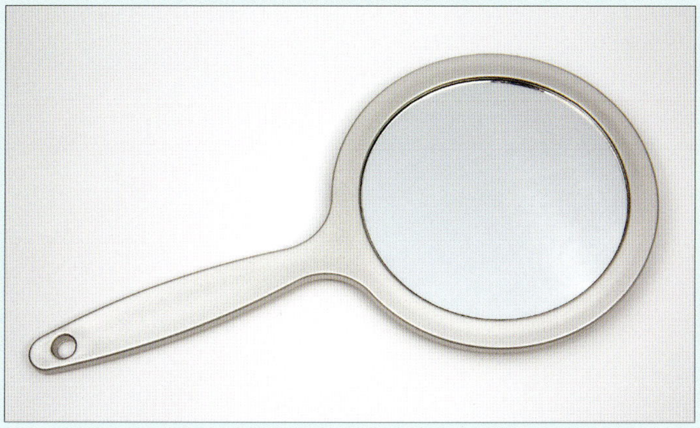

Fig. 7.13 Hand-held mirror – for optional use by the patient during the treatment.

Equipment used in Pre- and Post-Treatment Care (continued)

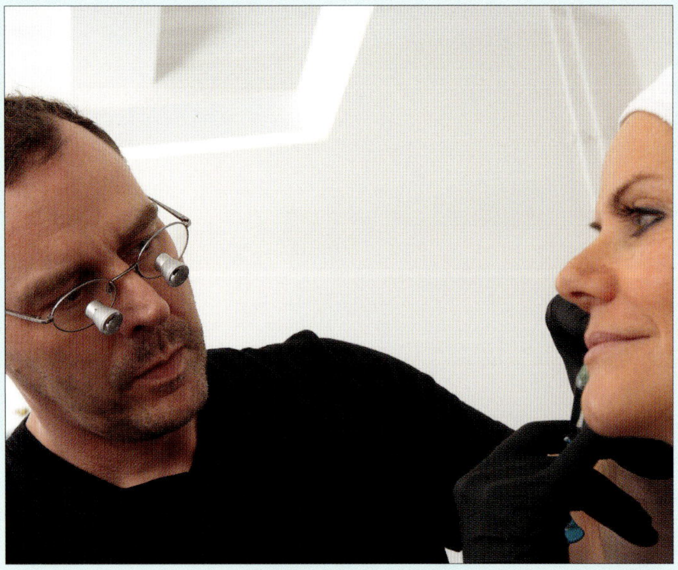

Fig. 7.14 Magnifying loupe glasses – These are recommended when treating the finest lines and for very superficial injections (e.g. for the blanching technique).

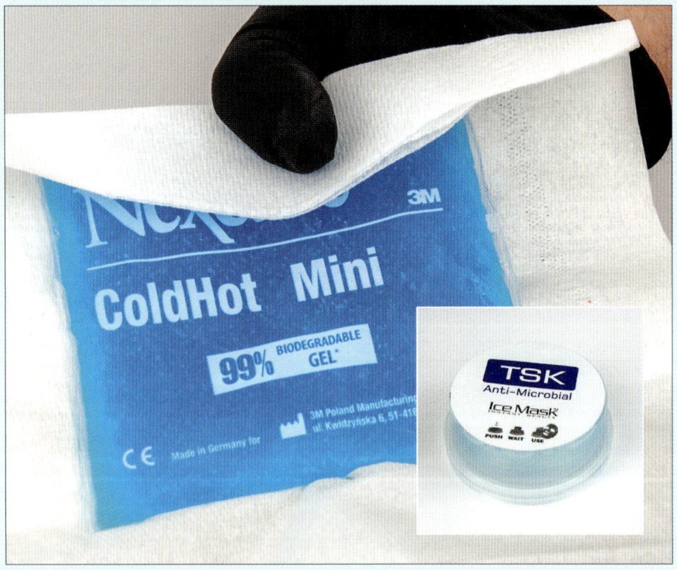

Fig. 7.15 Cooling pads and masks – for cooling pain relief after the treatment. They are available in various shapes and sizes, from a variety of manufacturers. For a lip treatment, the cooling pad needs to be bigger than the lip area.

Cooling masks (inset image) have a similar effect to cooling pads. These masks contain a variety of substances, such as aloe vera, HA, disinfectants, and substances that promote wound healing.

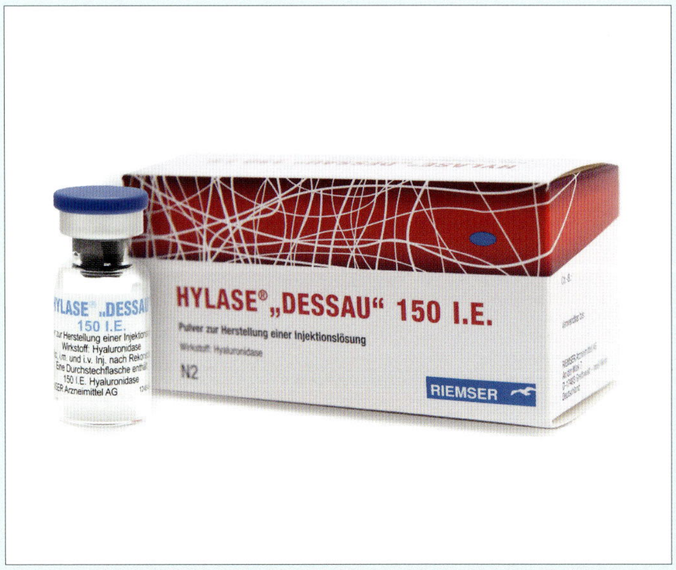

Fig. 7.16 Hyaluronidase – This can be used in cosmetic medicine after a treatment error or if an intolerance reaction to HA occurs, to dissolve the HA filler that was injected for cosmetic purposes.

Warning: This is a prescription-only product!

Equipment used in Pre- and Post-Treatment Care (continued)

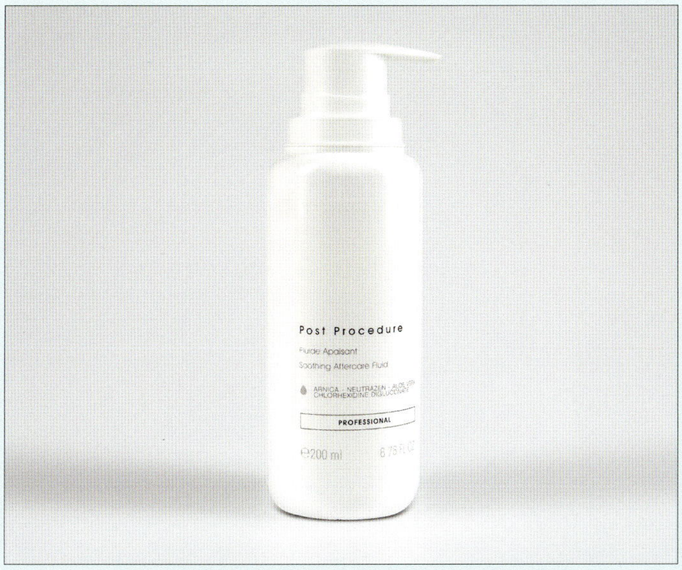

Fig. 7.17 Post-treatment cream – After each treatment, the wound should be cleansed and treated with a post-treatment cream. These creams or ointments that have an anti-inflammatory effect, reduce swellings, and accelerate the breakdown of hematomas. Of the many products available from pharmaceutical manufacturers, this image shows an example supplied by the company Teoxane.

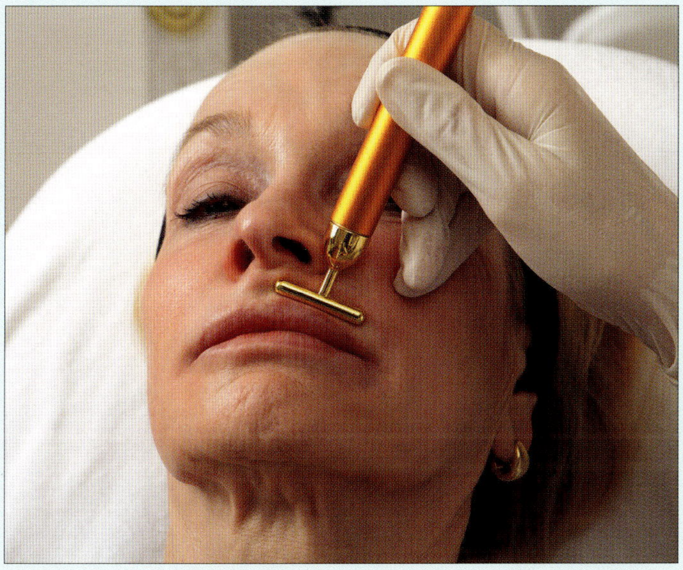

Fig. 7.18 24 K Gold Beauty Bar – This device is made of brass and aluminum, with gold plating. It has a T-shaped head and may be used by the assistant to evert the lip, thus leaving the therapist's hands free for administering the injection (when wearing gloves, the lubricant effect of the disinfectant often makes it difficult to evert the lip uniformly). Another advantage of the 24 K Gold Beauty Bar is that it gently clamps off the vessels that serve this region, slightly reducing the risk of intravascular injection.

The 24 K Gold Beauty Bar's T-shaped head produces an activating micro-vibration. This can be used after a treatment to better distribute the HA material, to massage out any irregularities, and to encourage perfusion of any small areas where an unwanted blanching effect was produced.

Checklist – Equipment used in Pre- and Post-Treatment Care for a Lip Treatment with Dermal Fillers

- Camera
- Documentation + ballpoint pen
- Sharps disposal box
- Single-use gloves
- Cleaning agent for the hands
- Disinfectant for the skin
- Disinfectant for the hands
- Skin-marker pencil
- Makeup remover wipes
- Spatulas, cotton buds (Q-tips)
- Kidney dishes
- Swabs
- Anesthetic cream containing lidocaine
- Local anesthetic, single-use syringe, needle
- Loupe glasses or magnifier light
- Hairband
- Cooling pads, masks
- Mirror
- Waste basket
- HA syringes
- Spare needles
- Cannulas
- Nokor needles
- Post-treatment cream
- Hyaluronidase
- Medical masks to cover the nose and mouth

7.5 Patient Management during the Treatment (→ Figs. 7.19–7.38)

Preparatory Measures and Adjustments

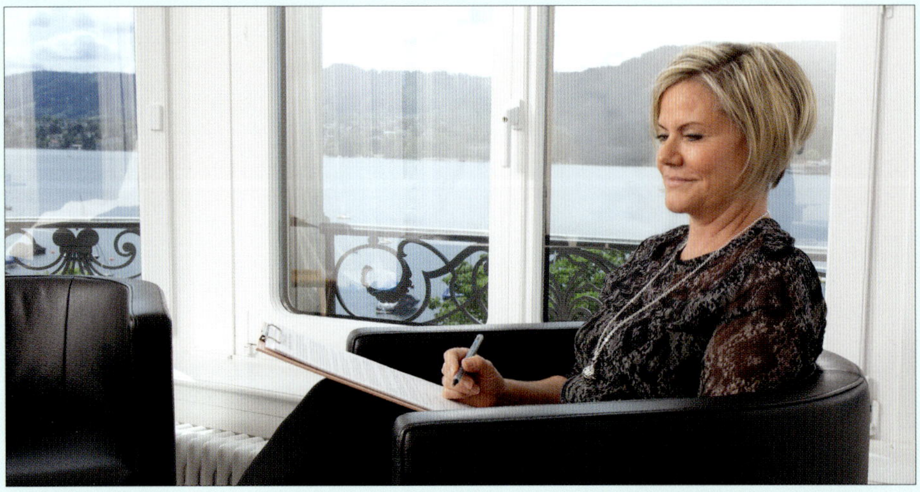

Fig. 7.19 After the welcome, the patient should be asked to complete the medical history questionnaire in the waiting area.

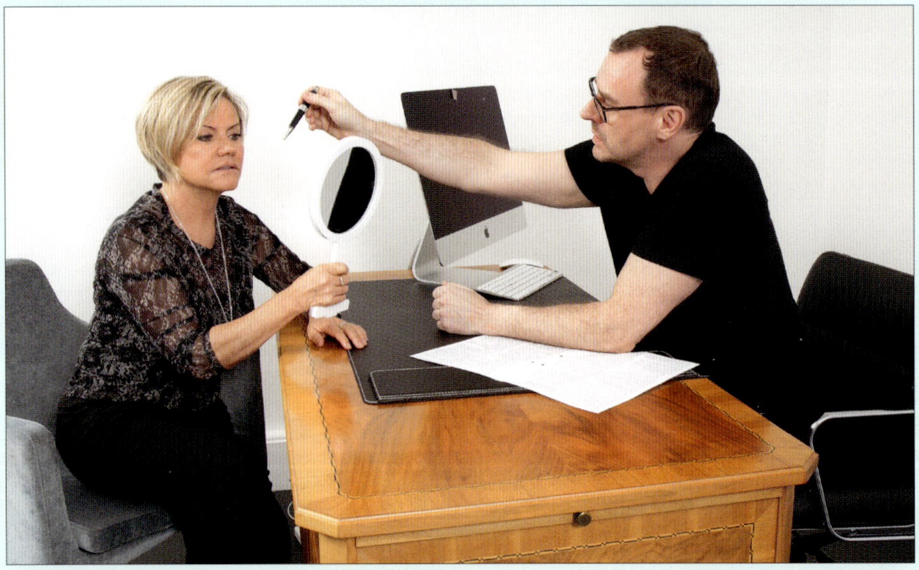

Fig. 7.20 The patient's wishes regarding the treatment are discussed. The therapist then conducts the consultation and informs the patient about the potential effects and side effects of an esthetic treatment.

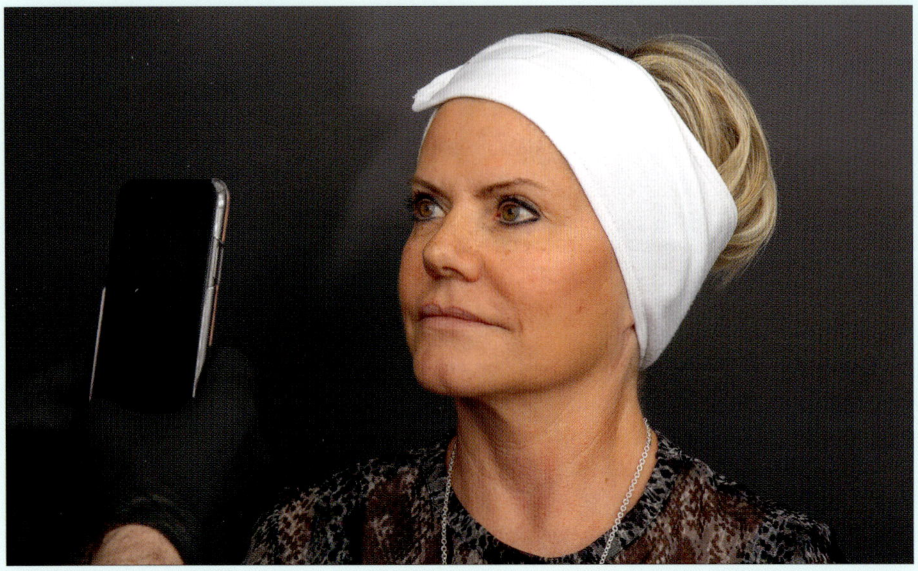

Fig. 7.21 This is followed by the photographic documentation. After this, the patient is invited into the treatment room and asked to sit in the treatment chair.

Preparatory Measures and Adjustments (continued)

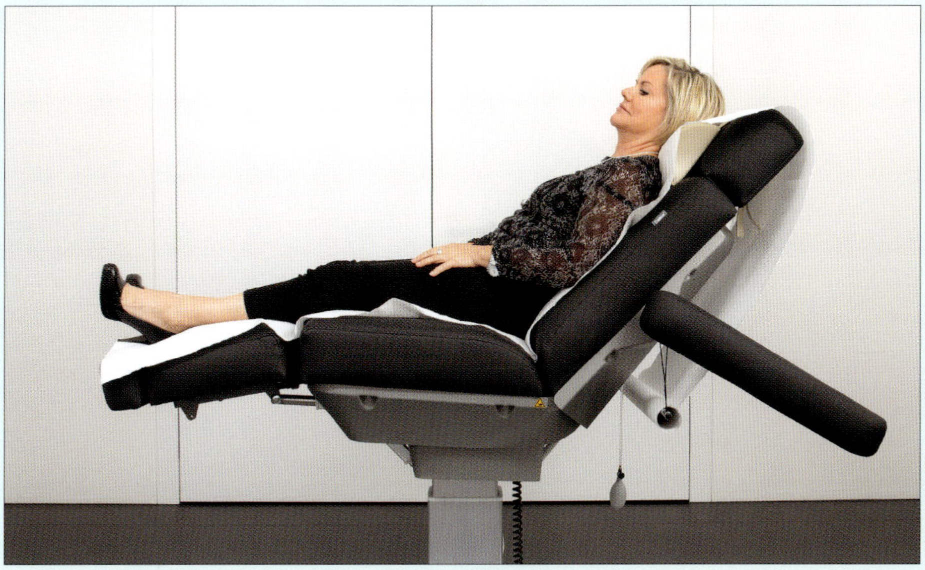

Fig. 7.22 Position of the chair during the analysis: For a lip augmentation, it is a good idea for the patient to be analyzed while sitting almost upright. In this position, the tissues sag downward, clearly showing how the corners of the mouth and the perioral region behave. The injection itself, especially into the vermillion, can be administered with the patient in a supine position. When treating the marionette lines and chin region, we recommend administering the injection with the patient seated.

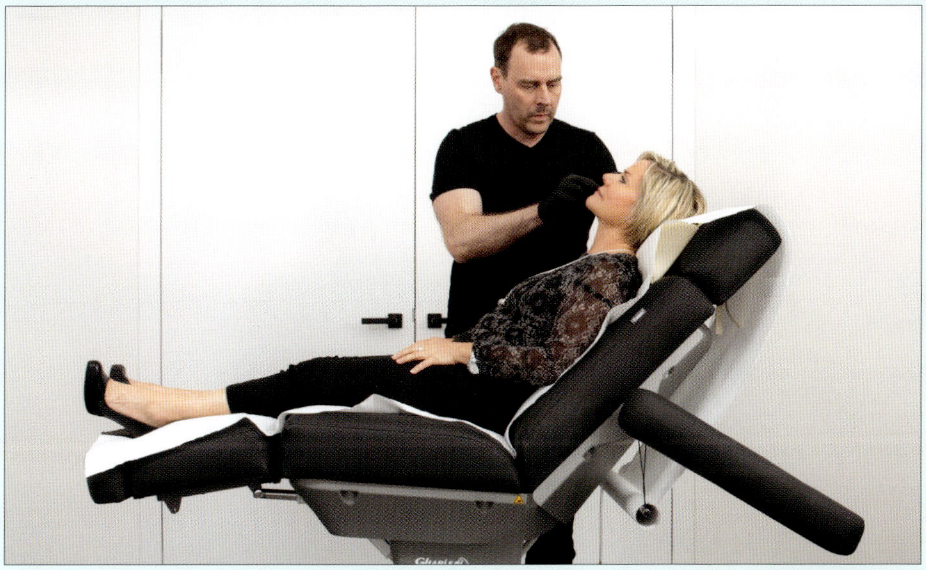

Fig. 7.23 The chair should be adjusted so that the patient is sitting comfortably and the therapist can adopt a relaxed position in which to carry out the treatment.

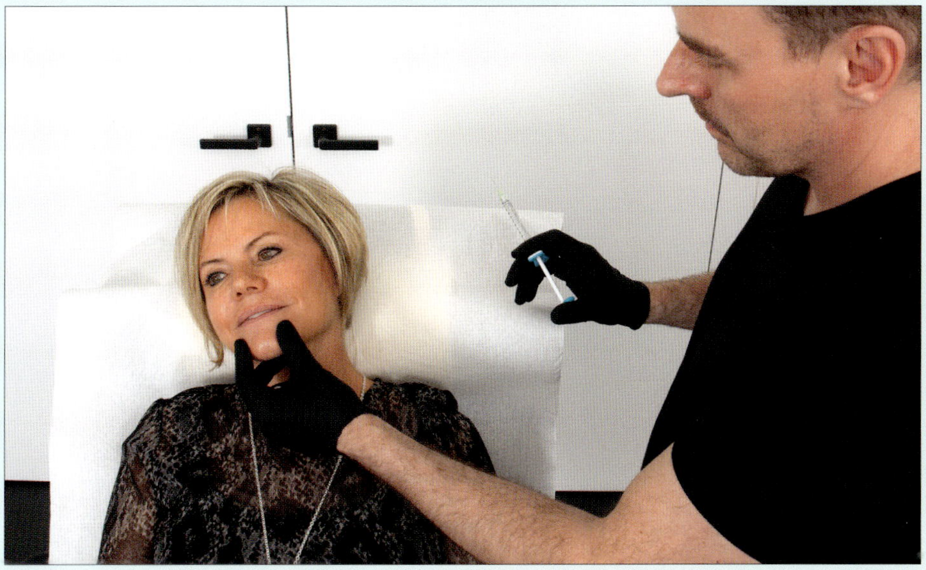

Fig. 7.24 The therapist needs to be able to reach all the areas being treated while maintaining a near-upright posture.

Preparatory Measures and Adjustments (continued)

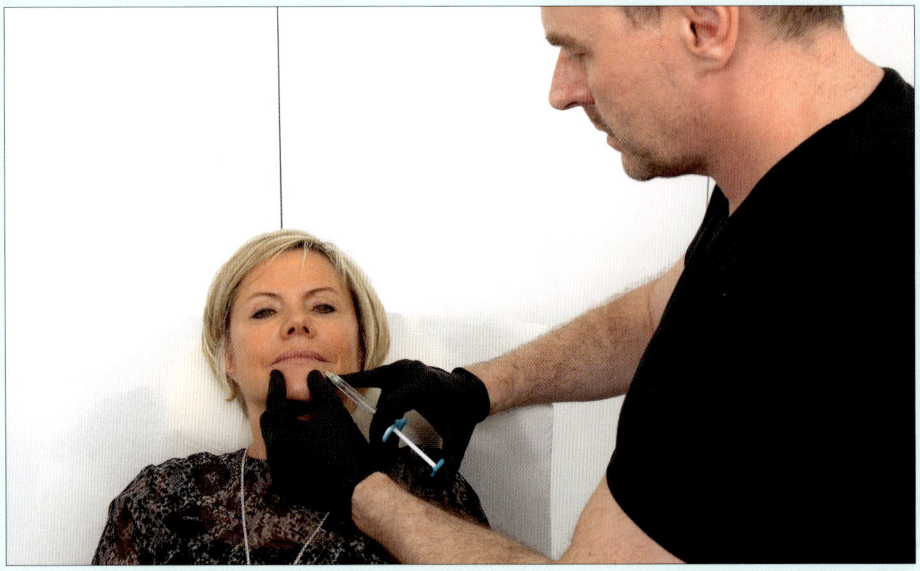

Fig. 7.25 The therapist should stand or sit up straight throughout the treatment.

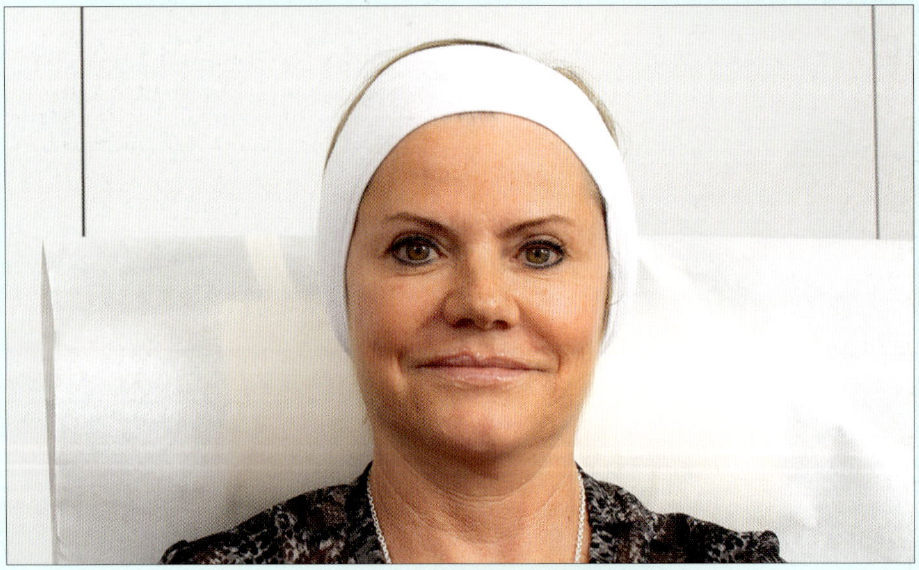

Fig. 7.26 A hairband, hair net or surgical cap should be fitted to keep the patient's hair out of the treatment zone.

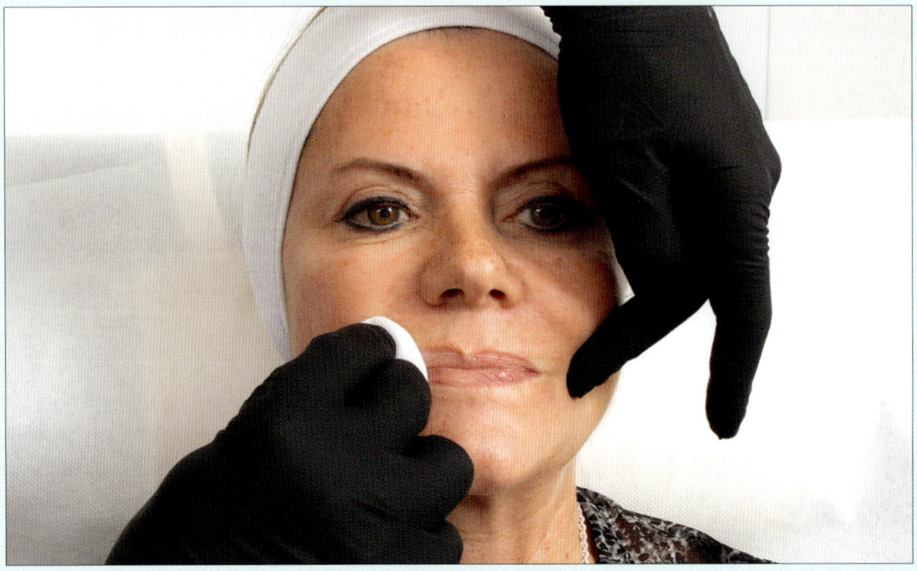

Fig. 7.27 Thorough makeup removal is essential.

Preparatory Measures and Adjustments (continued)

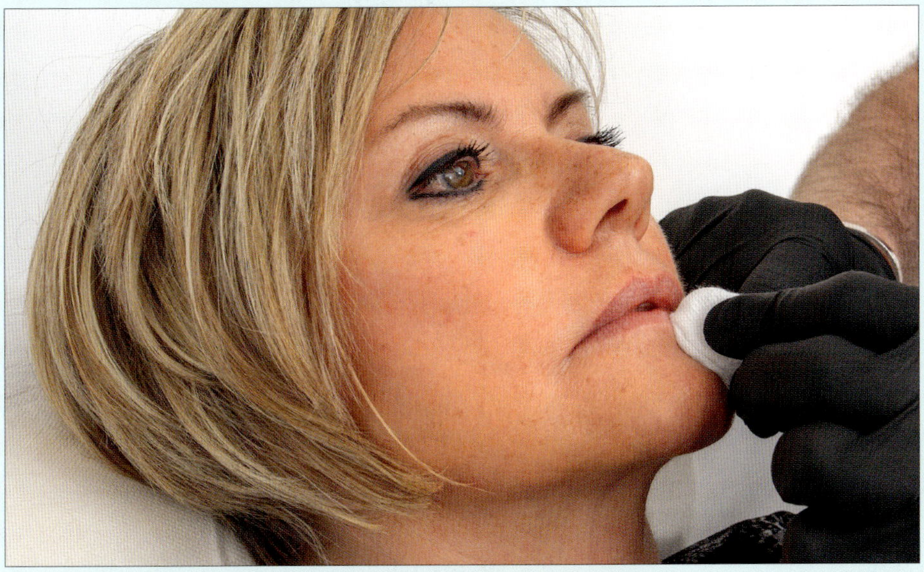

Fig. 7.28 Cleaning and infection control: The skin should be extensively disinfected before the treatment by cleansing the area being treated with a solution of chlorhexidine or alcohol (70%). The recommended way of offering the patient the maximum possible protection from infection is to use sterile single-use gloves and sterile pads (Becker-Wegerich 2016).

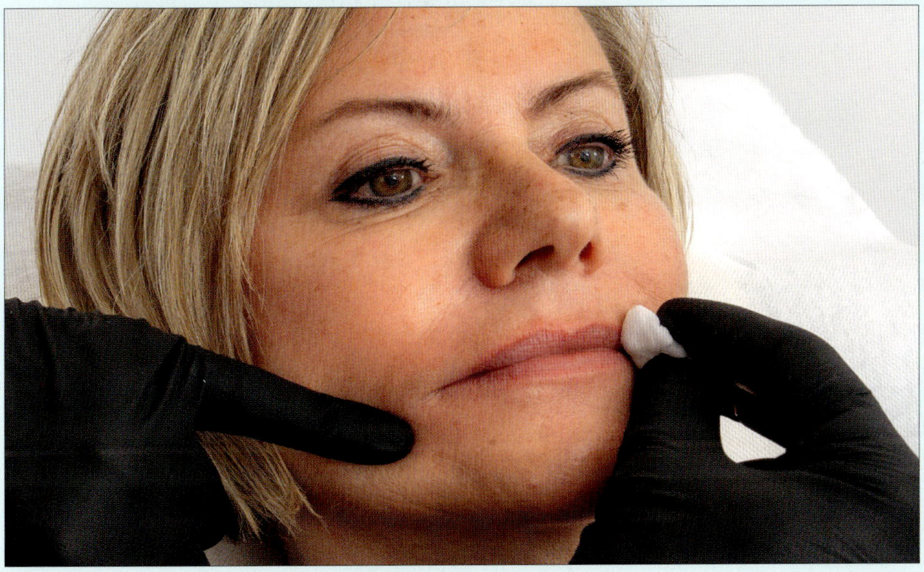

Fig. 7.29 Disinfect by rubbing each site to be treated with at least three consecutive swabs soaked in disinfectant. The patient's hands should also be disinfected, as there is a common tendency for patients to inadvertently touch the treatment area during the treatment.

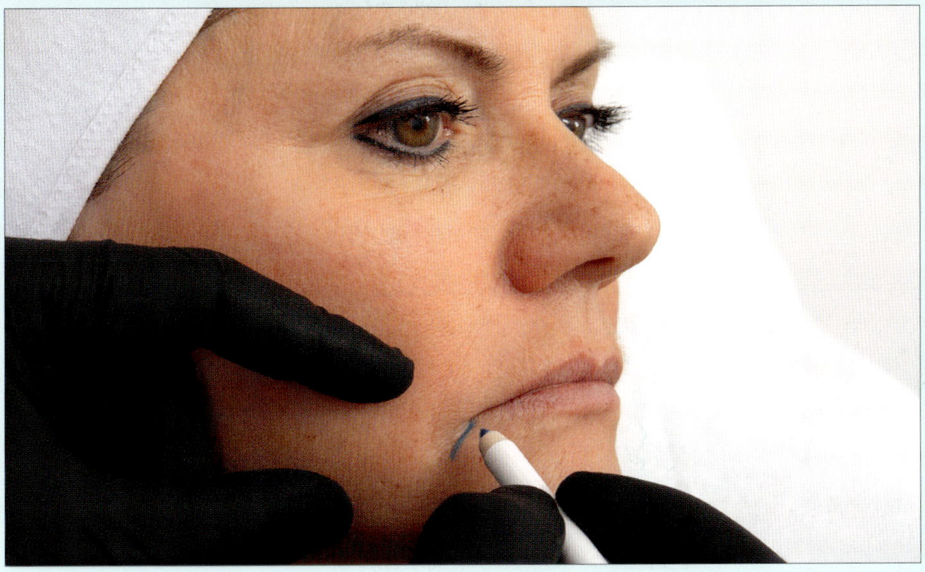

Fig. 7.30 All the sites being treated should be marked with the patient standing or sitting, before starting with the injections. The shadows and lines that need to be injected are marked with a colored or white eyeliner or similar skin-marker pencil.

Preparatory Measures and Adjustments (continued)

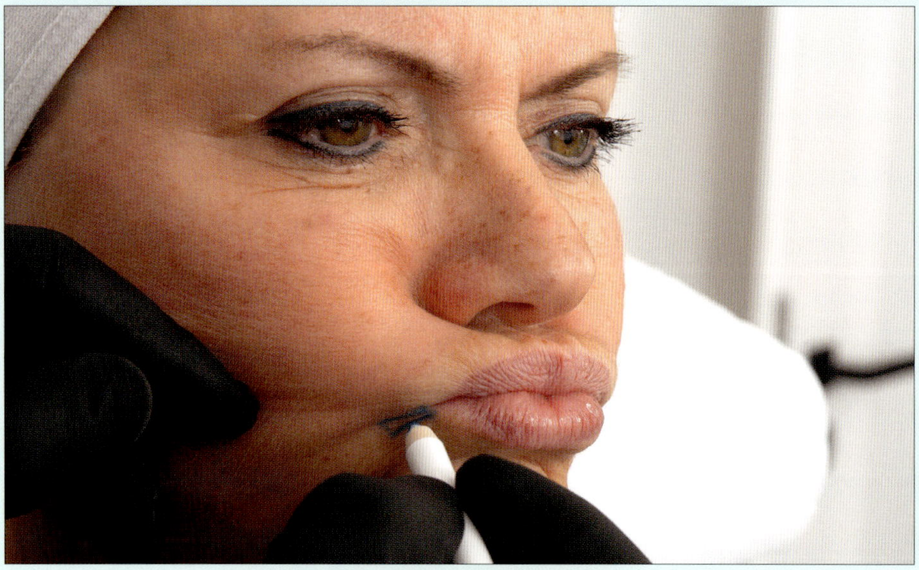

Fig. 7.31 When marking the skin, it is important for the patient to move the face into different expressions, so that the therapist can capture the problem zones accurately. The areas being treated should be drawn in with the eyeliner/skin-marker pencil and confirmed by the patient – and also photographed if appropriate.

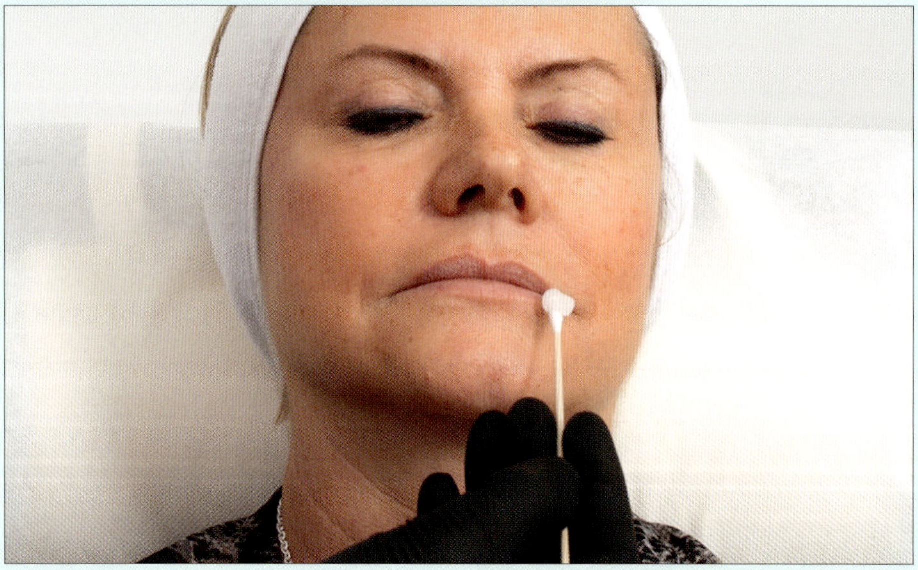

Fig. 7.32 The area being treated should be numbed with a cream containing lidocaine or by using another anesthetic method (see Chap. 5, p. 78). This procedure may even be preferable, as it may take 15–30 minutes for the anesthetic to act. If desired, the area being treated could even be pre-cooled with cold compresses, as the cold stimulus will make the skin less sensitive to pain (Sattler & Sommer 2015).

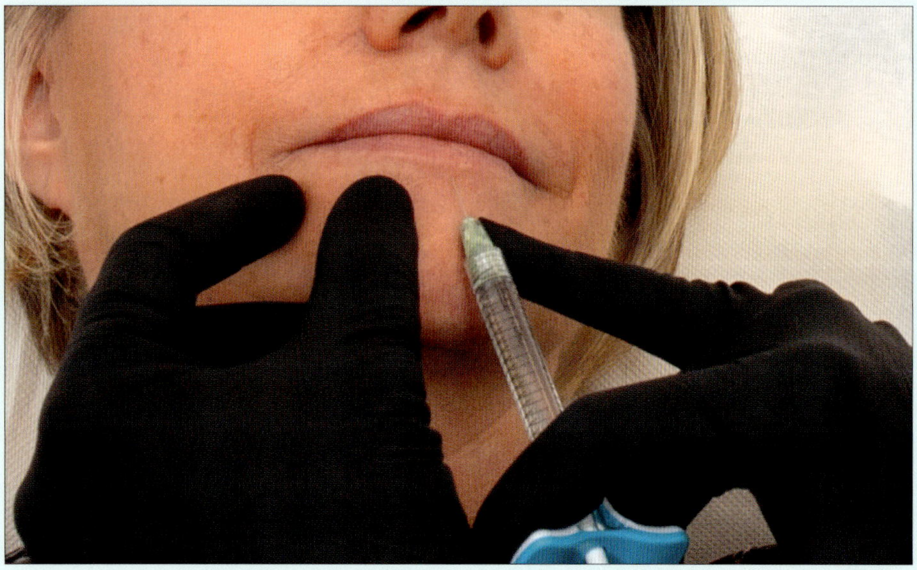

Fig. 7.33 To keep a steady hand while performing tasks that require fine motor coordination, it helps if the therapist's hand is supported against the patient.

The agreed lip treatment, as recorded in the documentation record, can now take place according to the treatment plan (see Chap. 9, p. 127 ff.).

Immediate Post-Treatment Measures after the Lip Augmentation

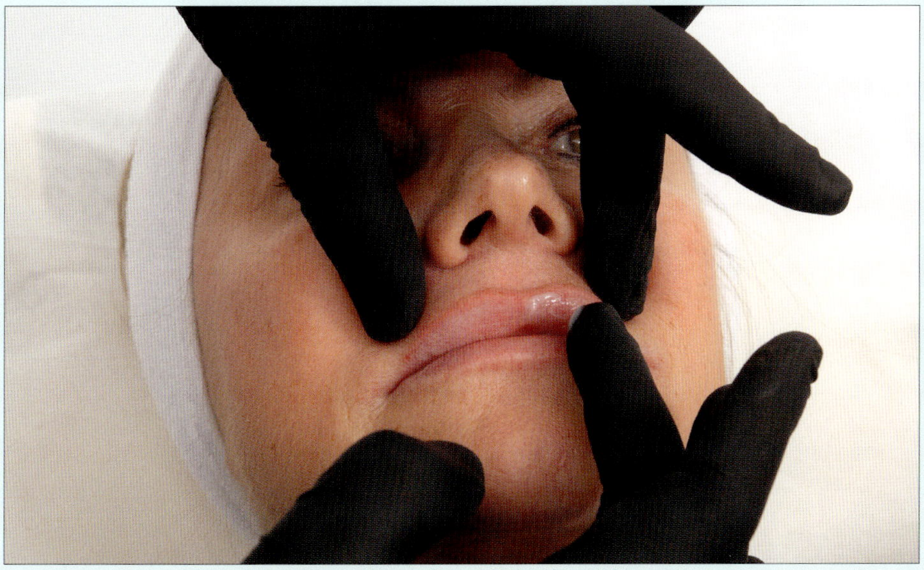

Fig. 7.34 A post-treatment cream should be applied and spread over the skin after the lip augmentation.

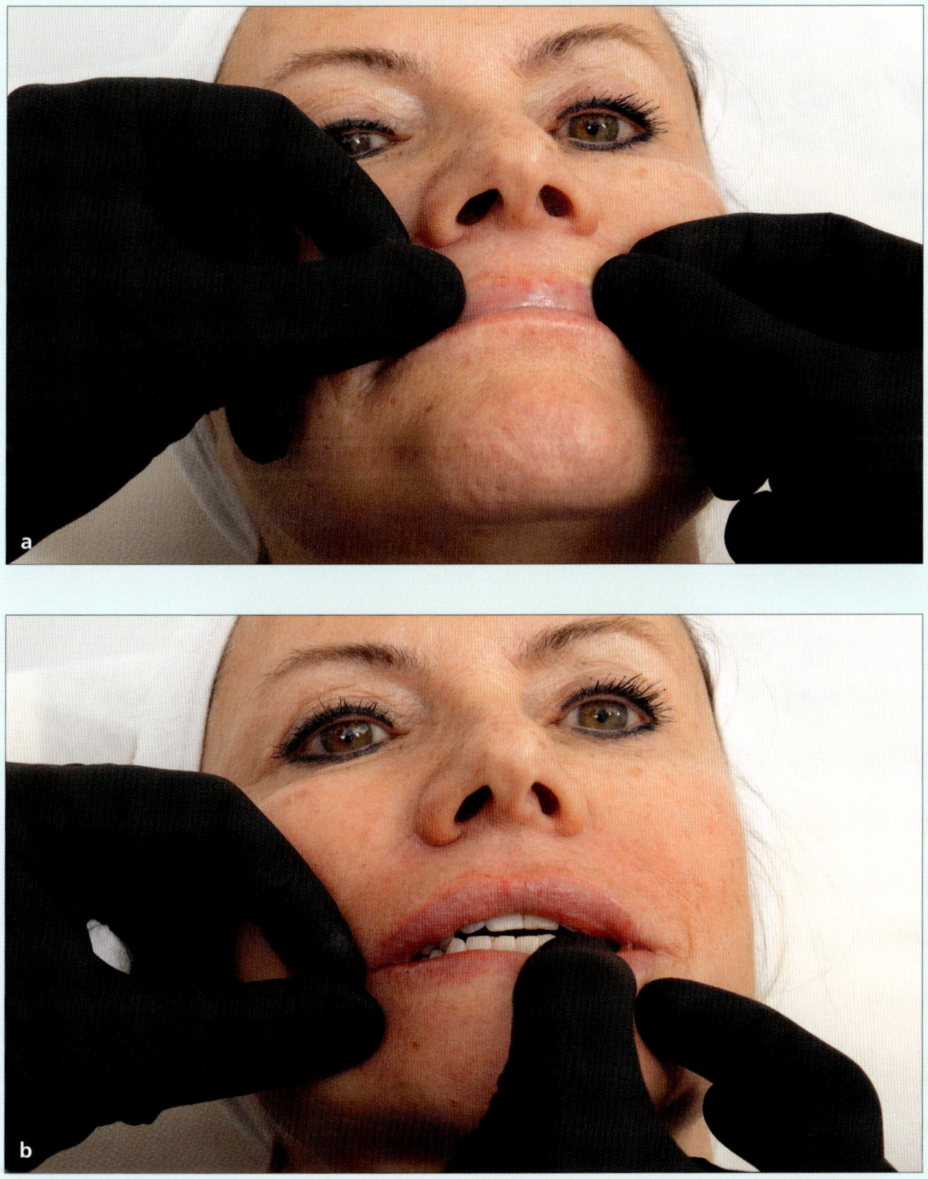

Fig. 7.35 a+b Gentle massage and stroking of the lip is a good way to visibly and palpably reveal any irregularities that have resulted from the excess accumulation of filler. The upper and lower lip should be palpated using a gentle stroking motion.

Immediate Post-Treatment Measures after the Lip Augmentation (continued)

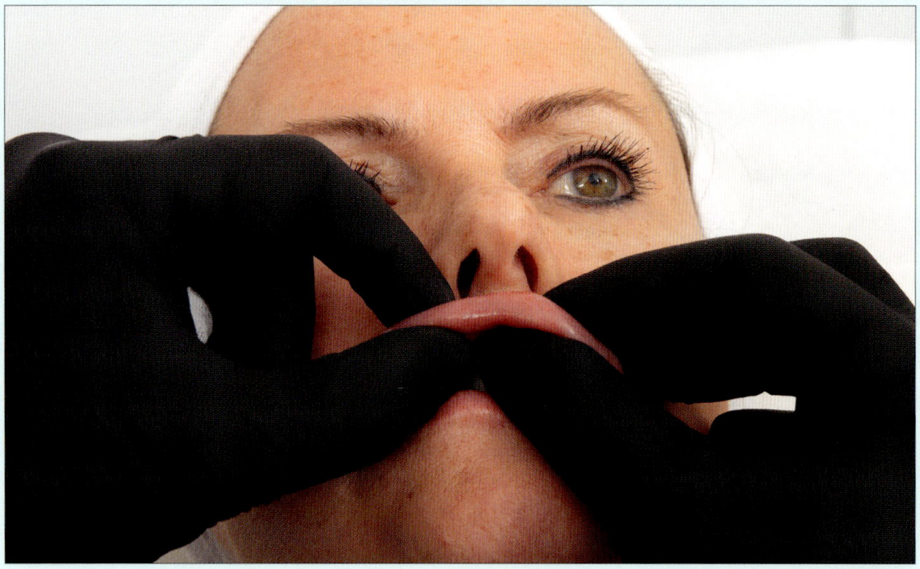

Fig. 7.36 Whether the lip should be massaged after a lip augmentation or not is disputed. We recommend massage after use of the cannula technique, to ensure uniform distribution of the material. If the lip has been treated with a sharp needle, it should only be massaged in the case of asymmetry or if there are visible nodules. This should be done carefully and gently, to redistribute the material slightly better, taking care not to cause further stress to the already traumatized tissue.

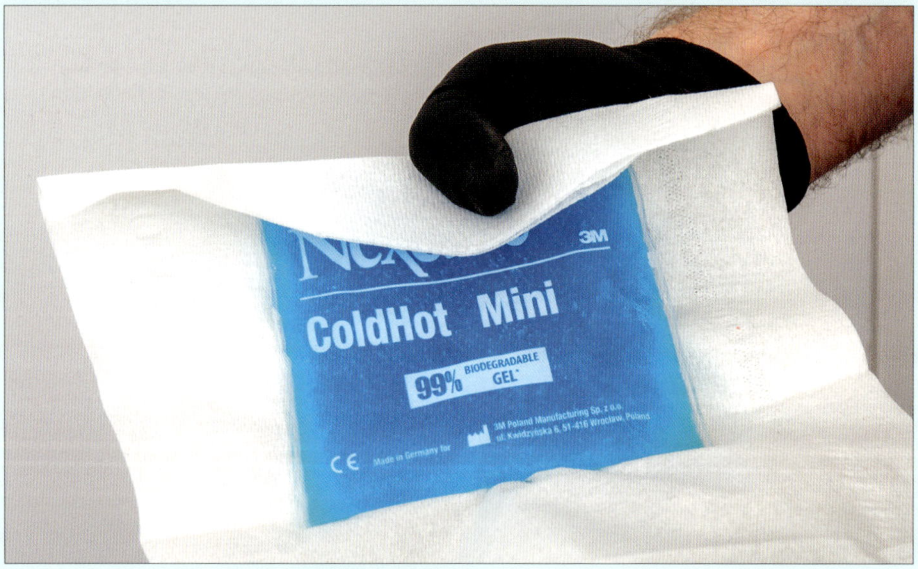

Fig. 7.37 Cold compresses should be offered after the treatment to cool the treated mouth region and counter any swelling. The compresses should be larger than the lip area.

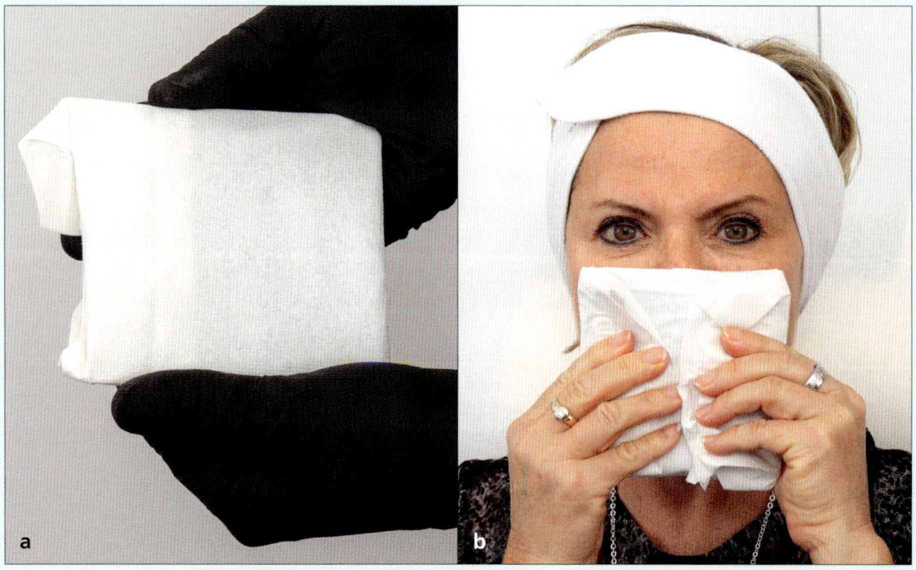

Fig. 7.38 a+b With the cooling pads wrapped in a cloth (a), the patient can hold them in place to cool the lips (b).

An "after" photo is then taken for the photographic documentation. The treatment should be logged and documented in detail, including the product, batch number, indication, special features, follow-up treatment, etc. A follow-up appointment needs to be made to check on the treatment result, to document it photographically, and to administer any repeat injections, if required. At the end of the session, the patient should receive one more information sheet that contains advice on how to care for the freshly injected lips.

Checklist – Treatment Course at a Glance

- Patient check-in
- Welcome the patient
- Investigate any previous treatments
- The patient's wishes and expectations
- Investigate if there is any lidocaine intolerance
- Documentation
- Agree a fee
- Photographic documentation
- Analysis
- Treatment goal, treatment planning
- Mark the treatment area
- Clean the patient's skin
- Anesthesia (plan in 20–40 minutes for anesthetic to work)
- Adjust treatment chair
- Wash and disinfect your own hands
- Put on single-use gloves
- Disinfect the patient
- Open the material pack
- Assemble the syringe, prepare Nokor needle, if appropriate
- Prepare swabs, prepare swab with hydrogen peroxide (to be used to stop any minor bleeding more quickly)
- Disinfection
- Injection
- Disinfect repeatedly
- Post-treatment cream
- Massage gently if appropriate
- Cool the treated area
- Prescribe Arnica globuli or ibuprofen, as appropriate
- Take "after" photograph
- Make follow-up appointment
- Hand out information sheet with after-treatment care instructions

Illustrated Atlas "The Lips"

8 Injection Techniques

8 Injection Techniques

8.1 Introduction

It is our objective to provide the reader with a practical overview of all the injection techniques known to us for use in lip augmentation. There is a multitude of technical variants that can produce the desired result. In the chapters that follow, we explain in which situations a specific technique is recommended. In Chapter 9, we demonstrate 45 techniques in detail, and also list these in a table that shows the degree of difficulty, the technical details of the needle, and the indication (see Chap. 10, p. 312 ff.), providing an at-a-glance guide to the practical applications of these techniques. Fundamentally, the principle of injection is clear: a defined volume of dermal filler needs to be injected accurately into a specific location in the region being treated to achieve a particular effect. The aim is rejuvenation and/or beautification. The following four factors define the success of a treatment:

- The patient's age and skin consistency
- The selected tools (needles, cannulas)
- The selected hyaluronic acid (HA) product
- The therapist's anatomical knowledge and technical skill

The interplay of these factors, within the framework of the requirements set by the patient and the patient's budget, provides a varying degree of leeway.

The lip, especially its soft, red part, i.e. the vermillion, is covered with a very thin dermis and is highly perfused with blood. For this reason, the choice of injection method used for augmentation, hydration, and reshaping needs to be made with the appropriate degree of care. It involves selecting the injection needles, products, and procedures that are consistent with the best possible treatment outcome. The issues of skin layer and injection direction will be explored in detail in the sections that deal with specific injection techniques for the lips (see Chap. 9, p. 127 ff.).

Various different needles are available for the lip techniques that we describe, depending on indication and also on the therapist's experience. Either the sharp hypodermic needle or the blunt cannula may be used.

8.2 Injection according to Skin Layer

(→ Figs. 8.1–8.5)

8.2.1 Intradermal Injection (Superficial Augmentation)

When administering very superficial injections, the bevel of the needle should face upward. The needle is slightly visible through the skin. Once the material has been delivered, the tissue at the injection site may blanch briefly, but the blanching will disappear again after a few seconds. This layer is suitable for the treatment of the finest superficial wrinkles and lines, and for skin revitalization and hydration. Intradermal injection into the red part of the lip is not possible because the three layers of lip skin are very thin in this region, and there is no fat layer.

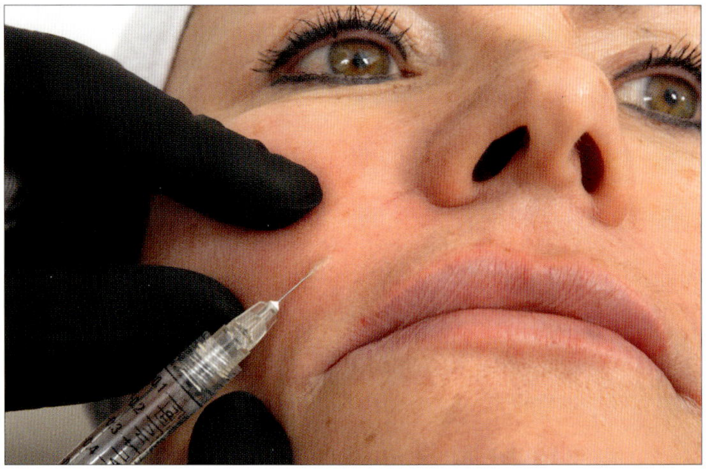

Fig. 8.1 Intradermal injection. The needle is visible through the skin. If the pores of the skin are too large, the material will leak out through them. Unwanted blanching is a common undesirable side effect (see Chap. 6.1.3, p. 86).

8.2.2 Subdermal Injection (Medium-Depth Augmentation)

The subdermal injection method may also be described as superficial subcutaneous injection. In this technique, the skin forms a slight bulge when the needle is lifted, so that it is no longer visible through the skin, although the injection is still considered to be superficial. The bevel of the needle may be turned to face upward or downward, depending on the indication. This technique is commonly used. Overcorrection causes worm-like bulges. In this layer, augmentation with highly crosslinked HA that is administered too superficially may produce a Tyndall effect (see Chap. 6.1.2, p. 86). Subdermal injection of the vermillion with a sharp needle is virtually impossible because the skin is too thin and the risk of perforation too high. For this reason, the cannula technique is used in such a case.

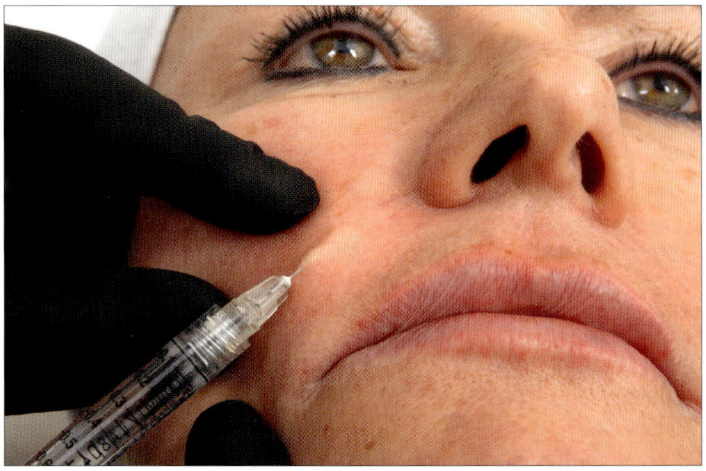

Fig. 8.2 Subdermal intracutaneous injection. The needle is no longer visible, and conspicuous augmentation is apparent.

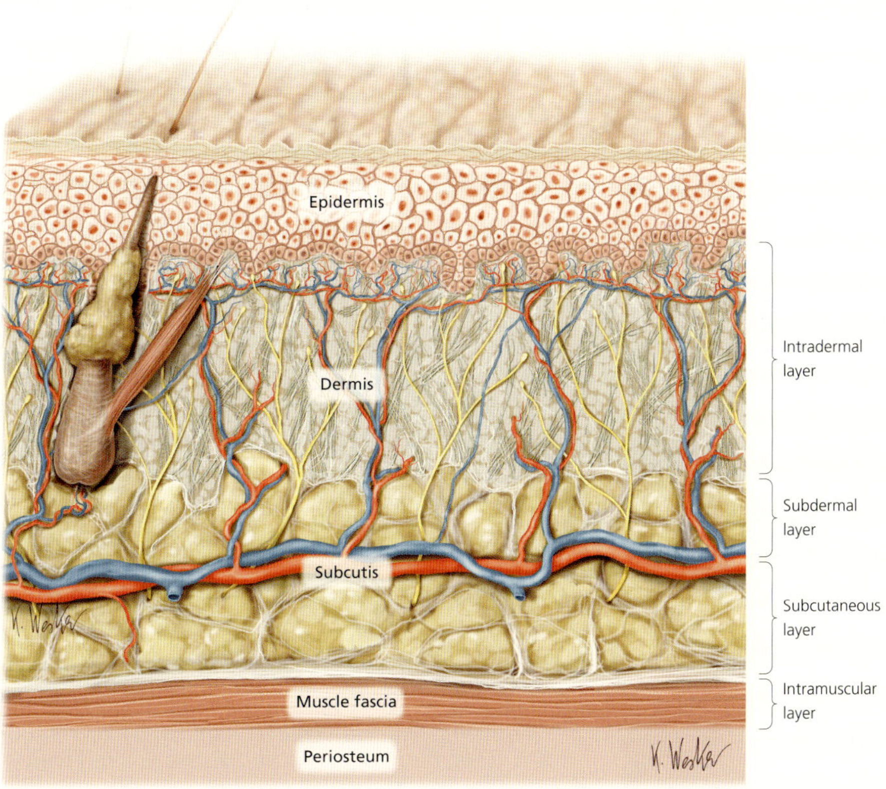

Fig. 8.3 The skin layers shown here relate to the perioral region.

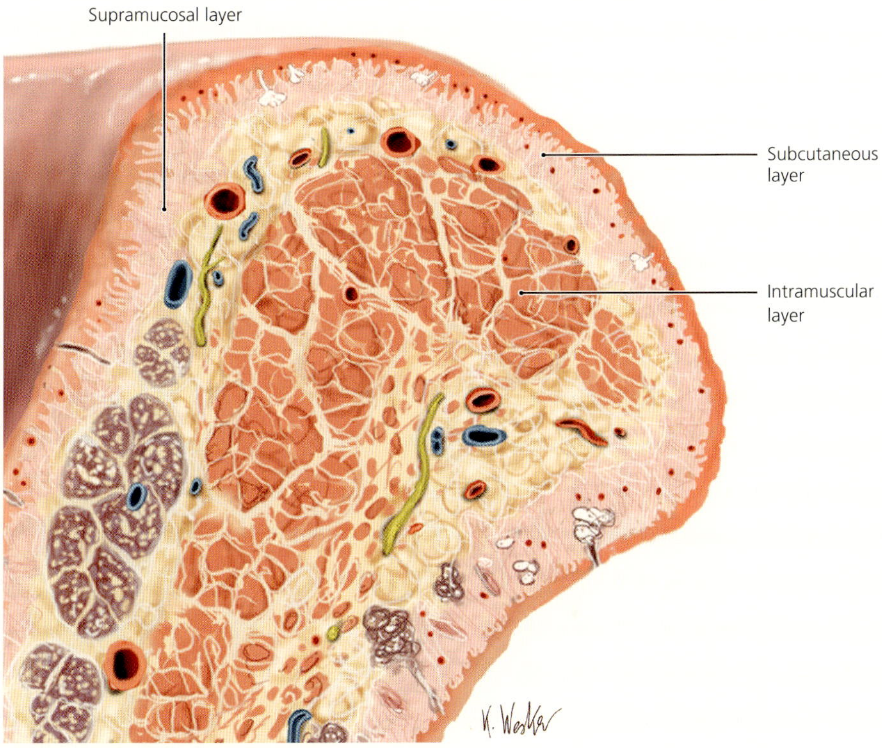

Fig. 8.4 The skin of the vermillion (red part of the lip) is very thin, and the three skin layers cannot be distinguished when administering an injection. Here, we talk of a subcutaneous, an intramuscular, and a supramucosal layer.

8.2.3 Subcutaneous/Supramucosal Injection (Deeper Augmentation)

Subcutaneous injection into the mucosa is also referred to as supramucosal. A slight bulge is visible when the needle is lifted. This layer is suitable mainly for volume build-up and deep lines. The thickness of the skin, which can amount to 2–5 mm outside the lips, can vary greatly in this area, depending on the proportion of subcutaneous tissue, which in turn influences the treatment procedure.

The deeper the injection, the more tissue lies above the material, and the more softly the tissue will be augmented. In the vermillion, "subdermal" and "subcutaneous" mean the same thing, because the skin is very thin, and the individual layers cannot be distinguished in practice.

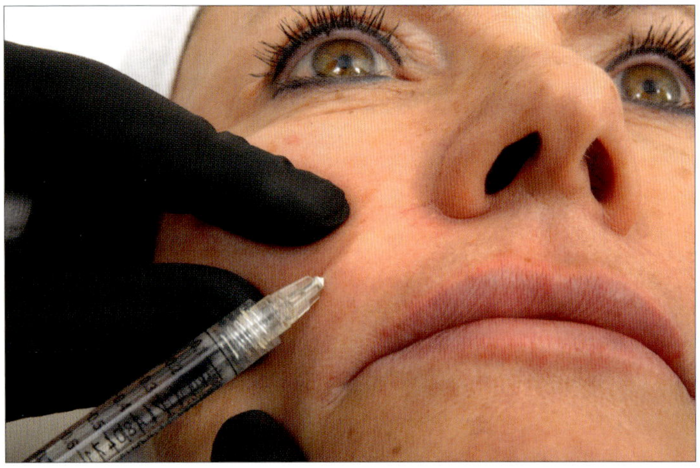

Fig. 8.5 Subcutaneous injection. The needle is no longer visible, and gentle, extensive augmentation is apparent.

8.2.4 Intramuscular Injection

This method involves injecting the material directly into the muscle. In lip augmentation, this situation is encountered when HA is injected into the orbicularis oris muscle.

8.2.5 Supraperiosteal Injection

In lip treatments, a supraperiosteal injection is administered only in the outer, perioral part of the lip when treating labiomental lines.

8.3 Injection Techniques and Effects – Sharp Needle

8.3.1 Characteristics of the Sharp Needle

The advantage of the sharp hypodermic needle is that it penetrates the tissue very easily and places the HA into the target area with the required precision. It is highly suitable for intradermal augmentation treatments and fine correction. The size most commonly used for the lip technique is 27–30G (gauge). In certain techniques, it is advisable to vary the length of the needle.

The disadvantage of the sharp needle is that it causes greater tissue trauma, making the treatment more painful for the patient. More hematomas and swellings are also produced. The sharp needle carries the risk of intravascular obstruction with an irreversible loss of blood supply. Caution is therefore needed when such needles are used.

In general, sharp injection needles of the correct size are supplied together with the HA. Should it be necessary for therapists to use their own needles, care must be taken to select the gauge appropriate for the HA, to ensure that the HA particles are not destroyed by a lumen that may be too narrow.

Once a sharp needle is used several times, it becomes blunted, which would cause more pain for the patient. For this reason, the needle needs to be changed more often if more frequent insertion is needed, e.g. in treatments using the micropuncture technique.

Whether the bevel of the needle faces up or down is generally up to the therapist. If the bevel faces up, the HA will be delivered toward the superficial dermis; this technique is used intentionally if the aim is to hydrate the skin superficially with a low- or non-crosslinked gel. With highly crosslinked HA, however, the potential disadvantage of this is that it can produce a Tyndall effect or irregularities on the skin surface. If the bevel faces down, the material is delivered downward, which is the correct procedure in treatments such as lip contour modeling: this technique stops the material from migrating into the cutaneous part of the lip if any previously damaged septa are present.

8.3.2 Point Technique

The point technique describes the precise placement of individual, adjacent injection points at short intervals. Synonyms and variants include the following: droplet technique, micro-droplet technique, multipuncture technique, multiple microinjections, micro-wheal injections, serial puncture technique. The angle of insertion is 30–45 degrees, with the needle bevel facing up. Intradermal or subdermal injection is the standard method. The technique is particularly suitable for superficial treatments or for the minor correction of irregularities.

■ Serial Point Technique (→ Fig. 8.6)

The delivery of a series of injection points placed one after the other, e.g. along a skin line or wrinkle, is referred to as the serial point technique. The serial intracutaneous delivery of small points of HA allows the lower dermis to be built up uniformly, thus correcting the tiniest hollows or other minor deficits.

■ Micropuncture Technique (→ Fig. 8.7)

This technique, also called the multi-point or nappage technique, is suitable for the superficial injection of very small volumes of HA, especially in younger skin. Tiny lines of HA are delivered sequentially at regular intervals into the intra- or subdermal layer. This technique is used with less highly crosslinked material to hydrate the tissue.

■ Micropapule Technique

The micropapule technique is a modification of the point technique, the difference being that the needle bevel faces down and the points are delivered as superficially as possible using the smallest volumes, at a distance of 2 to 3 mm. This technique is used to hydrate older skin.

Note

If highly crosslinked HA products are injected superficially into the dermis in the form of wheals, these may remain visible as irregularities and persist for up to four months or even longer. Less highly crosslinked materials should be selected for superficial injections using the point technique.

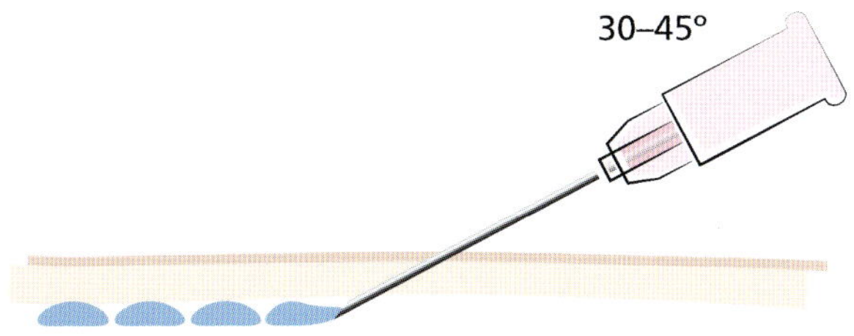

Fig. 8.6 Serial point technique.

Angle of insertion: 30–45 degrees
Needle bevel: facing up
Layer: intradermal, subdermal
Injection volume: 0.01–0.05 ml per point

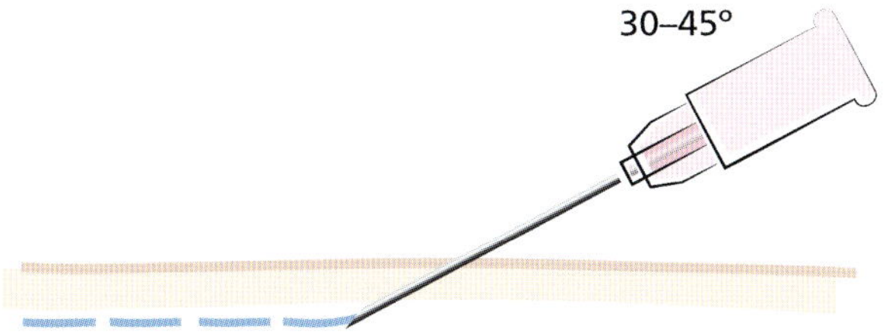

Fig. 8.7 Micropuncture technique.

Angle of insertion: 30–45 degrees
Needle bevel: facing up
Layer: intradermal, subdermal
Injection volume: 0.01 ml per point

8

8.3.3 Linear Technique

■ Tunnel Technique (→ Fig. 8.8)

The tunnel technique (linear/serial technique) consists of injections delivered along a straight line, either directly into skin lines or into the tissue. This technique may be applied in every skin layer, using any product, depending on indication.

The technique is suitable for deep injection with a gentler result, since fewer punctures with the needle are required. The full length of the needle is inserted into the apex of the wrinkle or the region that supports it. These injected lines form a single strand, which raises the wrinkle to the desired level in the skin.

■ Linear Droplet Technique (→ Fig. 8.9)

The linear droplet technique is a variant of the linear technique, the only difference is that considerably more material is delivered at the start of the linear injection than at the end, i.e. the material is injected in the form of elongated, tapering droplets.

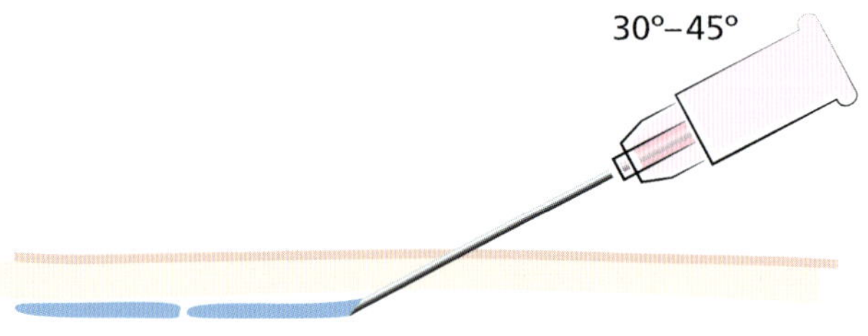

Fig. 8.8 Linear technique.

Angle of insertion: 30–45 degrees
Needle bevel: facing up
Layer: intradermal, subdermal
Direction of insertion: The "line" (approximately 10 mm) is injected along the length of the line or wrinkle in the skin.

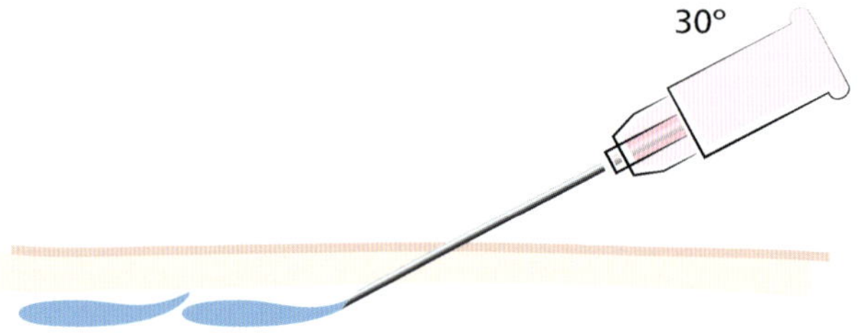

Fig. 8.9 Linear droplet technique.

Angle of insertion: 30 degrees
Needle bevel: facing up
Layer: subdermal
Direction of insertion: The material is injected into the wrinkle in a line of elongated, tapering droplets.

Note

Delivering highly crosslinked HA too superficially may produce the Tyndall effect (see Chap. 6.1.2, p. 86).

8.3.4 Fanning Technique

(→ Fig. 8.10)

The fanning technique is suitable for the coverage of a relatively large area with a limited number of puncture sites. As the name indicates, the material is introduced into the skin in a triangular fan shape. In doing so, the needle is not withdrawn fully from the skin until the treatment has been completed. The point of needle insertion forms the apex of the triangle.

As in the linear technique, the needle is introduced at the periphery of the region being augmented. Once a line of material has been injected, the needle is not withdrawn fully. Instead, its direction is changed, once again injecting the material in a linear fashion. This procedure is repeated to form a fan.

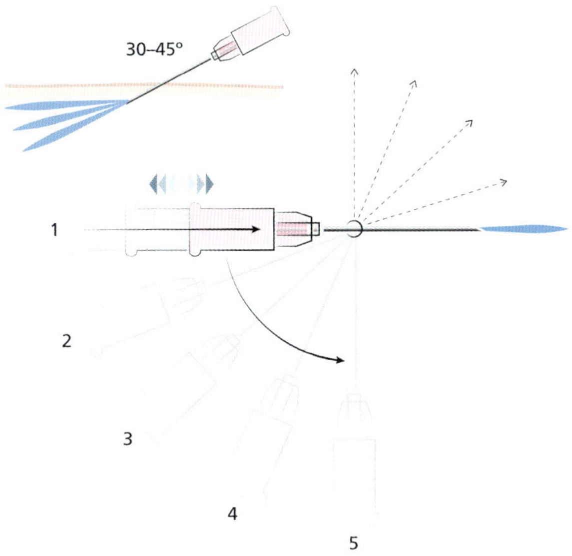

Fig. 8.10 Fanning technique.

Indication: nasolabial line, wrinkles at the oral commissures
Angle of insertion: 30–45 degrees
Needle bevel: facing up
Layer: intradermal, subdermal
Direction of insertion: "Lines" of material are injected into the area using the retrograde method (i.e. injecting the material while withdrawing the needle) in various directions.

8.3.5 Criss-Cross Technique

(→ Fig. 8.11)

The criss-cross technique is suitable for larger areas and deeper injections. It is used for the stabilization of slack tissue and for facial shaping. As in the linear technique, the needle is introduced at the periphery of the area being treated. A number of parallel lines of material are injected side by side at intervals of 5–10 mm to cover the desired area. Using the same method, additional parallel lines are injected at a 90-degree angle to the first set of lines to form a grid that reinforces the tissue.

This technique is highly suitable for the perioral lip region, i.e. for subtle volume build-up/firming of the cheeks, fine skin creases, and the revitalization of dry skin with low- or non-crosslinked HA.

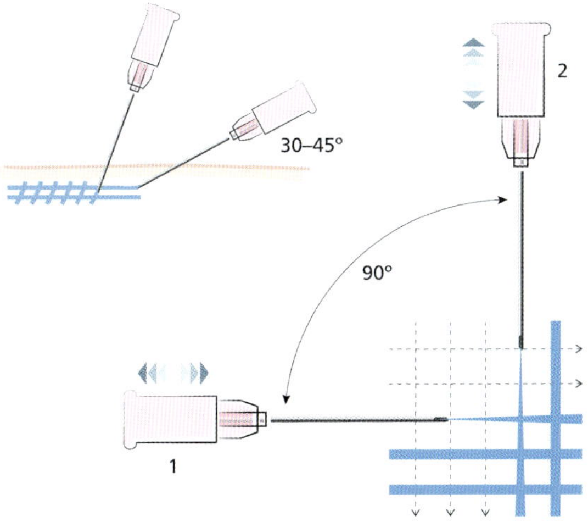

Fig. 8.11 Criss-cross technique.

Angle of insertion: 30–45 degrees
Needle bevel: facing up
Layer: intradermal, subdermal
Direction of insertion: Parallel "lines" of HA are injected at intervals of 3–5 mm along the length of the area being treated using the retrograde method. Using the same method, HA lines are then injected crossways (at a 90-degree angle to the original lines) into the area so that a grid is formed.

8

8.3.6 Bolus and Depot Technique

(→ Figs. 8.12, 8.13)

Bolus technique: The HA is injected into the skin vertically and delivered as a bolus into the center of the target area. This raises the tissue and corrects the shadow. It is advisable to grasp the area being injected between thumb and forefinger, which produces counterpressure that prevents the HA from spreading too far.

Depot technique: Volume can be built up by placing a number of boluses side by side, or the tissue stabilized by placing several depots into the target area. For larger treatment areas, distributing several small depots side by side or on top of each other can prevent the material from being encapsulated with connective tissue.

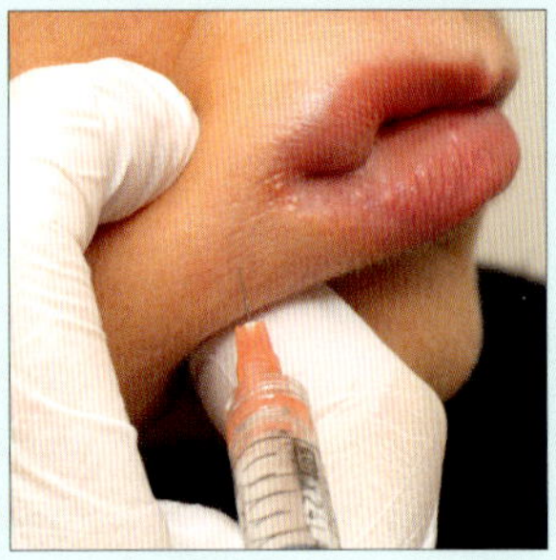

Fig. 8.13 If the therapist squeezes the outside of the cheek between the thumb and forefinger, thus producing a degree of resistance to the injection, supramucosal depots can be accurately placed into the target area where there has been a loss of substance (vertical depot technique). It is advisable to aspirate beforehand to prevent the infiltration of larger blood vessels.

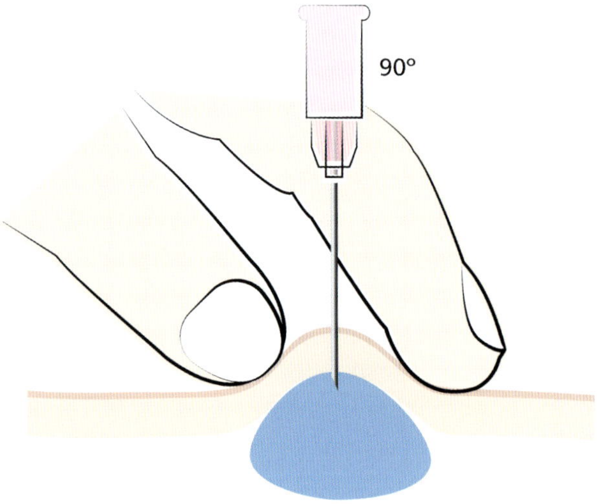

Fig. 8.12 Bolus and depot technique.

Angle of insertion: 90 degrees
Needle bevel: specified
Layer: deep and middle dermis, intracutaneous
Injection volume: 1–2 boluses of 0.05–0.1 ml using the retrograde method.

8.3.7 Sandwich Technique

(→ Fig. 8.14)

The sandwich technique is suitable for the placement of material into various tissue layers, to raise the tissue, to arrest any muscle effects or to correct shadows.

This is a form of the bolus technique involving the placement of depots in several layers. To do this, the tissue (e.g. along a marionette line) is raised between the thumb and forefinger, and the depots then injected one over the other. Different HA strengths can also be injected in layers in a similar fashion.

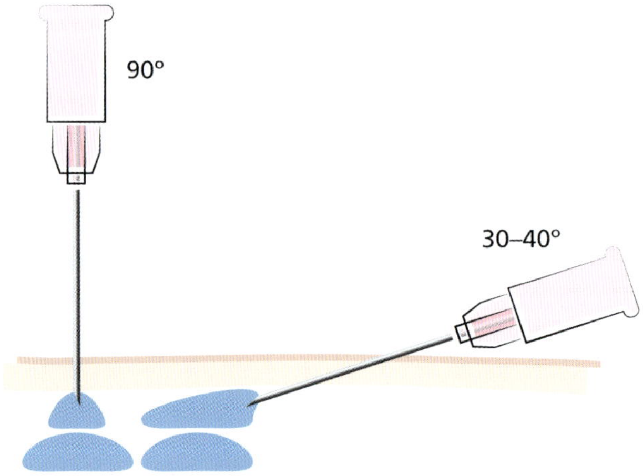

Fig. 8.14 Sandwich technique.

Angle of insertion: 30–40 and 90 degrees, respectively
Needle bevel: facing up
Layer: deep and middle dermis
Direction of insertion: The material is injected along the area in two layers, one above the other. Several depots are placed in this way.

8.3.8 Stretching Technique

(→ Fig. 8.15)

The stretching technique applies to the linear and point injection techniques for superficial correction. During the injection, the skin is stretched transversely to the direction of insertion, and as much as possible. The counterpressure of the stretched skin can prevent overcorrection and help the HA distribute more widely into the tissue. Asking an assistant to help with this can be useful.

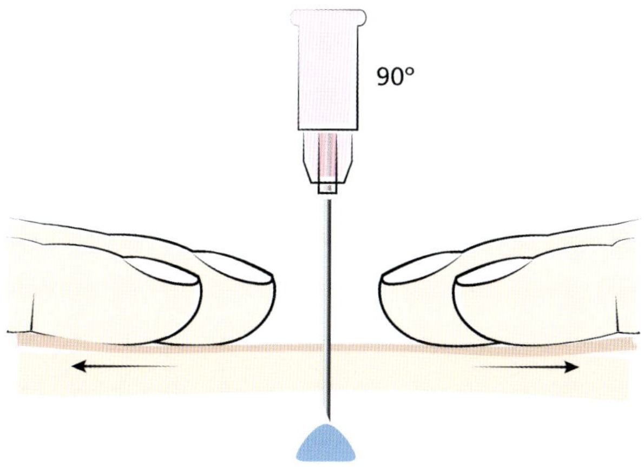

Fig. 8.15 Stretching technique.

Angle of insertion: 90 degrees

8.3.9 Compression Technique

(→ Fig. 8.16)

The compression technique applies to the linear, point, and bolus injection techniques. During the injection, the skin around the area being treated is compressed between the thumb and fore-finger. This changes the tissue pressure, limiting the distribution of the HA. The material can thus be "forced" into a specific area.

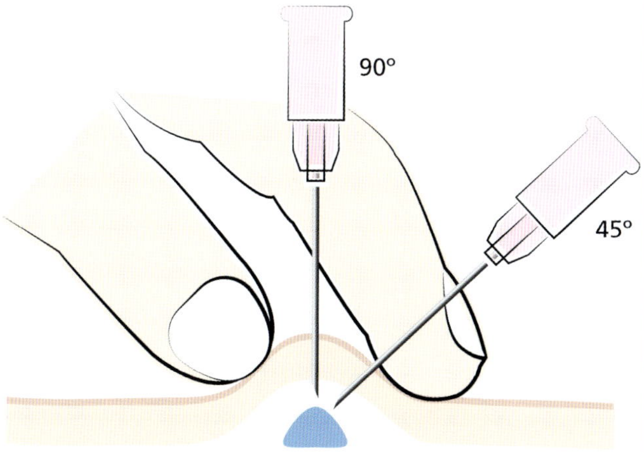

Fig. 8.16 Compression technique.

Angle of insertion: 45–90 degrees

8.3.10 Blanching Technique

(→ Fig. 8.17)

The blanching effect is when the skin turns pale under the pressure of the injected product. It is achieved by extremely superficial injection using the linear technique, with the material administered intradermally. This technique is performed only with non-crosslinked or low-crosslinked HA. The spread of the HA and the resultant displacement cause compression of the superficial vessels, resulting in skin blanching.

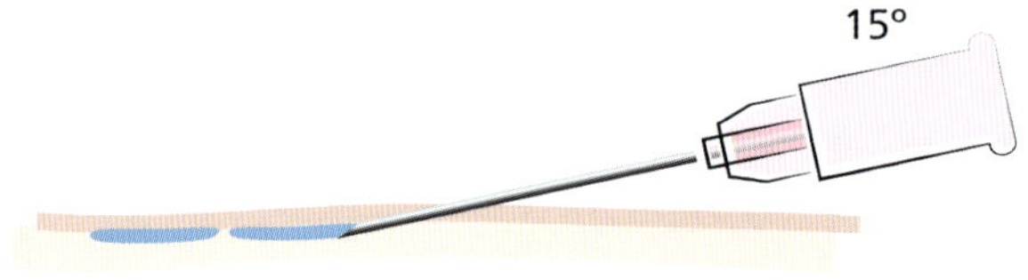

Fig. 8.17 Blanching technique.

Angle of insertion: 15 degrees
Needle bevel: facing up
Layer: intradermal
Direction of insertion: The material is delivered very superficially, longitudinally, and using the retrograde technique.

8.3.11 Fold Technique

(→ Fig. 8.18)

This technique describes the targeted application of the superficial blanching technique into the deepest cornified indentation of a skin line (see also Chap. 9.3.3, p. 178 ff.).

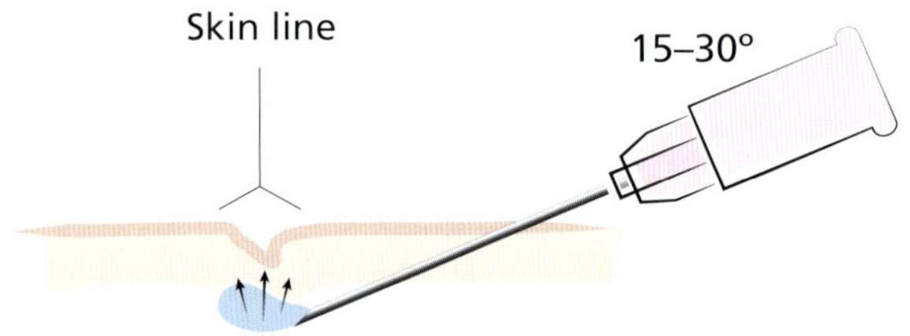

Fig. 8.18 Fold technique.

Angle of insertion: 15–30 degrees
Needle bevel: facing up
Layer: intradermal
Direction of insertion: Along the course of the apex of the skin line. The material is delivered as required.

8.3.12 Fern Pattern Technique (Tom van Eijk)

(→ Fig. 8.19)

This technique is an arrangement of the intradermal injection lines in the shape of a fern leaf, with the needle always inserted from the center of the skin line, wrinkle or linear dermal weakness (see Chap. 9.3.4, p. 182 ff.). The aim of the Fern Pattern Technique is to strengthen the dermis without adding unnecessary volume.

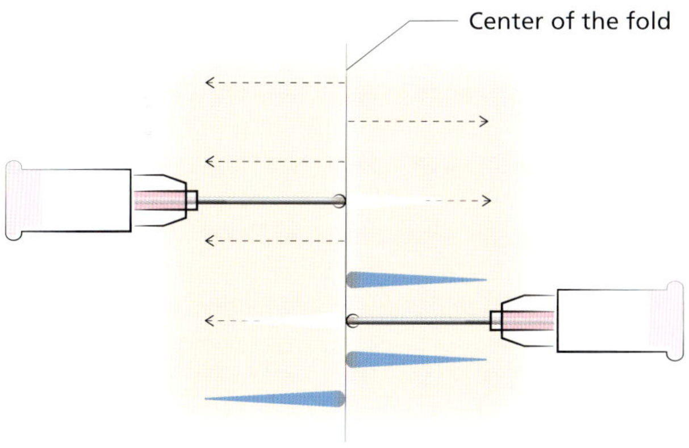

Fig. 8.19 Fern pattern technique (Tom van Eijk).

Angle of insertion: 90 degrees, turn to 0 degrees at the desired plane
Needle bevel: facing down
Layer: middermal
Direction of insertion: Across the skin line or wrinkle.

8.3.13 Fishbone Technique

(→ Fig. 8.20)

This technique blocks the force of the facial expression muscles that act on a skin line or wrinkle. It consists of an injection along the length of the wrinkle, accompanied by the injection of smaller, arcuate lines of material across the wrinkle, placed at intervals of 1 mm, to distribute the pressure that acts on the wrinkle. The result is a fishbone-shaped framework of material.

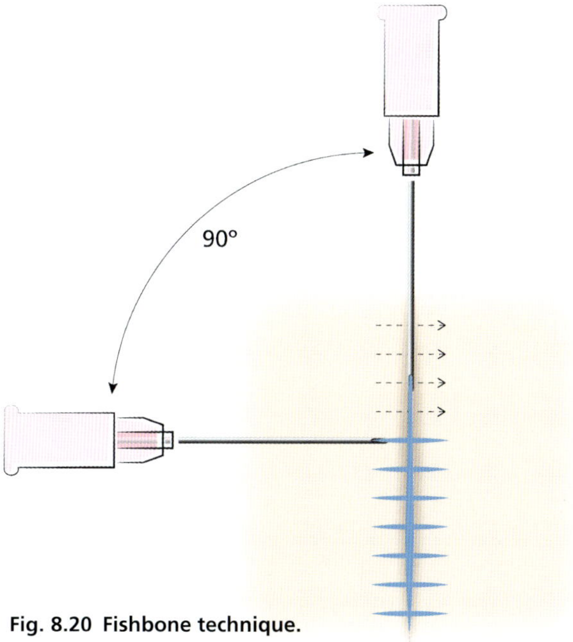

Fig. 8.20 Fishbone technique.

Angle of insertion: 30–45 degrees
Needle bevel: facing up
Layer: subdermal
Direction of insertion: Across the skin line or wrinkle.

8.4 Injection Techniques and Effects – Blunt Cannula

8.4.1 Characteristics of the Blunt Cannula

As its name indicates, the blunt cannula (→ Figs. 8.21, 8.22) is an injection needle with a rounded, blunt end and an exit hole at the side, allowing less painful penetration into tissue and muscle. As it penetrates, the cannula glides through the links between the fibers instead of cutting through tissue. This enables atraumatic tissue mobilization with a reduced risk of injuring larger blood vessels. There are several suppliers of blunt cannulas, which are available in varying sizes and different levels of flexibility (e.g. the products TSK STERi-GLIDE, Pix'L, SoftFil, Magic Needle; see manufacturers' webpage links, p. 339). Blunt cannulas differ with respect to the following features:

- **Rounding of the needle tip** (→ Fig. 8.23) – The less pointed or the more rounded the tip, the less trauma is caused by the injection; however, a rounded tip means that the cannula does not glide as well through the tissue.
- **Lumen** (→ Fig. 8.23) – The lumen opening may be located at varying distances from the tip. The advantage of an opening that is close to the tip is that the material can be placed precisely where the needle ends. This makes it possible to bring the material to the target area with greater accuracy.
- **Flexibility** – The thinner the cannula, the more flexible it is, although this can make it more difficult to change direction or to guide the needle reliably. There are also qualitative differences between the manufacturers in this respect. It is up to the therapist to decide which cannula to use for which indication. For example, we recommend a more stable, less flexible cannula for lip contour definition because it is more difficult to direct a flexible cannula along a set line against resistance.
- **Length** – Cannulas are supplied in various lengths. The length should be chosen according to the size of the area being treated. For the lips, we recommend a cannula that is not too long (25–30 mm) for better needle guidance, while a longer cannula (50 mm) is recommended for perioral treatment, so that the therapist will need as few entry points as possible.

8.4.2 Cannula Technique

The principle of injection with the cannula technique consists of treating a large area with as few entry points as possible. Figure 8.24 shows how the entire lip area on one side can be reached from just one entry point, without having to puncture a new access (windmill technique). The linear and fanning techniques are used for HA lip treatment with a cannula. The following treatments can be performed:

- Hydration/revitalization
- Contouring
- Volume build-up/hydration
- Treatment of marionette lines

Notes

Patient comfort with the blunt cannula

- The treatment is virtually painless and may therefore make anesthesia unnecessary
- Insertion is simple, as the cannula is coated with silicone
- The results are precise
- There is a low risk of swellings and hematomas.
- No downtime

Combination of the cannula technique and injection with a sharp needle

A combined method is also used. In certain indications, part of the lip is treated with a cannula and another with a sharp needle. One combination that often occurs in practice is when the lip has been augmented with the cannula technique (see Technique 20, p. 206 ff.) and small asymmetries have developed. These are then corrected with a sharp needle (see Technique 44, p. 302 ff.). The lip can also be hydrated with the cannula technique (see Technique 3, p. 136 ff.) and then augmented through the cutaneous part of the lip using a sharp needle (see Technique 26, p. 230 ff.).

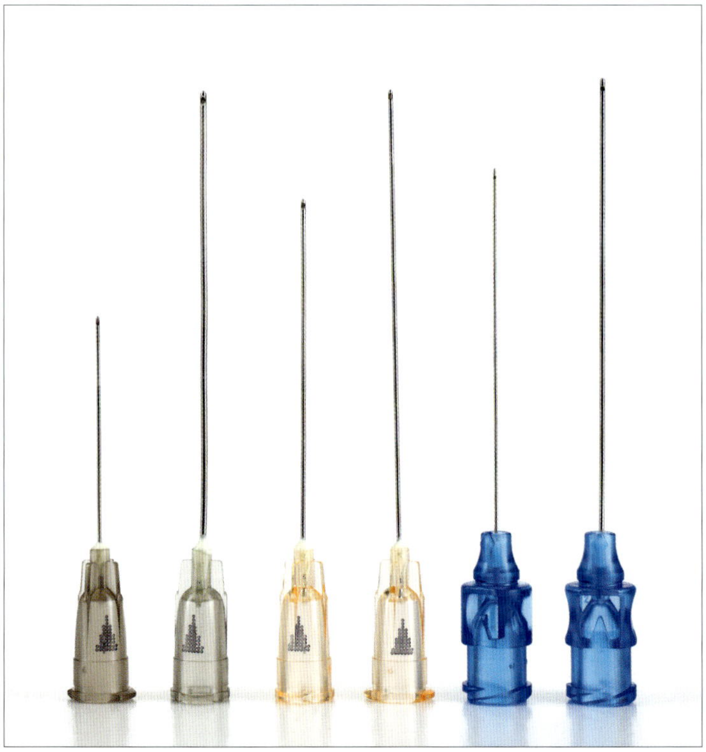

Fig. 8.21 Different qualities of blunt cannula are available from various manufacturers.

8

Characteristics of the Blunt Cannula

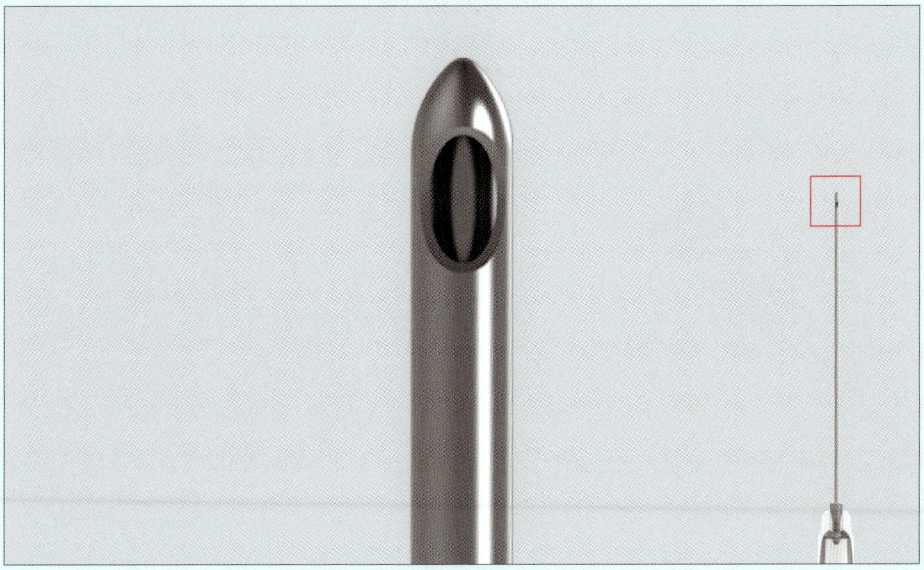

Fig. 8.22 With its blunt tip, the cannula enables atraumatic penetration and progression through the subcutaneous tissue, which is also virtually painless for the patient.

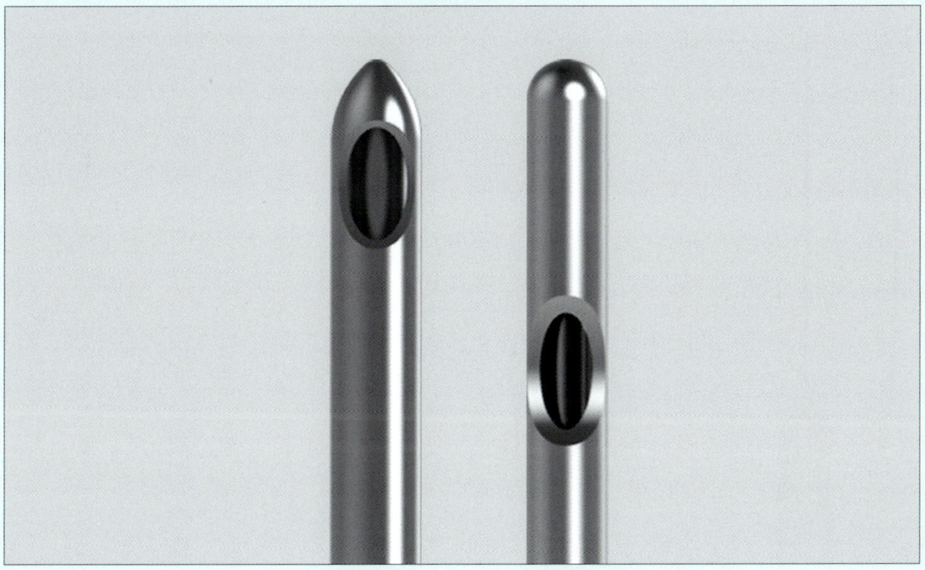

Fig. 8.23 Differences in head and lumen opening in a blunt cannula: the more pointed cannulas (left) are easier to guide because they glide through the tissue with greater ease, while the rounded cannula heads (right) cause fewer tissue injuries. The citing of the exit hole on the cannula also plays a part: the further forward this opening is located at the head of the cannula, the more precisely the material can be placed.

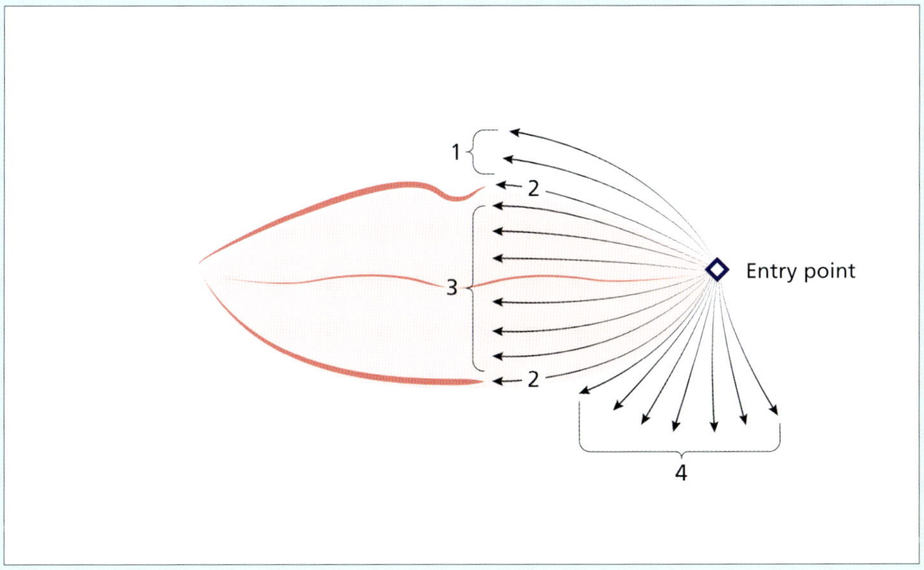

Fig. 8.24 The entire lip area on one side can be reached through a single entry point (windmill technique).

1 Hydration, revitalization
2 Contour
3 Volume, hydration
4 Marionette lines

Procedure with the Cannula Technique (→ Figs. 8.25–8.31)

- Measure the area.
- Pre-prick the cannula insertion site with a Nokor needle.
- Introduce the cannula.
- Deliver the material by either anterograde or retrograde injection.
- Change the direction of insertion of the cannula without leaving the insertion site.

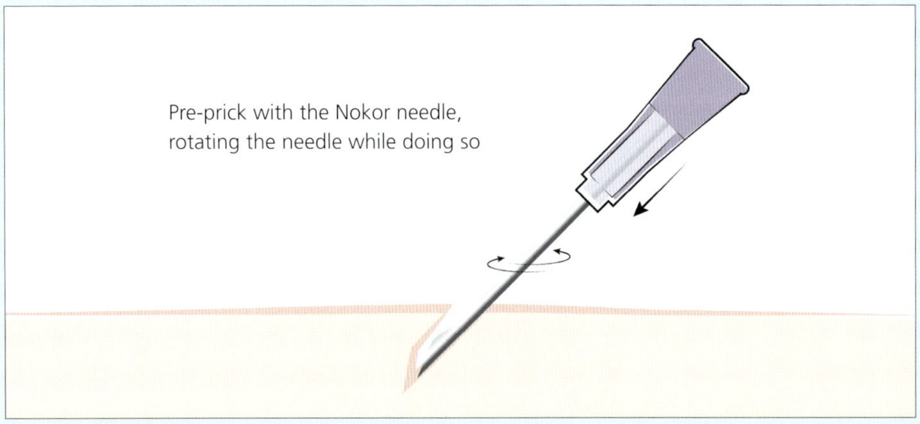

Fig. 8.25 To reach the tissue with the blunt cannula, the skin at the entry point needs to be perforated by making a point incision with a sharp needle (1–2-mm deep using a Nokor needle). Enlarge the insertion site by rotating the Nokor needle to allow the cannula to glide in more easily.

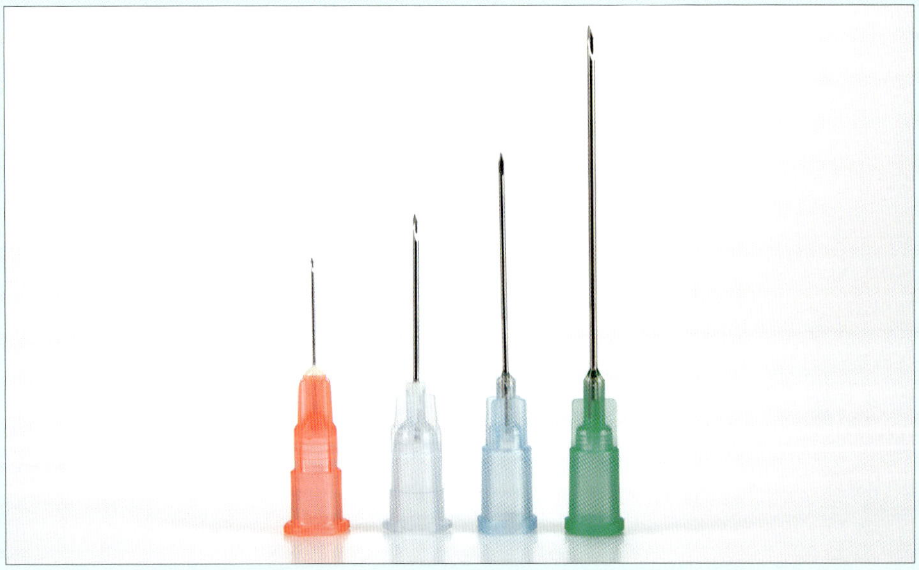

Fig. 8.26 Select a suitable Nokor needle depending on the size of the cannula. The gauge of the Nokor needle should always be one unit higher than that of the cannula, for greater ease of entry into the pre-pricked entry point.

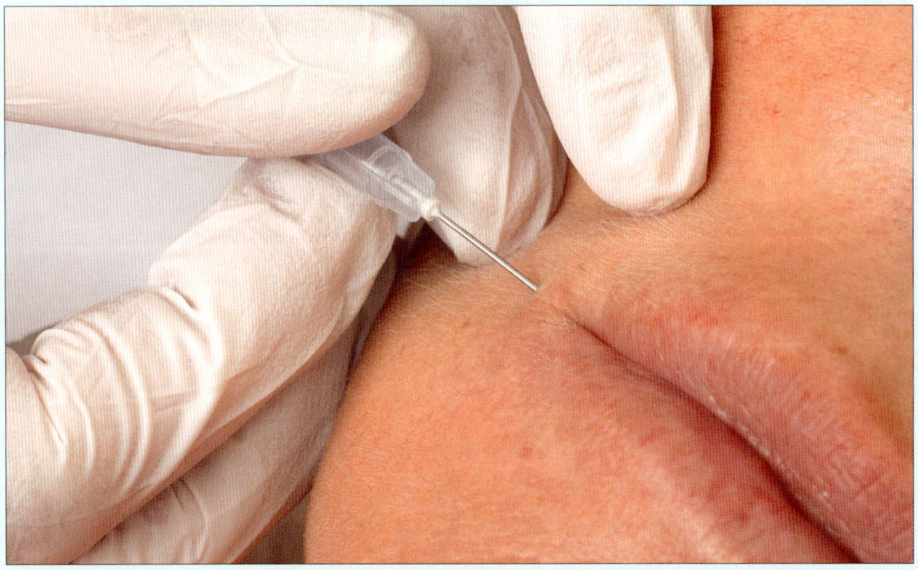

Fig. 8.27 Plunge in the tip of the Nokor needle to a depth of approximately 1–2 mm and rotate gently. To ensure that as few blood vessels as possible are damaged when pre-pricking with the Nokor needle, do not insert it any further than 2 mm into the tissue. However, it is not always possible to prevent a hematoma.

Procedure with the Cannula Technique (continued)

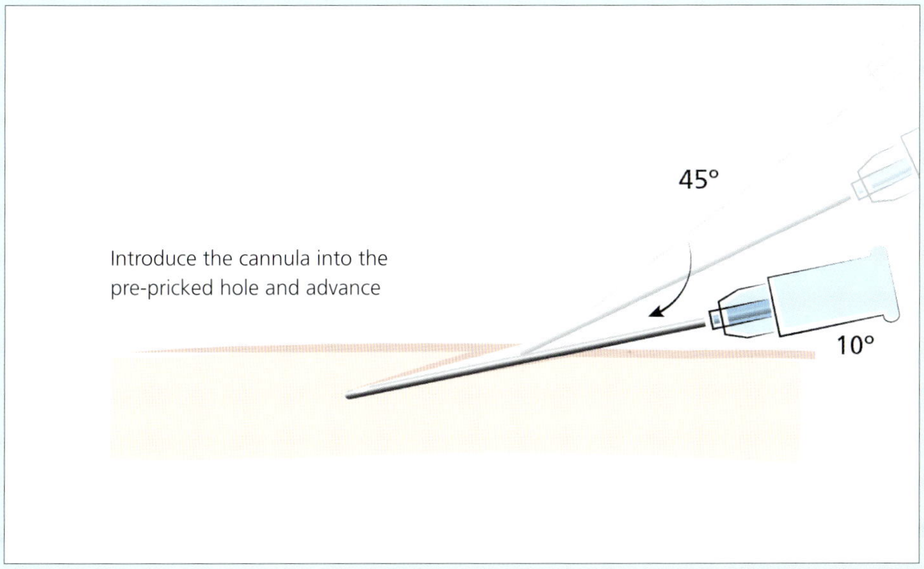

Fig. 8.28 Introduce the cannula by advancing it gently into the pre-pricked hole. Insert the first 2 mm of the cannula tip at a 45-degree angle. After this, slowly reduce the angle of insertion to 10 degrees, and then advance the cannula below the skin.

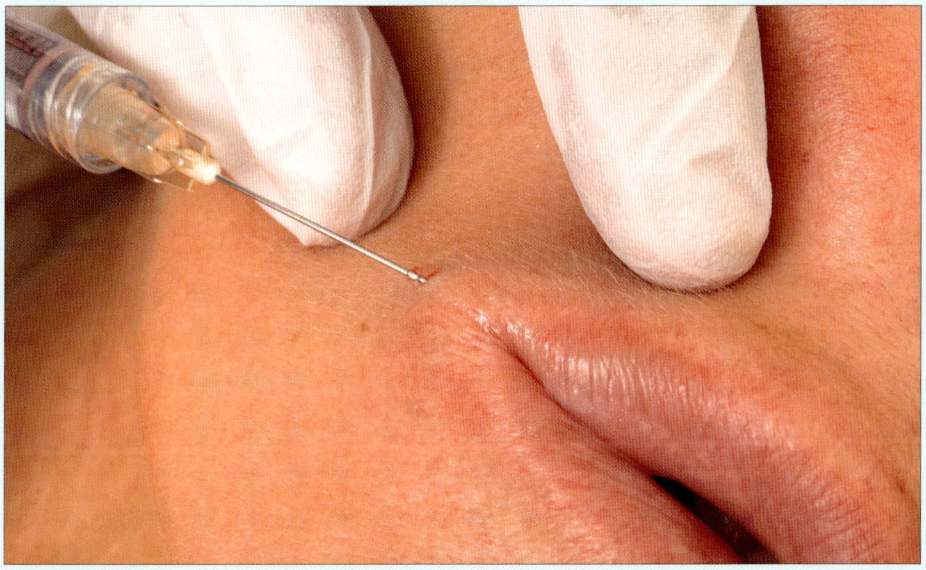

Fig. 8.29 Stretch the skin slightly with the thumb and forefinger, and the cannula will glide into the lip.

If the cannula is difficult to introduce, i.e. if there is any resistance, this should not be overcome by force. Instead, look for another layer. The cannula will glide easily through the tissue in the "correct" layer.

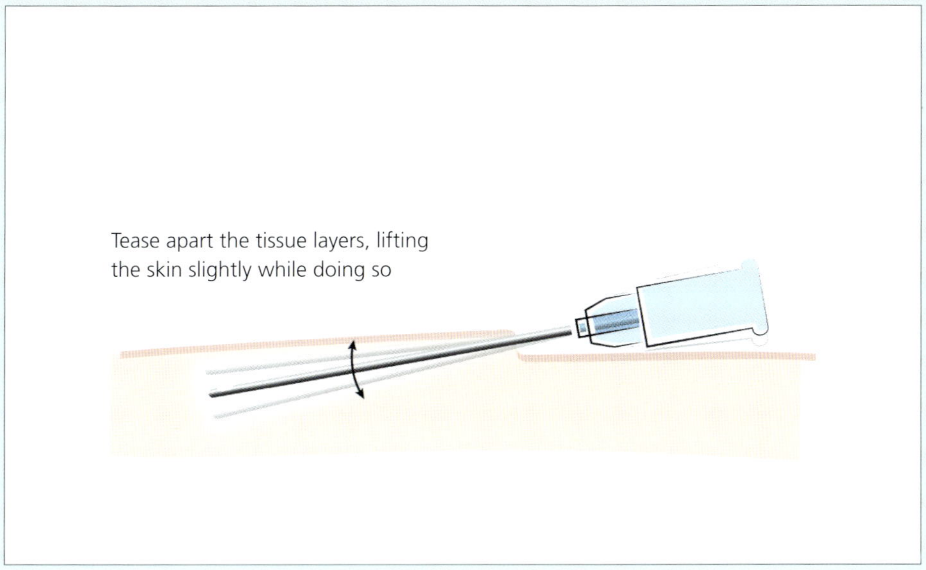

Fig. 8.30 Insert the tip of the cannula like a spatula to separate the dermis of the vermillion or the cutaneous part of the lip. This action causes the skin to be raised slightly. We call this procedure "teasing apart."

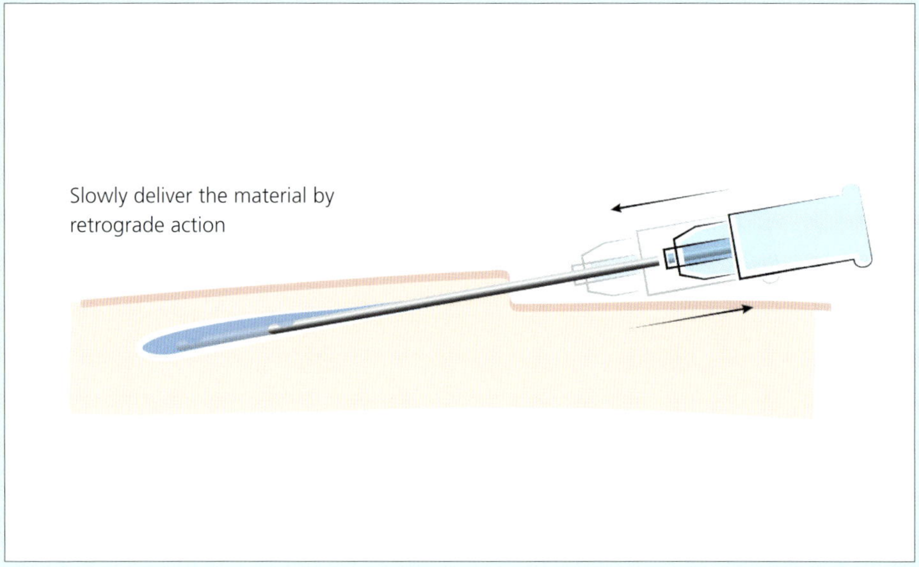

Fig. 8.31 Once the cannula has reached the target area, deliver the HA uniformly using the retrograde method.

Notes

Teasing apart the tissue layers

To treat a large area of the lip, the tip of the cannula is inserted like a spatula and moved gently backward and forward to separate the dermis of the vermillion or the cutaneous part of the lip. We refer to this as "teasing apart" the tissue layers.

Pain relief with HA containing lidocaine

Once the cannula has entered the skin, patients who are sensitive to pain may benefit from an anterograde injection of a small volume of HA with lidocaine to numb the tissue in advance. Having done this, wait for at least one minute to allow the lidocaine to act.

8.5 Technical Notes, Experience-Based Observations, and Practical Tips

Stretching – To stretch the tissue being treated, use the forefinger to take hold of the cheek and pull the tissue toward yourself. This stretches the tissue, making it easier to place the material accurately into small target areas.

Entry point (→ Figs. 8.32, 8.33) – If the opening that is pre-pricked with the Nokor needle is very small, closes up again rapidly, and is thus no longer visible, it helps to press the tissue slightly so that a droplet of blood emerges from the wound and makes the hole visible.

Apex of a skin line or wrinkle (→ Fig. 8.34) – The visible center of a wrinkle is generally associated with necrotized epithelium. Since the skin at this point kinks repeatedly, it forms what is called the fold or the apex of the wrinkle.

Avoiding blood vessels (→ Fig. 8.35) – It is virtually impossible not to injure any vessels when injecting with a sharp needle. Every injection will injure a blood vessel.

To avoid intravascular injections, it is helpful to compress the afferent vessels with a finger and to aspirate. Another thing to be avoided is the placement of oversized boluses of highly crosslinked HA in the vicinity of afferent vessels, since these boluses can cause underperfusion or even necrosis by exerting pressure on a vessel.

Cannula size – A 27–30G cannula is recommended for the underpinning of the perioral lip tissue and for augmentation of the vermillion, while a 25G cannula is recommended for the thicker dermis of the lower chin region. The thicker the cannula, the less pain it causes when gliding through the tissue.

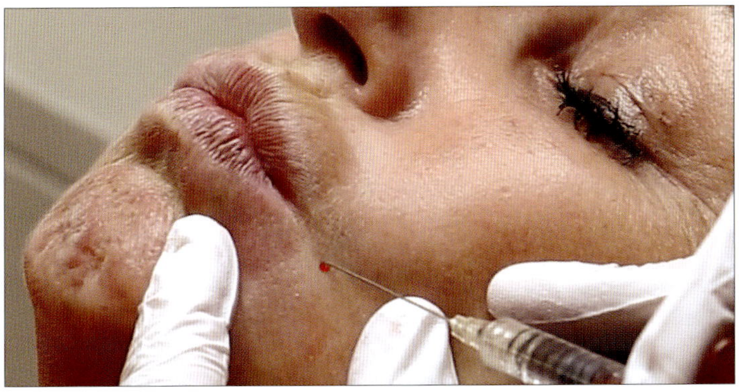

Fig. 8.32 The entry point for the cannula is revealed by a blood droplet.

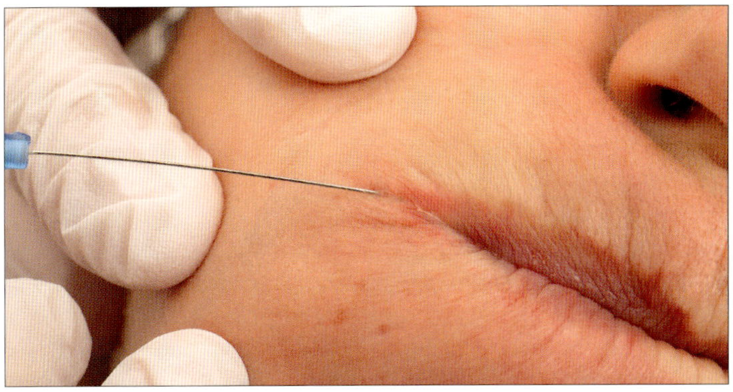

Fig. 8.33 Another option is to ask the patient the puff up the cheeks tightly. The hole becomes readily visible in the stretched tissue. With the cheek puffed up, the blunt cannula glides easily into the pre-pricked channel.

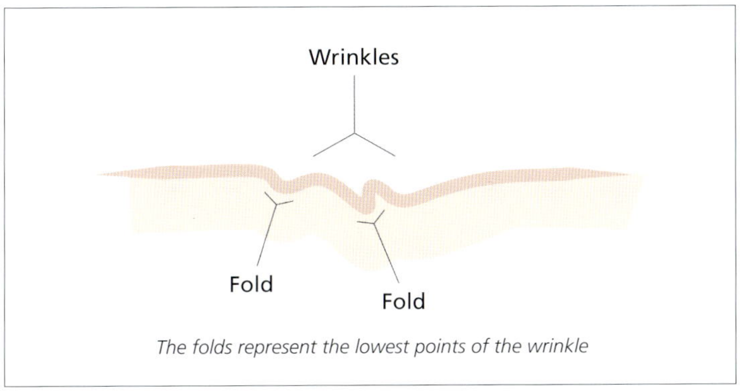

Fig. 8.34 Wrinkles of varying depth with their apices (folds).

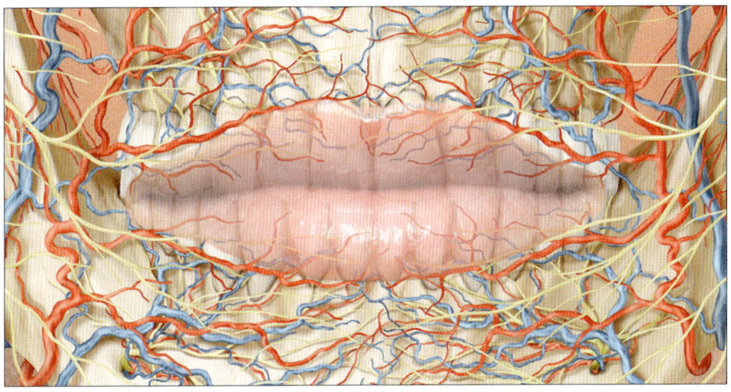

Fig. 8.35 Vascular and neural networks in the mouth region.

It is common to use fine cannulas with the intention of making the needle stab incision as small as possible, so as not to cause any unnecessary permanent scarring. The disadvantage of a fine cannula (27G–30G) is that it is difficult to insert it accurately into the pre-pricked hole. Similarly, it is not always a simple task to glide into the correct layer with a fine cannula, as it is more flexible and more difficult to control.

HA delivery – The volume of HA being delivered needs to be controlled accurately. The best way is to observe the movement of the plunger while delivering the material, and to use the scale on the syringe to record the amount of material that has been delivered into each zone of the lips. The material needs to be delivered precisely and uniformly.

Material delivery (retrograde/anterograde) (→ Fig. 8.36) **–** The material is usually delivered using the retrograde method: insert the needle, advance it up to the end of the treatment target area (1), and deliver the material uniformly while withdrawing the needle (2). No material should be delivered just before the needle is fully withdrawn, since the needle is located in the upper dermis at this point and any material delivered here would cause visible irregularities. The anterograde injection technique is used to exploit the anesthetic action of lidocaine in the filler by pre-injecting it into the tissue. To do this, insert the needle or cannula a few centimeters into the tissue, deliver one to two microdroplets (3), wait a few minutes, and then slowly advance the needle further in order to deliver a few more droplets (4), up to the end of the line to be injected. This procedure is quite prolonged, but less painful for the patient.

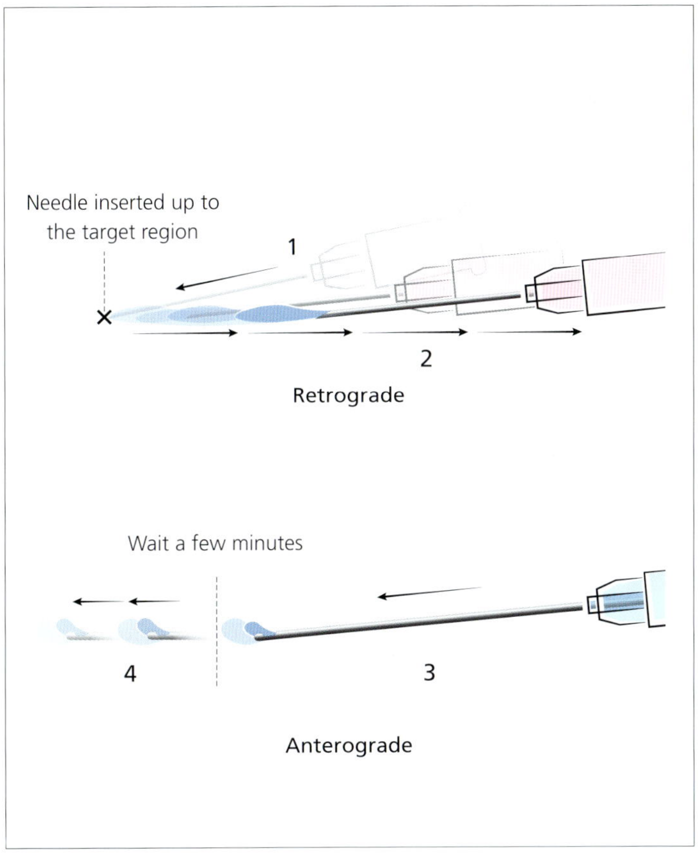

Fig. 8.36 Retrograde and anterograde delivery of material.

Loss of material – To avoid loss of material, care should be taken to stop the injection before the needle is withdrawn. Doing so can also prevent visible, unsightly bumps at the end of the needle exit hole.

Needle bevel – During the injection, the needle bevel may face either up or down, depending on what the therapist is trying to achieve: if the bevel faces up, the material migrates into the peripheral regions. Examples of how this method is used include raising tissue or hydration, and when injecting the material subdermally or intradermally. The orientation of the needle bevel plays a less significant role in the deeper skin layers. The needle bevel should face down if the therapist wants to stop the material from migrating into the cutaneous part of the lip, for example when performing a lip contouring treatment (this problem is more common if the septa have been destroyed by actinic skin damage).

Needle tip – The material is delivered at the point where the needle tip is located; the therapist needs to know this precise location if the filler is to be accurately placed. This can be checked by palpating with a finger, or visually by lifting the needle gently in the tissue.

Needle changes – Since sharp needles become blunt after several insertions, making the process more painful for the patient, the needle should be changed after 10 insertions.

Pinching – The tissue is grasped between thumb and forefinger and pinched (→ Fig. 8.37) so that the needle can be inserted into the tissue along a clear guiding line between the two digits, ensuring that neither the needle nor the material is diverted.

Calipers – This instrument is used to measure the proportions of different areas of the face relative to each other. It is also used to analyze the lips (→ Fig. 1.54, p. 35).

Tension – It is easier to inject skin that is under slight tension. It is therefore advisable to tighten the skin between the thumb and forefinger.

Sweet spots – This term is used for areas that describe the deepest point of the tissue being injected. They may include the deepest point of a skin line or wrinkle, or of an area where volume has been lost.

The injecting hand – The active hand holding the syringe should be stable while administering the injection, since the risk of non-uniform delivery is considerably greater when this hand hovers unsupported. To ensure the required stability, the little finger may be used to brace the hand against the patient's face. Figures 8.38–8.44 show various ways of supporting the active hand when treating different areas of the lip.

Support by the opposite hand – If the cannula or sharp hypodermic needle are to be guided safely and accurately through the tissue, it is important to hold the tissue in place with the opposite hand. Figures 8.37–8.44 demonstrate various ways of doing this.

Visual check – Constant visual checking during the treatment provides the therapist with a reliable way of ensuring that the treatment is proceeding as planned. For this reason, the therapist should inspect the patient repeatedly in an upright position as the treatment progresses.

Supporting the Injecting Hand with the Opposite Hand when treating Different Areas of the Lip

(→ Figs. 8.37–8.44)

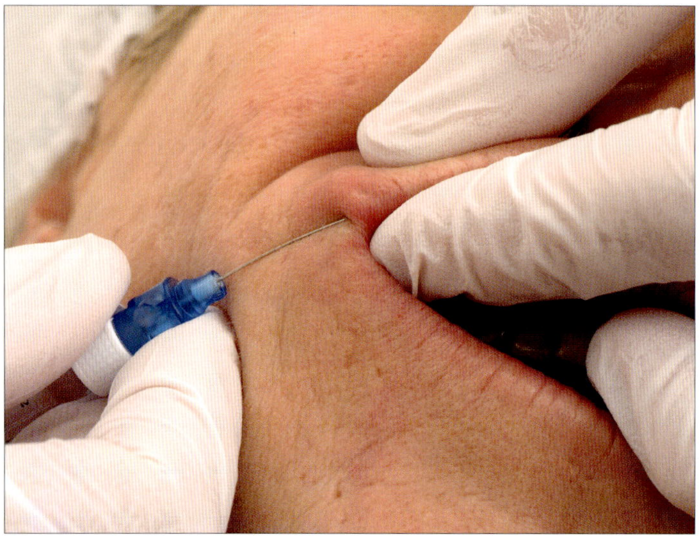

Fig. 8.37 To provide a guiding line for the cannula when it is being inserted into the lip, it is helpful to allow it to run between the thumb and forefinger.

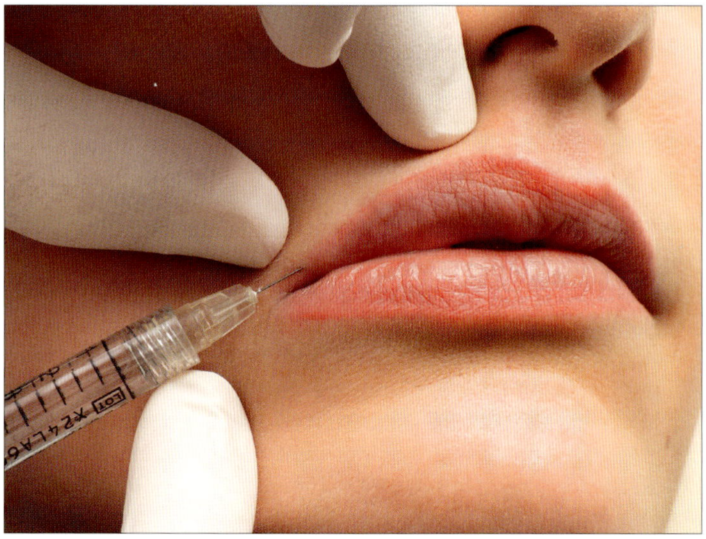

Fig. 8.38 The little finger of the active hand is supported on the patient's chin, allowing the sharp needle to be guided smoothly and securely.

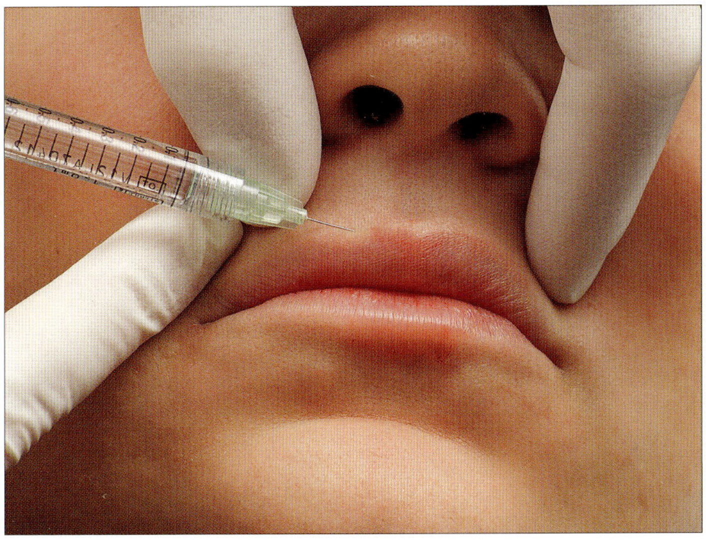

Fig. 8.39 Upper lip treatment: The little finger is supported against the lateral upper lip margin, while the other hand is used to stretch the lips until they are taut.

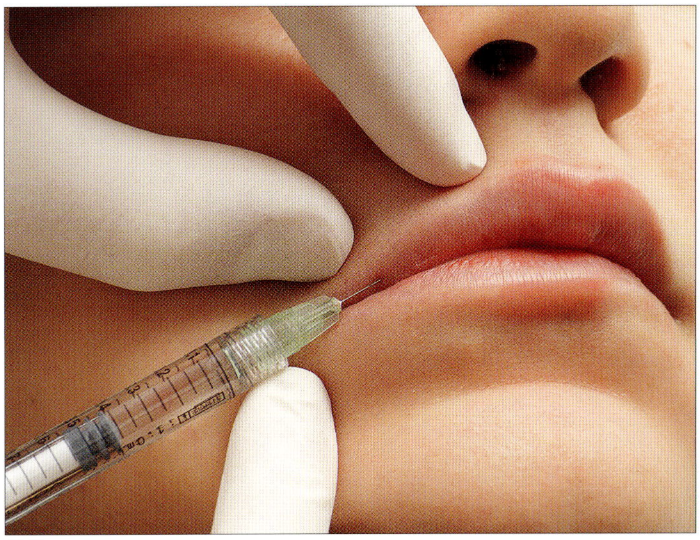

Fig. 8.40 Mouth corner treatment (upper lip): The little finger is supported against the lateral lower lip margin, while the other hand is used to stretch the lips until they are taut.

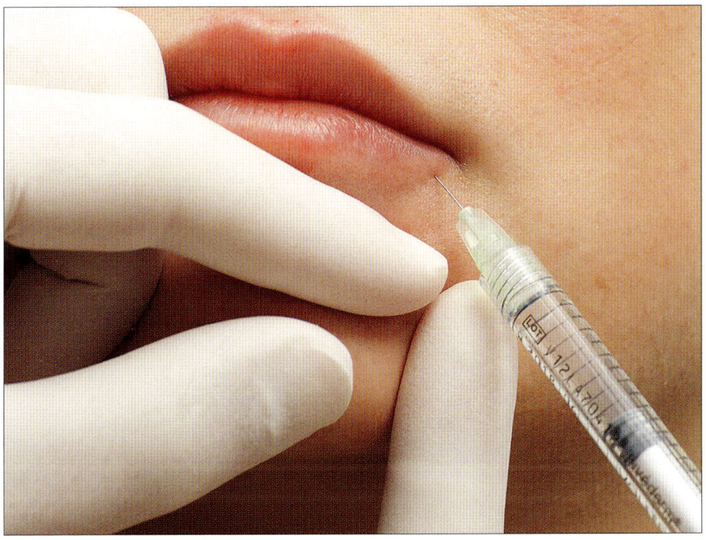

Fig. 8.41 Mouth corner treatment (upper lip): The little finger is supported against the lateral lower lip margin, while the other hand is used to stretch the skin downward until it is taut.

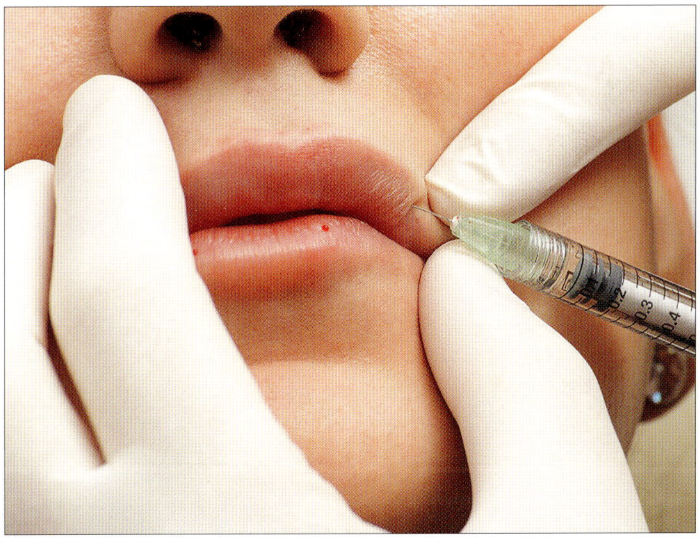

Fig. 8.42 The little finger presses gently against the upper lip margin, making the lip bulge out gently and revealing the dry/wet boundary.

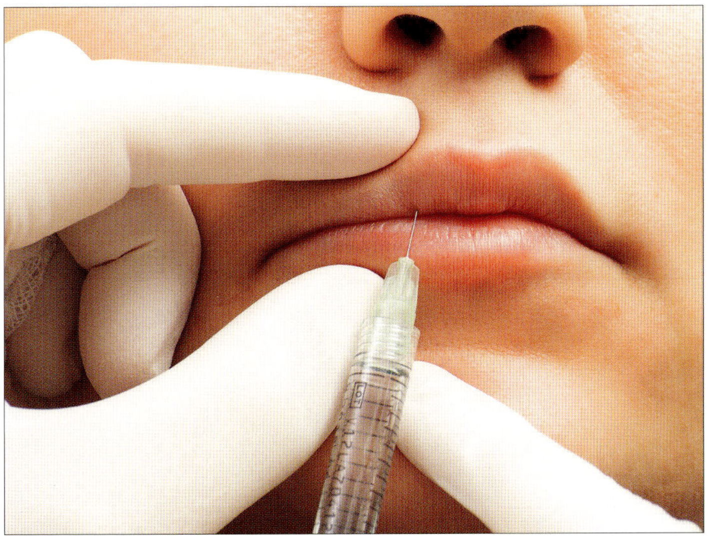

Fig. 8.43 Treating the lips near the oral fissure: The little finger is supported against the chin, while the other hand is used to gently part the lips.

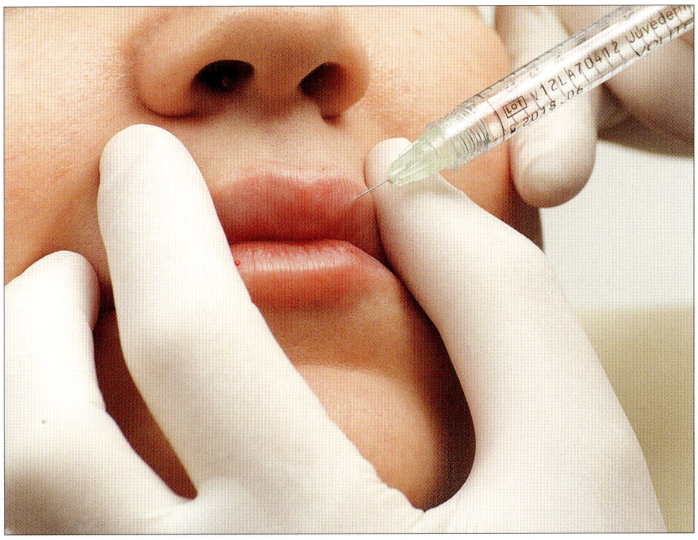

Fig. 8.44 The little finger is supported lengthways against the cheekbone, while the other hand holds the lips in place.

Illustrated Guide "The Lips"

9 45 Techniques for Lip Treatment

When treating the lips, no area can be considered in isolation; instead, the whole lip region should always be included. Here, we present a total of 45 techniques, arranged according to the following six topics:

Based on our practical experience, the particulars regarding volume of material and depth or direction of insertion as well as layer are variable by definition and should thus be interpreted only as ballpark figures. These particulars should be individually tailored according to anatomical conditions, the patient's wishes, and the treatment goal. All the techniques and particulars provided are simply recommendations and provide a demonstration of different approaches.

Our aim is to present a wide range of injection techniques and, with the aid of the many different approaches shown, to motivate therapists to find their own "best practice," to reflect on it, and to continue developing it, since esthetic work is as dynamic and ever-changing as the patient face itself.

9.1 Hydration, Revitalization

To refresh the skin, it may be hydrated and/or revitalized. Specific injection techniques are used for this. Revitalization differs from the other injection techniques in that the hyaluronic acid (HA) is injected very superficially and intradermally, and a low- or non-crosslinked HA is used. Multiple perforations of the tissue with a fine, sharp needle result in fibroblast formation with subsequent neocollagenesis (Kercher et al. 2008). If a long-term effect is to be achieved, the treatment needs to be repeated two to three times. In addition, the HA aids this tissue-rejuvenating process through its water-binding capacity. These two properties in combination "boost" the skin and revitalize it. The products used are also referred to as skin boosters. However, the skin can also be hydrated subdermally using a cannula. This results in tissue hydration only, not in fibroblast formation. The hydrating effect may be reinforced with a low-crosslinked filler, so that very subtle tissue augmentation is also achieved.

9.1.1 TECHNIQUE 1
Hydration and Revitalization – Cutaneous Part of the Lip (Sharp Needle)

The treatment goal is rehydration of the perioral region (cutaneous part of the lip), restoring its freshness and youthful vitality. Moisture depots are injected in the form of microdroplets of low- or non-crosslinked HA. This technique is performed using a sharp needle. It enables precise hydration of the lip through targeted administration of HA over an extensive area. The resultant neocollagenesis is initiated by causing multiple, minor tissue injuries with a sharp needle, which has a positive effect on general skin regeneration.

Patient Selection

- In age-related dryness and actinic skin damage of the perioral region, due to a lack of sebaceous glands or genetic factors; extrinsic and intrinsic factors also play a major role
- Younger patients who want to refresh and improve their complexion

Injection Scheme and Planning (→ Technique 1 – Figs. 1, 2)

The injections are given with a sharp needle. The tiniest amounts of HA are delivered intradermally with numerous, small injections at 1-mm intervals. This stimulates neocollagenesis and fibroblast formation, allowing the tissue to regenerate. The treatment should be repeated two to three times at intervals of 2–3 weeks.

Technique: point technique

Direction of insertion: along or across skin lines or wrinkles, regardless of their course

Layer: intradermal

Material: class "XS soft" product

Volume: 0.01 ml per point

Needle: 30–33G sharp needle

Anesthesia: lidocaine cream

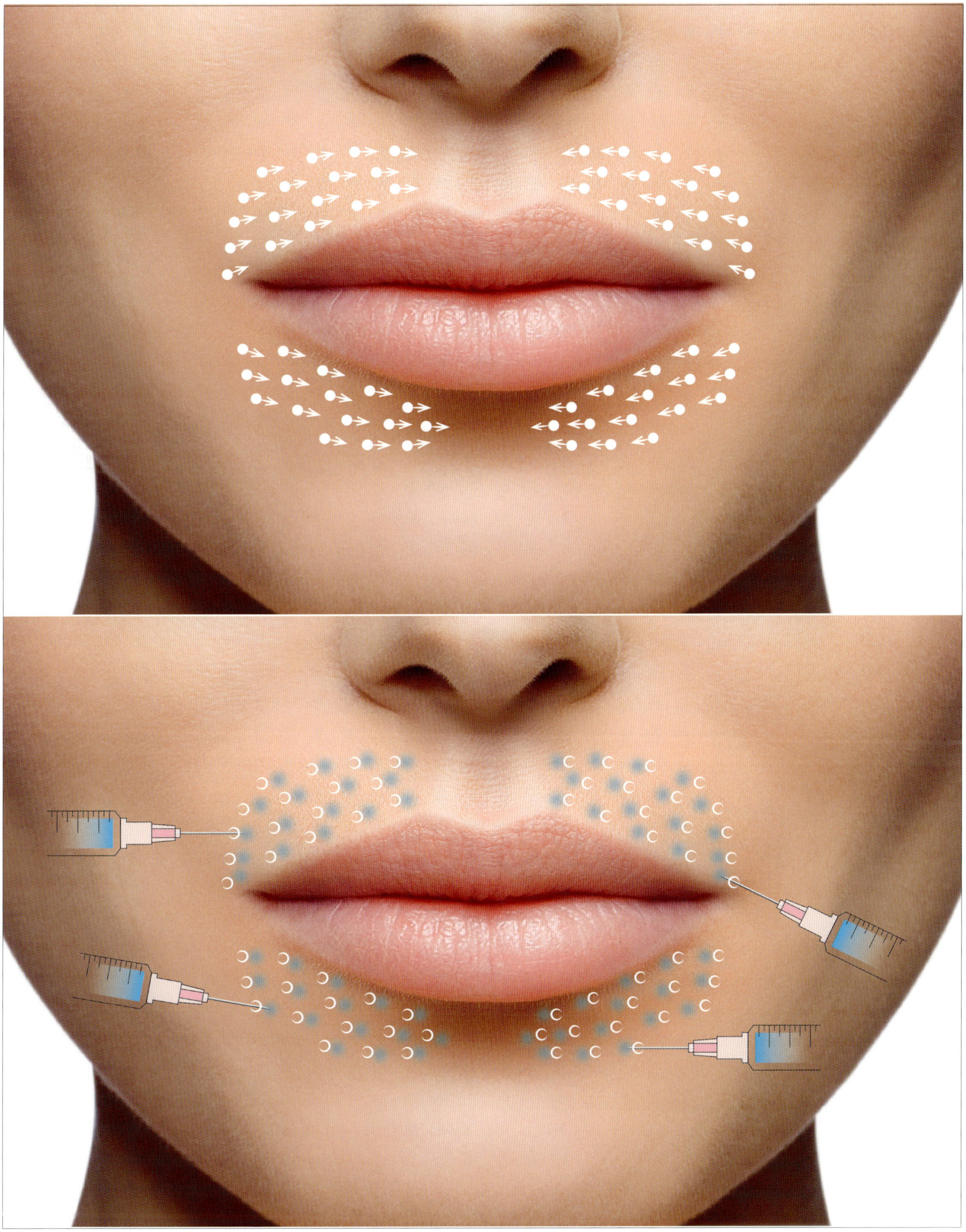

Technique 1 – Figs. 1, 2 Injection scheme and planning for hydration and revitalization – cutaneous part of the lip (sharp needle).

Treatment Method (→ Technique 1 – Figs. 3–6)

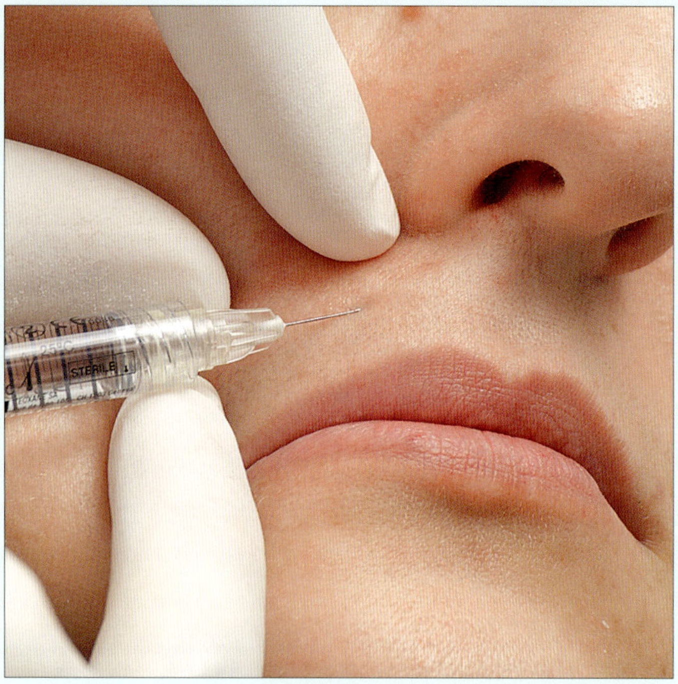

Technique 1 – Fig. 3 Insert the needle with the bevel facing up and at an angle of 15 degrees. Plunge the bevel to a depth of 1 mm. Using the point technique, inject the tiniest depots intradermally into the cutaneous region above the lip.

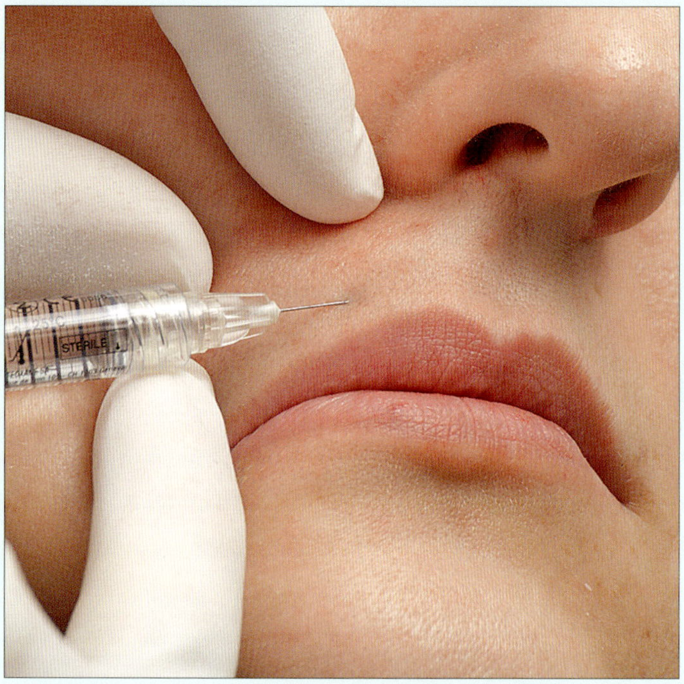

Technique 1 – Fig. 4 Inject the material into each quadrant, regardless of the course of any wrinkles or lines, since the product has no lifting capacity and merely revitalizes and hydrates the tissue.

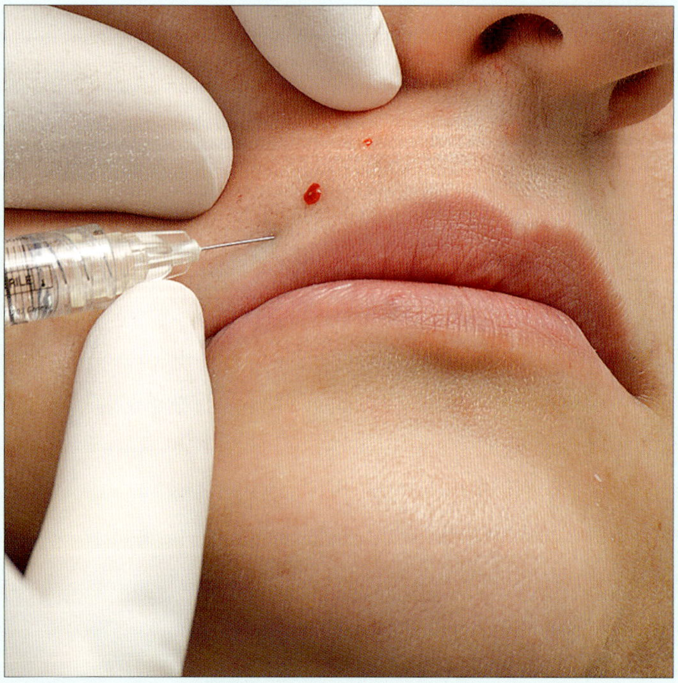

Technique 1 – Fig. 5 Repeat the procedure at intervals of 2–4 mm. Around 15–20 injections should be delivered per quadrant.

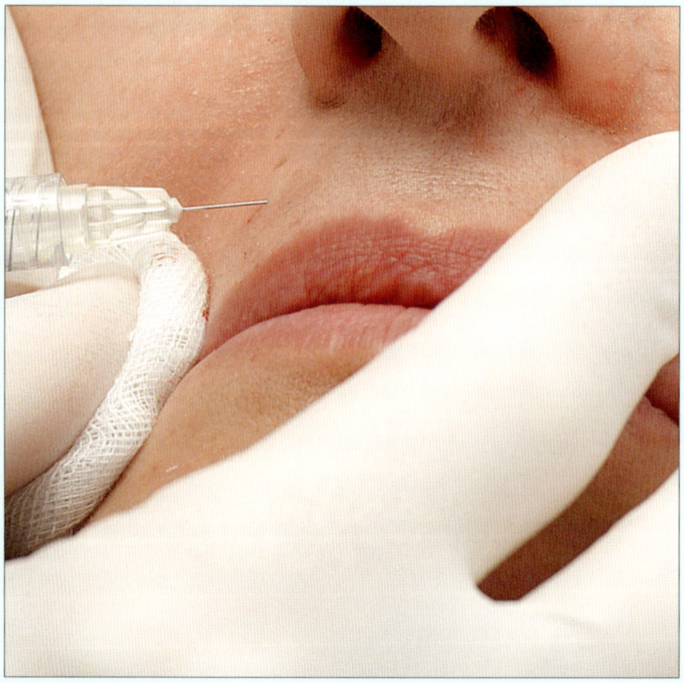

Technique 1 – Fig. 6 Stretching the skin makes the injection less painful for the patient.

Important Notes

The patient should not be on anticoagulant treatment.

Possible Side Effects

Slight reddening, rarely inflammation, mild swellings, depending on the water-binding capacity of the material

Undesirable Side Effects

Inflammation, nodules

Treatment Protocol at a Glance

- History, evaluation, and patient information
- Informed consent form
- Photo documentation: "before" images
- Analysis and marking of the areas to be treated
- Cleaning
- Thorough disinfection
- Local anesthesia if required (lidocaine cream)
- Injection technique: point technique
- Layer: intradermal
- Material: class "XS soft" product
- Volume: max. 1 ml in total
- Needle: 30–33G sharp needle
- No massage
- Cooling if required
- Heparin cream for hematomas, ibuprofen p.o., arnica
- Photo documentation: "after" images
- Advice on dos and don'ts after the procedure
- Follow-up appointment for a check-up after 8–14 days

9.1.2 TECHNIQUE 2

Hydration – Cutaneous Part of the Lip (Blunt Cannula)

The treatment goal is rehydration of the perioral region (cutaneous part of the lip), restoring its freshness and youthful vitality. The fine actinic lines are mitigated, and the skin texture improved. This is achieved by loosening the skin from the underlying orbicularis oris muscle, reducing its traction forces on the skin. The hydration with HA and the stimulation of neocollagenesis have a positive effect on skin regeneration. The effect generally sets in within 3–6 weeks, after two to three treatments.

Patient Selection

- In age-related dryness and actinic skin damage of the perioral region, due to a lack of sebaceous glands or genetic factors; extrinsic and intrinsic factors also play a major role

Injection Scheme and Planning (→ Technique 2 – Figs. 1, 2)

The injections are given with a cannula. Only one entry point is needed per side, located laterally of the mouth corner. This entry point should be selected so that all the required areas are easily accessible through it. The size of the area to be injected requires accurate calculation. The material is placed subdermally above the lip contour using the linear technique. For less damaged skin, a 27–30G cannula is used to inject the marked area with 4–6 lines of material using the fanning technique. If the skin is more severely damaged, the tissue layers throughout the area being treated should be teased apart (see Fig. 8.30, p. 121) in order to distribute the HA evenly.

Technique: fanning technique
Direction of insertion: along or across the lines produced by the orbicularis oris muscle, regardless of their course
Layer: subdermal
Material: class "XS soft" product
Volume: c. 0.1 ml per injection line, 4–6 injection lines per upper lip half
Needle: 27–30G cannula, > 25G Nokor needle
Anesthesia: lidocaine cream

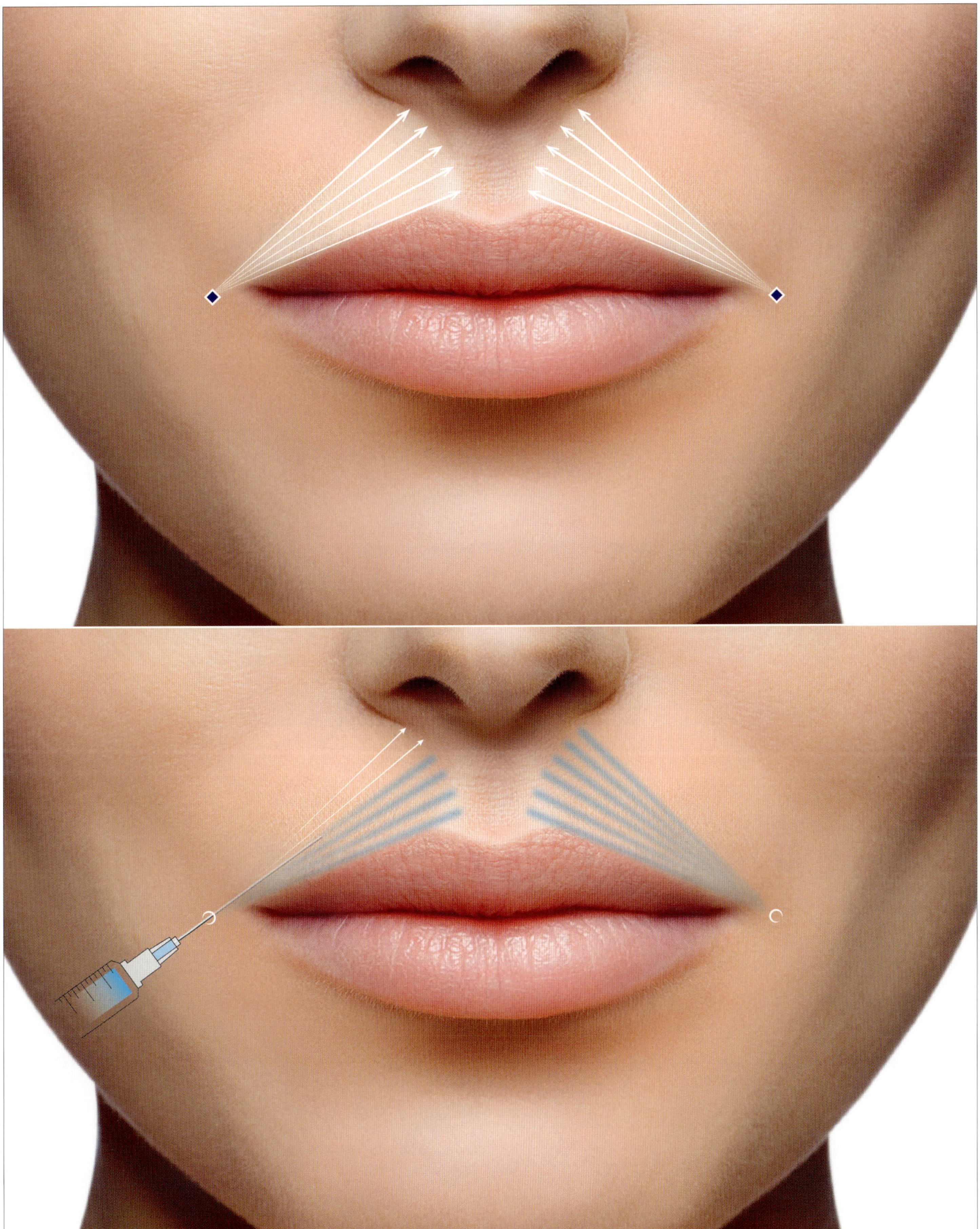

Technique 2 – Figs. 1, 2 Injection scheme and planning for hydration – cutaneous part of the lip (blunt cannula).

Treatment Method (→ Technique 2 – Figs. 3–6)

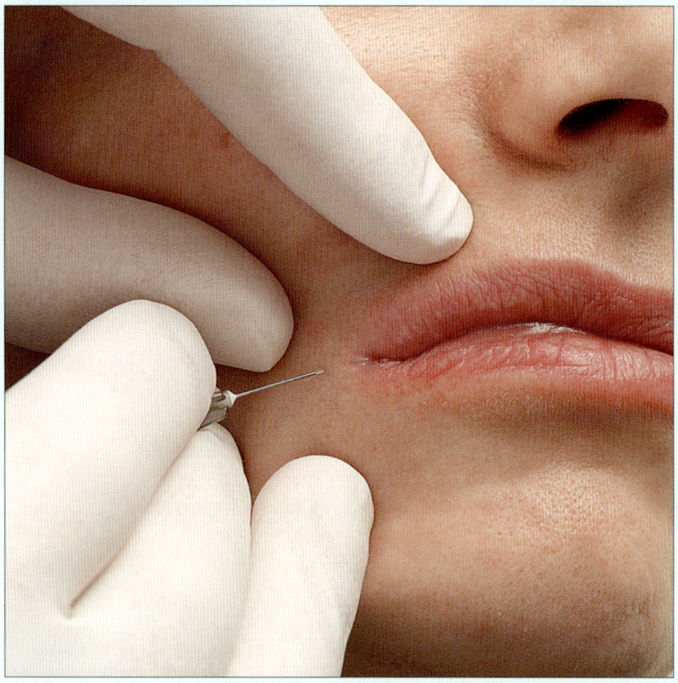

Technique 2 – Fig. 3 Stretch the skin gently, plunge the bevel of the Nokor needle to a depth of 2–3 mm, and rotate slightly to produce a round hole.

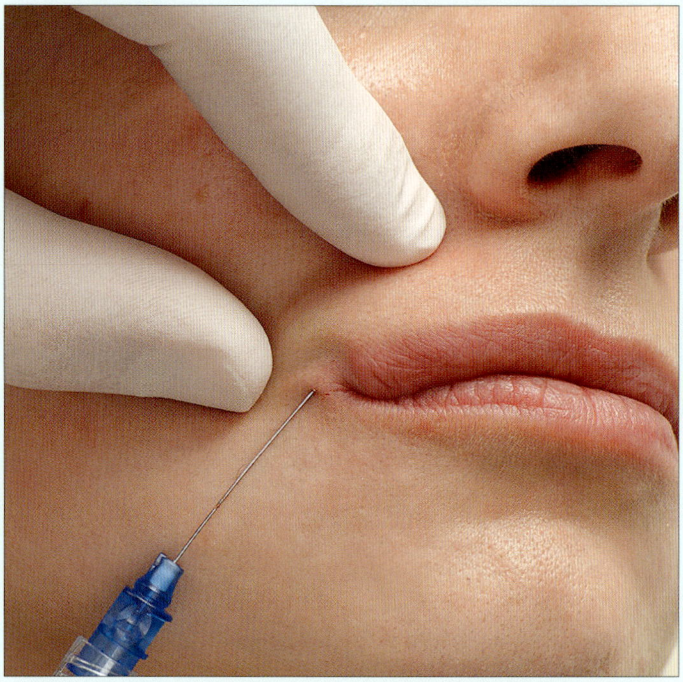

Technique 2 – Fig. 4 Carefully introduce the cannula with the skin stretched. The more flexible the cannula, the more difficult it is to control where it goes.

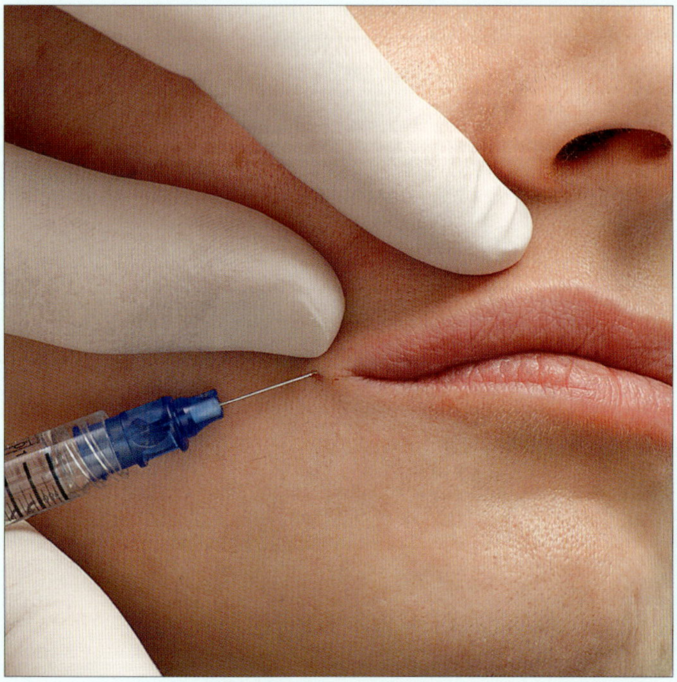

Technique 2 – Fig. 5 Advance the cannula forward up to the philtrum and tease apart the skin layers.

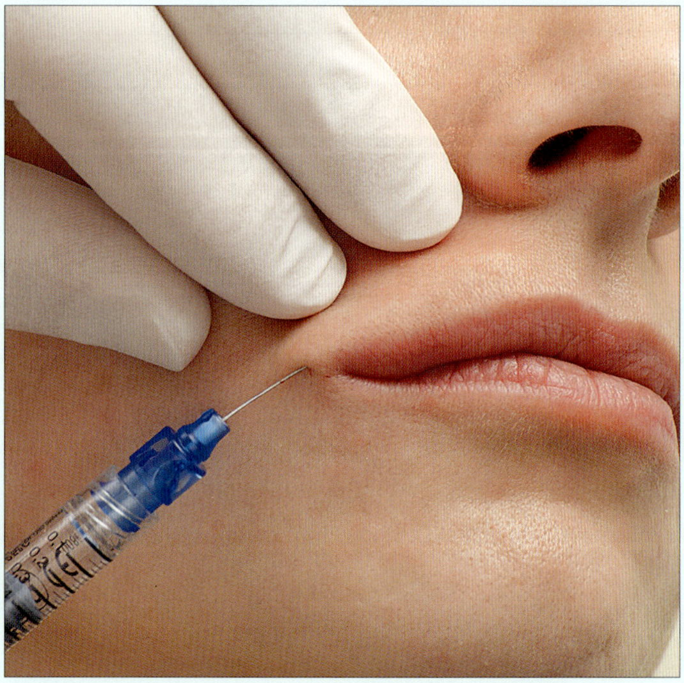

Technique 2 – Fig. 6 Deliver the material uniformly by retrograde injection in several adjacent lines, then massage the entire treatment area gently. Due to the water-binding capacity of the HA, the tissue will swell for up to 1–4 days after the treatment.

Important Notes

Possible Side Effects

Slight reddening, rarely inflammation, mild to more severe swellings for 1–4 days

Undesirable Side Effects

Overcorrection with resultant alteration of the oral region, non-uniform delivery of material with resultant asymmetry

Treatment Protocol at a Glance

- History, evaluation, and patient information
- Informed consent form
- Photo documentation: "before" images
- Analysis and marking of the areas to be treated
- Cleaning
- Thorough disinfection
- Local anesthesia if required (lidocaine cream)
- Injection technique: fanning technique
- Layer: subdermal
- Material: class "XS soft" product
- Volume: 1–1.5 ml in total
- Needle: 27–30G cannula, > 25G Nokor needle
- Gentle massage may be applied
- Cooling if required
- Heparin cream for hematomas, ibuprofen p.o., arnica
- Photo documentation: "after" images
- Advice on dos and don'ts after the procedure
- Follow-up appointment for a check-up after 8–14 days

9.1.3 TECHNIQUE 3
Hydration – Vermillion (Blunt Cannula)

The treatment goal is rehydration and revitalization of the entire surface of the vermillion. Lip dryness manifests as flaking, wrinkling, and sometimes also cracks in the skin surface. Hydration greatly improves the texture of the skin of the lips.

Patient Selection

- Patients with age-related lip dryness due to a lack of sebaceous glands or genetic factors; extrinsic and intrinsic factors also play a major role

Injection Scheme and Planning (→ Technique 3 – Figs. 1, 2)

The injections are given using the cannula technique. The first puncture is made c. 5 mm from the mouth corner. After pre-pricking with the sharp needle (Nokor needle), the therapist carefully introduces the blunt cannula into the pre-pricked opening. The injections with the cannula are delivered very superficially into the subcutaneous layer. The skin layers are teased apart carefully to form an extensive hollow space below the vermillion. The material is introduced under mobilization and placed throughout the vermillion (horizontal mobilizing technique with the cannula). The low-crosslinked HA is delivered slowly and uniformly and is distributed with the aid of gentle massage.

Technique: linear technique
Direction of insertion: along the body of the muscle
Layer: subcutaneous throughout the vermillion
Material: class "XS to S soft" product
Volume: max. 0.5 ml per upper and lower lip, 1.0 ml in total
Needle: 27–30G cannula, > 25G Nokor needle
Anesthesia: lidocaine cream, conduction anesthesia

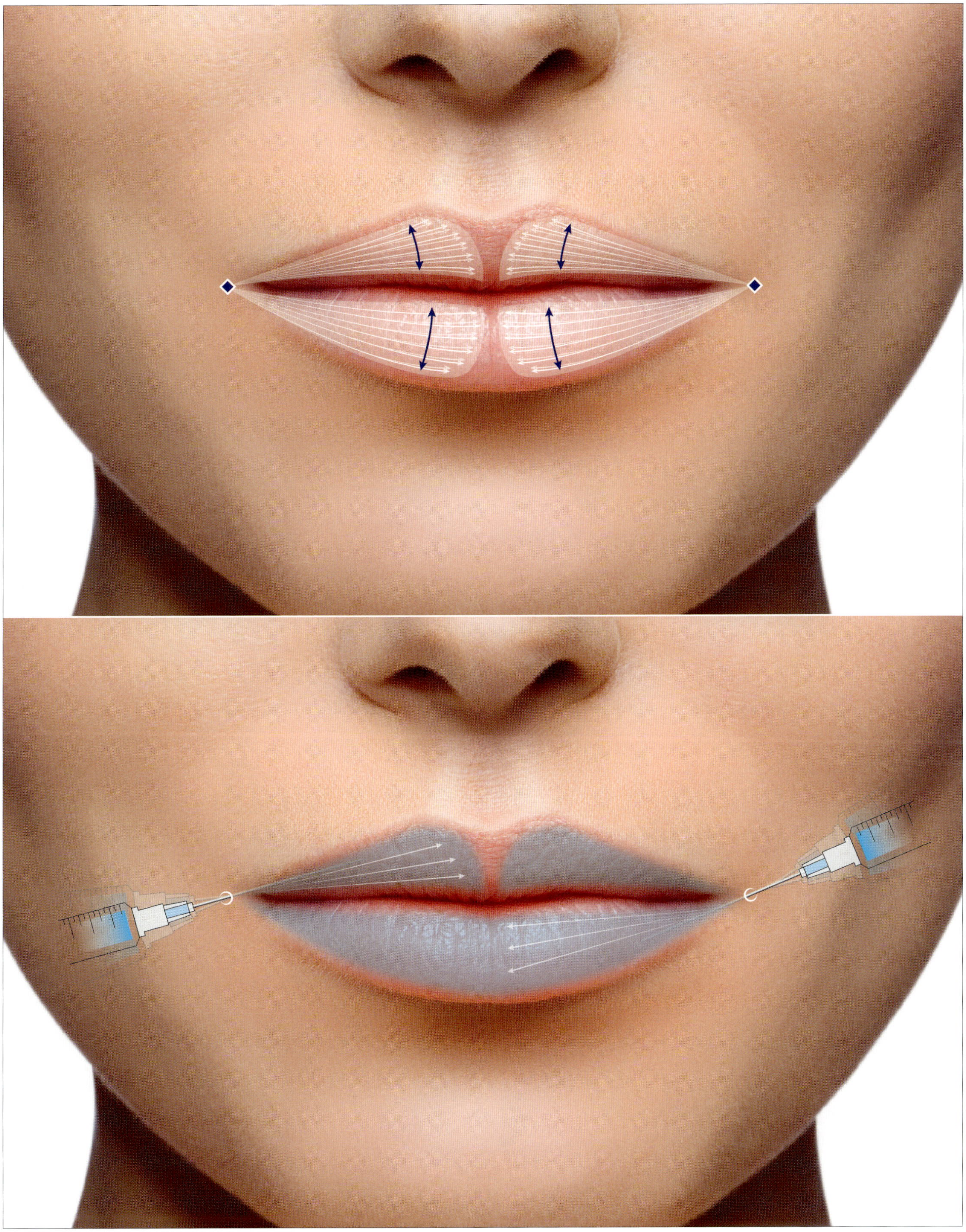

Technique 3 – Figs. 1, 2 Injection scheme and planning for hydration – vermillion (blunt cannula).

Treatment Method (→ Technique 3 – Figs. 3–7)

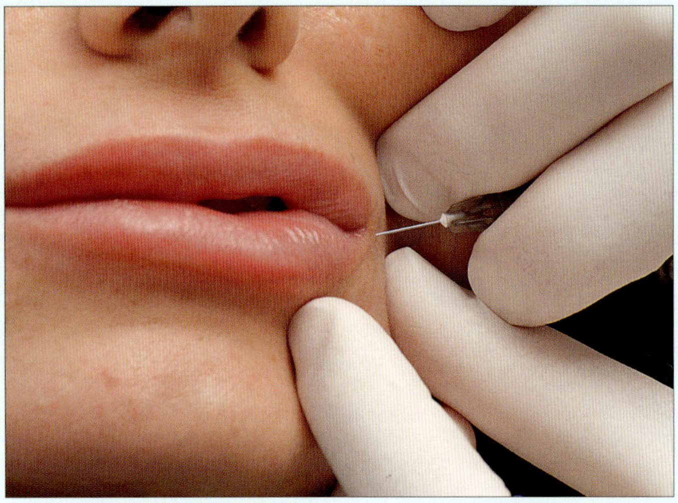

Technique 3 – Fig. 3 Pre-prick with the Nokor needle c. 3–5 mm from the mouth corner. Plunge in the Nokor needle to a depth of 2–3 mm.

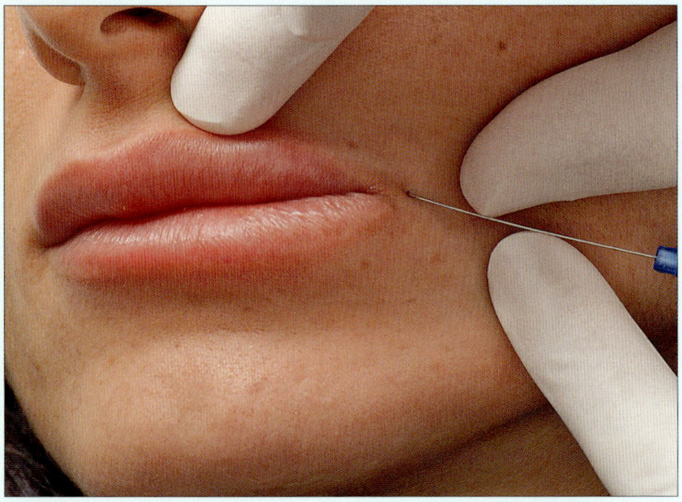

Technique 3 – Fig. 4 Stretching the lip makes it easier to guide the cannula up to the center of the lip. If the cannula is pushed against the skin of the lip, the therapist can check the location of its tip.

9

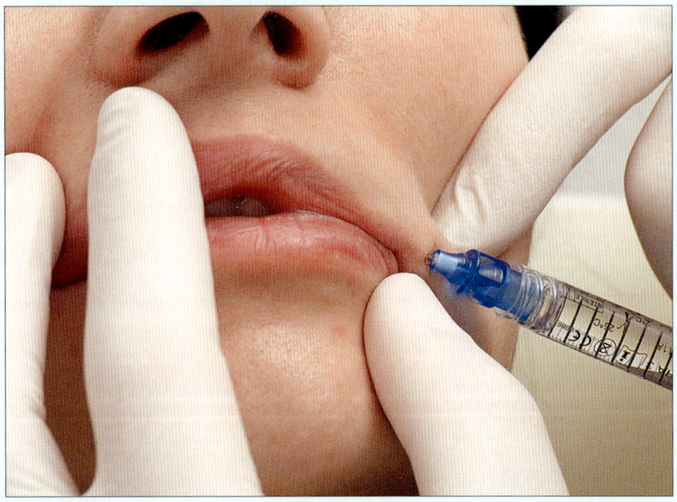

Technique 3 – Fig. 5 Scrape the cannula tip against the skin of the lip to detach it from the muscle along several parallel lines. After this, inject the material very superficially and uniformly, with continuous visual monitoring.

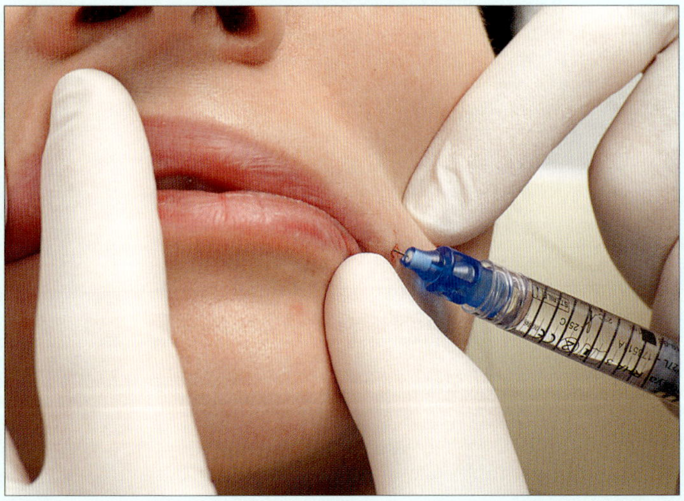

Technique 3 – Fig. 6 The bulge produced by the delivered HA allows the therapist to see exactly where the material is located.

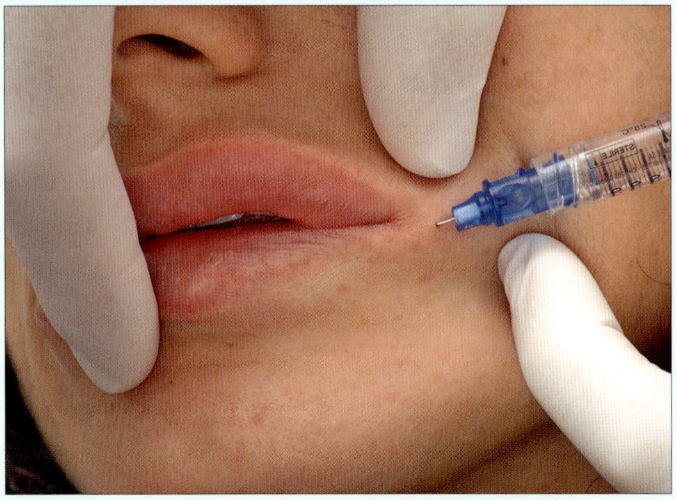

Technique 3 – Fig. 7 Use the same procedure in the lower lip. Gently pushing the cannula tip against the tissue indicates its location.

Important Notes

Since a fine, and thus very flexible, cannula (27–30G) is used in this technique, it is slightly more difficult to maintain the direction of insertion. We therefore recommend squeezing the lip gently between thumb and forefinger and delivering the material into the channel formed in this way. This stops the cannula from escaping. The procedure should be repeated until the whole of the desired target area has been treated. Several adjacent channels should be created to form an extensive hollow area below the skin of the lip, which is then filled with low-crosslinked HA.

Possible Side Effects

Slight reddening, rarely inflammation, rarely hematomas, mild to more severe swellings

Undesirable Side Effects

Overcorrection with resultant alteration of the oral region, asymmetry due to non-uniform delivery of material

Treatment Protocol at a Glance

- History, evaluation, and patient information
- Informed consent form
- Photo documentation: "before" images
- Analysis and marking of the areas to be treated
- Cleaning
- Thorough disinfection
- Local anesthesia (lidocaine cream), conduction anesthesia
- Injection technique: linear technique, several lines per upper and lower lip
- Layer: subcutaneous
- Material: class "XS to S soft" product
- Volume: max. 1 ml in total
- Needle: 27–30G cannula, > 25G Nokor needle
- Gentle massage may be applied
- Cooling if required
- Heparin cream for hematomas, ibuprofen p.o., arnica
- Photo documentation: "after" images
- Advice on dos and don'ts after the procedure
- Follow-up appointment for a check-up after 8–14 days

9.1.4 TECHNIQUE 4

Revitalization – Vermillion (according to Patrick Trevidic, Sharp Needle)

The goal is to supply moisture to the lips, to intensify the shape of their contours, and, as a secondary effect, to reduce the fine perioral wrinkles slightly. This technique is performed using a sharp needle. It enables precise hydration of the lips by the targeted administration of HA over the whole area. Furthermore, it induces neocollagenesis, resulting from the multiple, minor tissue injuries produced by perforation with the sharp needle.

Patient Selection

- In age-related lip dryness due to a lack of sebaceous glands or genetic factors; extrinsic and intrinsic factors also play a major role

Injection Scheme and Planning (→ Technique 4 – Figs. 1, 2)

The lips are treated using the fanning technique. The Cupid's bow is only included in the treatment if it exhibits tiny wrinkles due to dryness. Each fan consists of three lines with one entry point. These lines should be marked during the preoperative analysis. In this procedure, it is essential to ensure uniform distribution of the material.

The technique is painful for the patient and causes severe swellings. For this reason, we recommend conduction anesthesia in highly sensitive patients. Low-crosslinked HA may also be injected if the patient wants a more long-term result.

Technique: fanning technique
Direction of insertion: along and across the body of the muscle
Layer: subcutaneously over the orbicularis oris muscle
Material: class "XS soft" product
Volume: max. 0.1 ml per fan, 1.0 ml in total
Needle: 27G sharp needle, 20 mm
Anesthesia: lidocaine cream, conduction anesthesia

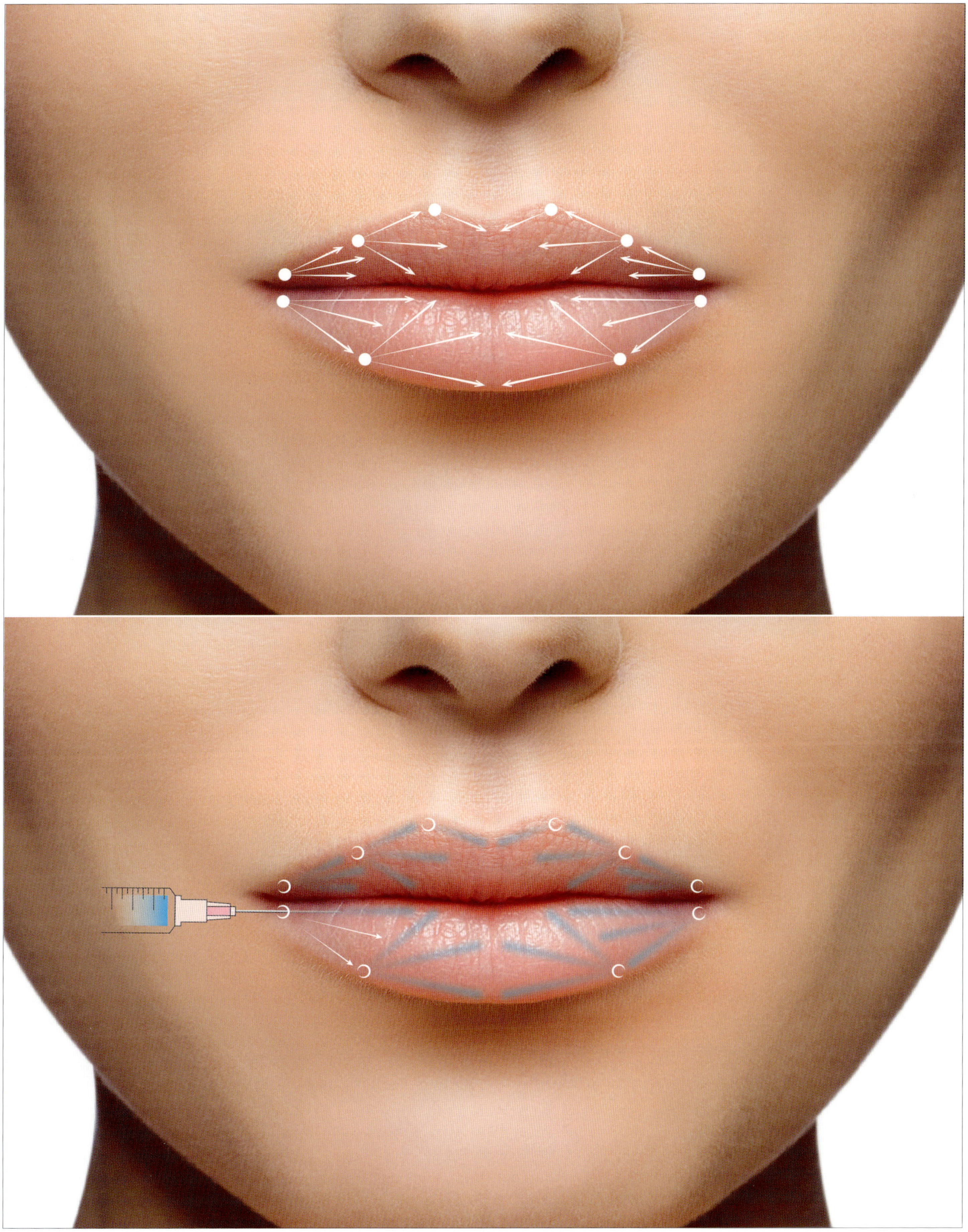

Technique 4 – Figs. 1, 2 Injection scheme and planning for revitalization – vermillion (according to Patrick Trevidic, sharp needle).

Treatment Method (→ Technique 4 – Figs. 3, 4)

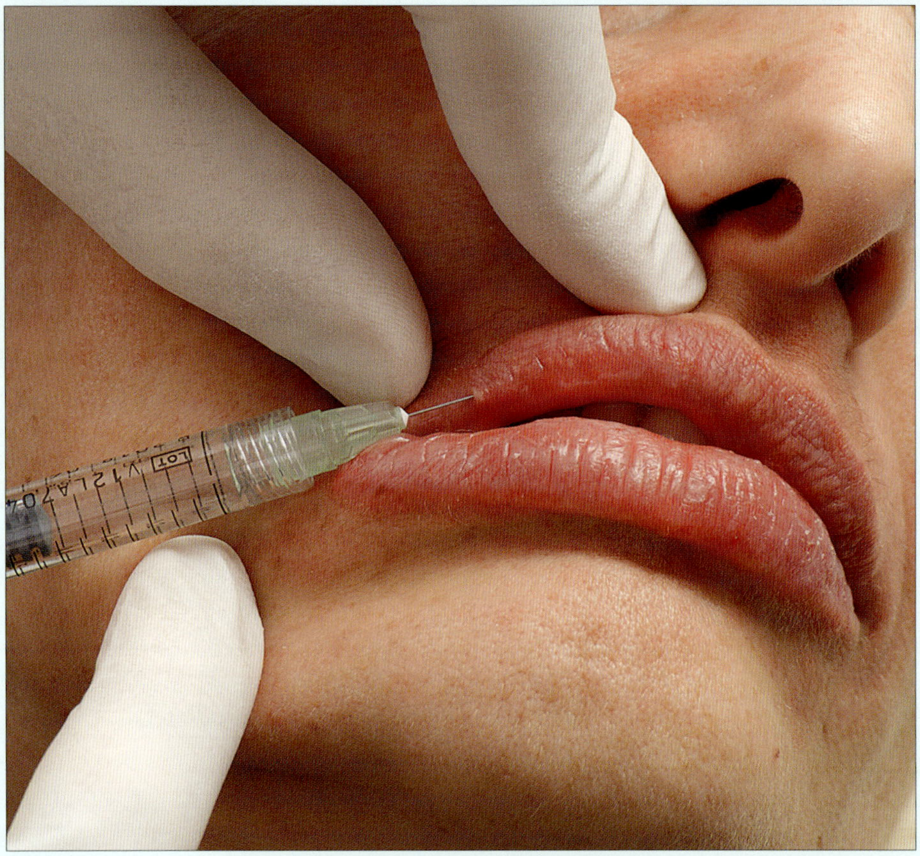

Technique 4 – Fig. 3 Since the injections are given very superficially, the therapist needs to ensure that the lip is not perforated when applying the fanning technique, and that the needle does not emerge again.

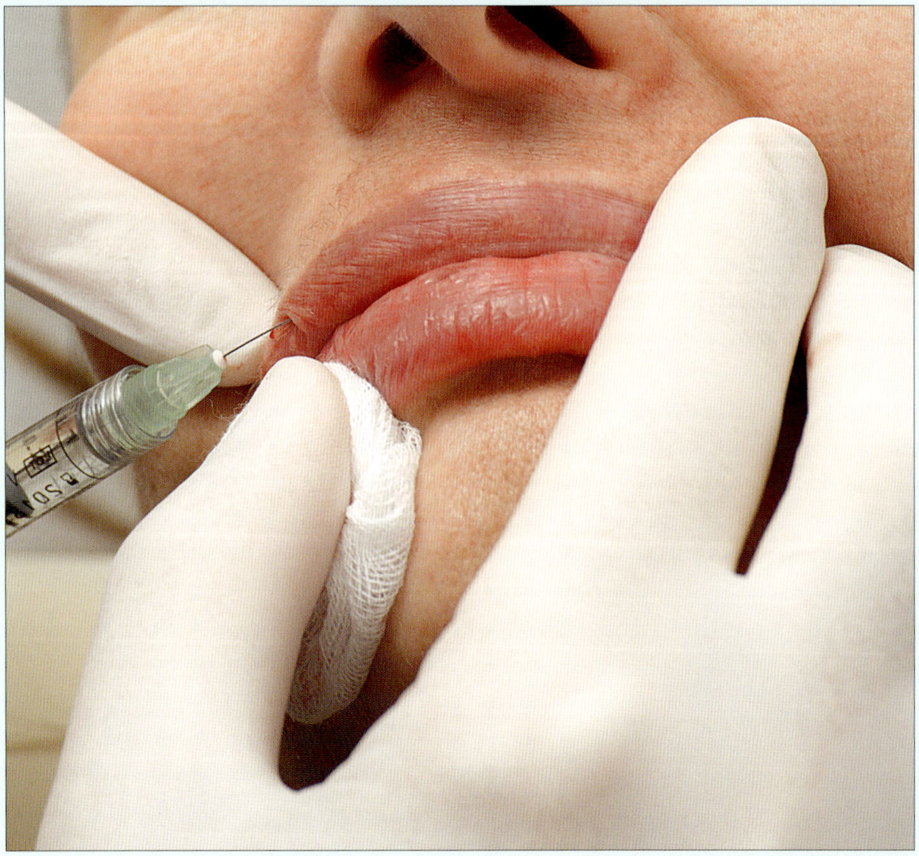

Technique 4 – Fig. 4 Performing the treatment 2–3 times is recommended for a more lasting result. Since the treatment is painful, the use of conduction anesthesia is advisable or, at the very least, the local application of a strong anesthetic cream.

Important Notes

This technique is very uncomfortable for the patient, as it is highly traumatizing, and thus less advisable than hydration with the cannula (see Technique 3, p. 136).

Hematomas and swellings may persist for several days.

Possible Side Effects

Slight reddening, commonly hematomas, severe swellings, pain persisting for up to several days

Undesirable Side Effects

Inflammation, asymmetry due to non-uniform delivery of material, necrosis

Treatment Protocol at a Glance

- History, evaluation, and patient information
- Informed consent form
- Photo documentation: "before" images
- Analysis and marking of the areas to be treated
- Cleaning
- Thorough disinfection
- Local anesthesia (lidocaine cream) or conduction anesthesia if required
- Injection technique: fanning technique
- Layer: subcutaneous
- Material: class "XS soft" product
- Volume: max. 1 ml in total
- Needle: 27G sharp needle
- No massage
- Cooling if required
- Heparin cream for hematomas, ibuprofen p.o., arnica
- Photo documentation: "after" images
- Advice on dos and don'ts after the procedure
- Follow-up appointment for a check-up after 8–14 days

9.2 Accents

The lip contours, the philtrum, the Cupid's bow, and the mouth corners define the shape of the lips. This section describes the finest accentuation treatment, designed only to freshen up the lips subtly with tiny amounts of HA. These treatments involve gentle contouring, the injection of microvolumes into the lips, and minimal correction for patients who only want minor accents rather than major changes.

9.2.1 TECHNIQUE 5

Fresh Up (Sharp Needle)

The term "fresh up" refers to the minimal delivery of HA into selected points of the lip contours (along the vermillion border) only. The goal is the very subtle accentuation of the lips, thus freshening them up without changing their shape. This technique can be used specifically to correct the tiniest irregularities or deficits at various places on the lips. The four examples of fresh up treatment shown here represent commonly chosen entry points in routine practice.

Patient Selection

- Patients who decline treatments that produce excessive, visible changes to the lips and only want a subtle result
- Ideal for patients who are having a treatment with HA fillers for the first time

Injection Scheme, Planning and Method (→ Technique 5 – Figs. 1–7)

Injection scheme for a fresh up (sharp needle) – four examples of prominent points at various sites of the lips, into which the tiniest amounts of HA can be injected to achieve a subtle freshening up. These points may be varied as required.

Technique: point technique

Direction of insertion: into the centers of the defined points, from the front

Layer: subcutaneous

Material: class "S/M viscous" product

Volume: max. 0.03 ml per point

Needle: 27–30G sharp needle

Anesthesia: lidocaine cream

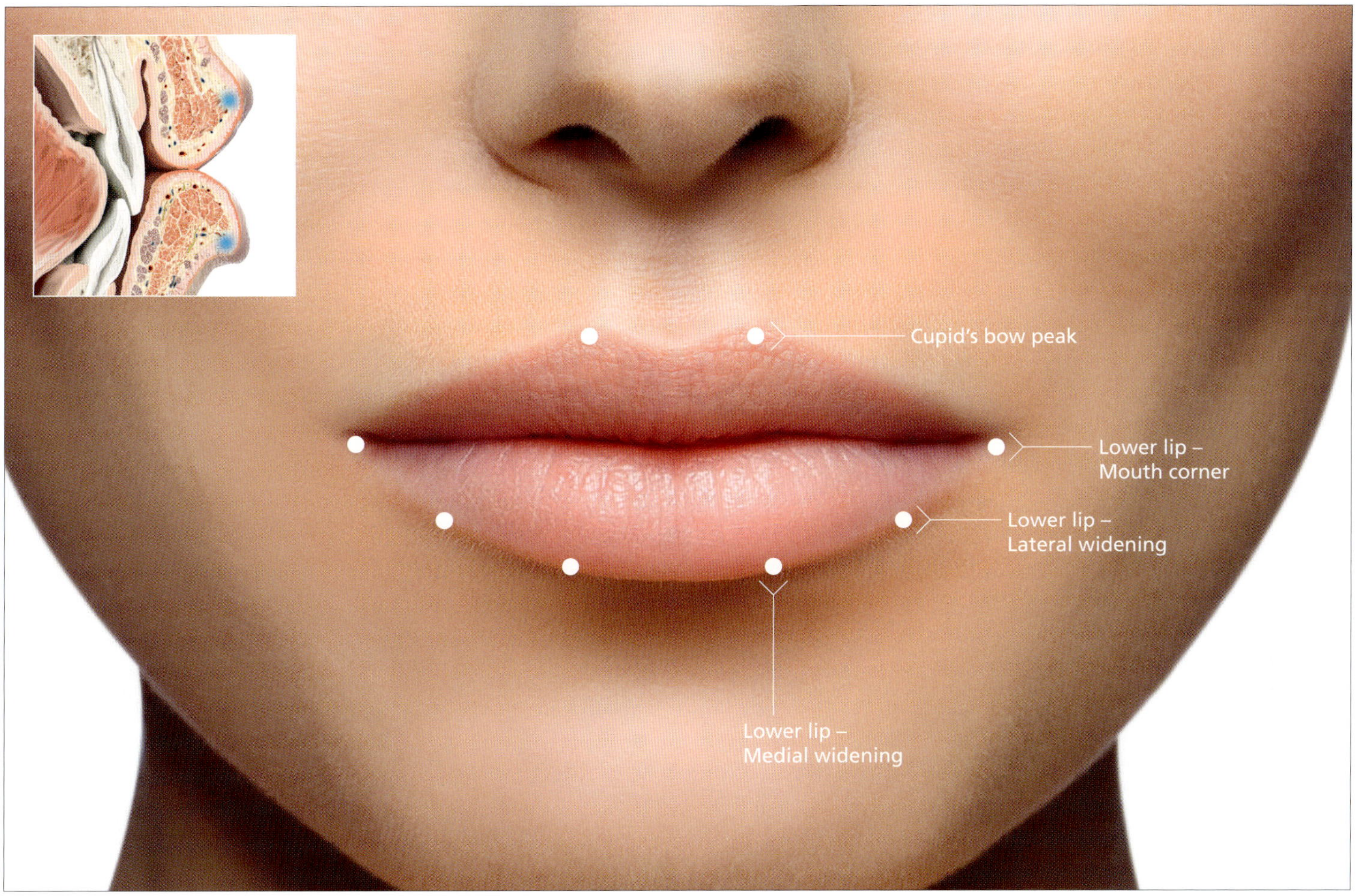

Technique 5 – Fig. 1 Injection scheme for a fresh up treatment (sharp needle) at various sites on the lip.

Cupid's Bow and Mouth Corners (→ Technique 5 – Figs. 2–5)

Depending on the direction from which the injection is given, the therapist can affect lip shape in different ways. Three procedures for injecting the Cupid's bow peak are demonstrated here.

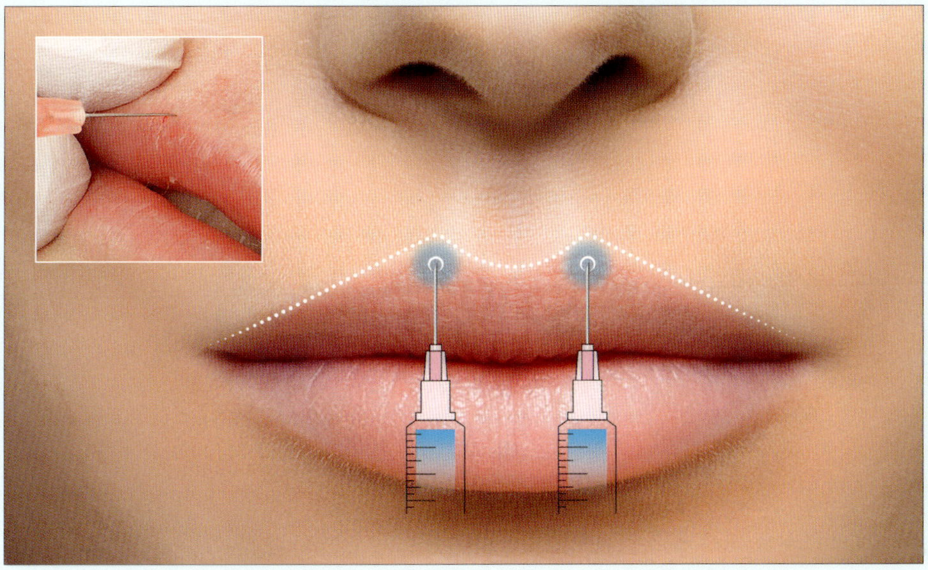

Technique 5 – Fig. 2

Variant 1: The needle insertion points show that the material is being injected precisely into the contour. Each point represents the delivery of a pinhead-sized micro depot of 0.03 ml HA. The procedure is performed using a sharp needle. To accentuate the shape of the Cupid's bow, plunge the needle bevel into the area where the edge of the philtrum meets the vermillion of the lip. Deliver the material into the subdermal layer using the point technique.

Cupid's Bow and Mouth Corners (continued)

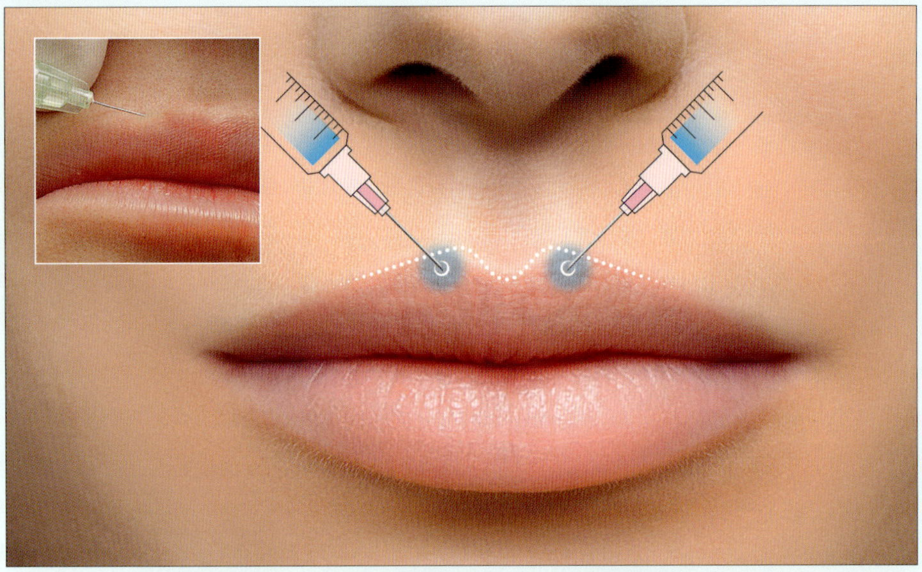

Technique 5 – Fig. 3

Variant 2: Approaching the lip from the lateral side, inject points into the Cupid's bow peak. This enhances the indentation of the Cupid's bow. When injecting this area using a lateral approach, it is helpful to stretch the lip between thumb and forefinger.

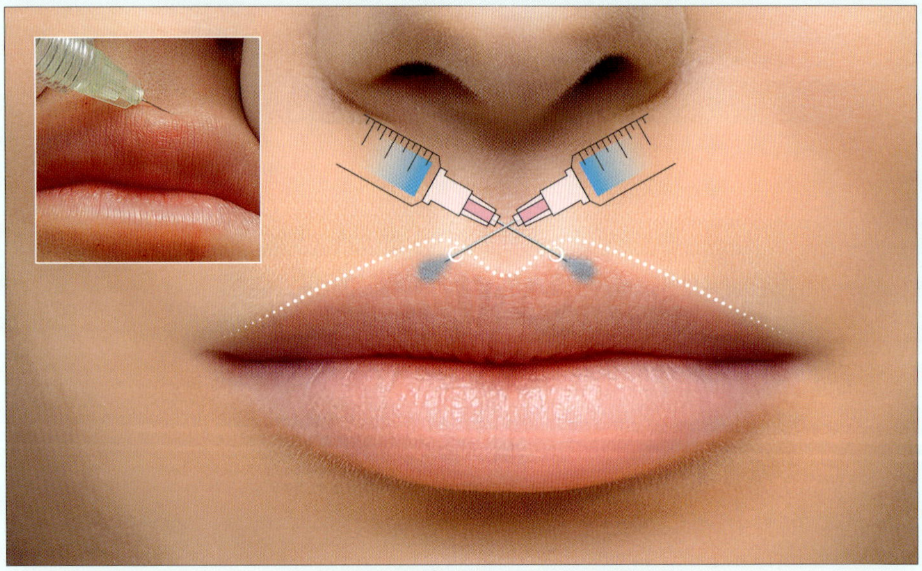

Technique 5 – Fig. 4

Variant 3: Approaching the lip from the medial side, inject points into the Cupid's bow peak in the direction of the lip margin. This widens the prominent curvature of the Cupid's bow, so that the butterfly shape of the lip is enhanced. When injecting from the medial side, take care to deliver a small volume because the lip contour would otherwise be altered to an unnatural extent.

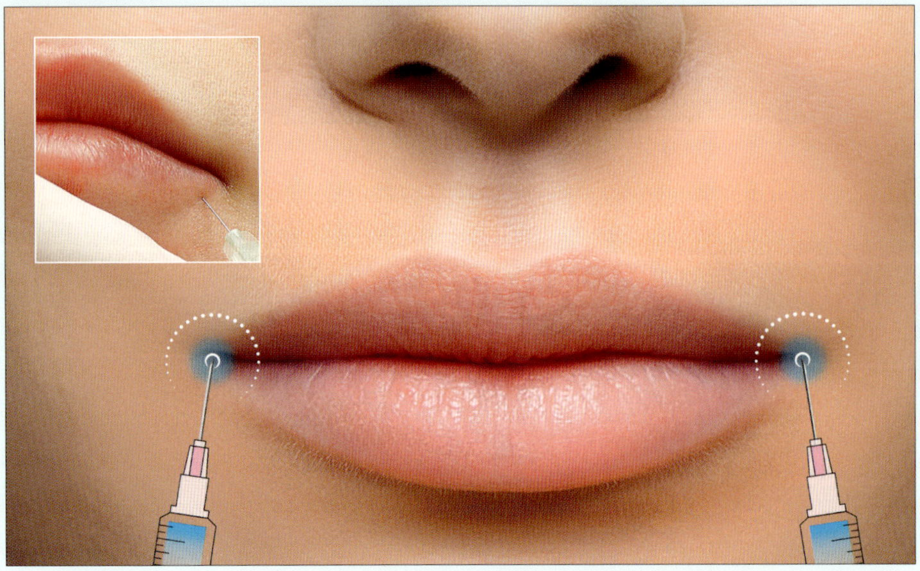

Technique 5 – Fig. 5

Approaching from the front, place points of material into the mouth corners to stabilize them, preventing them from drooping. This produces gentle pressure against the upper lip, giving the mouth a rather more cheerful expression. Hold the skin in place with the left hand (if right-handed), gently everting the lower margin of the lip. The direction of insertion is vertically from the front, introducing the needle into the lower lip c. 3 mm on the medial side of the mouth corner.

Lower Lip (→ Technique 5 – Figs. 6, 7)

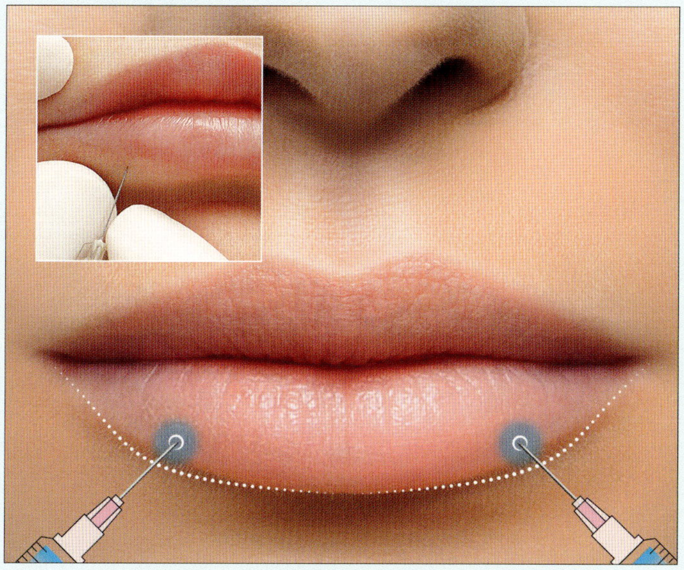

Technique 5 – Fig. 6

Lateral widening: Inject 1 point at a distance of 1–1.5 from each mouth corner. This causes subtle outward widening of the lip. The shape of the lip changes according to the amount of material delivered. For this reason, it is advisable to proceed at a moderate rate if a change in shape is required; it is preferable to reinject in a second treatment session.

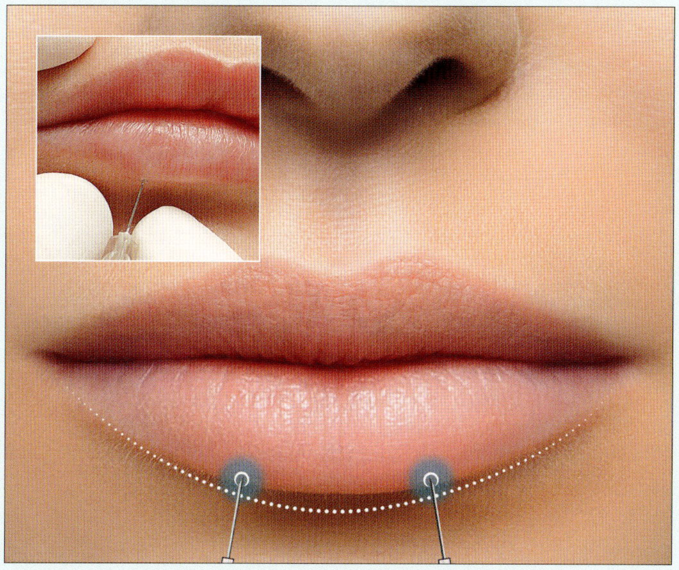

Technique 5 – Fig. 7

Medial widening: Inject material at the two points of the medial region of the lower lip which lie opposite the peaks of the philtrum. This causes very subtle downward enlargement of the lower lip. Plunge the tip of the needle to a depth of 0.5 cm. Deliver the material slowly as a small bolus, with visual monitoring.

Important Notes

Placing accents at the contours or making very minor corrections

Possible Side Effects

Slight reddening, rarely inflammation, rarely hematomas, rarely swellings

Undesirable Side Effects

Inflammation, overcorrection, asymmetry, blanching if the injection is too superficial, necrosis

Treatment Protocol at a Glance

- History, evaluation, and patient information
- Informed consent form
- Photo documentation: "before" images
- Analysis and marking of the areas to be treated
- Cleaning
- Thorough disinfection
- Local anesthesia if required (lidocaine cream)
- Injection technique: point technique, 1 point at each site
- Layer: subcutaneous
- Material: class "S/M viscous" product
- Volume: max. 0.03 ml per point
- Needle: 27–30G sharp needle
- No massage
- Cooling if required
- Heparin cream for hematomas, ibuprofen p.o., arnica
- Photo documentation: "after" images
- Advice on dos and don't after the procedure
- Follow-up appointment for a check-up after 8–14 days

9.2.2 TECHNIQUE 6

Contouring and Enhancement (Sharp Needle)

The vermillion border of the lip is also referred to as the lip contour or lip margin (see Fig. 1.5, p. 5). This contour defines the shape of the lips and varies greatly from one person to another. As a result of aging – especially in women as hormone levels decrease – and also due to extrinsic factors, the lip contour can change in accordance with available volume: it can become more irregular, drawn through with radial wrinkles or change shape asymmetrically.

Lip contouring treatment models the lip margin, treating the perioral wrinkles at the same time. This also gives the lips a little more freshness and volume without changing them. Targeted treatment of the contour can accentuate the Cupid's bow.

Patient Selection

- In cases of age-related atrophy of the lip margin with blurred contours
- Slight accentuation of full or young lips
- Lip shape reconstruction
- Preventive enhancement of the lip margin

Injection Scheme, Planning and Method (→ Technique 6 – Figs. 1–4)

The treatment is performed with a sharp needle and the material is delivered by subdermal, retrograde injection in 2–3 segments (depending on lip length) per quadrant, using the linear technique (from mouth corner to Cupid's bow/philtrum edge).

There are two possible approaches:

Starting from the corner of the mouth, the second needle insertion point is placed at the end of the first, while the third insertion point is placed at the end of the second one.

The advantage of this procedure is that the material cannot leak out from a previous needle insertion point.

However, it is also possible to start from the middle and work outward. Starting from the Cupid's bow makes it easier to place the material seamlessly by linear injection because the needle insertion point marks the end of the first line.

Where the material is placed depends on the treatment goal.

Technique: linear technique

Direction of insertion: in 2–3 segments, upper lip ending 3 mm short of the corner of the mouth, so that the corner does not push downward. The needle bevel should face up toward the vermillion. Retrograde material delivery.

Layer: subdermal

Material: class "S/M viscous" product; a more viscous material to produce a sharply defined contour is recommended, and a less viscous material if the contour needs to be softer

Volume: c. 0.1 ml per quadrant, max. 0.5 ml in total

Needle: 27–30G sharp needle

Anesthesia: lidocaine cream

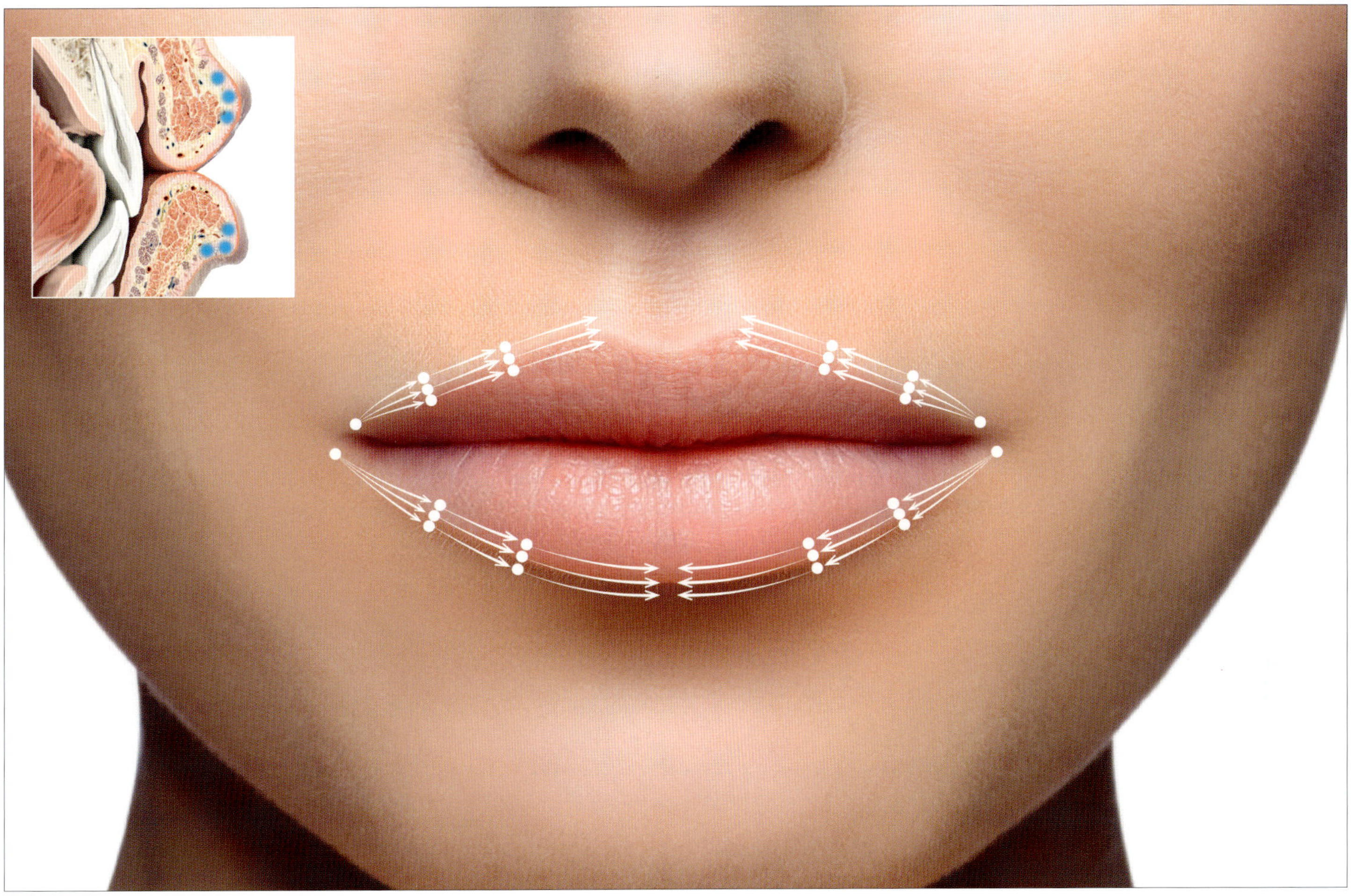

Technique 6 – Fig. 1 Injection scheme for contouring and enhancement (sharp needle).

Variant 1: Injection into the Vermillion Border – Contouring and Enhancement of the Lip Margin

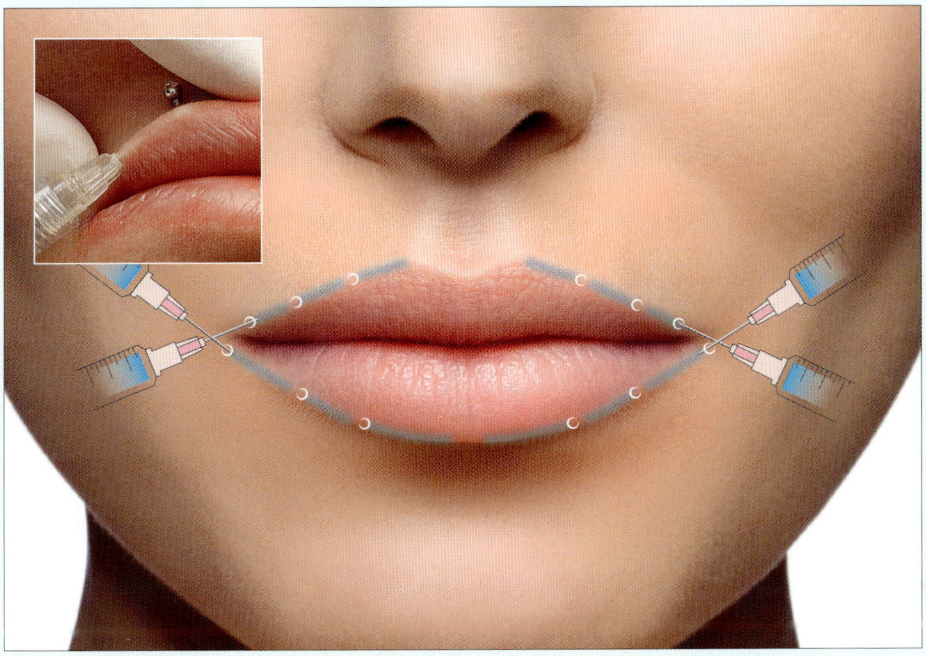

Technique 6 – Fig. 2 Inject the HA precisely into the vermillion border; this reinforces the lip margin, defines the contours, and prevents fine mimic wrinkles. The lip should be stretched gently when injecting into the vermillion border. This technique is used particularly for young lips and those showing incipient, slight volume loss from the Cupid's bow; the needle bevel should be plunged into the region where the philtral peak reaches the vermillion. Inject into the subdermal layer, delivering the material using the point technique.

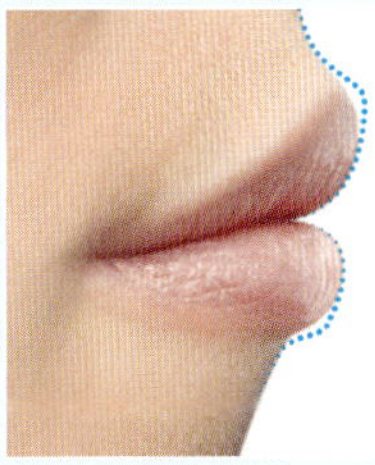

Variant 2: Injection outside the Vermillion – Enhancing the Prominence of the Lips

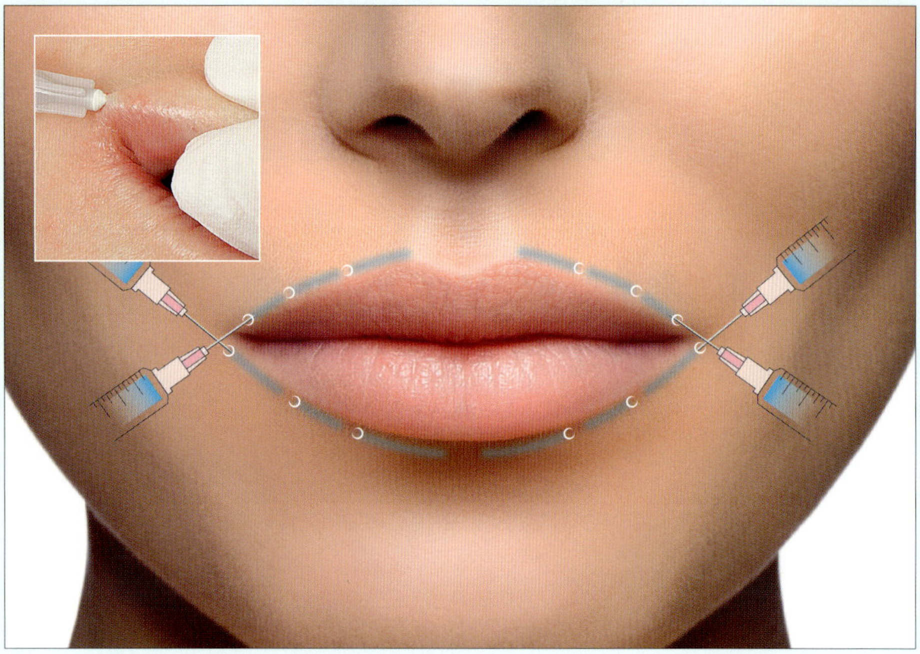

Technique 6 – Fig. 3 Inject the HA above and below the vermillion border, respectively. This causes gentle, convex upward enlargement of the lips, raising them gently and making them appear softer. The injection should be given outside the vermillion, along the contour. When doing this, it is important not to use a filler that is too thick, so that the lip does not bulge outward ("duck's bill" effect). Holding the lip between the thumb and forefinger along its contour and rolling it downward gently helps ensure accurate material placement.

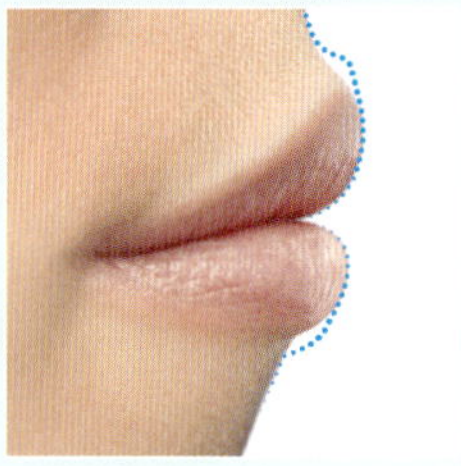

9

Variant 3: Injection within the Vermillion – Enhancing the Curvature and Volume of the Lips

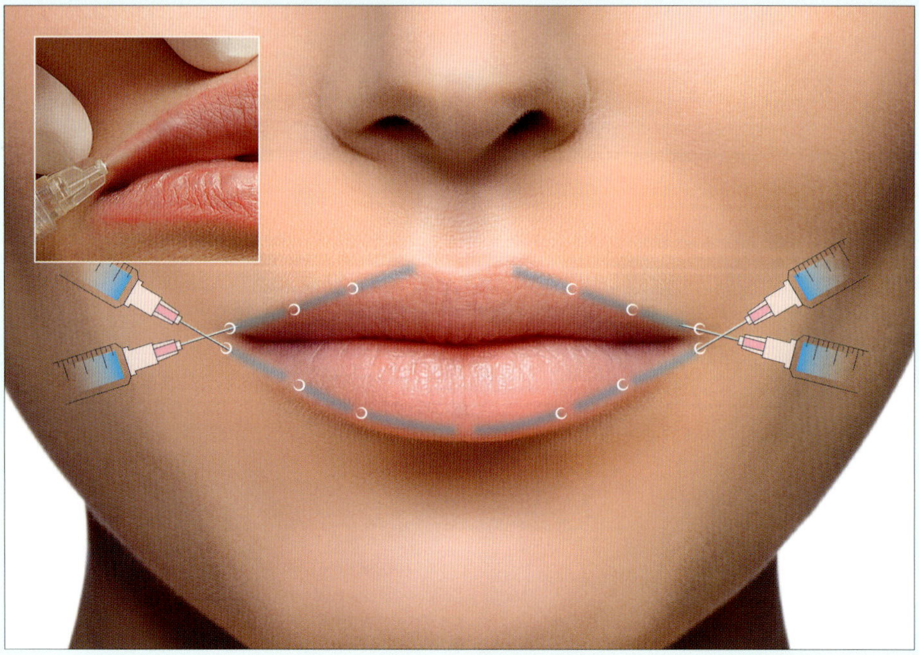

Technique 6 – Fig. 4 Inject the material just inside the vermillion. This enhances the curvature of the lip gently, raising it without causing a "duck's bill" effect. Give the injection below and above the lip contour, respectively. This is the preferred technique if the lips have already atrophied slightly, if they are naturally thin or if only a small amount of added volume is desired. By lifting the needle, the therapist can check that the material is being delivered into the correct layer.

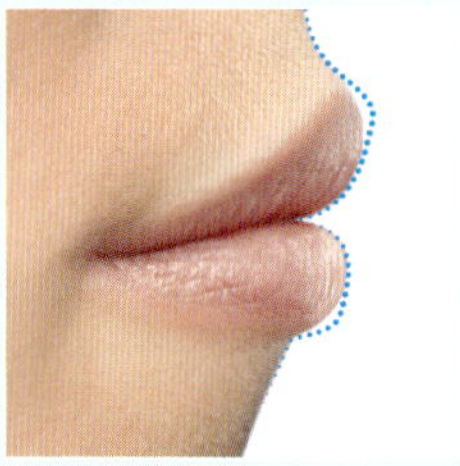

Important Notes

- In older patients, the region between the lower lip and the chin is reduced in height, and this feature would be exaggerated by the lip accentuation that is produced when filler is placed in or above the contour of the lower lip. In this case, therefore, the filler is injected directly into the vermillion of the lower lip. On the other hand, the cutaneous part of the upper lip increases in height in older patients and the lip flattens inward, making it appear thinner; for this reason, the filler should be injected above the vermillion, to produce a gentle, convex increase in the upward curvature of the slightly flattened upper lip (Verner 2013).
- Since a sort of channel runs between the vermillion and the cutaneous part of the lip, the delivered material may occasionally run right up into the edge of the philtrum – especially when starting the injections from the mouth corner.
- If too much material gets into the channel at the lip margin, the contour may show some white discoloration. If this happens, the lip needs to be massaged gently until the tissue regains its original color.
- Grasping the contour between the thumb and forefinger during the injection, and squeezing/pinching it together tightly, can force the material out of the lip contour channel. This also prevents the material from escaping into unwanted areas, something that can occur in the presence of septum damage in older or previously treated lips.
- It is advisable to inject firmer, crosslinked HA products if the treatment goal is to achieve a clearly defined contour.

Possible Side Effects

Slight reddening, rarely inflammation, swellings, the Tyndall effect (a blue line that occurs when a material of excessive particle size has been injected into the contour)

Undesirable Side Effects

Inflammation, overcorrection, asymmetry, blanching if the injection is too superficial, necrosis, Tyndall effect

Treatment Protocol at a Glance

- History, evaluation, and patient information
- Informed consent form
- Photo documentation: "before" images
- Analysis and marking of the areas to be treated
- Cleaning
- Thorough disinfection
- Local anesthesia (lidocaine cream) or conduction anesthesia if required
- Injection technique: linear technique, 2–3 lines per quadrant
- Layer: subdermal
- Material: class "S/M viscous" product
- Volume: 0.1 ml per quadrant, max. 0.5 ml in total
- Needle: 27–30G sharp needle
- No massage
- Cooling if required
- Heparin cream for hematomas, ibuprofen p.o., arnica
- Photo documentation: "after" images
- Advice on dos and don'ts after the procedure
- Follow-up appointment for a check-up after 8–14 days

9.2.3 TECHNIQUE 7
Contouring (Blunt Cannula)

Injecting with a blunt cannula allows the lip contours to be treated with a less traumatizing technique, i.e. the technique is less painful for the patient, and very popular for first-time treatment in particular. The risk of injuring blood vessels is considerably lower than when injecting with a sharp needle, which also reduces the risk of necrosis.

Since there is only one needle insertion point at each mouth corner, which is pre-pricked with a sharp needle (Nokor needle), tissue injuries are considerably less severe and there are few hematomas. Compared with injection with a sharp needle, a contour injected using the cannula technique is much softer in shape. The cannula technique should not be used if the contour has been severely damaged by scarring or extreme wrinkling.

Patient Selection

- Placement of subtle accents on a full lip
- Preventive reinforcement of the lip margin
- More freshness and volume without changing lip shape
- If the lips are irregular, have radial wrinkles or show asymmetric deformities: correction of the lip margin and tissue firming
- Comment: The selfie trend should not be underestimated. An increasing number of people in the 18 to 30 age group present to esthetic practices because they do not want any wrinkles or shadows to show up on photographs when taking selfies with puckered lips. The cannula technique described here is suitable for this purpose.

Injection Scheme and Planning (→ Technique 7 – Figs. 1, 2)

The procedure is performed with a blunt cannula. The entry point is on the lateral side of the mouth corner, starting with the right upper lip. This is followed by the left upper lip, and then the right and left lower lip.

The entry point is pre-pricked with the sharp Nokor needle, c. 1 mm away from the mouth corner, so that all the desired areas of tissue being injected can be accessed. A line of HA is injected subcutaneously from the mouth corner to the Cupid's bow/philtrum. It is important to advance the cannula gently and to place the material into the correct layer. Small amounts of material should be delivered by anterograde injection, to exploit the anesthetic effect of products that contain lidocaine. This is then followed by the retrograde delivery of material, constantly checking (by monitoring the syringe plunger and the volume of the lip) whether the material is being delivered uniformly on both sides. The lip may also be stretched with a finger inserted inside the mouth. Any irregularities can be distributed by gentle massage.

Technique: linear technique, entry point c. 5 mm on the lateral side of the mouth corner
Direction of insertion: along the lip margin up to the Cupid's bow
Layer: subcutaneous
Material: class "S/M viscous" product
Volume: max. 0.2 ml into the upper lip, 0.3 ml into the lower lip, 0.5 ml in total
Needle: 27–30G cannula c. 38–40 mm, sharp 25G Nokor needle
Anesthesia: lidocaine cream

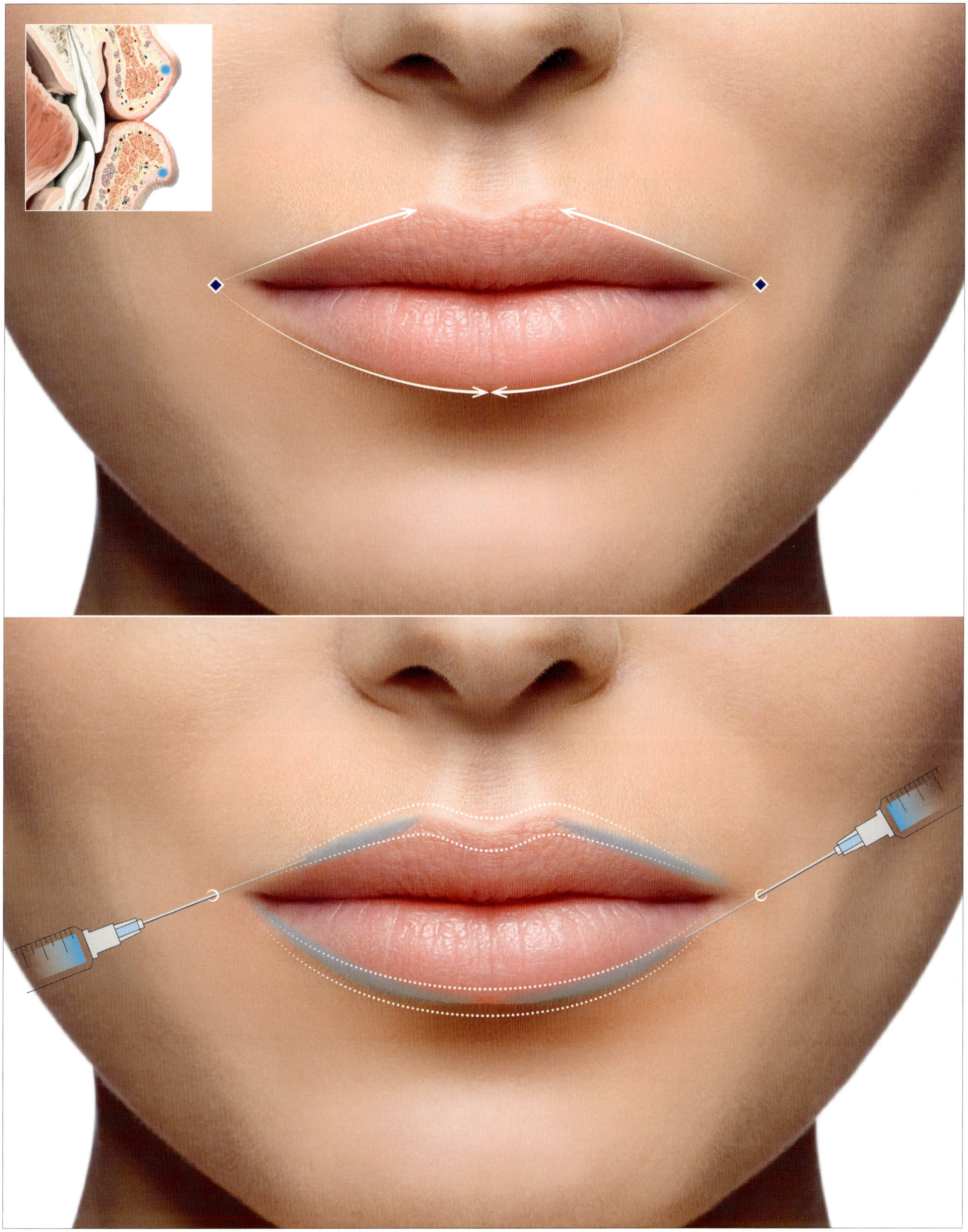

Technique 6 – Figs. 1, 2 Injection scheme and planning for contouring (blunt cannula).

9

Treatment Method (→ Technique 7 – Figs. 3–5)

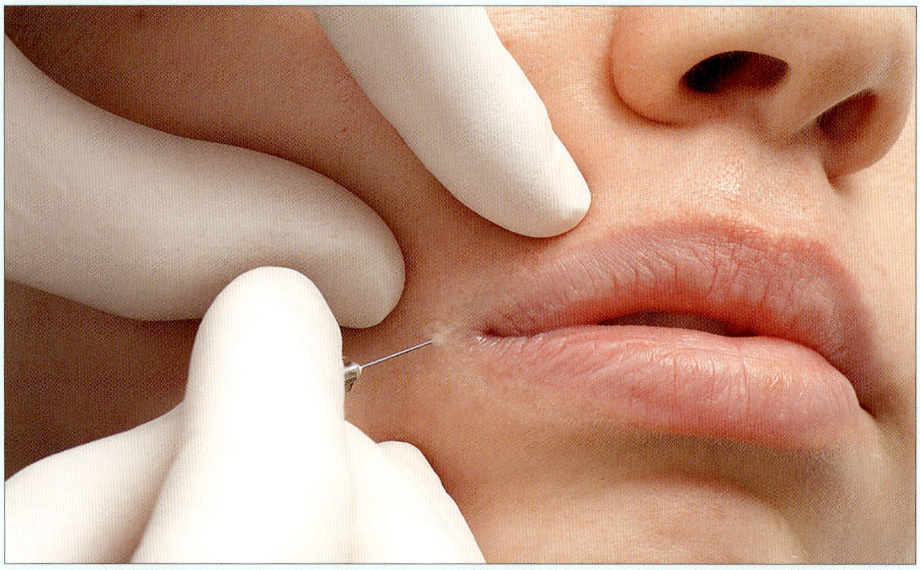

Technique 7 – Fig. 3 Pre-pricking the skin with a sharp Nokor needle: the bigger the hole, the easier it is to inject with the cannula. For this reason, it is advisable to always select a Nokor needle of slightly larger gauge than the cannula.

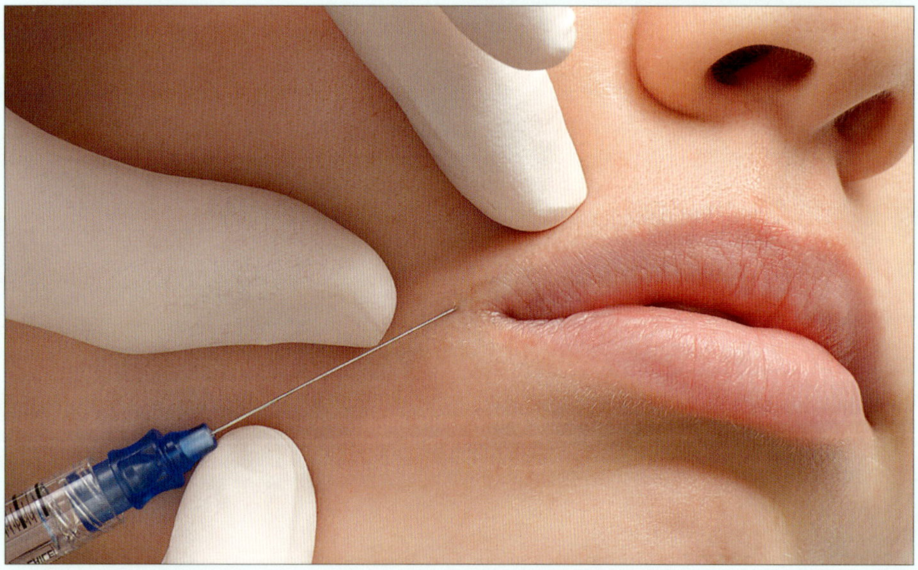

Technique 7 – Fig. 4 Gently stretching the skin makes it easier to introduce a blunt cannula. Angle of insertion: 15 degrees, shallow. Skin layer: parallel to the dermis, subcutaneous.

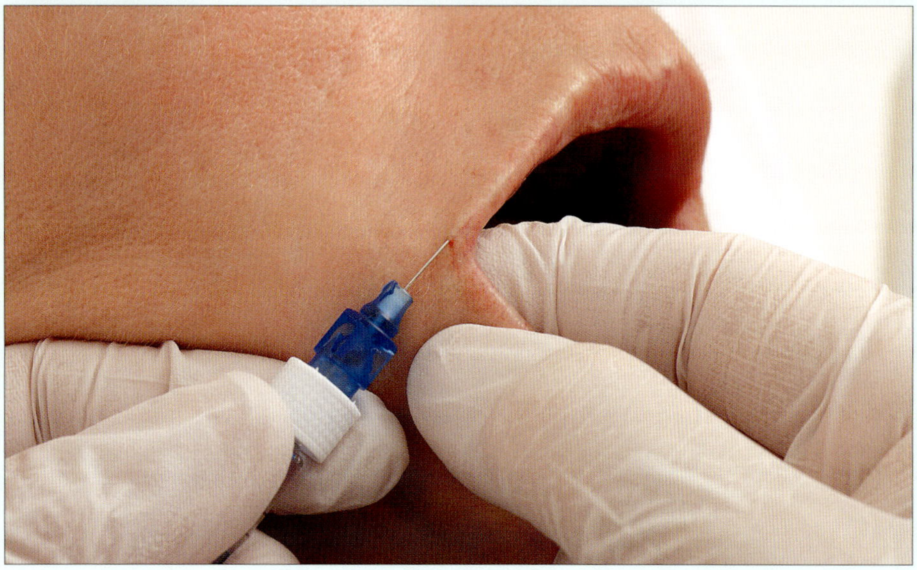

Technique 7 – Fig. 5 The overlying skin has been raised gently to check in which layer the needle is located.

Important Notes

- Due to the risk of infection, the therapist's hand and the patient's hair or skin should not come into contact with the cannula. Ideally, the cannula should be changed after each side. Lifting the cannula slightly shows where its tip is located.
- It is not always easy to get the cannula into the pre-pricked hole. Asking the patient to inflate the cheeks so that the skin is stretched helps to enlarge the hole and makes it easier to locate.
- Depending on the manufacturer, the fine 27G or 30G needles are very flexible. To place the material accurately into a contour, it helps to hold the lip between the thumb and forefinger and then insert the needle into this area.

Possible Side Effects

Blood vessel injuries resulting in local hematomas as a result of pre-pricking with the Nokor needle, slight reddening, rarely inflammation, hematomas, swellings

Undesirable Side Effects

Overcorrection, asymmetry

Treatment Protocol at a Glance

- History, evaluation, and patient information
- Informed consent form
- Photo documentation: "before" images
- Analysis and marking of the areas to be treated
- Cleaning
- Thorough disinfection
- Local anesthesia (lidocaine cream) or conduction anesthesia if required
- Injection technique: linear technique
- Layer: subcutaneous
- Material: class "S/M viscous" product
- Volume: max. 0.2 ml into the upper lip, 0.3 ml into the lower lip, 0.5 ml in total
- Needle: 27–30G cannula, 38–40 mm, sharp 25G Nokor needle
- Massage may be applied
- Cooling if required
- Heparin cream for hematomas, ibuprofen p.o., arnica
- Photo documentation: "after" images
- Advice on dos and don'ts after the procedure
- Follow-up appointment for a check-up after 8–14 days

9.2.4 TECHNIQUE 8

Contouring/Reshaping of the Cupid's Bow (Sharp Needle)

The Cupid's bow is located between the peaks of the heart shape of the upper lip. It gives the lips their characterful expression and can be accurately contoured using a fine needle (27–30G) and small amounts of a highly viscous, small-particle filler. Generally, the Cupid's bow is injected in combination with the philtrum, so that the latter is accentuated and emphasized. This can lead to the Cupid's bow becoming thicker and/or shallower, which can markedly alter the original shape of the lip.

Patient Selection

- Reconstruction of flattened or altered Cupid's bow peaks as a result of skin damage (due to herpes, actinic damage or aging processes)
- Reshaping to achieve a softer outline using a less viscous product, in patients with a very prominent and sharply delineated Cupid's bow

Injection Scheme and Planning (→ Technique 8 – Figs. 1, 2)

The injections are given using a sharp needle and the material is placed at the vermillion border. The needle is inserted subdermally at the highest point of the Cupid's bow peak, with retrograde delivery of the material up to the lowest point of the Cupid's bow, or vice versa. The lip margin being injected is grasped between the thumb and forefinger to prevent overcorrection by the application of gentle pressure onto the material being delivered and to place the material accurately.

Technique: linear technique

Direction of insertion: from the philtral ridge up to the center of the Cupid's bow, or vice versa from the center of the Cupid's bow up to the philtral ridge

Layer: subdermal

Material: class "S/M viscous" product

Volume: max. 0.1 ml per line, 0.2 ml in total

Needle: 27–30G sharp needle

Anesthesia: lidocaine cream, nerve block anesthesia

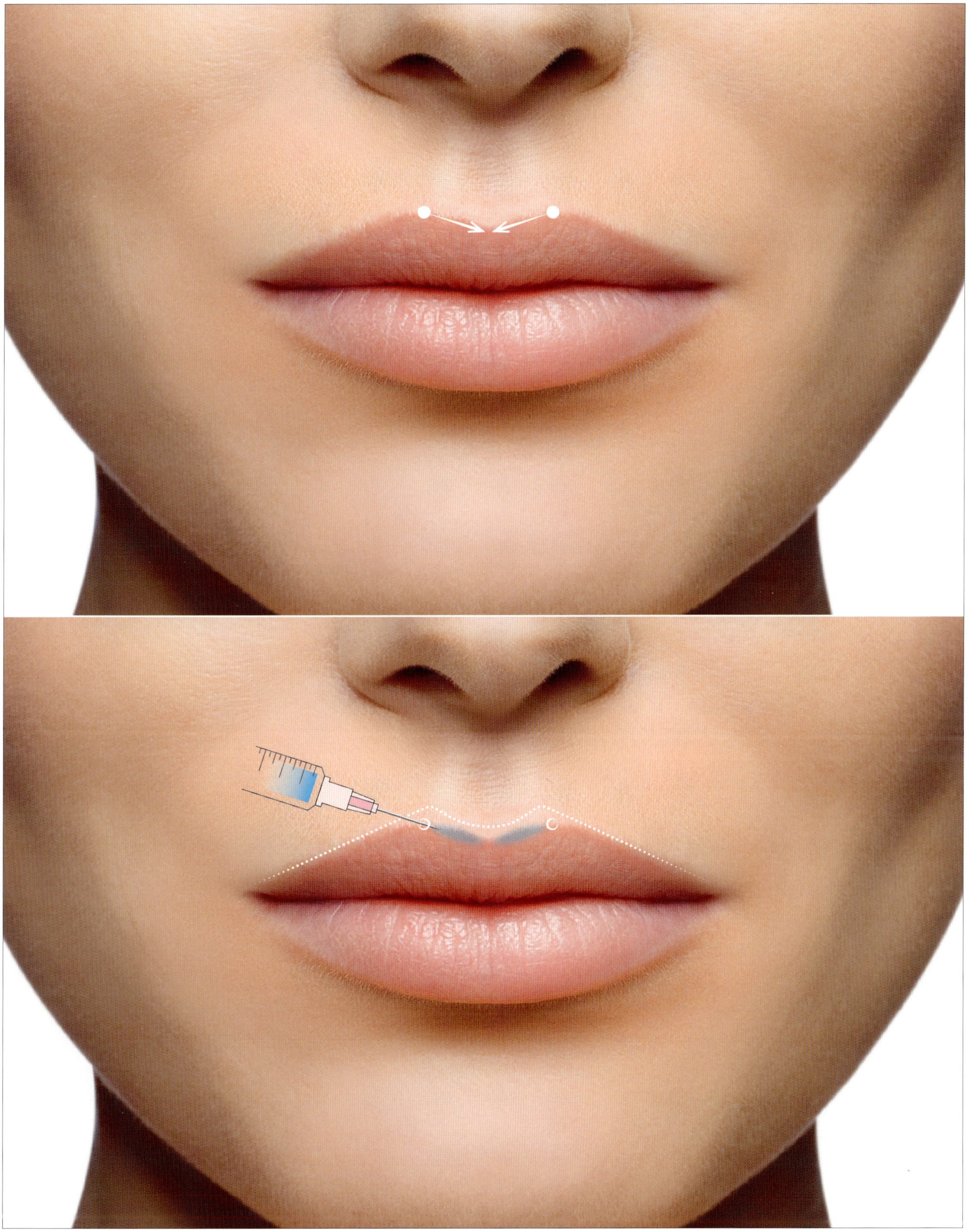

Technique 8 – Figs. 1, 2 Injection scheme and planning for contouring/reshaping of the Cupid's bow (sharp needle).

Treatment Method (→ Technique 8 – Figs. 3–5)

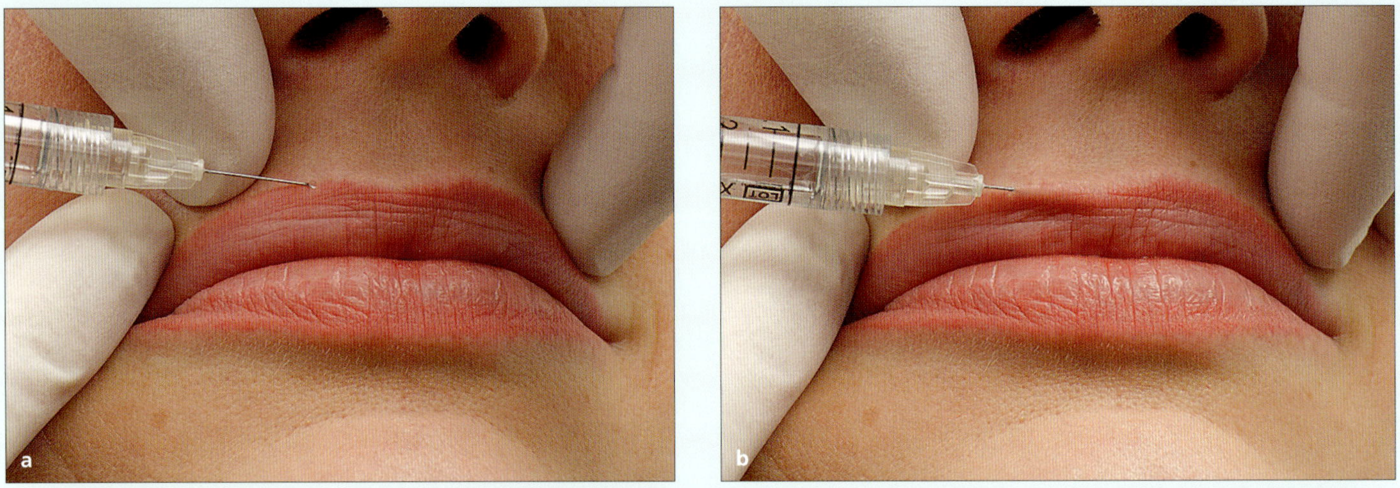

Technique 8 – Figs. 3 a+b Inject the material at the border between the vermillion and the cutaneous part of the lip, by retrograde linear delivery from the peak to the center of the lowest point of the Cupid's bow. Stretch the skin between the thumb and forefinger (a). By raising the needle, the therapist can check whether it is located in the correct skin layer (b).

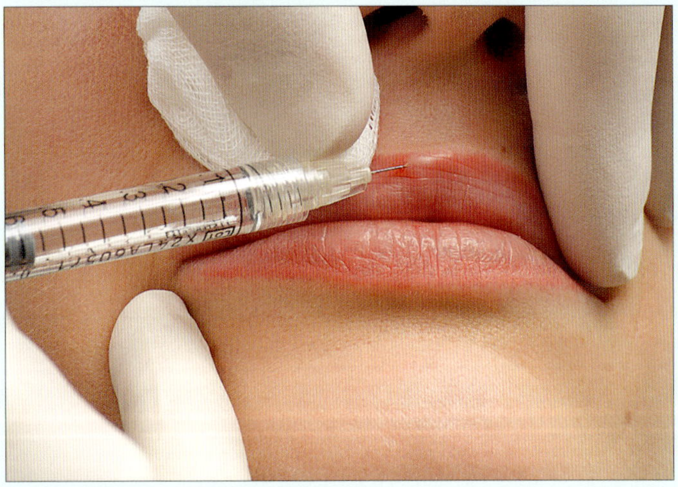

Technique 8 – Fig. 4 It is also possible to inject upward from the lowest point of the Cupid's bow. Droplet delivery of the material allows the shape of the Cupid's bow to be modelled and accentuated very nicely.

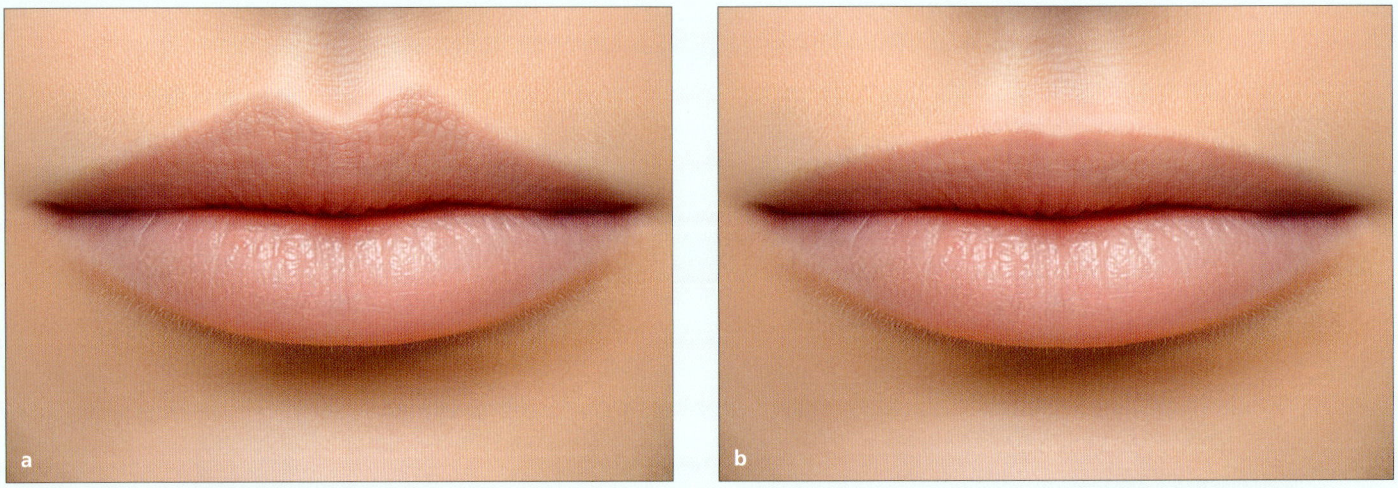

Technique 8 – Figs. 5 a+b Pronounced (a) and flat (b) Cupid's bow shape. There are limits as to how much the naturally determined Cupid's bow shape can be altered.

Important Notes

- The material should be used in small amounts, as overcorrection can occur very rapidly in this indication.
- There is no point in injecting a Cupid's bow if this feature is not naturally present. Doing so could greatly alter the lip and produce an unnatural appearance.

Possible Side Effects

Slight reddening, rarely inflammation, rarely hematomas, rarely mild swellings

Undesirable Side Effects

Overcorrection, asymmetry, blanching if the injection is too superficial, necrosis

Treatment Protocol at a Glance

- History, evaluation, and patient information
- Informed consent form
- Photo documentation: "before" images
- Analysis and marking of the areas to be treated
- Cleaning
- Thorough disinfection
- Local anesthesia (lidocaine cream) or conduction anesthesia if required
- Injection technique: linear technique, 1 line per side
- Layer: subdermal
- Material: class "S/M viscous" product
- Volume: max. 0.1 ml per side, 0.2 ml in total
- Needle: 27–30G sharp needle
- No massage
- Cooling if required
- Heparin cream for hematomas, ibuprofen p.o., arnica
- Photo documentation: "after" images
- Advice on dos and don'ts after the procedure
- Follow-up appointment for a check-up after 8–14 days

9.2.5 TECHNIQUE 9
Contouring of the Philtrum (Sharp Needle)

The philtrum is located between the nose and the upper lip and varies in depth between individuals (see Fig. 1.43, p. 28). Treatment enhances the philtral ridge, giving the upper lip a more prominent shape.

Patient Selection

- Patients whose natural philtral ridges have receded or been lost due to aging processes, fat accumulation, elastosis, actinic skin damage or loss of volume
- Younger lips with less pronounced contouring of the philtrum

Injection Scheme and Planning (→ Technique 9 – Figs. 1, 2)

The philtral ridge starts from the medial edge of the nostril, on the lateral side of the bridge of the nose and runs slightly outward, down to the curvature of the upper lip. If the philtral ridge is no longer clearly visible, it is advisable to map the lip by dividing it into segments (see Chap. 1.6.2, p. 29). The needle is inserted below the Cupid's bow peak (if present) into the border between the vermillion and the cutaneous part of the lip. The material is delivered by retrograde injection below the philtral ridge, starting from the nostril.

Technique: linear technique
Direction of insertion: retrograde along the philtral ridge
Layer: subdermal
Material: class "M viscous" product
Volume: max. 0.05–0.1 ml per philtrum line, 0.2 ml in total
Needle: 27G sharp needle
Anesthesia: lidocaine cream, nerve block anesthesia

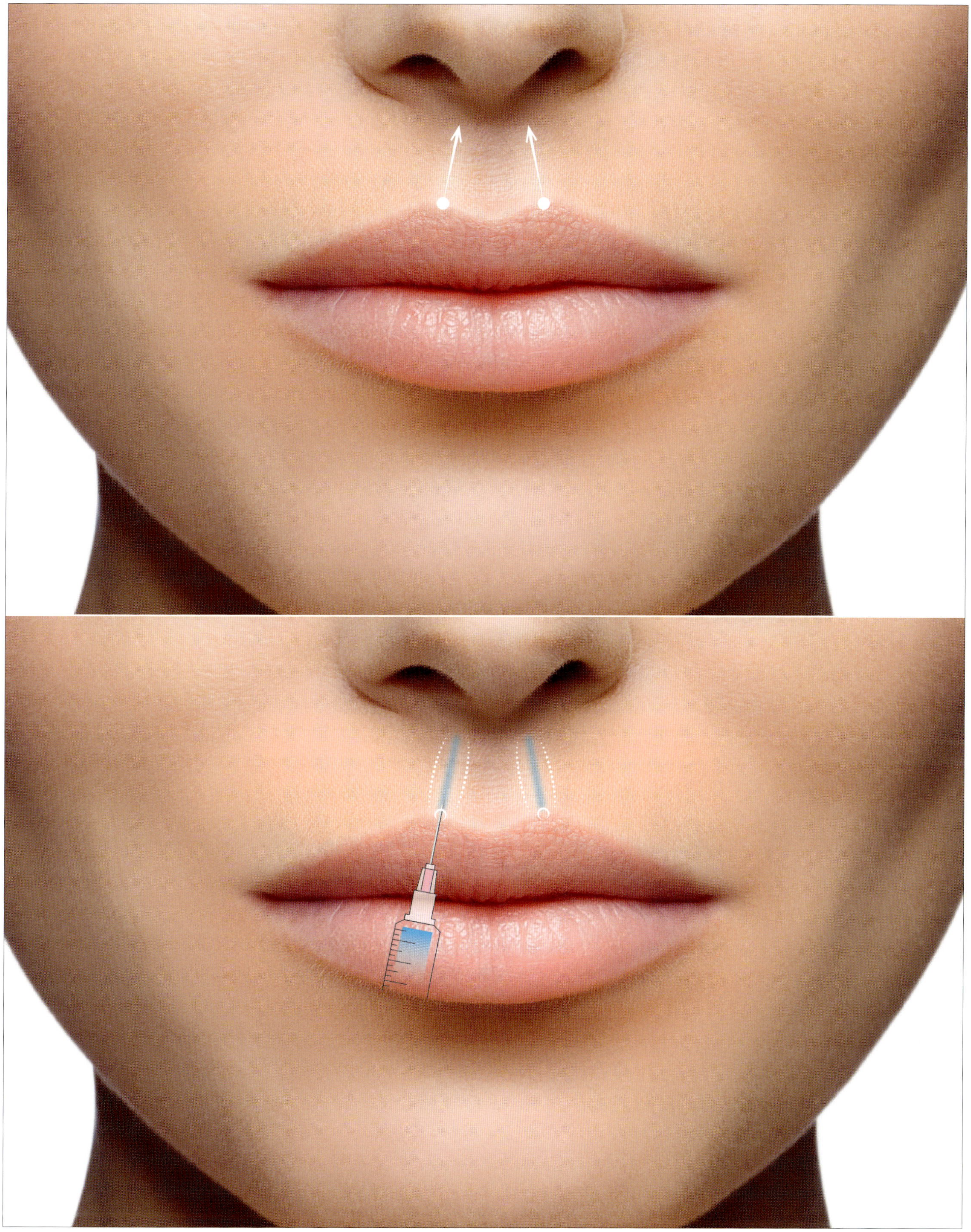

Technique 9 – Figs. 1, 2 Injection scheme and planning for contouring of the philtrum (sharp needle).

Treatment Method (→ Technique 9 – Figs. 3–5)

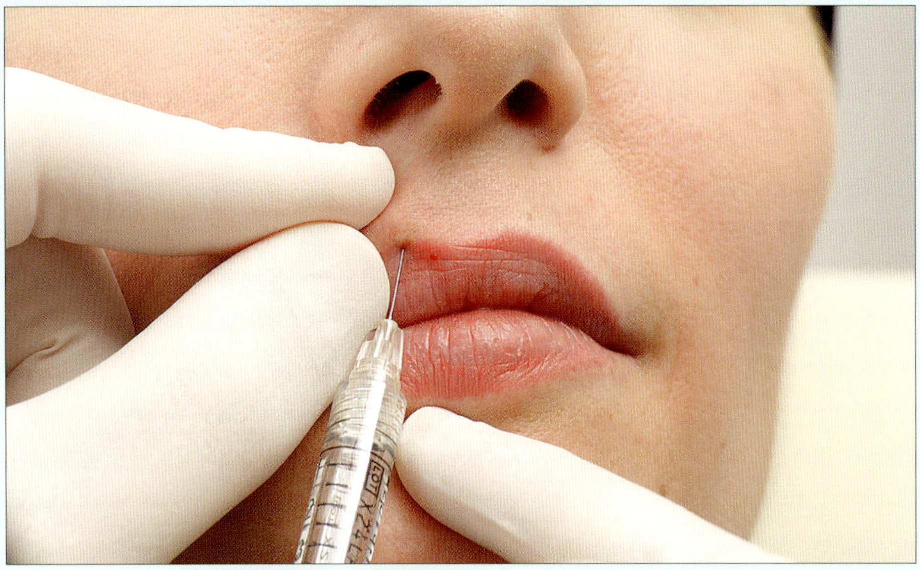

Technique 9 – Fig. 3 Insert the needle into the subdermal layer, starting from below at the lip margin and aiming up. Lift the needle to check whether it is in the correct layer. Deliver the material by retrograde injection using the linear technique, with visual monitoring of the injected volume.

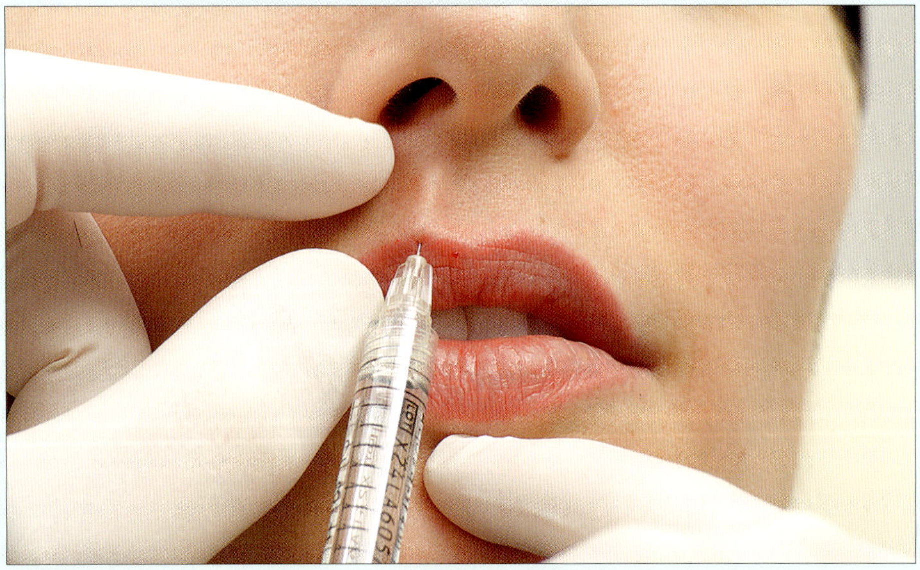

Technique 9 – Fig. 4 Advance the needle up toward the nostril, with gentle compression of the vertical upper lip curvature (the philtral ridge).

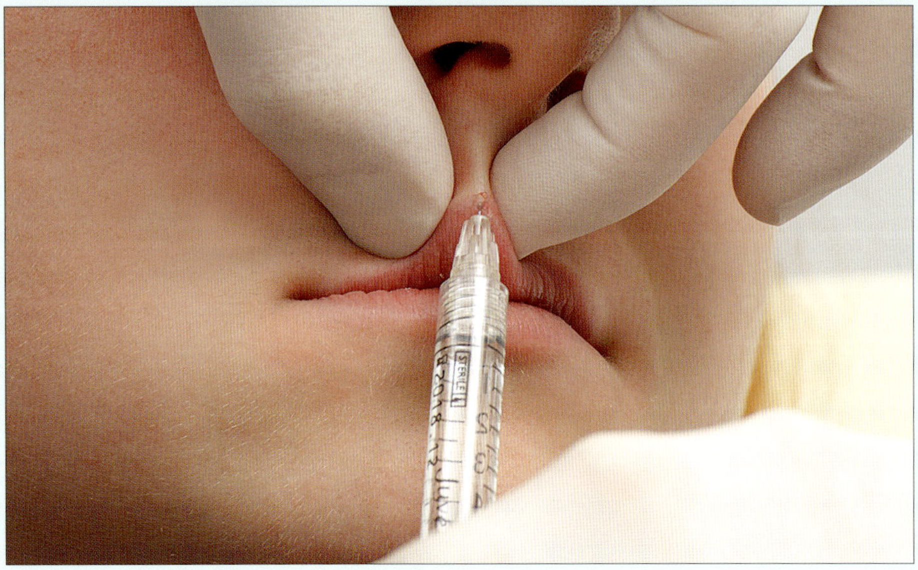

Technique 9 – Fig. 5 The philtrum should be contoured by palpation, achieved by applying pressure with the thumb and forefinger of the opposite hand. Delivering the material very slowly under compression is less painful for the patient. This compression is particularly important if the original shape of the philtrum has been lost or if the philtrum is shallow.

Important Notes

- The material should be delivered precisely along the correct line, to respect the natural shape of the lip.
- There is no point in modeling a philtrum if none was ever present naturally. This could produce a highly unnatural appearance and can easily lead to unwanted results, especially with less experienced therapists.
- It is important for the injection to be neither too deep, as the effect of the accentuation would be lost, nor too superficial, as this leaves small, unsightly bulges.

Possible Side Effects

Slight reddening, rarely inflammation, hematomas, swellings

Undesirable Side Effects

Overcorrection, asymmetry, blanching if the injection is too superficial, necrosis

Treatment Protocol at a Glance

- History, evaluation, and patient information
- Informed consent form
- Photo documentation: "before" images
- Analysis and marking of the areas to be treated
- Cleaning
- Thorough disinfection
- Local anesthesia (lidocaine cream) or conduction anesthesia if required
- Injection technique: linear technique, 1 line per philtral ridge
- Layer: subdermal
- Material: class "M viscous" product
- Volume: max. 0.05–0.1 ml per philtrum line, 0.2 ml in total
- Needle: 27G sharp needle
- No massage
- Cooling if required
- Heparin cream for hematomas, ibuprofen p.o., arnica
- Photo documentation: "after" images
- Advice on dos and don'ts after the procedure
- Follow-up appointment for a check-up after 8–14 days

9.2.6 TECHNIQUE 10

Modeling of the Philtrum and Cupid's Bow (Sharp Needle)

Here, the philtrum is injected in combination with the Cupid's bow, in order to gently raise the latter's peaks. Elevation of the philtral tip enhances this anatomically important region. The technique is particularly suitable for giving defined shape to a rather flat, undefined upper lip.

Patient Selection

- Where the shape of the upper lip is poorly defined due to age-related changes in lip shape, or where the contours of the upper lip are naturally flat

Injection Scheme and Planning (→ Technique 10 – Figs. 1, 2)

The injections are given with a sharp needle. The material is placed into the subdermal layer, directly into the Cupid's bow peaks and also into the philtrum. The philtral ridge starts from the medial edge of the nostril, on the lateral side of the bridge of the nose and runs outward slightly, down to the curvature of the upper lip.

Technique: linear technique

Direction of insertion: retrograde along the tip of the lip margin and in a line along the philtral ridge (applies to the upper lip only)

Layer: subdermal

Material: class "S/M viscous" product

Volume: max. 0.1 ml per tip, 0.1 ml per philtrum line, c. 0.4 ml in total

Needle: 27–30G sharp needle

Anesthesia: lidocaine cream, nerve block anesthesia

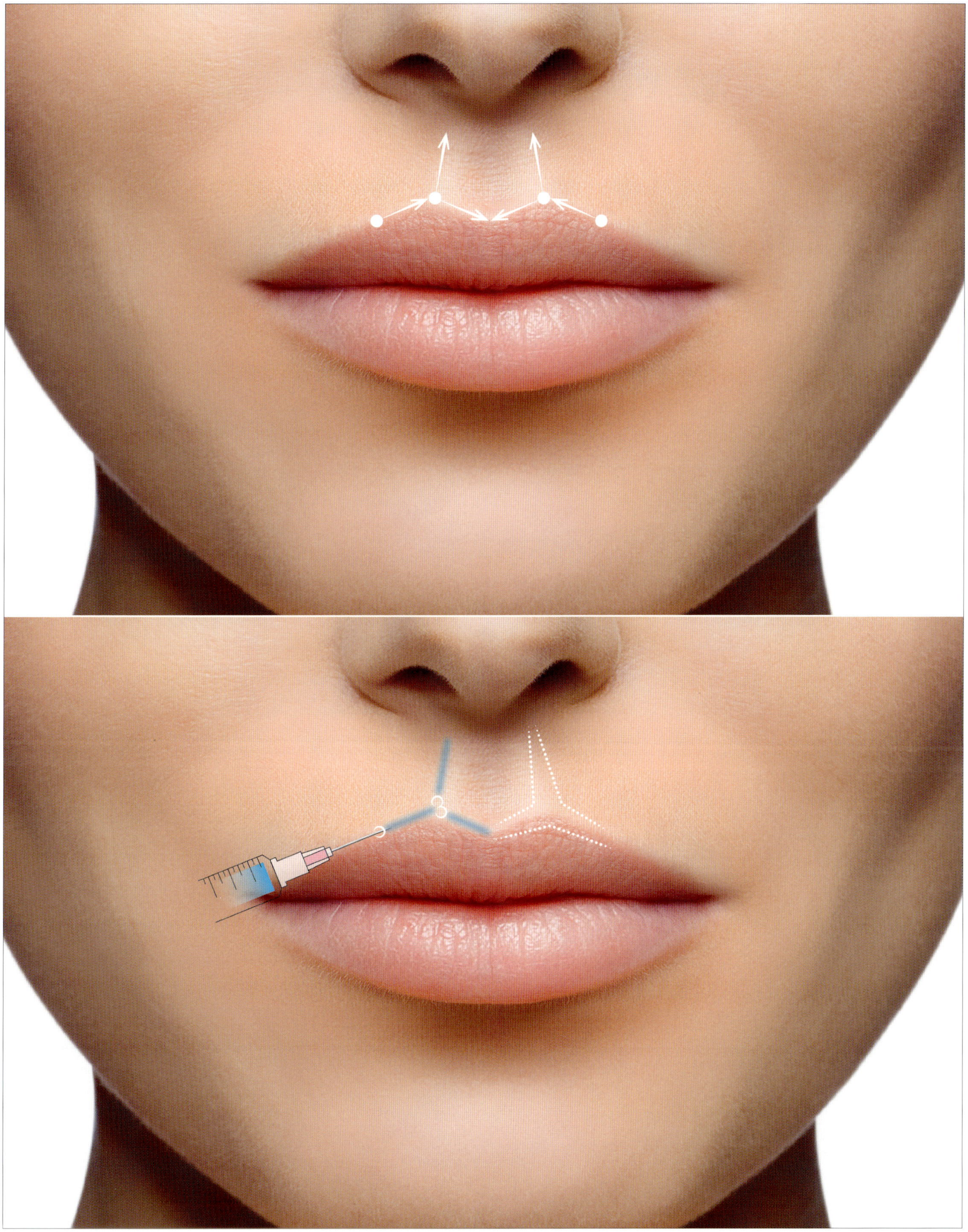

Technique 10 – Figs. 1, 2 Injection scheme and planning for modeling of the philtrum and Cupid's bow (sharp needle).

Treatment Method (→ Technique 10 – Figs. 3–5)

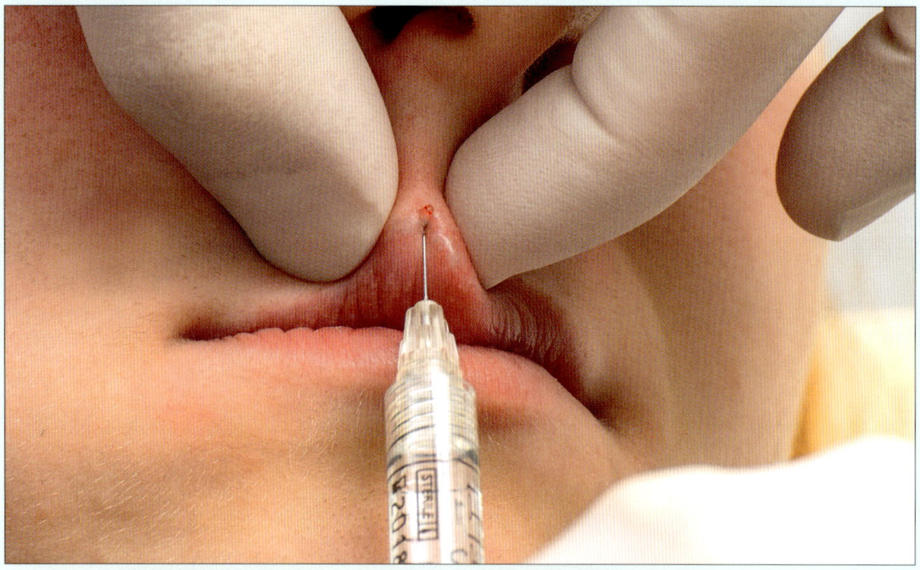

Technique 10 – Fig. 3 It is possible to accentuate the philtrum very slightly by injecting only one third of the length of the philtral ridge, starting from the Cupid's bow. We recommend this technique in patients who have never had a naturally prominent philtrum and in whom injection of the whole philtrum would give the mouth an alien appearance.

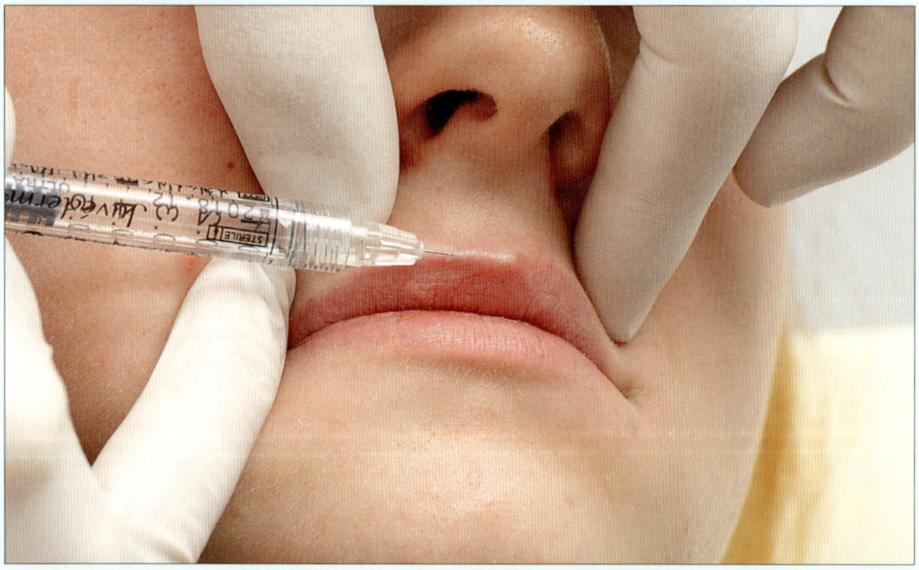

Technique 10 – Fig. 4 Stretch the lip between the thumb and forefinger of the left hand (if right-handed) and deliver the material into the subdermal layer, starting from the highest point of the Cupid's bow and working toward its lowest point.

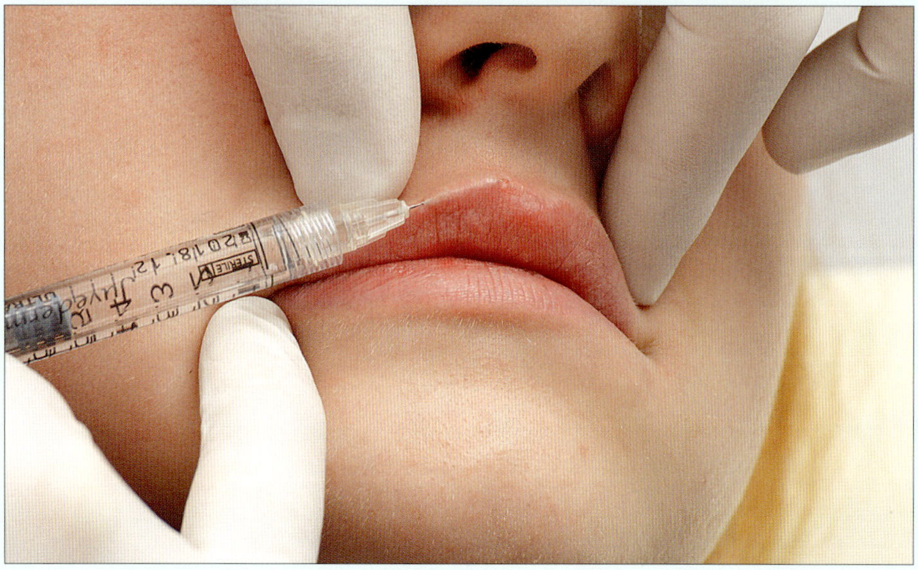

Technique 10 – Fig. 5 Stretch the lip between the thumb and forefinger of the left hand (if right-handed) and deliver the material into the subdermal layer by retrograde injection, starting 0.5 cm from the Cupid's bow peak.

Important Notes

- The material should be delivered precisely along the correct line, to respect the natural shape of the lip.
- There is no point in modeling a philtrum if none was ever present naturally. This could produce a highly unnatural appearance and can easily lead to unwanted results, especially with less experienced therapists.

Possible Side Effects

Slight reddening, rarely inflammation, hematomas, swellings

Undesirable Side Effects

Overcorrection, asymmetry, blanching if the injection is too superficial, necrosis

Treatment Protocol at a Glance

- History, evaluation, and patient information
- Informed consent form
- Photo documentation: "before" images
- Analysis and marking of the areas to be treated
- Cleaning
- Thorough disinfection
- Local anesthesia (lidocaine cream) or conduction anesthesia if required
- Injection technique: linear technique, 1 line per philtral ridge
- Layer: subdermal
- Material: class "S/M viscous" product
- Volume: max. 0.1 ml per peak, 0.1 ml per philtrum line, c. 0.4 ml in total
- Needle: 27–30G sharp needle
- No massage
- Cooling if required
- Heparin cream for hematomas, ibuprofen p.o., arnica
- Photo documentation: "after" images
- Advice on dos and don'ts after the procedure
- Follow-up appointment for a check-up after 8–14 days

9.3 Perioral Lines

It is common for patients of advanced age to come to the practice solely for treatment of the perioral zones of the cutaneous part of the lip. The aging process manifests itself most conspicuously in this region.

A number of approaches are available for the treatment of perioral lines (also known as radial lines). These treatments differ only slightly from one another and include the classic linear technique/fishbone technique as well as the stretching, compression, point, and blanching techniques. The treatment goal of the techniques shown here is to reduce or remove perioral lines that are produced by causes such as smoking, extrinsic or extrinsic damage, and aging processes, especially hormone deficits. It is also advisable to include the cutaneous part of the lip in any lip augmentation treatment, as this helps it integrate into the face more harmoniously. The more advanced the depth of the perioral lines, the more prolonged and difficult the treatment will be – and not always with satisfactory results.

9.3.1 TECHNIQUE 11 Linear and Fishbone Technique for Perioral Lines (Sharp Needle)

9

The treatment goal is rehydration of the perioral region (cutaneous part of the lip), restoring its freshness and youthful vitality. Moisture depots are injected in the form of microdroplets of low- or non-crosslinked HA. This technique is performed with a sharp needle. It enables accurate hydration of the lips by the targeted administration of HA over an extended area. The resultant neocollagenesis is caused by multiple, minor tissue injuries with a sharp needle, which has a positive effect on the general regeneration of the skin.

Patient Selection

- In age-related dryness of the lips due to a lack of sebaceous glands or genetic factors; extrinsic and intrinsic factors also play a major role
- Younger patients who want to refresh and improve their complexion

Technique: linear and fishbone technique

Direction of insertion: from the contour toward the nose and chin, respectively, and across the course of the perioral lines

Layer: subdermal in the cutaneous part of the lip

Material: class "XS/S soft" product

Volume: depending on the depth of the wrinkles, c. 0.5 ml

Needle: 27–30G sharp needle

Anesthesia: lidocaine cream

Injection Scheme and Planning (→ Technique 11 – Figs. 1–4)

The **linear technique along the course of a wrinkle** is a standard, basic technique used for the direct linear filling of fine perioral lines: they are filled, one by one, above the contour of the upper lip and below the contour of the lower lip. Low-crosslinked HA is used for this purpose to achieve a gentle lifting effect. The powerful mimic movements of the mouth rapidly squeeze the HA out again. The material is placed into the cutaneous part of the lip above (upper lip) and below (lower lip) the contour. A sharp needle is used in the upper lip in the part of the wrinkle close to the lip, inserting it into the subdermal layer and advancing it upward below the wrinkle. The HA is delivered by retrograde injection. In the lower lip, it can be easier to inject from below the lip and in the direction of the lip contour. Like the perioral point technique (see Technique 12, p. 172 ff.), this technique may be modified or supplemented by applying the stretching or compression method.

The **fishbone technique used across the course of a wrinkle** reinforces the effect of injecting along the course of the wrinkle. Low-crosslinked HA is first injected along the course of the wrinkle with a 30G needle using the linear injection technique. In the second step, the tissue is stretched between the thumb and forefinger of the opposite hand and the material injected very superficially across the wrinkle. This causes the compression that is the result of mimic activity to be distributed over a larger area. The injection may be given from either side. The volume of material delivered is very small.

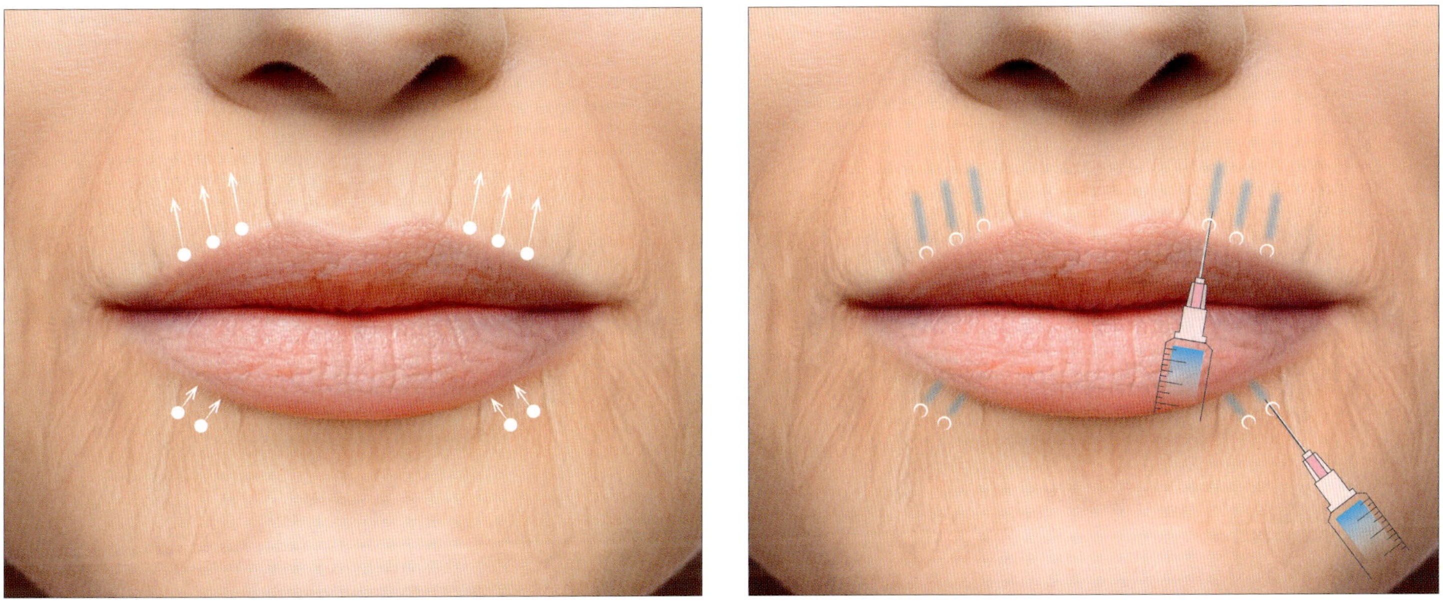

Technique 11 – Figs. 1, 2 Injection scheme and planning for **Variant 1: linear technique for perioral lines (sharp needle).**

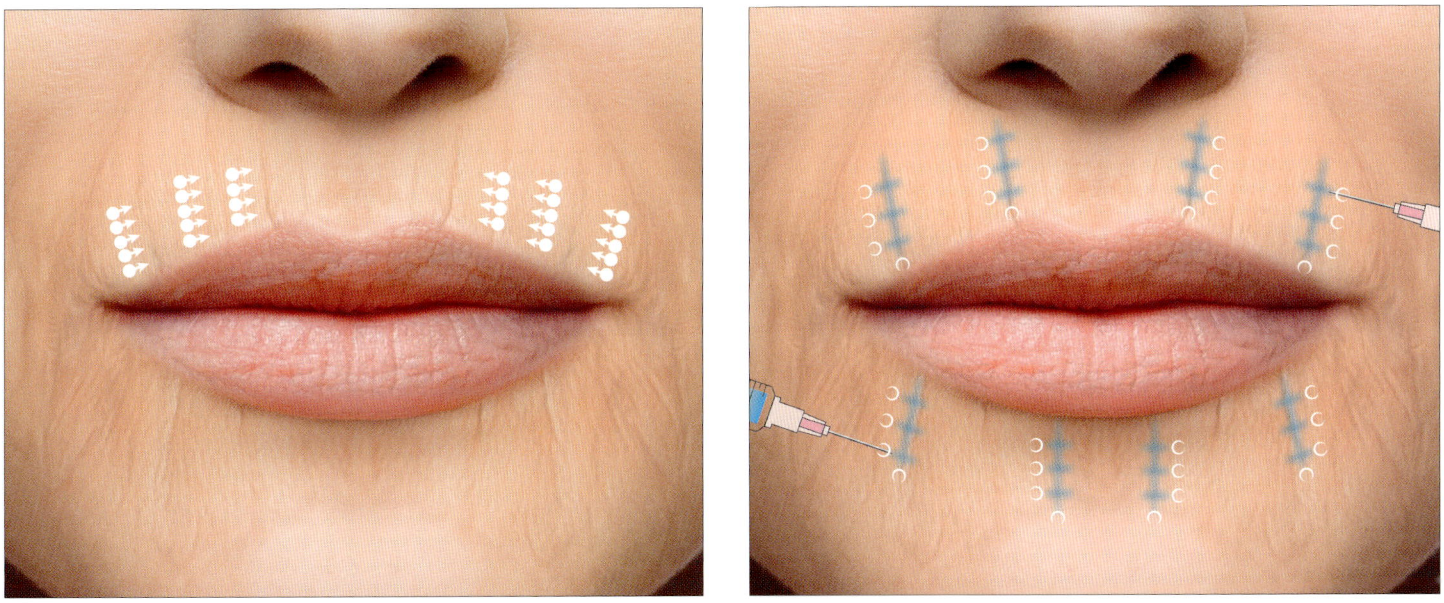

Technique 11 – Figs. 3, 4 Injection scheme and planning for **Variant 2: fishbone technique for perioral lines (sharp needle).**

Treatment Method (→ Technique 11 – Figs. 5–7)

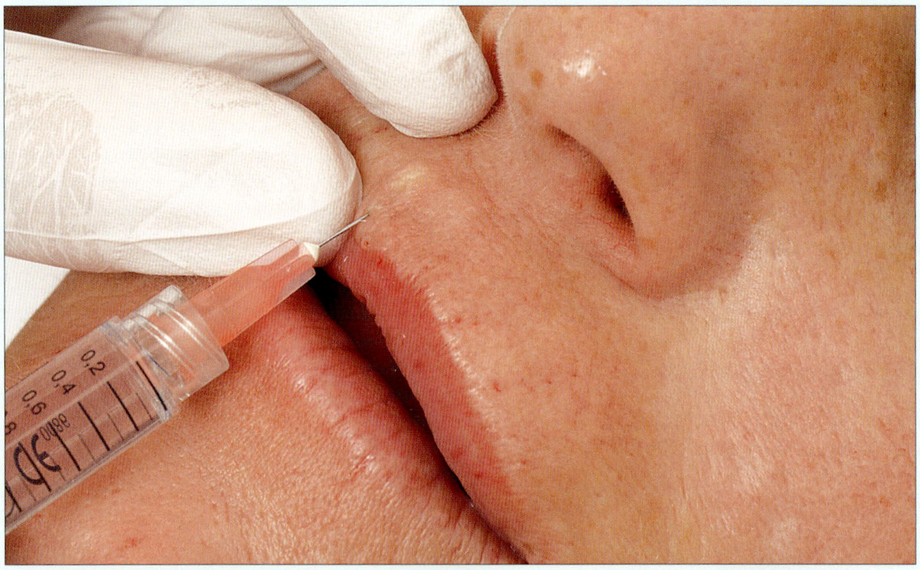

Technique 11 – Fig. 5

Variant 1 (linear technique): Inject the HA superficially, so that needle can be seen shimmering through the skin. Deliver the material by retrograde injection. It is important not to overcorrect the wrinkle, so that delivery of a small volume of material is recommended to begin with. The delivered material that can be seen in this image (white patch) can be levelled off by applying pressure with the thumb after the injection.

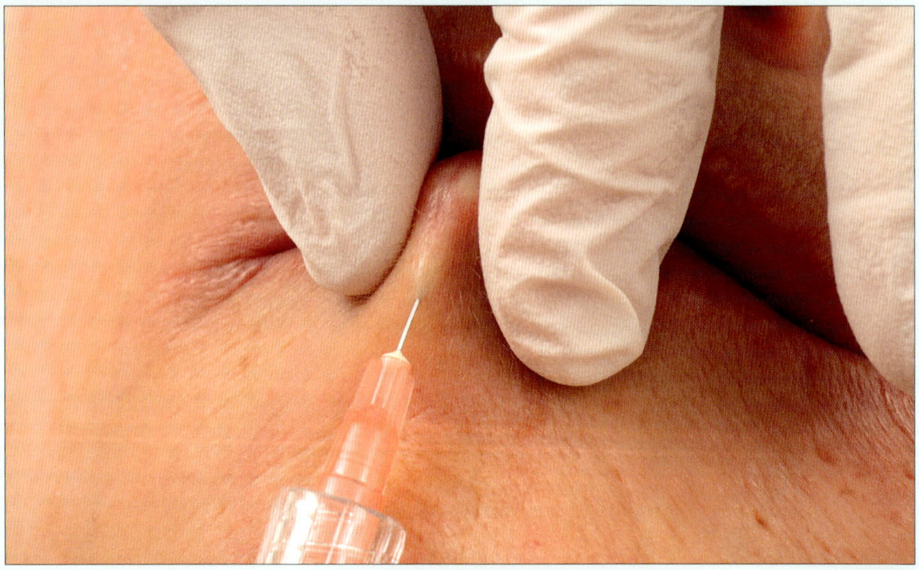

Technique 11 – Fig. 6

Variant 1 (linear technique): Holding the wrinkle in place gently makes it easier to control perioral linear injections, ensuring uniform delivery parallel to the surface of the skin.

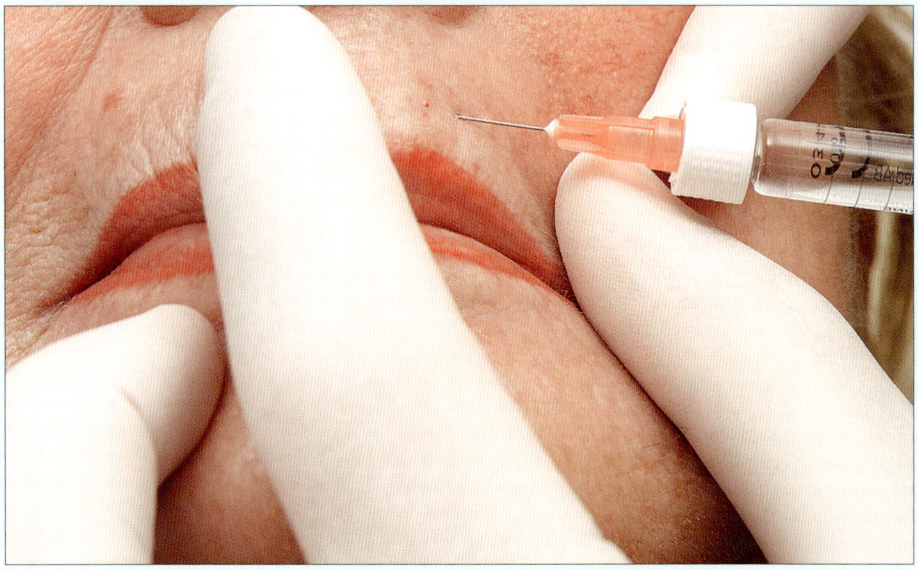

Technique 11 – Fig. 7

Variant 2 (fishbone technique): After injecting material along the wrinkle (see above), insert the needle c. 1 mm beside the wrinkle and across it, and advance the needle below the wrinkle up to c. 1 mm beyond it. Deliver tiny amounts of material by retrograde injection. This produces a gentle counterpressure to the compression produced by mimic activity.

Important Notes

- This technique is particularly suitable for the superficial augmentation of seborrheic skin.
- Overcorrection must be avoided at all costs, as it could easily lead to unwanted, visible irregularities or unsightly stripes.
- If too much material is used and if it is delivered too close to the surface, a bluish, glassy hue may become visible under the skin, known as the Tyndall effect. This effect can occur as a complication with all superficial injections.

Possible Side Effects

Slight reddening, rarely inflammation, rarely hematomas, mild to more severe swellings, Tyndall effect, blanching

Undesirable Side Effects

Inflammation, overcorrection with the resultant formation of stripes or nodules, non-uniform delivery of material resulting in asymmetry, necrosis

Treatment Protocol at a Glance

- History, evaluation, and patient information
- Informed consent form
- Photo documentation: "before" images
- Analysis and marking of the areas to be treated
- Cleaning
- Thorough disinfection
- Local anesthesia (lidocaine cream) or conduction anesthesia if required
- Injection technique: linear technique, 1 line of material per wrinkle, fishbone technique
- Layer: subdermal in the cutaneous part of the lip
- Material: class "XS/S soft" product
- Volume: depending on the depth of the wrinkles, c. 0.5 ml
- Needle: 27–30G sharp needle
- No massage
- Cooling if required
- Heparin cream for hematomas, ibuprofen p.o., arnica
- Photo documentation: "after" images
- Advice on dos and don'ts after the procedure
- Follow-up appointment for a check-up after 8–14 days

9.3.2 TECHNIQUE 12

Perioral Point Technique, Modification by Stretching or Compression (Sharp Needle)

Like the linear technique, the perioral point technique is a classic, basic injection technique for the treatment of lines in the perioral region (see Technique 11, p 168 ff.), which allows the tiniest depots to be placed into the effective zones (sweet spots) of these wrinkles. The vertical injection, placed into relaxed skin, produces a lift effect after the material is delivered, and smooths out the wrinkle. In addition, the bolus has a moderating effect on mimic activity in the area, so that the positive effect of the augmentation persists for a longer time.

To avoid undesirable side effects, both the stretching and compression techniques are used to modify the procedure when administering linear and point injections into the cutaneous part of the lip. In the relaxed state, side effects can include irregularities ranging up to bulging overcorrections, which can be prevented by increasing pressure on the tissue by either stretching or compression.

The stretching technique is recommended for the augmentation of superficial radial lines, and the stretching technique for deep lines in order to optimize the treatment results of perioral point and linear injections administered according to Technique 11.

Patient Selection

- For mimic, perioral or smoker's lines
- In patients with fine lines of varying cause (stretching technique)
- In patients with deep lines of varying cause (compression technique)

Technique: both point and linear technique, modified by stretching and compression

Direction of insertion: point technique: vertical or slightly lateral injection; linear technique: from the contour toward the nose and chin, respectively, or horizontally (angle of insertion 30 degrees, 45–90 degrees with the compression technique)

Layer: subdermal in the cutaneous part of the lip; intracutaneous, subcutaneous or intramuscular for deep wrinkles

Material: class "XS/S soft" product

Volume: depending on the depth of the wrinkles, c. 0.03–0.05 ml

Needle: 27–30G sharp needle

Anesthesia: lidocaine cream

Injection Scheme and Planning (→ Technique 12 – Figs. 1–6)

The apex of a wrinkle is the primary treatment target of the **perioral point technique**. Injection into the apex produces targeted soft tissue augmentation. The material is delivered until the tissue is lifted and, ideally, once the wrinkle has been smoothed out. Excellent lighting and accurate work are important, as any irregularities are clearly visible in the cutaneous part of the upper lip. The HA used should exhibit very low crosslinking to avoid the potential creation of wheal-like bumps. Should visible boluses still occur, these can be dispersed by massage.

In the **stretching technique**, the interstitial tissue pressure is increased by added maximum stretching in preparation for the augmentation (Sattler & Sommer 2015). The perioral wrinkles are filled by means of direct point injections or the tiniest linear injections, with an angle of insertion of 30 degrees. The best procedure is for an assistant to stretch the tissue powerfully during the injection. This causes the skin to exert counterpressure to the injected filler, influencing HA distribution during the injection and preventing bulgy overcorrection.

In the **compression technique**, the interstitial tissue pressure is altered by added maximum compression in preparation for the augmentation. The free hand should be used to grasp and compress the tissue powerfully between thumb and forefinger. The apex of the wrinkle is the target of the augmentation. Injection into the apex under compression produces targeted soft tissue augmentation. Here, the point technique is a vertical depot technique enabling the tiniest depots to be placed into the most effective point of the wrinkle, to augment it by adding volume. The injection depth varies with that of the wrinkle. If the wrinkles are very pronounced, an HA bolus may be injected as an intramuscular depot to counteract the mimic power generated in the muscle tissue.

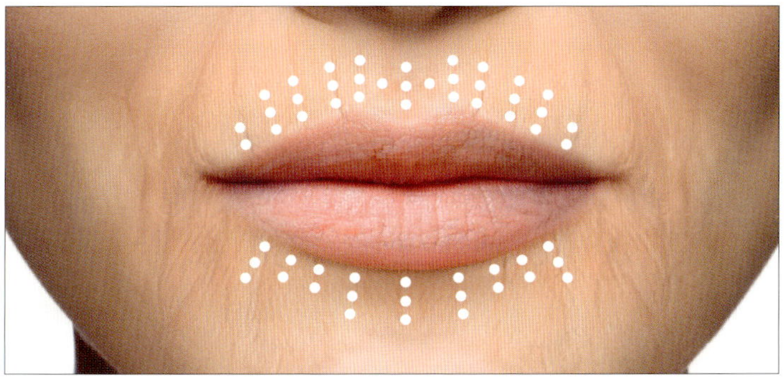
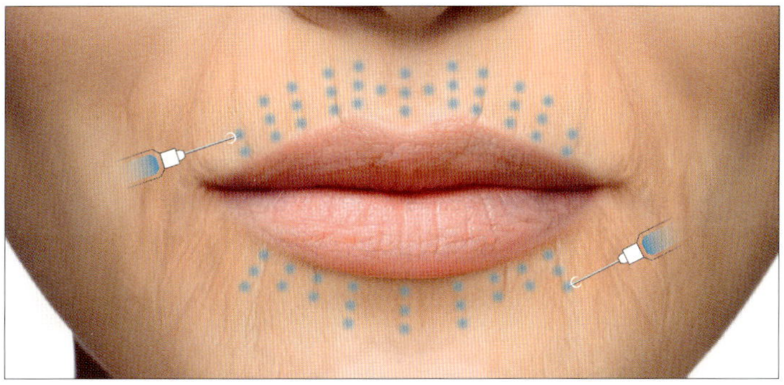

Technique 12 – Figs. 1, 2 Injection scheme and planning for **Variant 1: classic perioral point technique (sharp needle).**

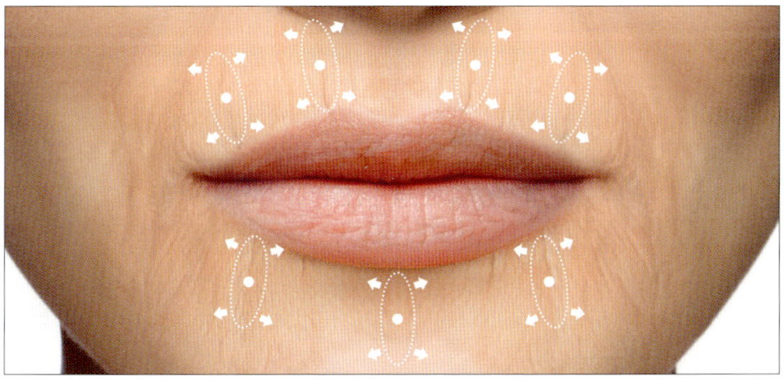
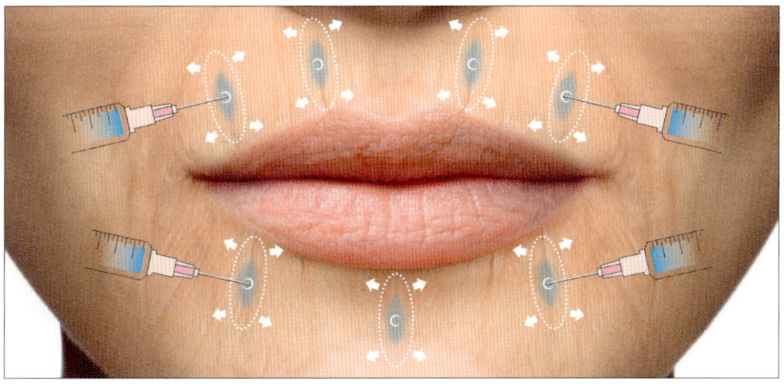

Technique 12 – Figs. 3, 4 Injection scheme and planning for **Variant 2: stretching technique for perioral injection (sharp needle).**

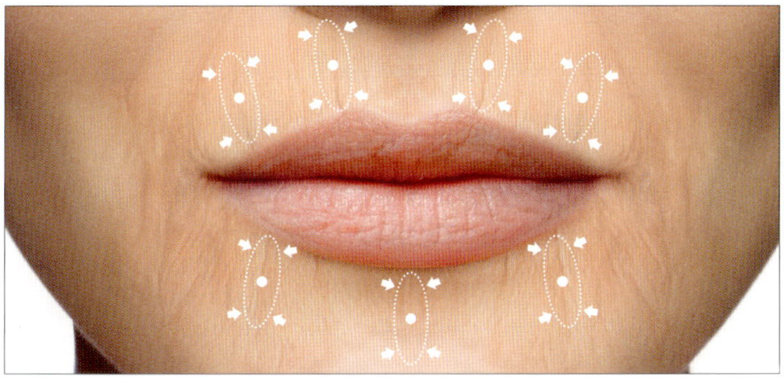
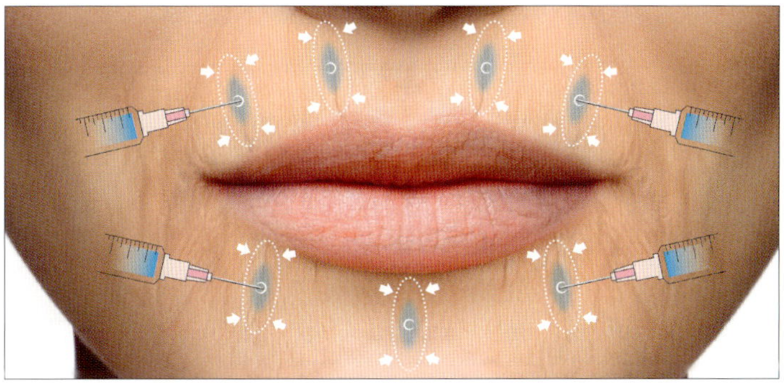

Technique 12 – Figs. 5, 6 Injection scheme and planning for **Variant 3: compression technique for perioral injection (sharp needle).**

Treatment Method (→ Technique 12 – Figs. 7–12)

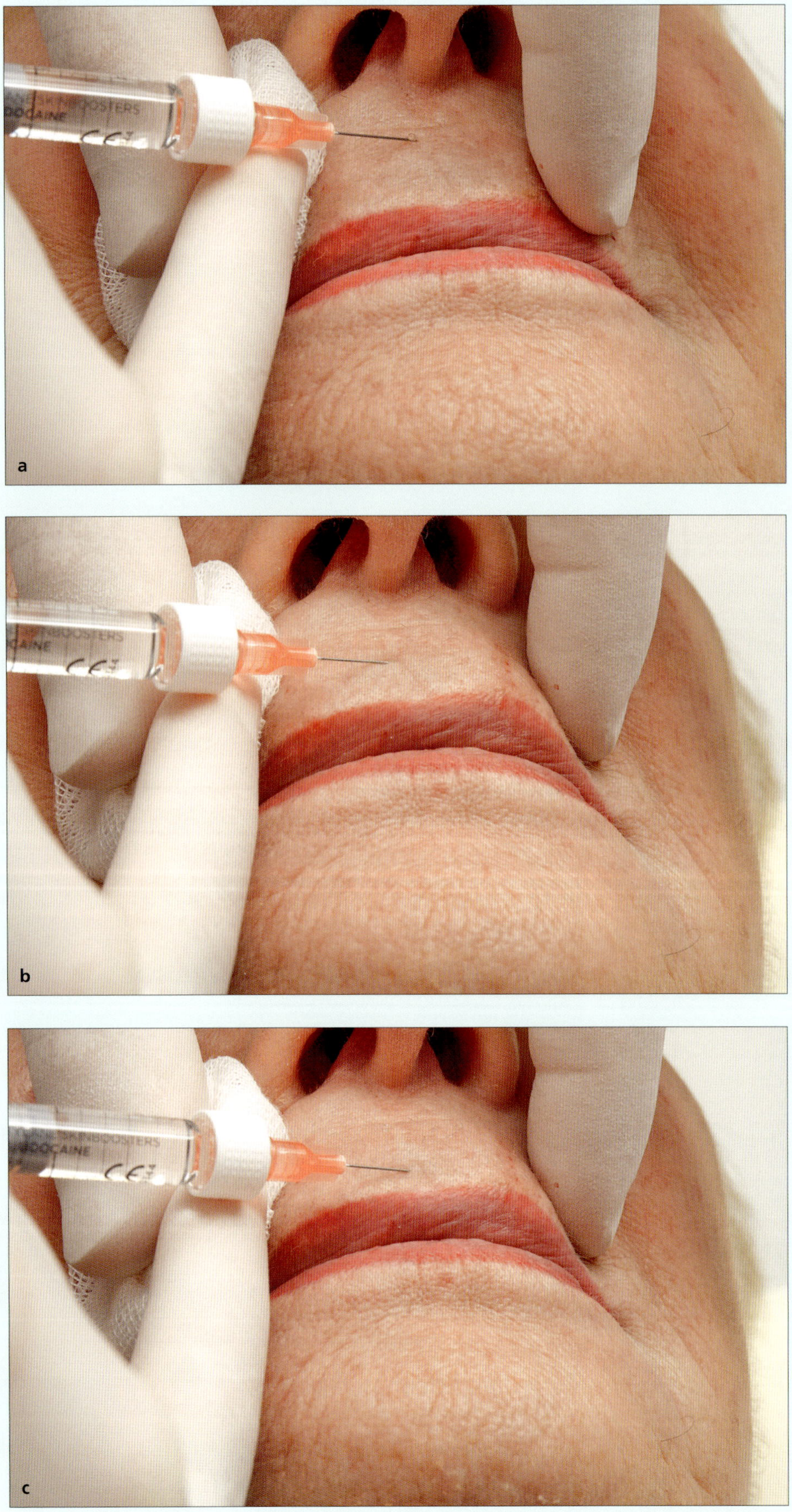

Technique 12 – Figs. 7 a–c

Variant 1 (point technique): Following thorough disinfection, stretch the skin gently and, with small, quick movements, place a pinhead-sized point of material into the center of the wrinkle. Treat each wrinkle with numerous small points placed along its course (a–c).

Point technique

Treatment Method (continued)

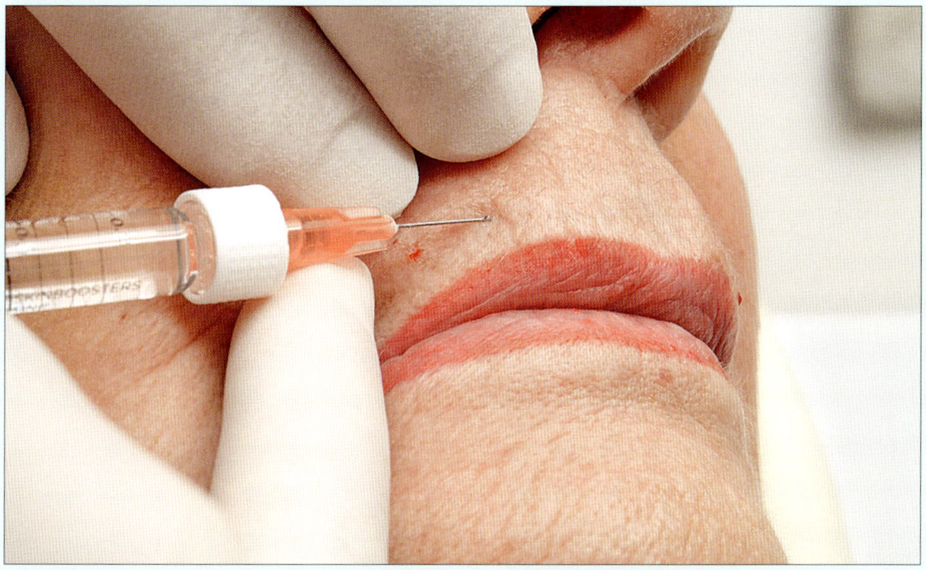

Technique 12 – Fig. 8

Variant 1 (point technique): Inject from the front or slightly from the side, directly into the center of the wrinkle.

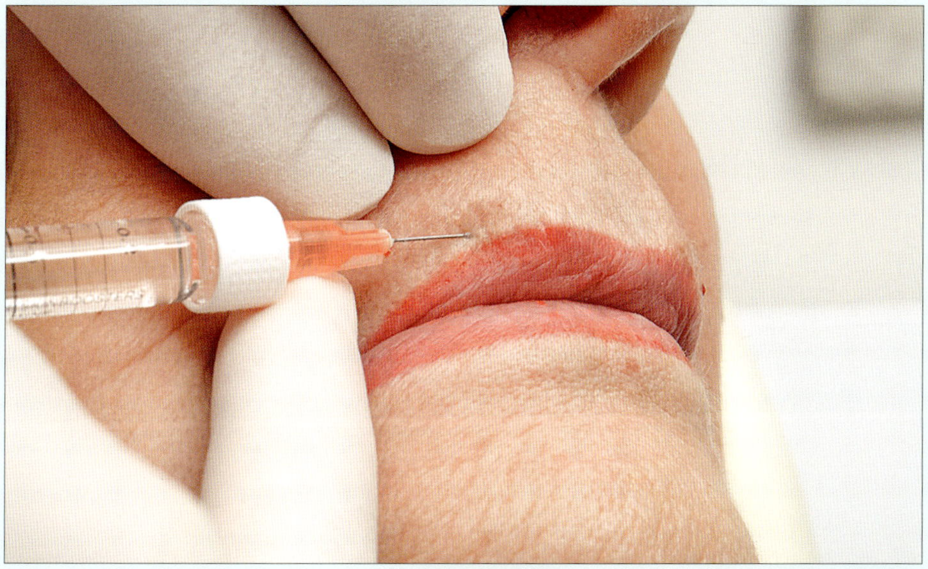

Technique 12 – Fig. 9

Variant 1 (point technique): For very fine perioral wrinkles that are located close to the contour, and which are thus exposed to extreme mimic movements, it is advisable to deliver slightly more material to generate resistance to the pressure of the mimic muscles on the wrinkle.

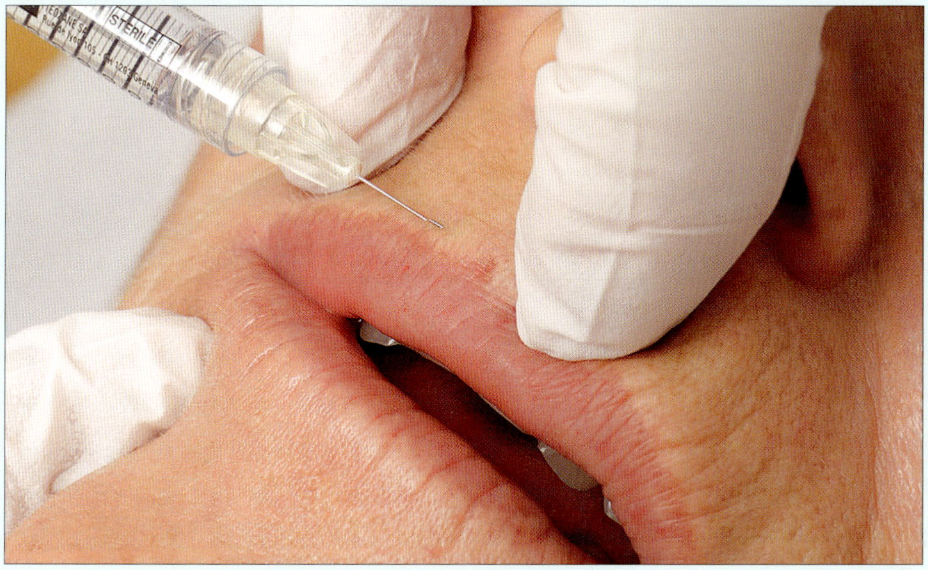

Technique 12 – Fig. 10

Variant 2 (stretching technique): Before the skin is stretched, the patient should be asked to pucker up the lips as much as possible, so that the therapist can see the exact course of the wrinkles. The skin should be stretched to a maximum immediately after this. If possible, this can be done by an assistant, leaving the therapist with both hands free. The skin can also be stretched by the therapist's free hand. The stretch needs to be powerful to allow the tissue to resist overcorrection. The needle bevel should face upward.

Stretching technique

Treatment Method (continued)

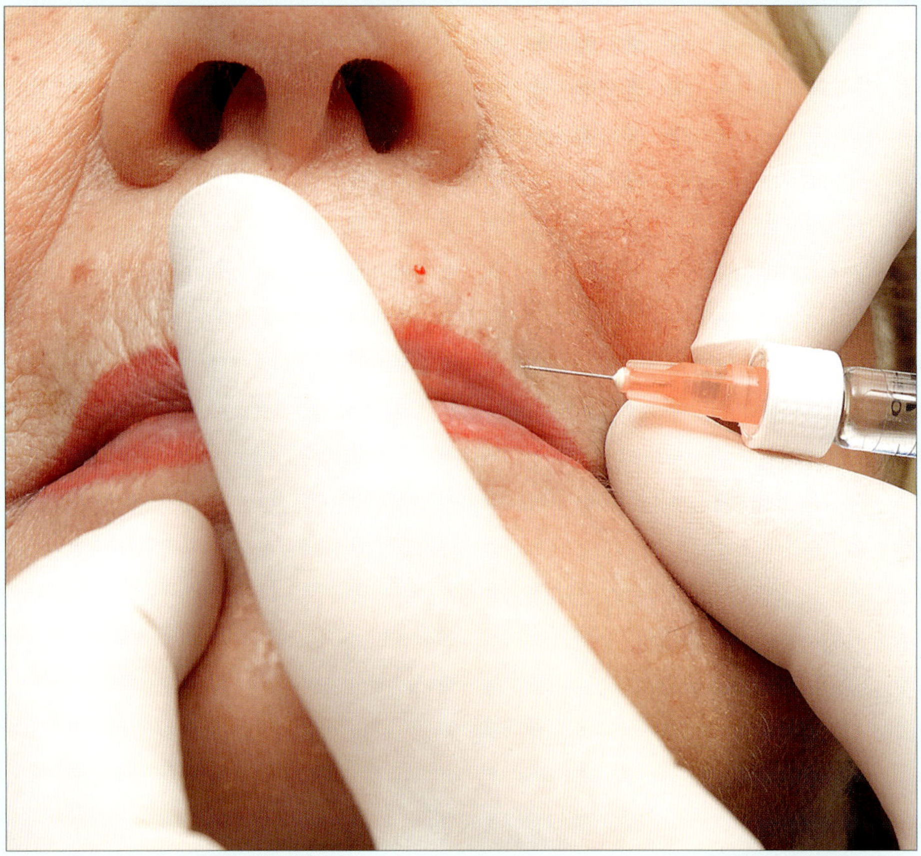

Technique 12 – Fig. 11

Variant 2 (stretching technique): Inject the HA superficially, placing the points next to each other along the entire wrinkle (as an alternative, the wrinkle may be injected using the linear technique). This treatment needs to be repeated 2–3 times to allow the tissue to regenerate by fibroblast formation.

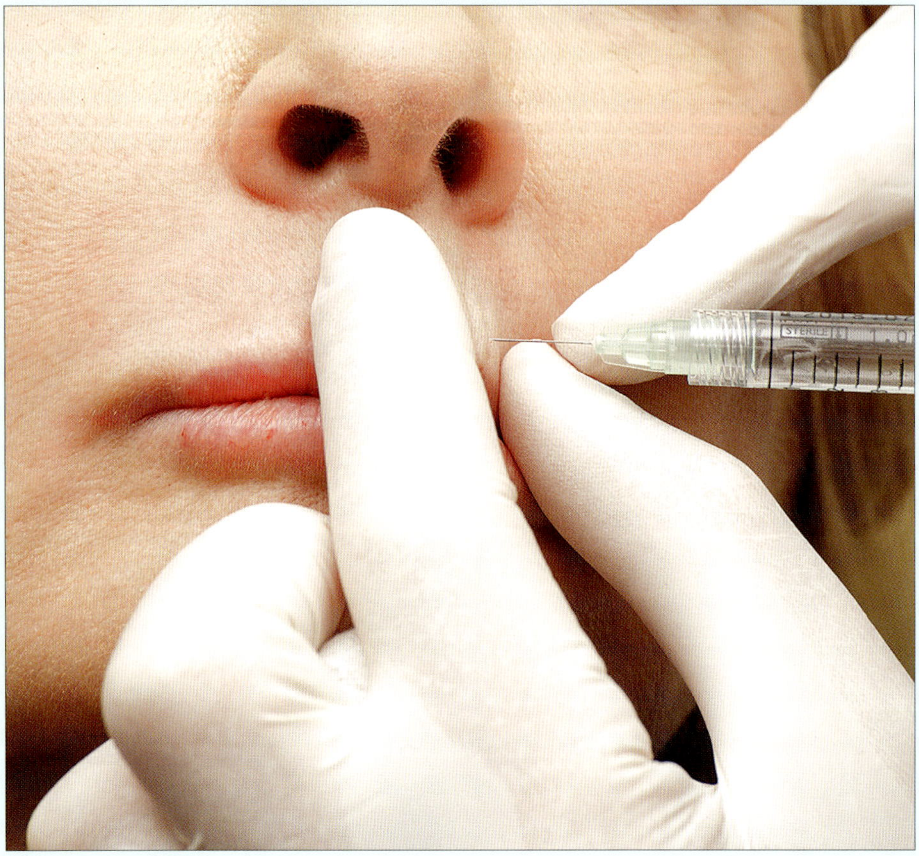

Technique 12 – Fig. 12

Variant 3 (compression technique): The compression needs to be powerful to generate enough pressure to allow the tissue to counteract overcorrection.

Compression technique

Important Notes

- If too much material is used and if it is delivered too close to the surface, a bluish, glassy hue may become visible under the skin, known as the Tyndall effect. If low-crosslinked materials are used, as recommended in this case, the risk of producing a Tyndall effect is very low.
- A bumpy, irregular appearance is easily produced if a lot of material is used, if it is delivered too close to the surface or if less pronounced wrinkles are overcorrected.
- Swellings may remain prominent for one to five days after the treatment. This should be discussed with the patient beforehand.

Possible Side Effects

Slight reddening, rarely inflammation, rarely hematomas, mild to more severe swellings, Tyndall effect, blanching effect

Undesirable Side Effects

Inflammation, overcorrection in the form of stripes or nodules, non-uniform delivery of material with resultant asymmetry, necrosis

Treatment Protocol at a Glance

- History, evaluation, and patient information
- Informed consent form
- Photo documentation: "before" images
- Analysis and marking of the areas to be treated
- Cleaning
- Thorough disinfection
- Local anesthesia (lidocaine cream) or conduction anesthesia if required
- Injection technique: both point and linear technique, modified by stretching and compression
- Layer: subdermal in the cutaneous part of the lip; intracutaneous, subcutaneous or intramuscular for deep wrinkles
- Material: class "XS/S soft" product
- Volume: dependent on the number of wrinkles treated: 0.03–0.05 ml per wrinkle
- Needle: 27–30G sharp needle
- No massage
- Cooling if required
- Heparin cream for hematomas, ibuprofen p.o., arnica
- Photo documentation: "after" images
- Advice on dos and don'ts after the procedure
- Follow-up appointment for a check-up after 8–14 days

9.3.3 TECHNIQUE 13

Perioral Blanching Technique (Sharp Needle)

The blanching technique differs from the preceding perioral point technique in that the injections are given into the most superficial skin layer, delivering extremely small amounts of material so that intentional blanching of the skin is produced.

Patient Selection

- In persistent fine and superficial perioral lines
- In age-related dryness of the lips due to a lack of sebaceous glands or genetic factors; extrinsic and intrinsic factors also play a major role

Injection Scheme and Planning (→ Technique 13 – Figs. 1, 2)

Use of this minimally invasive technique makes it possible to break up a wrinkle with HA injections in the uppermost skin layer. The injections are given along the apex of the wrinkle with a sharp needle and the point technique. The success of the treatment is evident when skin blanching (Sattler & Sommer 2015) occurs at each point.

The goal is to lift the tissue gently and to activate neocollagenesis through multiple, minor tissue injuries that have a positive effect on skin regeneration. The material is injected intradermally, either across the wrinkle or vertically, inserting the needle to a depth of 1–2 mm.

Technique: point blanching technique
Direction of insertion: along or across the wrinkle
Layer: intradermal in the cutaneous part of the lip
Material: class "XS/S soft" product
Volume: 0.01–0.02 ml per point
Needle: 27–33G sharp needle
Anesthesia: lidocaine cream

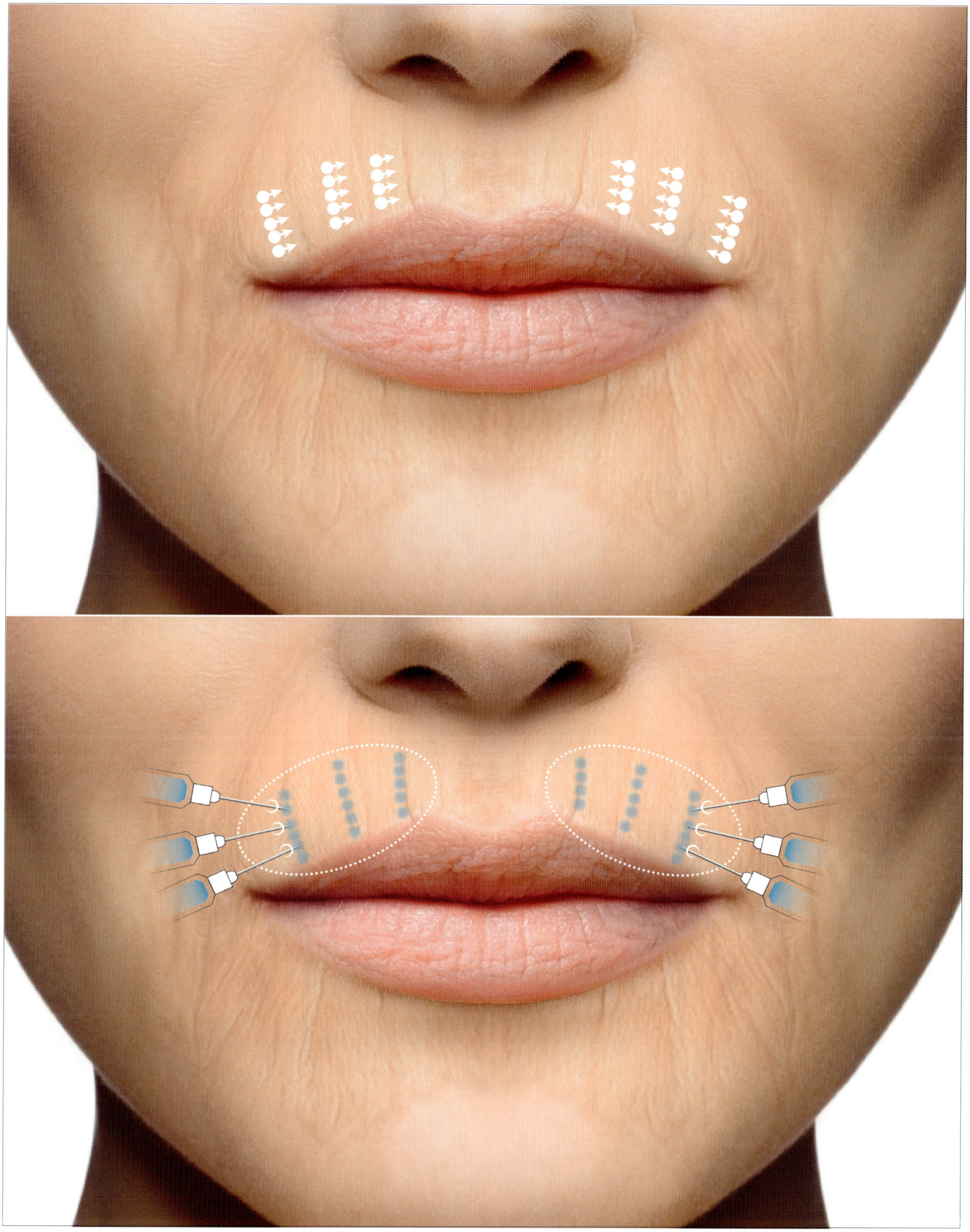

Technique 13 – Figs. 1, 2 Injection scheme and planning for the perioral blanching technique (sharp needle).

Treatment Method (→ Technique 13 – Figs. 3, 4)

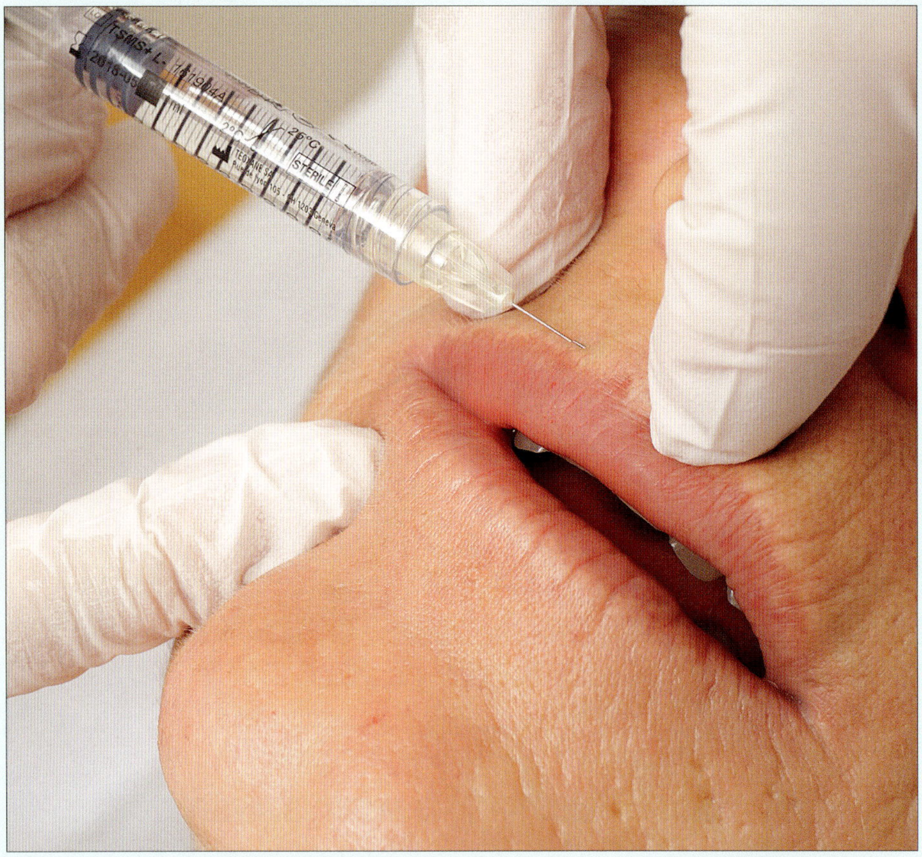

Technique 13 – Fig. 3 Stretch the skin gently, plunge in the needle bevel very superficially and parallel to the skin, advancing it 1 mm toward the front. Deliver points of material by retrograde injection, across the course of the wrinkle. The needle bevel should face upward and should be inserted superficially into the deepest part of each wrinkle. Proceed in this way along the entire length of the wrinkle.

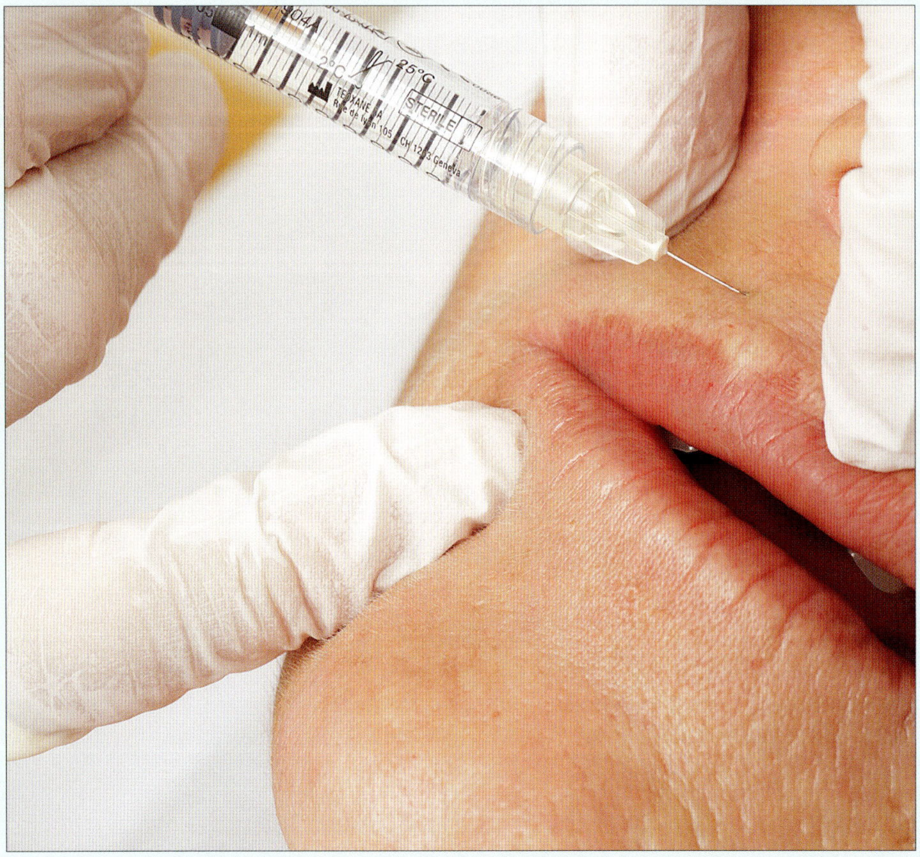

Technique 13 – Fig. 4 Repeat the procedure at intervals of 2–3 mm. Administer around 20–30 injections per quadrant into the cutaneous part of the lip. A possible variant is to inject into and along the course of the wrinkle using the linear technique.

9

Important Notes

- It is not easy to deliver such small amounts of material without wasting some of it when withdrawing the needle. It is therefore necessary to work slowly and accurately. However, if too much material is delivered, it is easy to massage it gently into the skin.
- The stretching technique is recommended to pull the wrinkle apart. An alternative is to insert a forefinger into the patient's mouth behind the lip and to use the thumb to pull at the lip to make the wrinkle bulge outward.
- The linear technique is recommended if the wrinkle is already somewhat more pronounced, i.e. if it is visible as a defined line. The point technique is preferable if the skin is uneven due to loss of elasticity, but no definite wrinkles are yet visible.
- If very pronounced lines are already present, 1–2 follow-up treatments will be necessary.

Possible Side Effects

Slight reddening, rarely inflammation, rarely hematomas, mild swellings

Undesirable Side Effects

Inflammation, overcorrection possible if using low-cross-linked HA with resultant bulges, necrosis

Treatment Protocol at a Glance

- History, evaluation, and patient information
- Informed consent form
- Photo documentation: "before" images
- Analysis and marking of the areas to be treated
- Cleaning
- Thorough disinfection
- Local anesthesia (lidocaine cream) or conduction anesthesia if required
- Injection technique: point blanching technique
- Layer: intradermal in the cutaneous part of the lip
- Material: class "XS/S soft" product
- Volume: 0.01–0.02 ml per point
- Needle: 27–33G sharp needle
- No massage required
- Cooling if required
- Heparin cream for hematomas, ibuprofen p.o., arnica
- Photo documentation: "after" images
- Advice on dos and don'ts after the procedure
- Follow-up appointment for a check-up after 8–14 days

9.3.4 TECHNIQUE 14
"Fern Pattern Technique" according to Tom van Eijk (Sharp Needle)

The aim of this technique is to injure the sweet spot (effective zone) of a wrinkle very superficially by making a direct incision with the tip of a needle (van Eijk 2007, van Eijk & Braun 2007). The long-term result is astonishingly good, even with stubborn wrinkles. The reason is that neocollagenesis is activated by the multiple minor tissue injuries, which has a positive effect on skin regeneration.

Patient Selection

- For smoker's wrinkles, mimic wrinkles, fine perioral (radial) lines, and a dry perioral region, caused by extrinsic and/or intrinsic factors, aging processes, and the hormone deficits associated with them.

Injection Scheme and Planning (→ Technique 14 – Figs. 1, 2)

During the treatment, the wrinkles need to be lit well to allow the deepest point, or apex, of each one to be accurately identified. The needle is placed into the apex with the bevel facing up, and the HA is injected c. 3 mm intradermally, going sideways in one direction (e.g. toward the right). This procedure is repeated along the wrinkle at 3-mm intervals. The therapist then moves to the other side and repeats the procedure along the same wrinkle, but in a staggered fashion (see the schematic diagram on the right): the needle should be placed into the apex of the wrinkle between two insertion sites on the other side, so that the injections are administered laterally in the opposite direction (toward the left), forming a fern pattern.

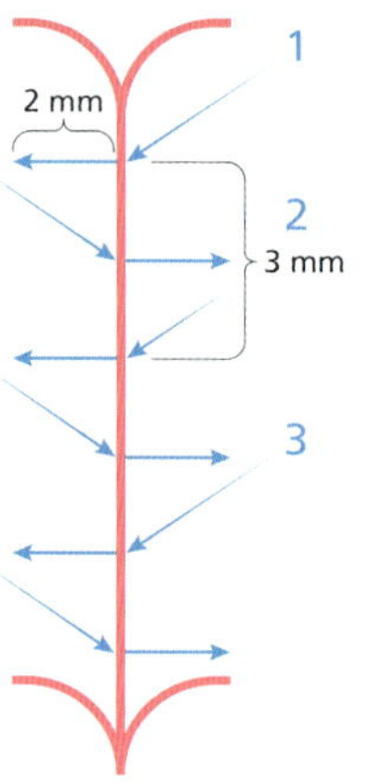

Schematic representation of the fern pattern technique

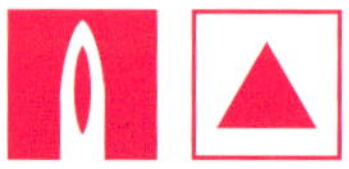

Technique: short linear technique
Direction of insertion: from the apex of the wrinkle toward the periphery
Layer: subdermal in the cutaneous part of the lip
Material: class "S viscous" product
Volume: max. 0.02 ml per line of material
Needle: 27–30G sharp needle
Anesthesia: lidocaine cream, conduction anesthesia if required

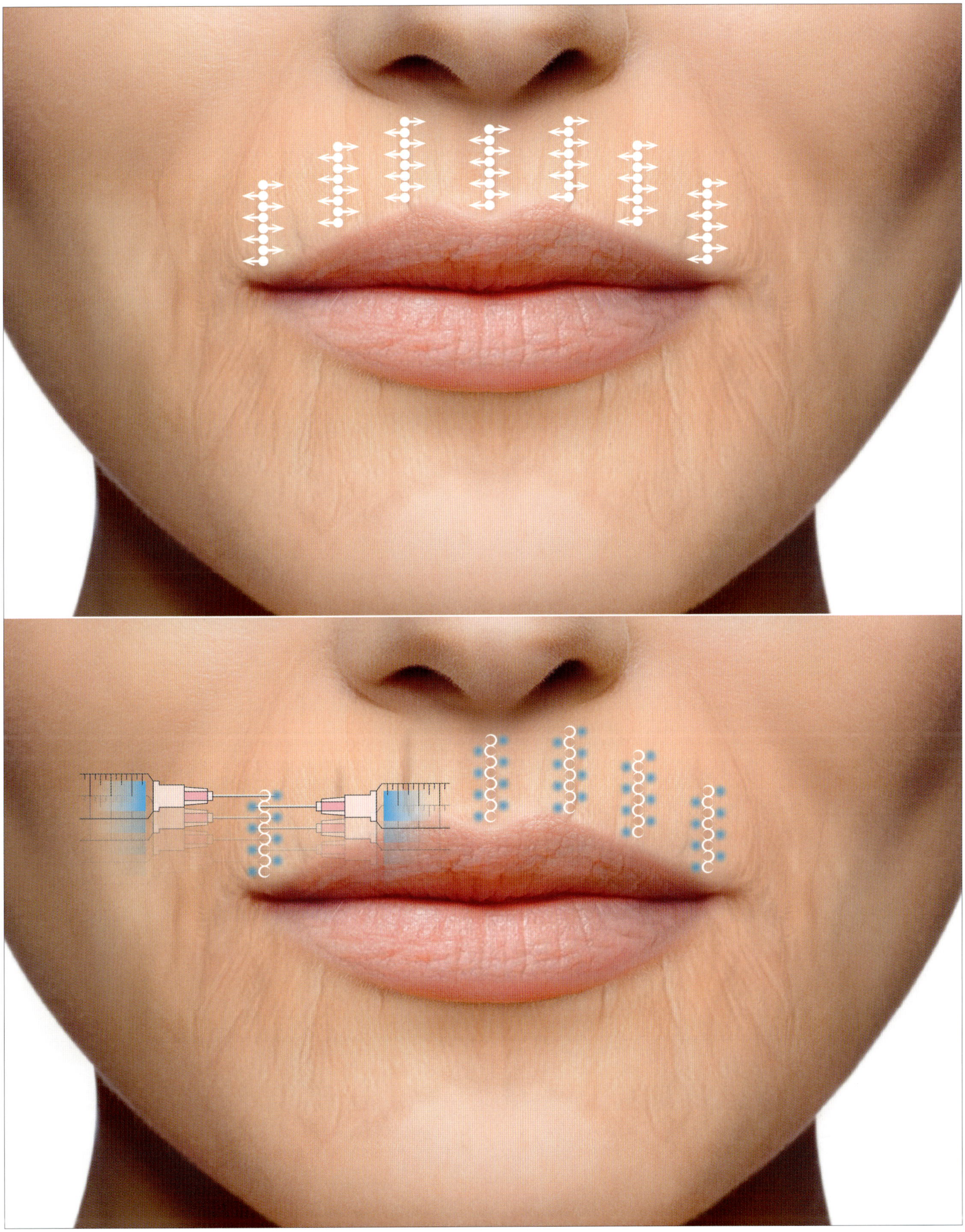

Technique 14 – Figs. 1, 2 Injection scheme and planning for the fern pattern technique according to Tom van Eijk (sharp needle).

Treatment Method (→ Technique 14 – Figs. 3–6)

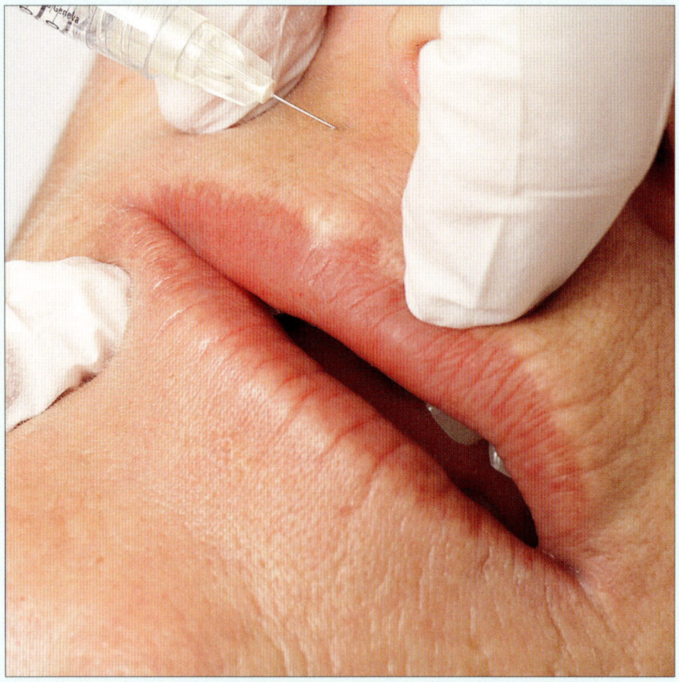

Technique 14 – Fig. 3 Practice and a good eye are needed to inject according to the fern pattern technique. The distance between the injection lines on each side should be no more than 3 mm.

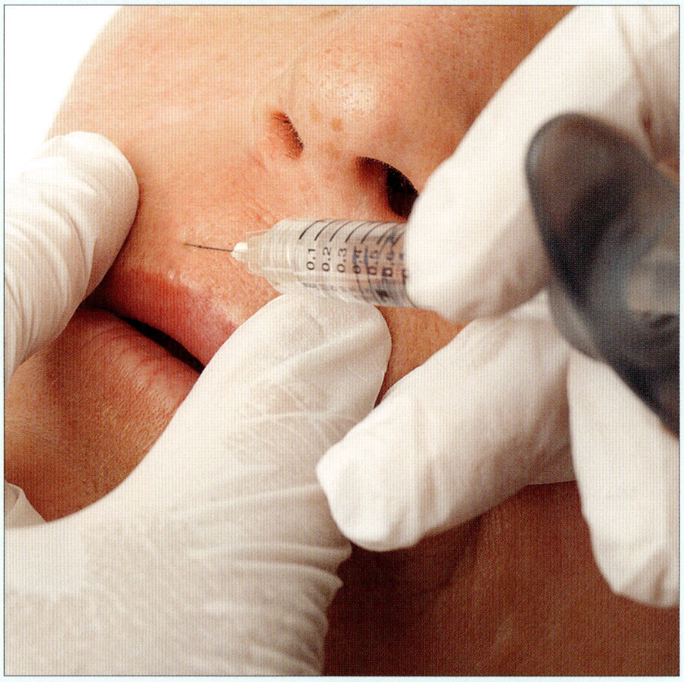

Technique 14 – Fig. 4 Inject the HA in the same way from the other side, staggering the needle insertion points so that they are located between the previously made punctures at intervals of 3 mm. A certain amount of practice and routine is needed for the therapist to be able to deliver minimal amounts at regular intervals.

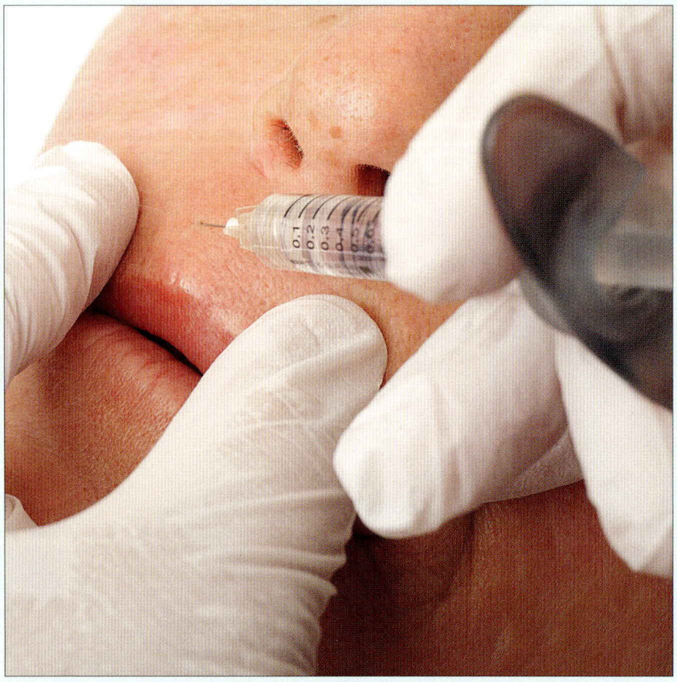

Technique 14 – Fig. 5 When stretching the upper lip between the thumb and forefinger, ensure that the tissue is not stretched out too smoothly and that the wrinkle relief is still visible.

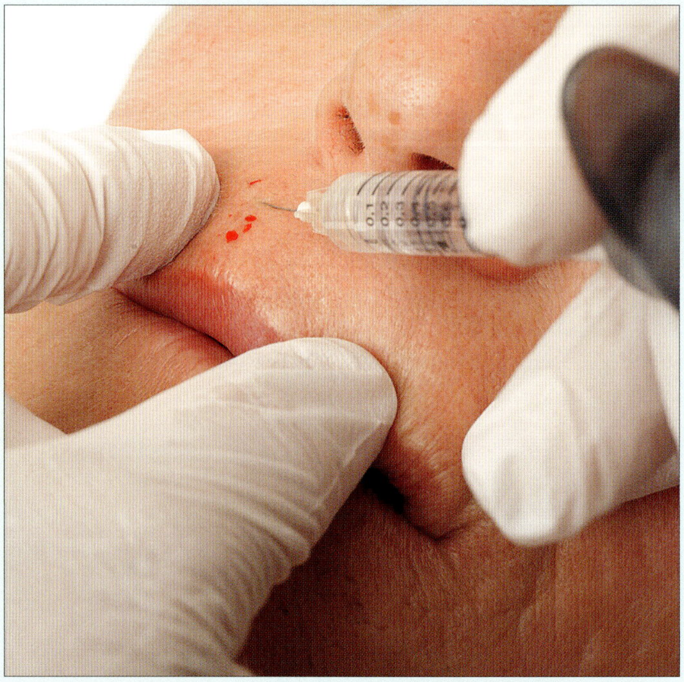

Technique 14 – Fig. 6 Since the punctures are very fine, it is often difficult to see the previous ones on the opposite side. For this reason, do not immediately swab away the blood from these punctures, but leave them in place as markers.

Important Notes

- Overcorrection must be avoided at all costs as this could easily lead to unwanted and visible irregularities. A "sausage-like" overcorrection can be avoided if the therapist generates counterpressure with the thumb while delivering the material, forcing it to remain at the required tissue level.
- If too much material is used and if it is delivered too close to the surface, a bluish, glassy hue may become visible under the skin, known as the Tyndall effect. This can occur with all superficial injections.
- If the therapist pinches the skin together loosely, the wrinkle becomes more visible. However, this makes it more difficult to insert the needle superficially with the required accuracy.

Possible Side Effects

Slight reddening, rarely inflammation, rarely hematomas, mild to more severe swellings, blanching

Undesirable Side Effects

Overcorrection causing stripes or nodules, asymmetry due to non-uniform delivery of material, necrosis

Treatment Protocol at a Glance

- History, evaluation, and patient information
- Informed consent form
- Photo documentation: "before" images
- Analysis and marking of the areas to be treated
- Cleaning
- Thorough disinfection
- Local anesthesia (lidocaine cream) or conduction anesthesia if required
- Injection technique: short linear technique, 1 line of material per wrinkle
- Layer: subdermal in the cutaneous part of the lip
- Material: class "S viscous" product
- Volume: dependent on the number of wrinkles treated, 0.02 ml per line of material
- Needle: 27–30G sharp needle
- Massage may be applied
- Cooling if required
- Heparin cream for hematomas, ibuprofen p.o., arnica
- Photo documentation: "after" images
- Advice on dos and don'ts after the procedure
- Follow-up appointment for a check-up after 8–14 days

9.4 Lip Volume

The techniques presented in this section involve filling the lips to differing degrees using various methods.

9.4.1 TECHNIQUE 15

Minimal Four-Point Volume Replacement (Sharp Needle)

This is a simple technique to refresh the lips subtly by delivering minimal volumes of material.

Patient Selection

- For lips showing mild age-related atrophy or lips that are a bit too thin, with the aim of refreshing them without making this directly obvious
- Patients who are having an injection treatment for the first time and are afraid of changing their appearance too much

Injection Scheme and Planning (→ Technique 15 – Figs. 1, 2)

The four-point technique refreshes the lips all over by delivering a minimal volume of material. This simple technique is also suitable for balancing out any asymmetry or to place additional, subtle accents following augmentation with a cannula. Using a sharp needle, the injections are given into four points, i.e. 1 point into each lip quadrant.

The material is injected into the center of the selected point. However, this can vary according to requirements. In the upper lip, the Cupid's bow peaks are used for orientation. Depending on lip shape, the material is placed 0.5–0.7 cm below the Cupid's bow peak, wherever there is a lack of volume.

Technique: point technique
Direction of insertion: from the front into the vermillion
Layer: intramuscular, 2–3 mm into the vermillion
Material: class "M soft" product
Volume: max. 0.05 ml per point, 0.2 ml in total
Needle: 27G sharp needle
Anesthesia: lidocaine cream

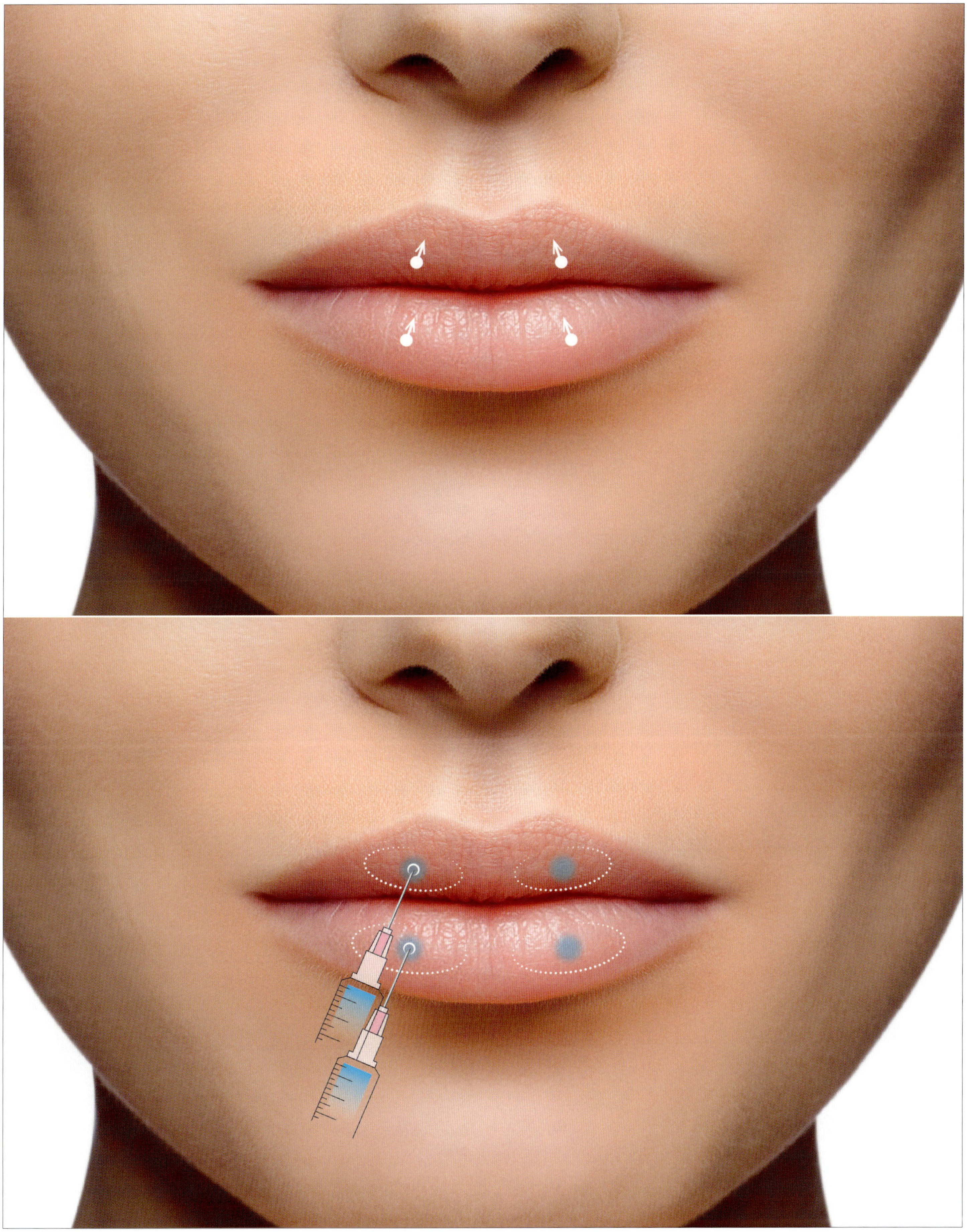

Technique 15 – Figs. 1, 2 Injection scheme and planning for minimal four-point volume replacement (sharp needle).

9

Treatment Method (→ Technique 15 – Figs. 3–6)

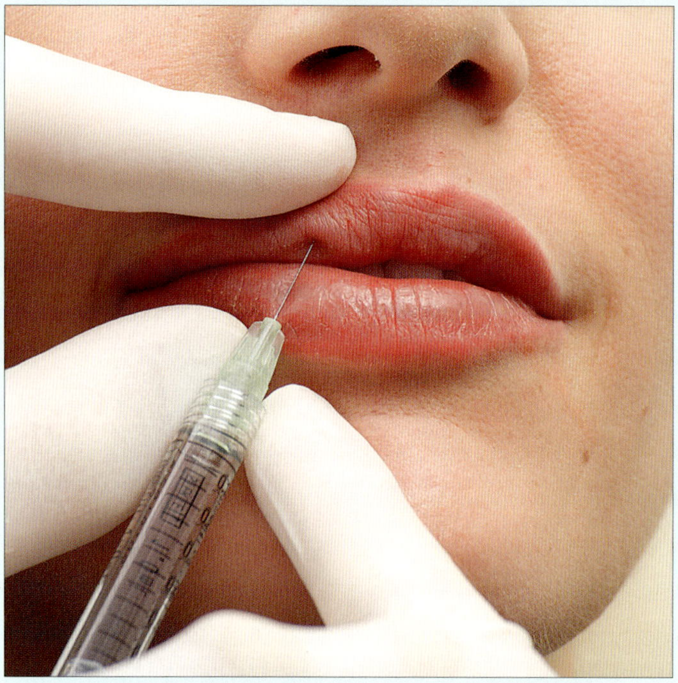

Technique 15 – Fig. 3 Roll the lip upward gently to find the center. Insert the needle very slowly as this is less painful for the patient. Plunge the needle to a depth c. 2–3 mm. Always deliver a very small amount of material.

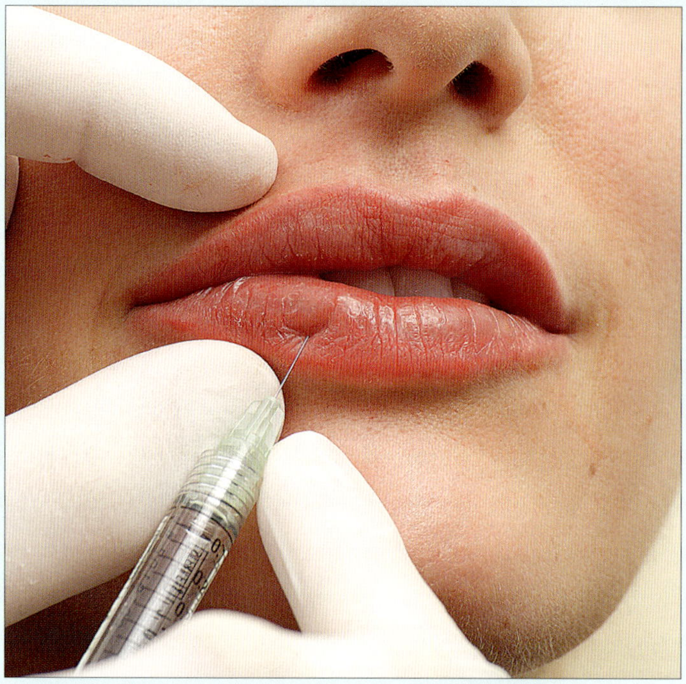

Technique 15 – Fig. 4 Roll the lower lip gently outward. Slightly more material should be injected into the lower lip than into the upper one.

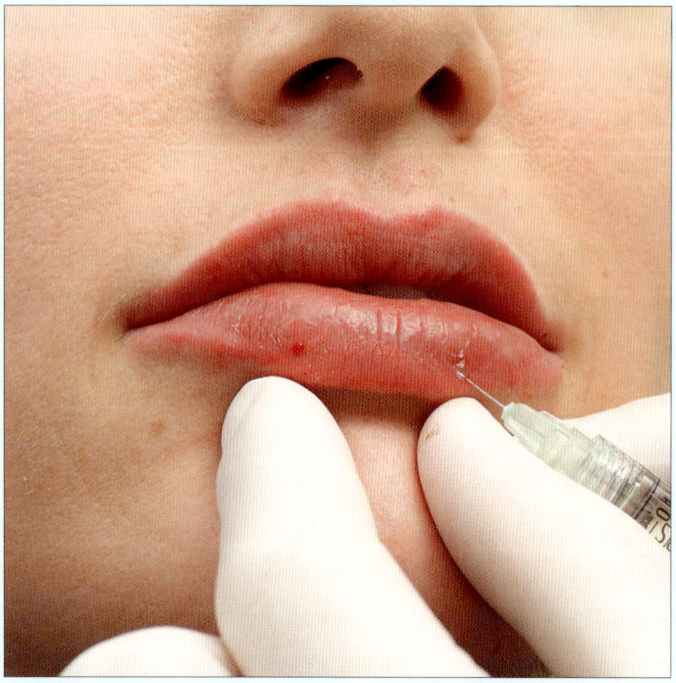

Technique 15 – Fig. 5 It is important to deliver the material symmetrically and to inject the same amount on each side.

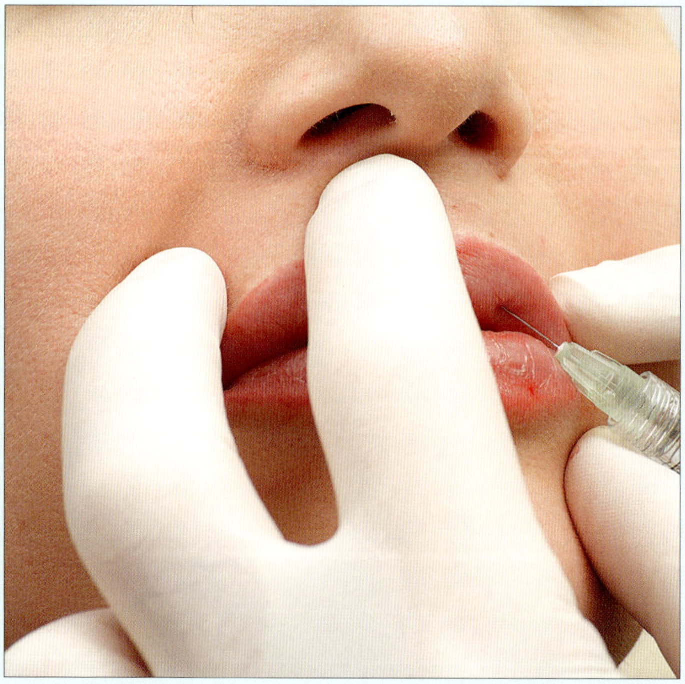

Technique 15 – Fig. 6 The closer the needle is to the dry/wet boundary when it enters, the more the lip will curve forward. However, these small volumes do not have a huge effect.

Important Notes

- It is important to keep observing the syringe and the delivered volume as well as the color of the skin.
- Even if small amounts of material are delivered with this technique, swellings can occur in the first 2–4 days, which may obscure the true result of the treatment.
- It is advisable to use low-crosslinked HA, which will make it easier to massage away any palpable or visible nodules.
- The immediate result of the injection can be seen if the patient is asked to stretch the mouth into a wide smile directly after the treatment.

Possible Side Effects

Slight reddening, rarely inflammation, hematomas, commonly swellings

Undesirable Side Effects

Overcorrection causing nodules in the lip, visible bumps if the injection was given too superficially, nodules that can be felt with the tongue if the injection was given at the mucous membrane border of the oral cavity, necrosis

Treatment Protocol at a Glance

- History, evaluation, and patient information
- Informed consent form
- Photo documentation: "before" images
- Analysis and marking of the areas to be treated
- Cleaning
- Thorough disinfection
- Local anesthesia (lidocaine cream) or conduction anesthesia if required
- Injection technique: point technique, 1 point per quadrant
- Layer: intramuscular, 2–3 mm into the vermillion
- Material: class "M soft" product
- Volume: max. 0.05 ml per point, 0.2 ml in total
- Needle: 27G sharp needle
- Massage if required
- Cooling if required
- Heparin cream for hematomas, ibuprofen p.o., arnica
- Photo documentation: "after" images
- Advice on dos and don'ts after the procedure
- Follow-up appointment for a check-up after 8–14 days

9.4.2 TECHNIQUE 16

Subtle Volume Replacement (Sharp Needle)

This simple technique produces subtle volume replacement, which is concentrated in the middle section of each lip.

Patient Selection

- For lips showing age-related atrophy
- Where there is a volume deficit in the middle section of the lips
- Following additional gentle lip augmentation, if desired

Injection Scheme and Planning (→ Technique 16 – Figs. 1, 2)

This technique is very simple. The injection is given with a sharp needle using the retrograde linear technique. The material is injected into the lower third of the upper lip and into the middle of the lower lip along a line about 1–1.5 cm in length. The exact length of the line of material injected depends on the width of the lip and on the desired treatment result. The length of the area to be injected is marked out in advance.

Technique: linear technique
Direction of insertion: along the body of the muscle
Layer: subcutaneous
Material: class "S/M soft" product
Volume: max. 0.05–0.15 ml per line, < 0.3 ml in total
Needle: 27G sharp needle, 20 mm
Anesthesia: lidocaine cream

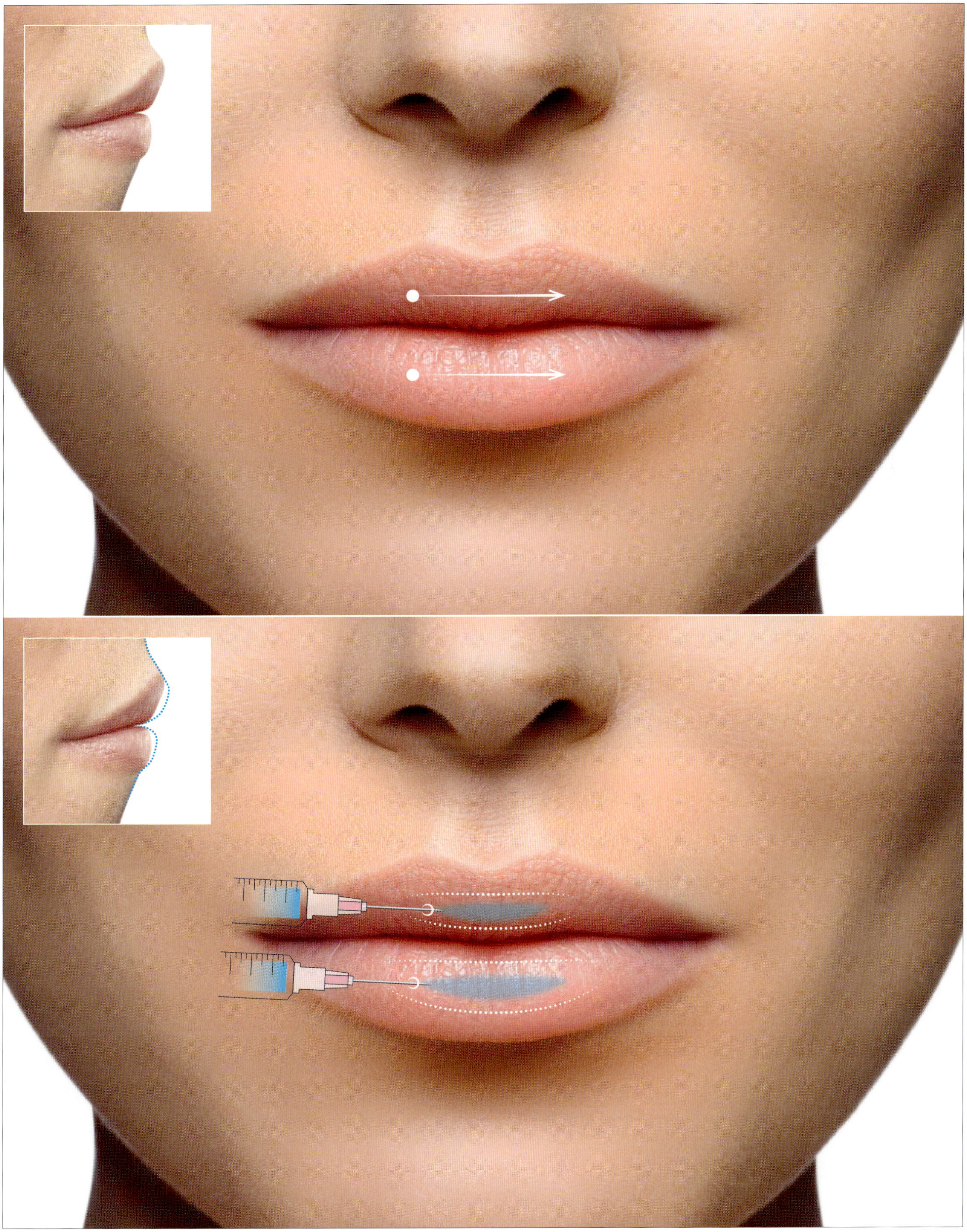

Technique 16 – Figs. 1, 2 Injection scheme and planning for subtle volume replacement (sharp needle).

Treatment Method (→ Technique 16 – Figs. 3–5)

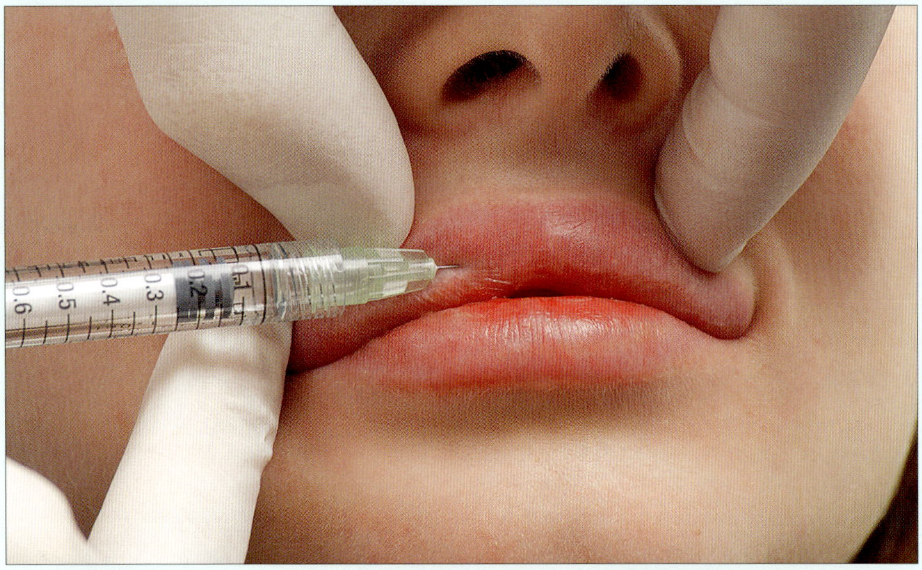

Technique 16 – Fig. 3 Stretch the lip between the forefinger and thumb to generate slight tension. It is essential to ensure symmetry and uniform injection volumes. Upper lip: the closer the injection is to the dry/wet boundary, the more the lip will protrude (see Technique 22, p. 214 ff.).

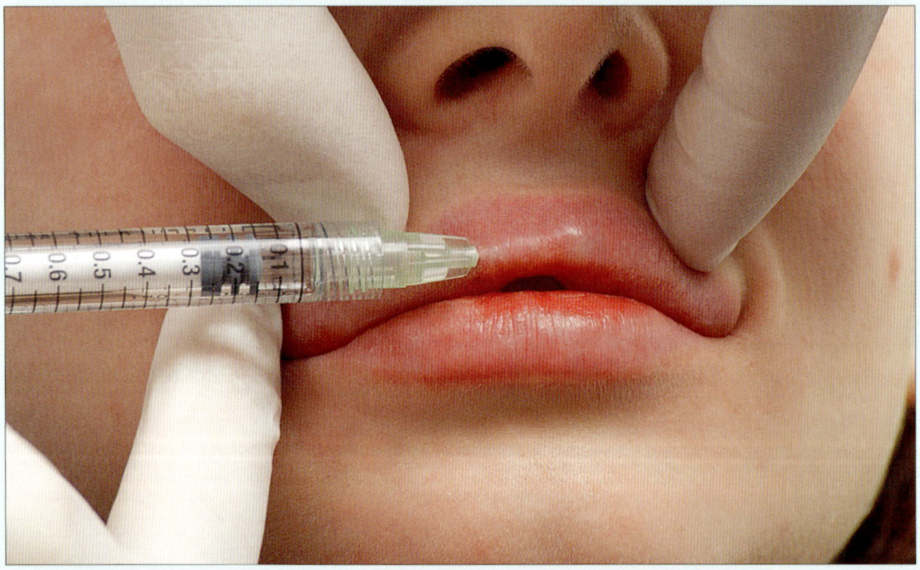

Technique 16 – Fig. 4 Lifting the needle reveals its position in the skin.

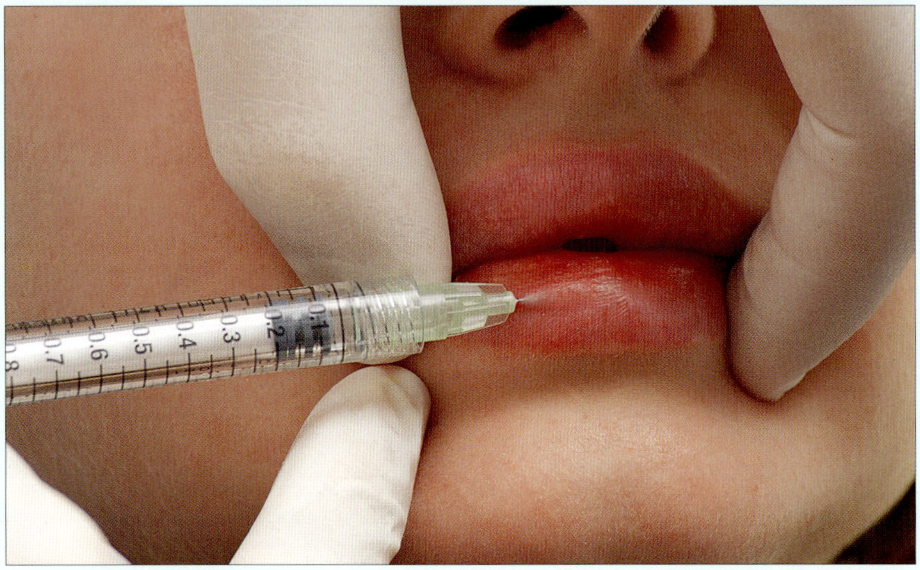

Technique 16 – Fig. 5 When delivering the material, ensure that it is tapered off slightly toward the end of the line being injected (toward the entry point). In general, no material should be injected at the point where the needle is withdrawn.

Important Notes

- According to the proportions dictated by the beauty code, the lower lip should always have a little more volume than the upper one. If this is not naturally the case, it can be balanced out by injecting more volume.
- The immediate result of the injection can be assessed by asking the patient to stretch the mouth into a wide smile directly after the treatment. In this way, the therapist can also check whether the injections have been given uniformly.

Possible Side Effects

Slight reddening, rarely inflammation, rarely hematomas, mild to more severe swellings

Undesirable Side Effects

Overcorrection with the resultant alteration of the shape of the lip or nodule formation, asymmetry due to non-uniform delivery of material, necrosis

Treatment Protocol at a Glance

- History, evaluation, and patient information
- Informed consent form
- Photo documentation: "before" images
- Analysis and marking of the areas to be treated
- Cleaning
- Thorough disinfection
- Local anesthesia (lidocaine cream) or conduction anesthesia if required
- Injection technique: linear technique, 1 line per upper and lower lip
- Layer: subcutaneous in the vermillion
- Material: class "S/M soft" product
- Volume: max. 0.3 ml in total
- Needle: 27G sharp needle
- No massage
- Cooling if required
- Heparin cream for hematomas, ibuprofen p.o., arnica
- Photo documentation: "after" images
- Advice on dos and don'ts after the procedure
- Follow-up appointment for a check-up after 8–14 days

9.4.3 TECHNIQUE 17
Subtle Lip Augmentation (Sharp Needle)

This technique has been used ever since fillers have been in existence and is suitable for mild augmentation of the lips. It is easy to use as the material can be placed with great accuracy. Uniform delivery of the material is the key factor in producing a harmonious lip shape.

Patient Selection

- For thinner lips, a small mouth or wrinkled lips
- If more lip volume is desired

Injection Scheme and Planning (→ Technique 17 – Figs. 1, 2)

Each lip quadrant is filled with one line of material. The viscosity of the HA and the length of the lines injected determine the lip shape. As there is a lot of leeway in this treatment, accurate planning is required regarding how the material is to be delivered. The material is injected into the selected, marked region. Frequent visual checks of the syringe plunger are important to monitor delivery of the material because the lips swell quickly. The technique offers a number of potential variations. It is also suitable for correcting any areas of asymmetry; this requires accurate pre-treatment planning of how much material to deliver. Following an accurate analysis, the curvature of the lips can be perfected in the side view by correcting any flattened sections.

Technique: linear technique
Direction of insertion: along the body of the muscle
Layer: subcutaneous in the vermillion over the orbicularis oris muscle
Material: class "S/M soft" product
Volume: max. 0.05 ml per injected line, 0.4 ml in total
Needle: 27G sharp needle, 20 mm
Anesthesia: lidocaine cream, conduction anesthesia if required

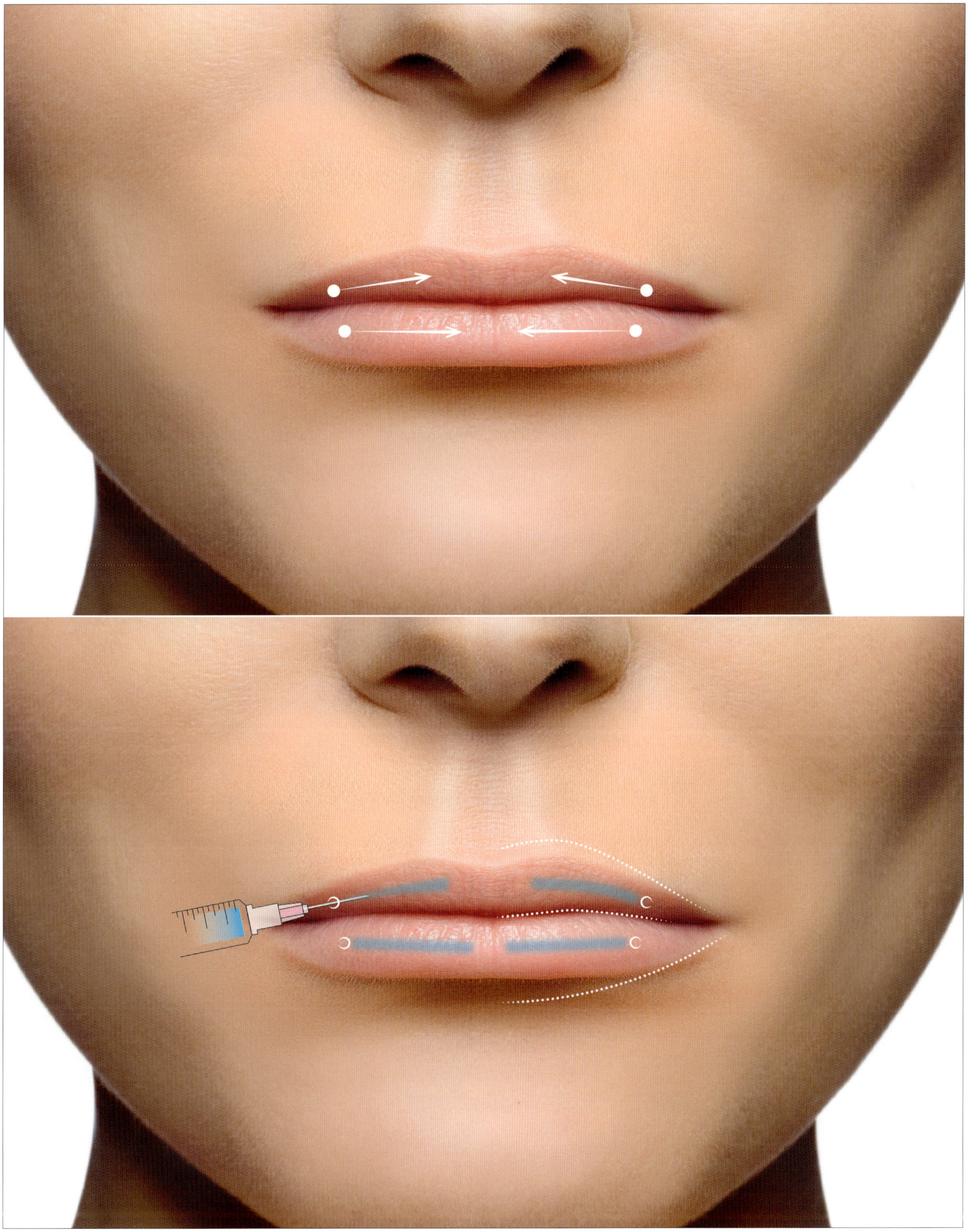

Technique 17 – Figs. 1, 2 Injection scheme and planning for subtle lip augmentation (sharp needle).

9

Treatment Method (→ Technique 17 – Figs. 3–6)

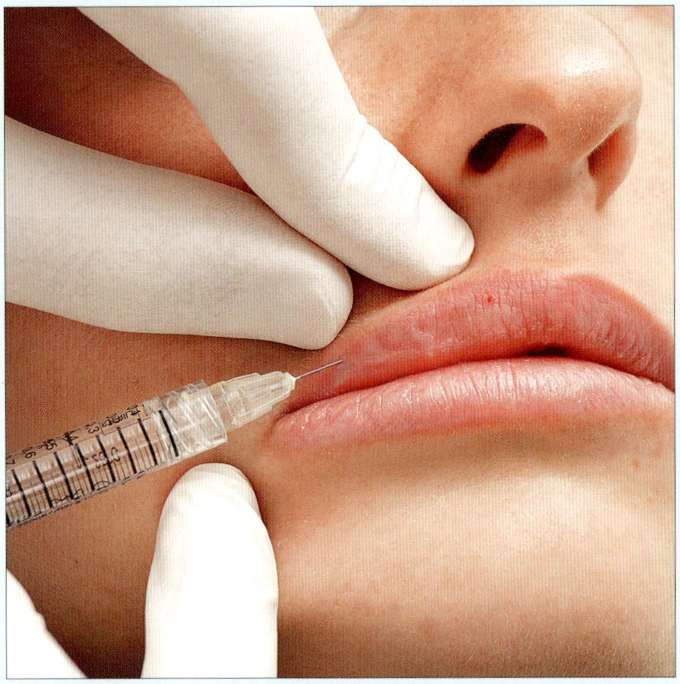

Technique 17 – Fig. 3 Hold the lip in place between the thumb and forefinger and roll it gently upward. Inject subcutaneously into the vermillion to a depth of 1–2 mm. Deliver the material by retrograde injection; it is essential to check the amount delivered.

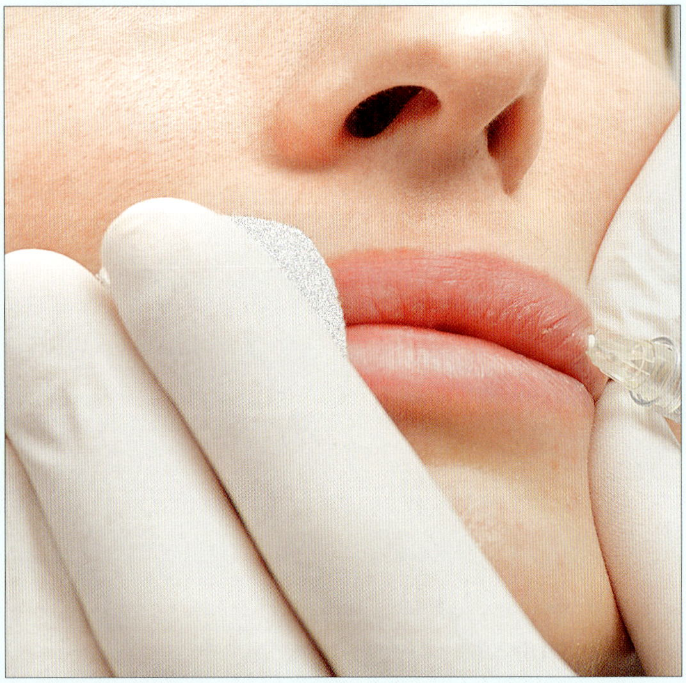

Technique 17 – Fig. 4 Since the tissue swells quickly, first inject the upper lip in full and then the lower lip in full.

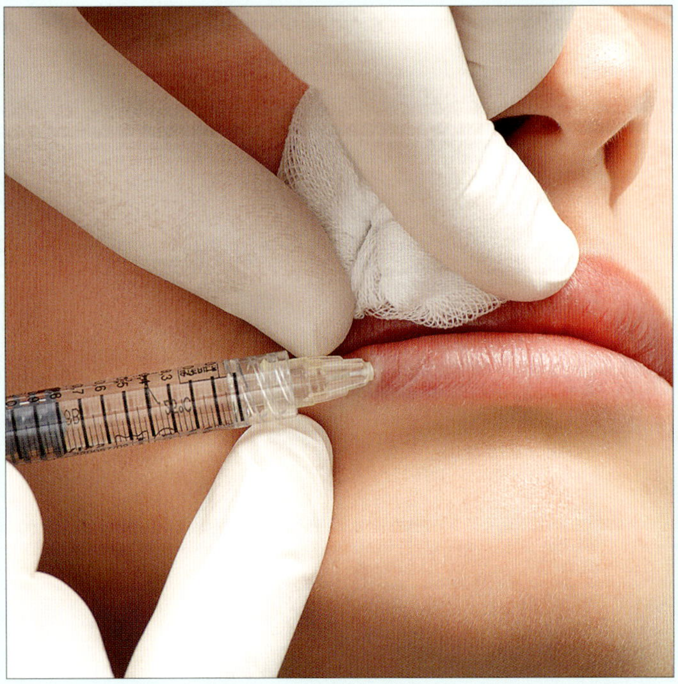

Technique 17 – Fig. 5 Advance the needle into the depth of the vermillion from the lateral to the medial side. This makes the shape softer, and any irregularities are better covered by the overlying tissue than if the injection is more superficial.

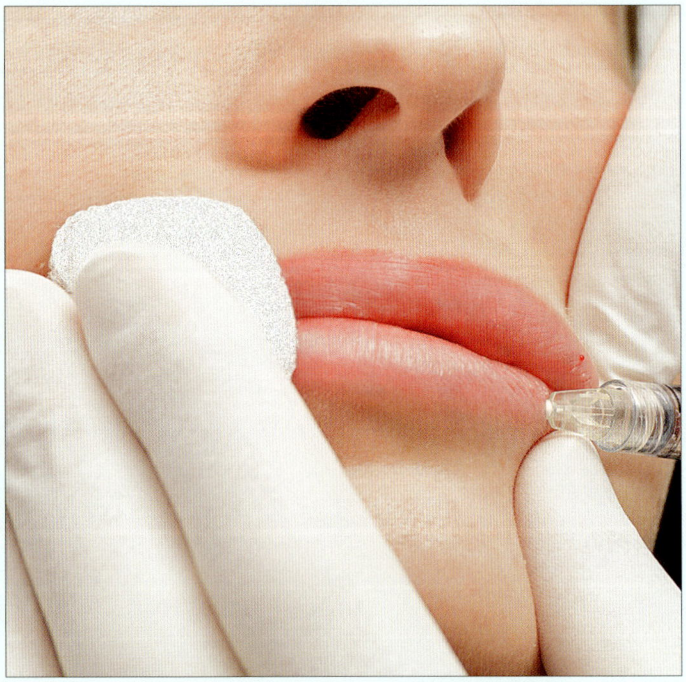

Technique 17 – Fig. 6 To enhance the lip slightly in the center, insert the needle into the ridge of the lip on each side (see Fig. 1.44, p. 29).

Important Notes

- If the injection is too superficial, the lips will show uneven areas.
- Injury to a vessel can cause a hematoma within the lip, resulting in an irregularity. If this happens, the therapist must not be tempted to inject more material into the side that is not swollen. The "say cheese" test (see p. 41) is a good way of checking whether any swelling has been caused due to excess HA or a hematoma.
- This technique is painful for the patient. The lips need to be adequately anesthetized, especially if the patient is sensitive.
- The immediate result of the injection can be assessed by asking the patient to stretch the mouth into a wide smile directly after the treatment. This can also be used to check if the injections have been given uniformly.

Possible Side Effects

Slight reddening, rarely inflammation, hematomas, mild to more severe swellings

Undesirable Side Effects

Overcorrection with resultant alteration of the shape of the lip or nodule formation, asymmetry due to non-uniform delivery of material, necrosis

Treatment Protocol at a Glance

- History, evaluation, and patient information
- Informed consent form
- Photo documentation: "before" images
- Analysis and marking of the areas to be treated
- Cleaning
- Thorough disinfection
- Local anesthesia (lidocaine cream) or conduction anesthesia if required
- Injection technique: linear technique, 2 lines each into the upper and lower lip
- Layer: subcutaneous in the vermillion over the orbicularis oris muscle
- Material: class "S/M soft" product
- Volume: max. 0.4 ml in total
- Needle: 27G sharp needle
- No massage
- Cooling if required
- Heparin cream for hematomas, ibuprofen p.o., arnica
- Photo documentation: "after" images
- Advice on dos and don'ts after the procedure
- Follow-up appointment for a check-up after 8–14 days

9.4.4 TECHNIQUE 18
Classic Augmentation (Sharp Needle)

This technique is a basic, classic one and aims to produce uniform – moderate or even strong – volumization of the lips by augmenting the substance of the vermillion. The treatment outcome depends on the volume and viscosity of the filler being used as well as on the number and length of the lines in each fan of injected material. In patients with naturally thin lips or in older patients, this technique can produce a "duck's bill" effect.

Patient Selection

- If the patient wants to increase general lip volume; this may range up to extreme lip volume augmentation
- If there are asymmetries and the patient wants a lip shaping treatment
- If the patient wants to balance out age-related lip volume deficits

Injection Scheme and Planning (→ Technique 18 – Figs. 1–4)

The material can be delivered in fine lines, producing gentle, moderate augmentation, but the delivery of bigger volumes in several lines can also result in strong plumping of the whole lip. Lines of material are injected using the fanning technique, starting from the lateral side. The first injection is given in the medial direction from this lateral needle insertion site, which then serves as the entry point for the 2–3 lines of material per quadrant.

The material needs to be delivered equally on both sides, unless asymmetry is a treatment indication. The lip area to be treated should be marked. Since the curvature of the lip plays a major part in the procedure, the lip should be viewed from the side. If the lip shows natural curvature, the material should be distributed extensively over the upper third; if the lip recedes without a curve, a thicker strand of material should be placed into the center of the flattened area to restore the convex shape.

The needle should be changed after each quadrant to ensure that it remains sharp and causes less pain. An appropriate anesthesia to block pain is also recommended (see Chap. 5, p. 78 ff.).

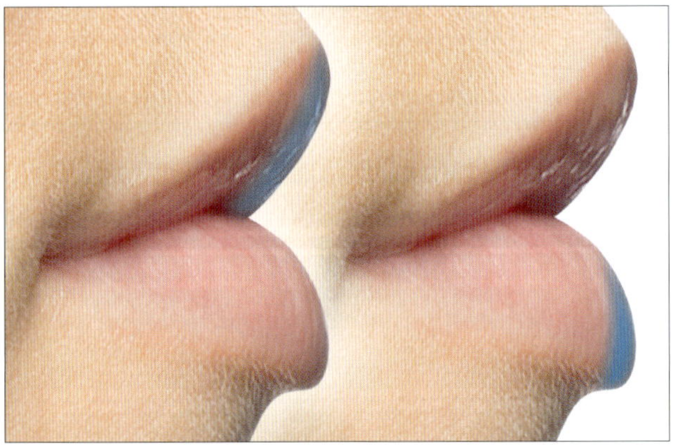

Upper and lower lip areas that need to be augmented (shown in blue).

Technique: fanning technique
Direction of insertion: along the body of the muscle
Layer: subcutaneous in the vermillion over the orbicularis oris muscle
Material: class "M/L soft" product, according to the desired extent of the augmentation
Volume: max. 0.08–0.1 ml per line, 1.0 ml in total
Needle: 27G sharp needle, 20 mm
Anesthesia: lidocaine cream, conduction anesthesia

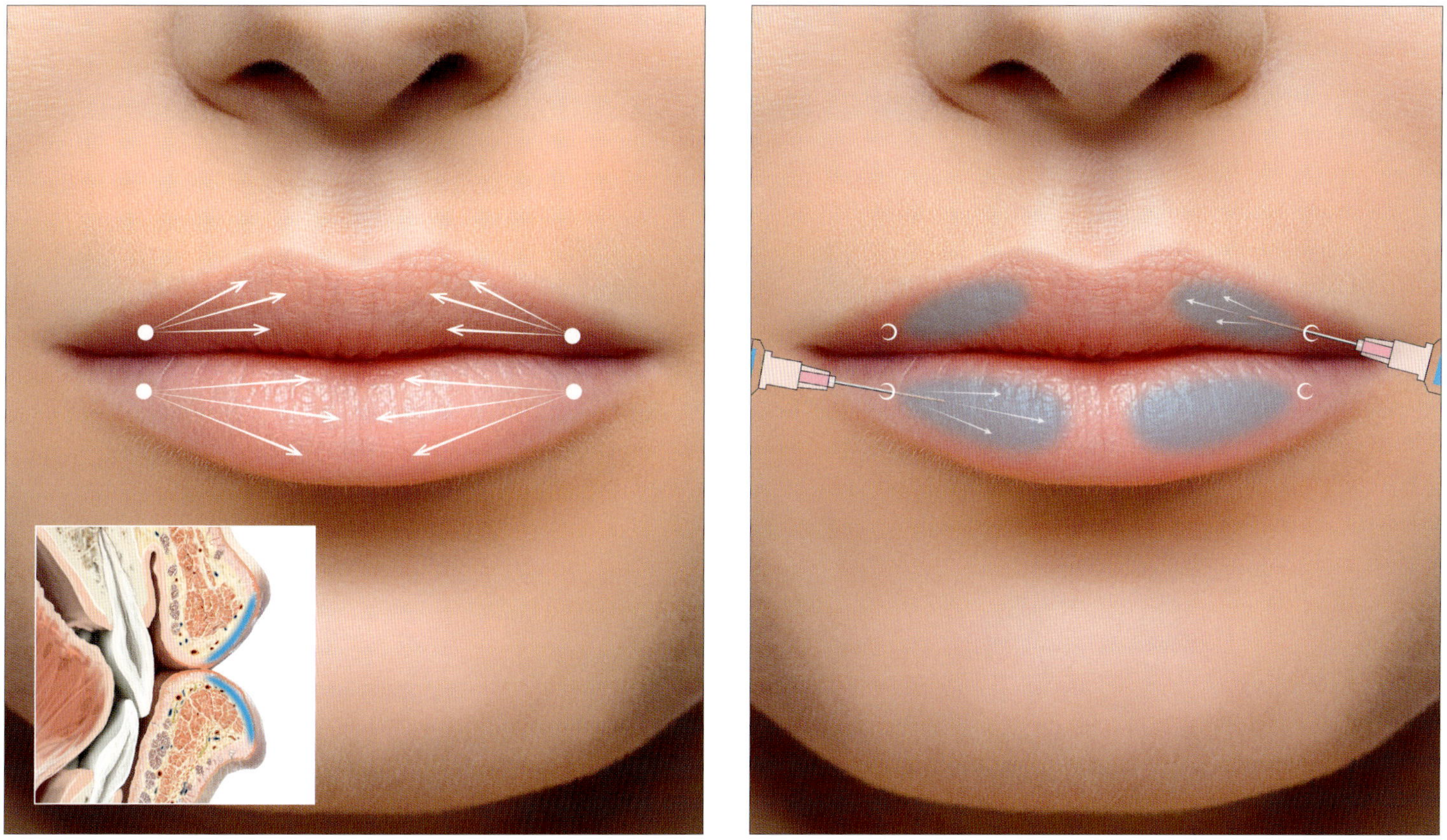

Technique 18 – Figs. 1, 2 Injection scheme and planning for moderate classic lip volume augmentation (sharp needle).

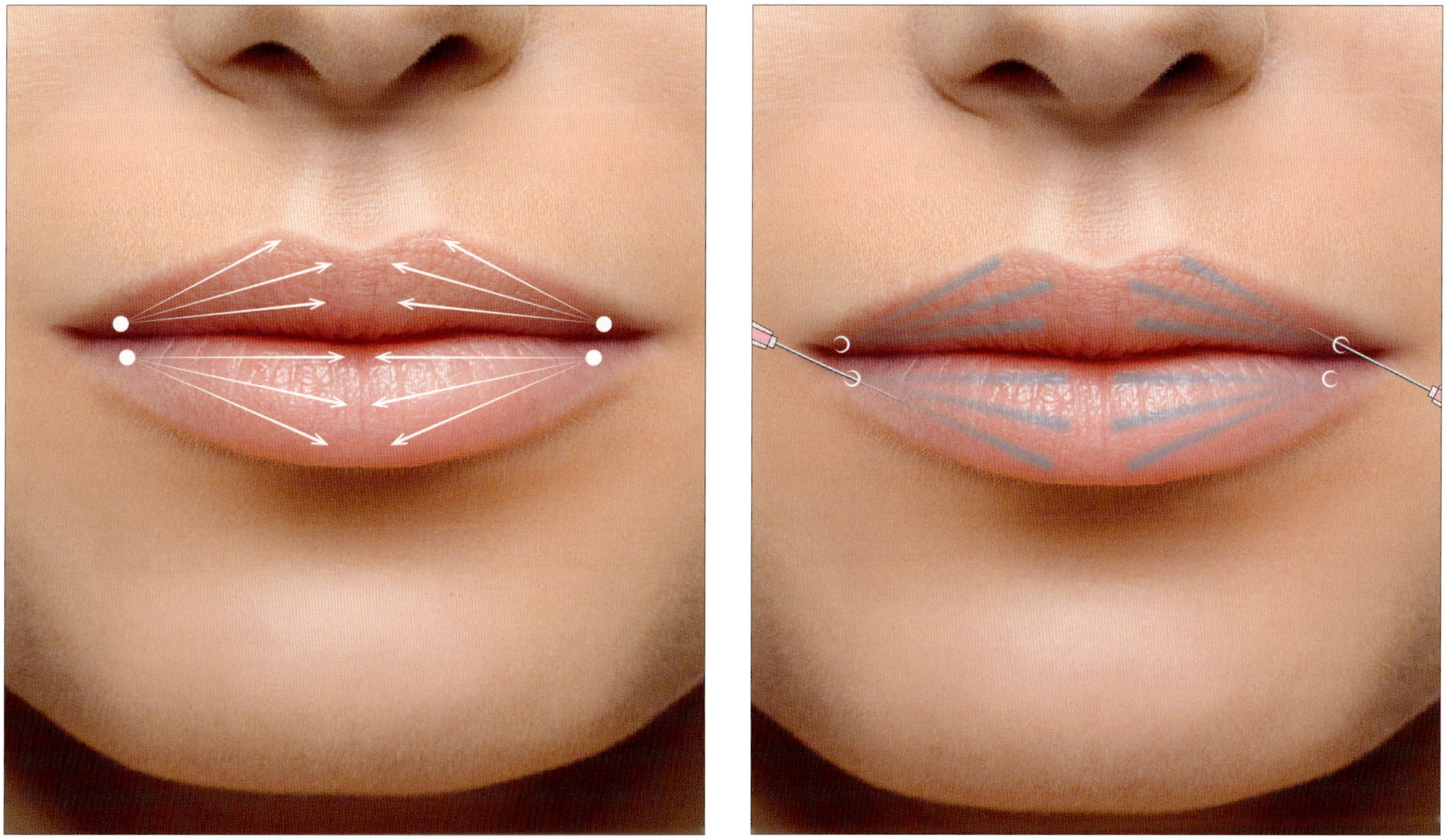

Technique 18 – Figs. 3, 4 Injection scheme and planning for strong classic lip volume augmentation (sharp needle).

Treatment Method (→ Technique 18 – Figs. 5–7)

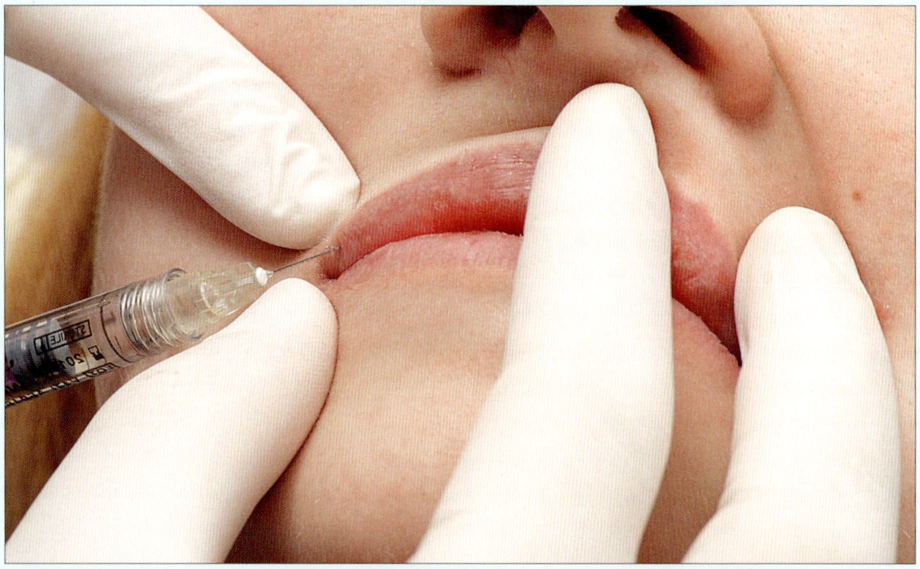

Technique 18 – Fig. 5 Applying gentle pressure with the forefinger above the lip causes it to evert slightly. This makes it easier to find the central line.

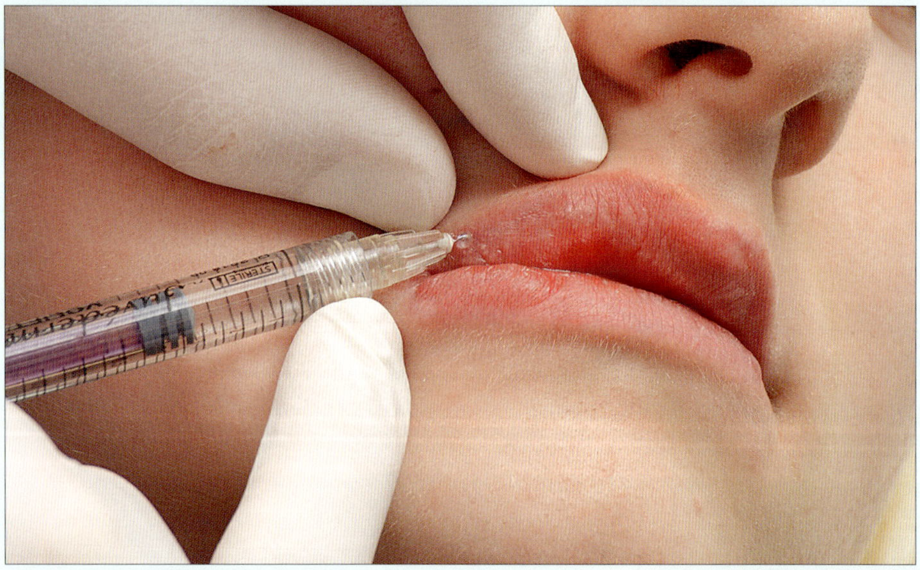

Technique 18 – Fig. 6 Stretch the lip while inserting the needle. Advance the needle and lift it gently to check whether it is in the correct layer. Deliver the material slowly and uniformly by retrograde injection.

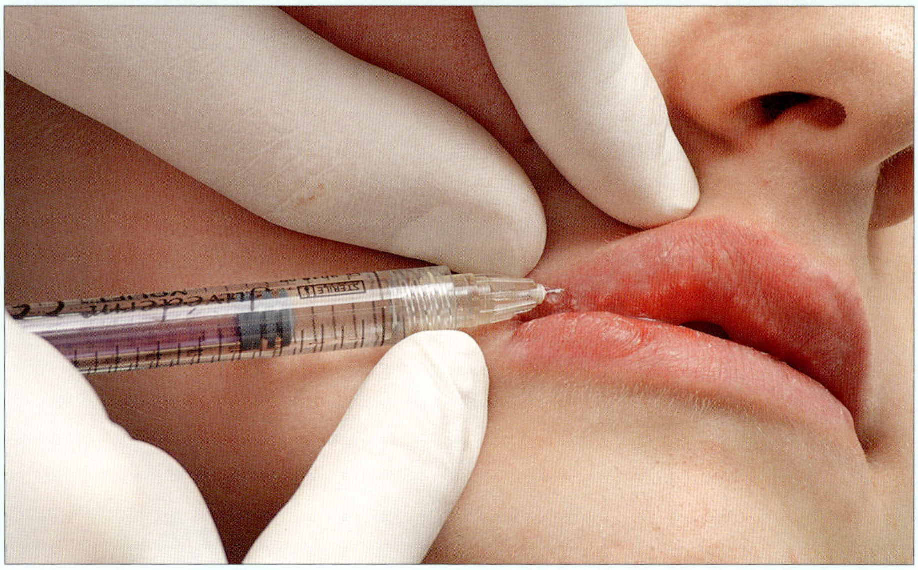

Technique 18 – Fig. 7 Inject 2–3 lines of material (fanning technique) into the lip using a sharp needle. While doing so, take great care to deliver the material uniformly on both sides. Frequent checks of the volume marks on the syringe are recommended because the lips swell quickly, making it appear that more volume has been delivered than is actually the case.

Important Notes

- The material and the volume to be delivered need to be adjusted to the patient's needs. Delivering too much material can quickly produce an unnatural appearance, which is particularly true in patients with a narrow gap between the lip and nose.
- Various combined techniques are recommended to prevent a "duck's bill" effect such as restoring the foundations in the cutaneous part of the lip to increase its natural surface area (Sattler & Sommer 2015).
- The trauma to the lips due to the multiple injections with a sharp needle is considerable and leads to severe swellings. For this reason, the tissue should not be stressed further by vigorous massage.

Possible Side Effects

Slight reddening, rarely inflammation, rarely hematomas, mild to more severe swellings, pain (2–4 days after the treatment)

Undesirable Side Effects

Overcorrection, asymmetry, altered lip shape, nodule formation, blanching if the injection is too superficial, necrosis

Treatment Protocol at a Glance

- History, evaluation, and patient information
- Informed consent form
- Photo documentation: "before" images
- Analysis and marking of the areas to be treated
- Cleaning
- Thorough disinfection
- Local anesthesia (lidocaine cream) or conduction anesthesia if required
- Injection technique: fanning technique, 2–3 lines per side in the upper and lower lip, respectively
- Layer: subcutaneous in the vermillion over the orbicularis oris muscle
- Material: class "M/L soft" product
- Volume: max. 0.08–0.1 ml per line, 1.0 ml in total
- Needle: 27G sharp needle, 20 mm
- No massage
- Cooling if required
- Heparin cream for hematomas, ibuprofen p.o., arnica
- Photo documentation: "after" images
- Advice on dos and don'ts after the procedure
- Follow-up appointment for a check-up after 8–14 days

9.4.5 TECHNIQUE 19
Moderate Augmentation (Blunt Cannula)

This involves a deep, horizontally mobilizing technique using a cannula. The treatment goal is the uniform, soft build-up of volume within the lip. Use of a blunt cannula is recommended for a particularly injury-free and less painful procedure. This treatment requires accurate planning to define how much material is to be delivered in which area. Even the slightest differences between the right and left halves of the lips lead to asymmetry.

Patient Selection

- Where there is a volume deficit
- If an increase in lip volume is desired

Injection Scheme and Planning (→ Technique 19 – Figs. 1, 2)

As there is only one entry point on each side, injury to the blood vessels is less likely than when a sharp needle is used. The first perforation is made with a sharp Nokor needle inserted adjacent to the mouth corners to make an entry point for the cannula. The blunt cannula is then advanced into the pre-pricked opening. It is sometimes difficult to find this hole; we therefore recommend using a Nokor needle of larger gauge than that of the cannula itself. The direction of insertion of the cannula is along the insertion points of the zygomaticus muscle above the depressor anguli oris muscle. If the cannula is not in the correct layer and resistance can be felt, it must not be advanced by force. If this happens, the therapist should withdraw the cannula and look for another layer. The needle needs to glide smoothly. The material is introduced up to the middle of the lip on each side, with mobilization. To make space for the material, the layers of lip skin are teased apart gently (see Fig. 8.30, p. 121). The material is placed into the vermillion over the orbicularis oris muscle. If the tubercles of the lip are very prominent, they should be avoided when placing the material. The therapist's discretion and the patient's wishes take priority here.

Technique: linear technique
Direction of insertion: along the course of the lip, from the mouth corner going medially to the center of the lip
Layer: subcutaneous, in the vermillion over the orbicularis oris muscle
Material: class "S/M soft" product
Volume: c. 0.5–1.0 ml in total
Needle: 27G blunt cannula, 38 mm, > 25G Nokor needle
Anesthesia: lidocaine cream

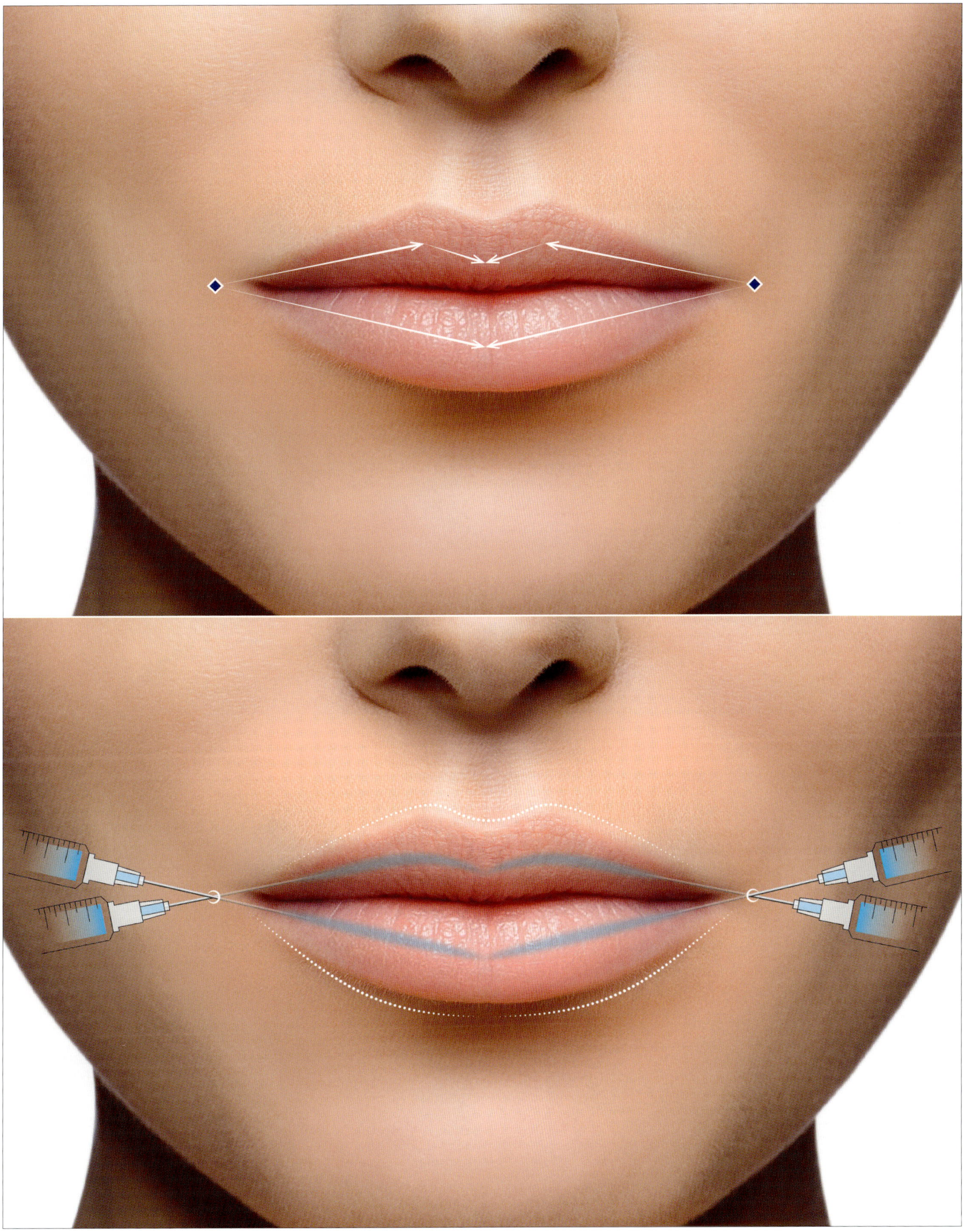

Technique 19 – Figs. 1, 2 Injection scheme and planning for moderate augmentation (blunt cannula).

Treatment Method (→ Technique 19 – Figs. 3–7)

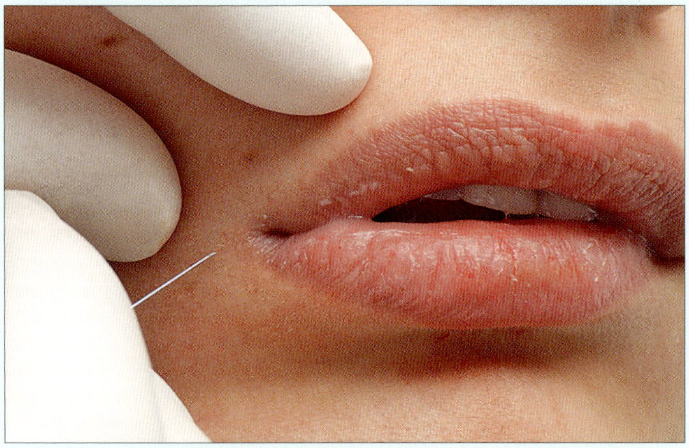

Technique 19 – Fig. 3 Before using the cannula, first perforate the skin with a pre-pricking needle (Nokor needle).

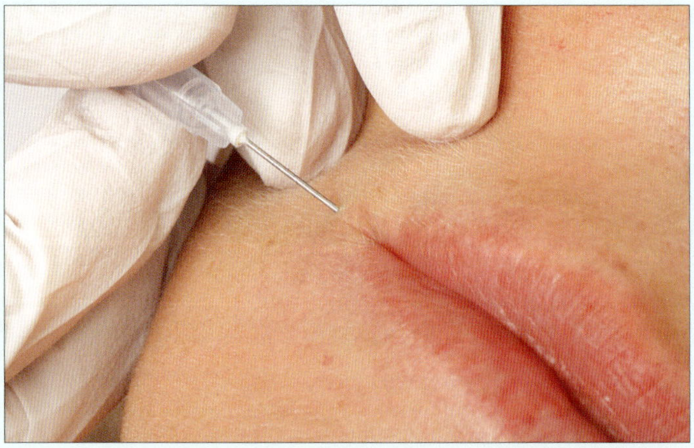

Technique 19 – Fig. 4 The insertion point should be chosen so that all the parts of the upper and lower lip being treated on each side can be reached with the cannula. Plunge the needle bevel into the skin to a depth of 1–2 mm at the entry point.

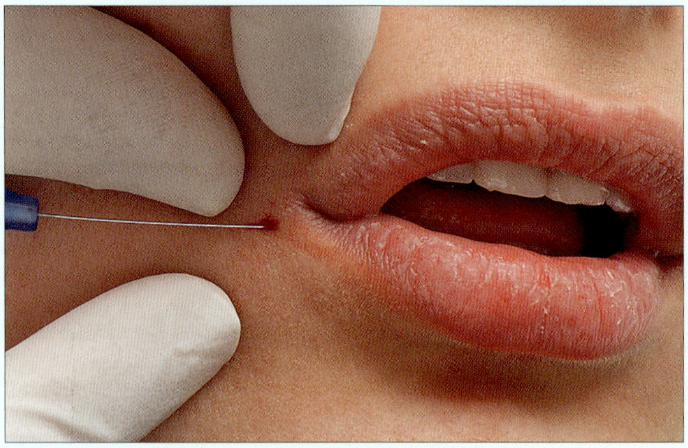

Technique 19 – Fig. 5 Insert the cannula into the pre-pricked hole and allow it to find a subcutaneous path through the tissue gently and without force. Always do this with visual and sensory checks. In the lower lip, the cannula needs to negotiate the tendon of the risorius muscle. If the going is difficult here, change the angle of insertion or the depth of the skin layer again.

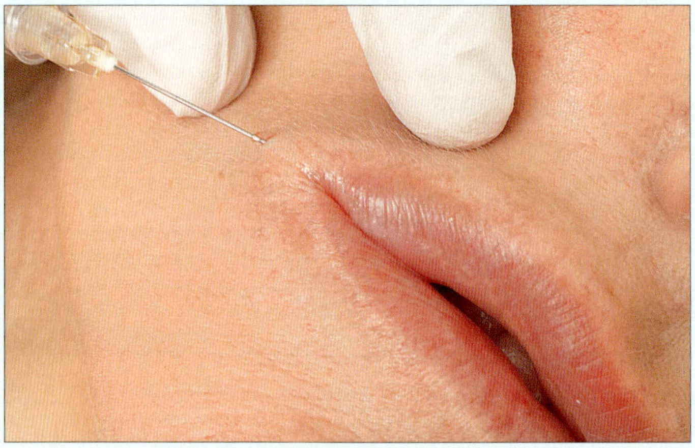

Technique 19 – Fig. 6 When changing direction, e.g. from the lower to the upper lip, the tip of the cannula should be left in the pre-pricked hole at a depth of c. 1 mm, to ensure that the hole does not close up and need re-puncturing. If it proves difficult to advance the cannula into the lower lip, repeat perforation with the Nokor needle may be necessary. The direction of insertion of the Nokor needle should be toward the lower lip.

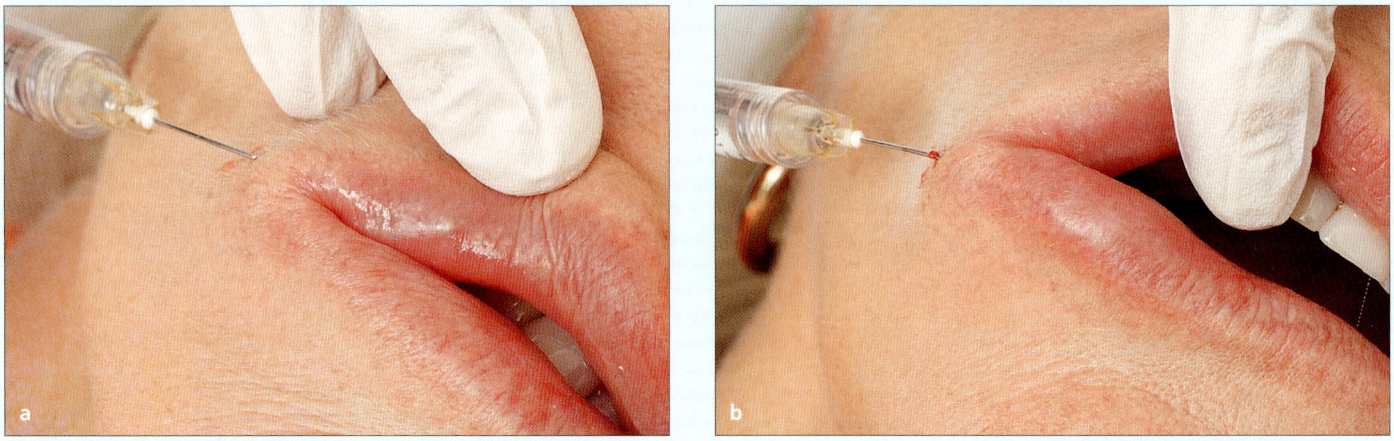

Technique 19 – Figs. 7 a+b Lifting the cannula reveals the location of its tip to ensure accurate delivery of material (a). In the upper lip, delivery should stop 1 cm from the corner of the mouth. In the lower lip (b), the pronounced bulge shows where the delivered material is located.

Important Notes

- The treatment result depends greatly on how symmetrically the filler has been delivered into the lip quadrants. The key factors here are the volume of material and its placement.
- The material should be injected sparingly, since overcorrection can lead to an unnatural result.
- The material can be readily distributed by gentle massage after the treatment.

Possible Side Effects

Rarely inflammation, very rarely hematomas at the insertion site of the Nokor needle, mild swellings

Undesirable Side Effects

Inflammation, overcorrection with resultant alteration of the shape of the lip, nodule formation, asymmetry due to non-uniform delivery of material, rarely necrosis

Treatment Protocol at a Glance

- History, evaluation, and patient information
- Informed consent form
- Photo documentation: "before" images
- Analysis and marking of the areas to be treated
- Cleaning
- Thorough disinfection
- Local anesthesia if required (lidocaine cream)
- Injection technique: linear technique, 1 line per quadrant
- Layer: subcutaneous in the vermillion over the orbicularis oris muscle
- Material: class "S/M soft" product
- Volume: c. 0.5–1.0 ml in total
- Needle: 27G blunt cannula, 38 mm, > 25G Nokor needle
- Massage may be applied
- Cooling if required
- Heparin cream for hematomas, ibuprofen p.o., arnica
- Photo documentation: "after" images
- Advice on dos and don'ts after the procedure
- Follow-up appointment for a check-up after 8–14 days

9.4.6 TECHNIQUE 20

Classic to Strong Augmentation (Blunt Cannula)

This involves a deep, horizontally mobilizing technique using a cannula to harmonize and augment the lips. This cannula technique is less traumatizing and highly suitable for building up the lips uniformly in different dimensions.

Patient Selection

- If the patient wants increased volume; this may range up to extreme lip volume augmentation
- If there are asymmetries and the patient wants the lips to be shaped and any deficits balanced out

Injection Scheme and Planning (→ Technique 20 – Figs. 1, 2)

As there is only one entry point on each side, injury to the blood vessels is less likely than when a sharp needle is used. Therefore, the technique has fewer side effects than augmentation with a sharp needle, but it requires skill and practice from the therapist. The first perforation is made with a Nokor needle (sharp needle) around 5 mm laterally of the mouth corner, to make an entry point for the cannula. The blunt cannula is then advanced into the pre-pricked opening. It is sometimes difficult to find this hole; we therefore recommend using a Nokor needle of a larger gauge than that of the cannula itself. The direction of insertion of the cannula is along the insertion points of the zygomaticus muscle above the depressor anguli oris muscle. If the cannula is not in the correct layer and resistance can be felt, it must not be advanced by force. If this happens, the therapist should withdraw the cannula and look for another layer. The needle needs to glide smoothly. The material is introduced with mobilization. If any retractions or irregularities are encountered, the skin should be loosened from its attachments by carefully moving the cannula to and fro (teasing apart the tissue layers). The material is placed into the vermillion over the orbicularis oris muscle. Irregularities should be massaged into the correct shape.

Technique: fanning technique
Direction of insertion: along the course of the lip, from the mouth corner going in the medial direction to the center of the lip
Layer: subcutaneous in the vermillion over the orbicularis oris muscle
Material: class "M/L soft" product
Volume: max. 0.3 ml per quadrant, 1–1.2 ml in total
Needle: 27G cannula, 40 mm, > 25G Nokor needle
Anesthesia: lidocaine cream

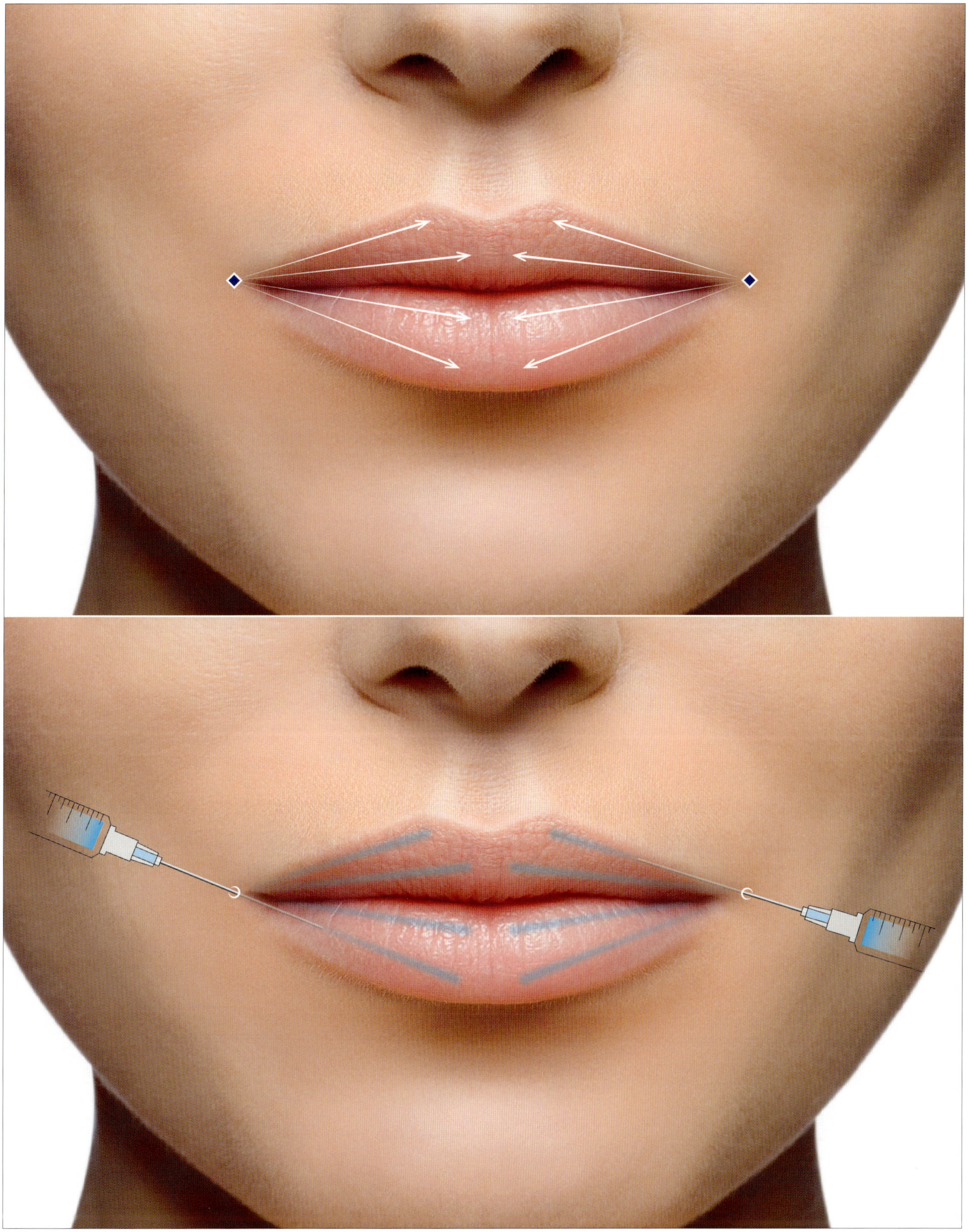

Technique 20 – Figs. 1, 2 Injection scheme and planning for classic to strong augmentation (blunt cannula).

Treatment Method (→ Technique 20 – Figs. 3–7)

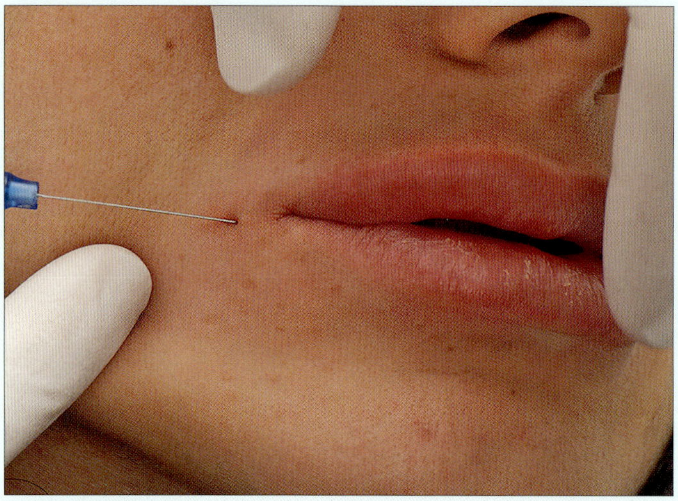

Technique 20 – Fig. 3 Pre-prick the skin with the Nokor needle close to the corner of the mouth, to provide the maximum possible range from the entry point.

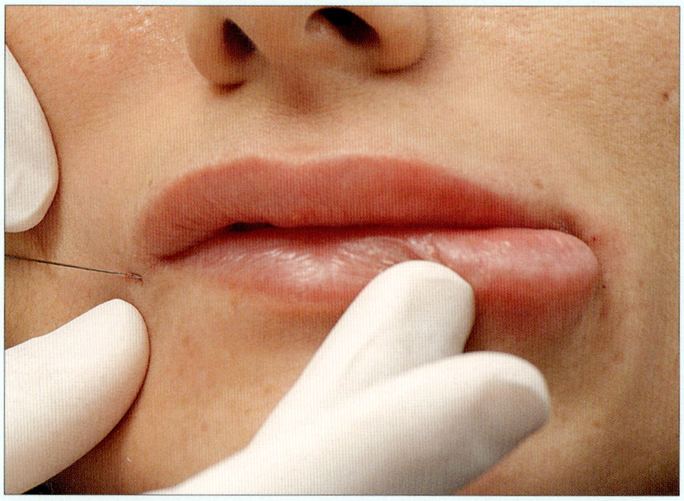

Technique 20 – Fig. 4 Stretch the lip with the opposite hand and carefully advance the cannula into the lip through the pre-pricked opening. The cannula should move along the skin of the lip.

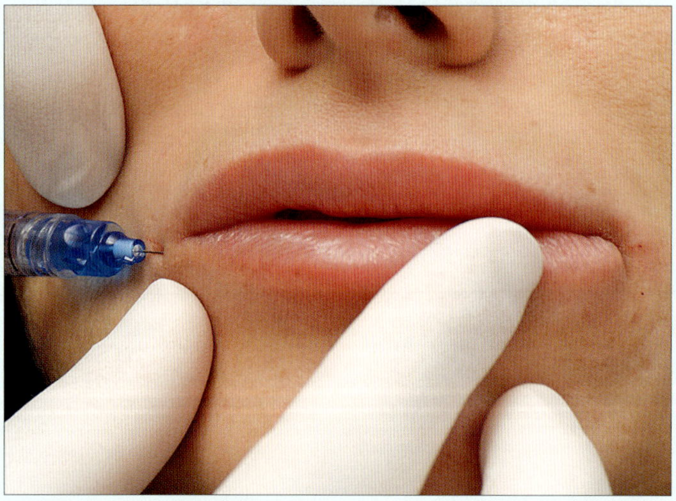

Technique 20 – Fig. 5 Stretching the lip during the injection makes it easier to control and guide the cannula.

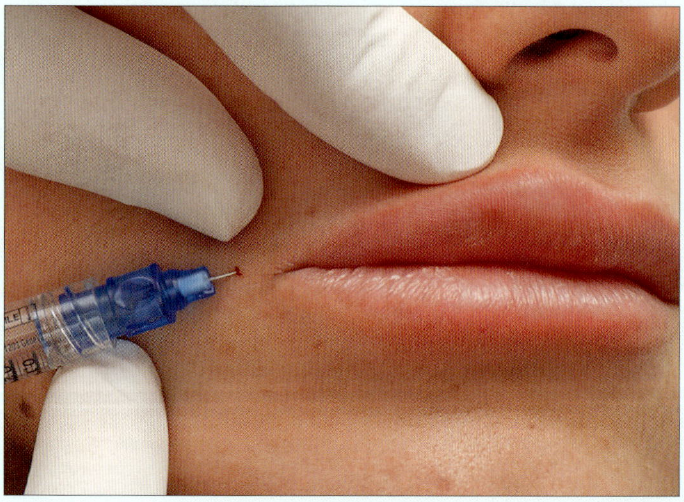

Technique 20 – Fig. 6 The tip of the cannula should not be advanced any further than the philtrum. To check where the end of the cannula is located at any point during the infiltration, raise the cannula gently and push it against the lip. Repeat the procedure until the desired volume is achieved.

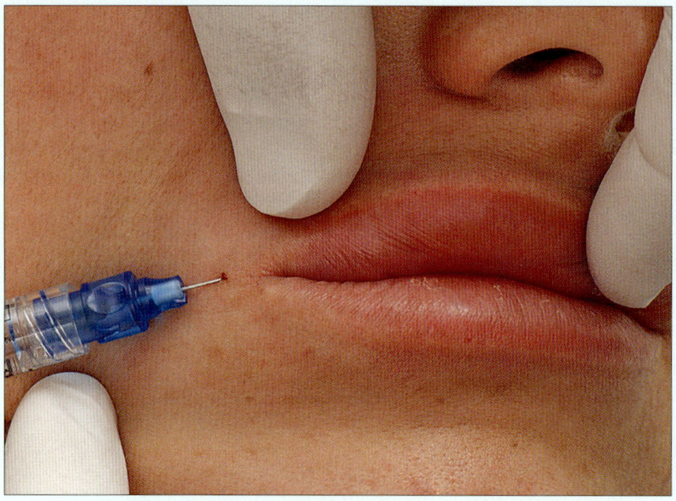

Technique 20 – Fig. 7 Proceed in this way in all four quadrants. It will be necessary to record exactly how much material was delivered in the individual quadrants, as the lips swell quickly, making it seem that more volume has been injected. No further material should be delivered in the last 5 mm before the exit point, as the needle channel would otherwise remain open.

Important Notes

- While advancing the cannula, the therapist can deliver small volumes by anterograde injection and wait for a few minutes until the numbing effect of the lidocaine in the product sets in. This means that the therapist can work in a more relaxed way because the patient will experience less pain.
- The material can be readily distributed by gentle massage after the treatment.

Possible Side Effects

Slight reddening, rarely inflammation, rarely hematomas, mild to more severe swellings, pain in the lips for 2–3 days

Undesirable Side Effects

Inflammation, overcorrection with resultant alteration of the shape of the lip, nodule formation, asymmetry due to non-uniform delivery of material, necrosis

Treatment Protocol at a Glance

- History, evaluation, and patient information
- Informed consent form
- Photo documentation: "before" images
- Analysis and marking of the areas to be treated
- Cleaning
- Thorough disinfection
- Local anesthesia if required (lidocaine cream)
- Injection technique: fanning technique, 2–3 lines per quadrant
- Layer: subcutaneous in the vermillion over the orbicularis oris muscle
- Material: class "M/L soft" product
- Volume: max. 0.3 ml per quadrant, 1–1.2 ml in total
- Needle: 27G cannula, 40 mm, > 25G Nokor needle
- Massage may be applied
- Cooling if required
- Heparin cream for hematomas, ibuprofen p.o., arnica
- Photo documentation: "after" images
- Advice on dos and don'ts after the procedure
- Follow-up appointment for a check-up after 8–14 days

9.4.7 TECHNIQUE 21

Extreme Augmentation – Bolus and Fanning Technique (Sharp Needle)

In this technique, the lips are built-up through the extreme administration of volume. Use of a sharp needle means that hematomas and swellings are likely.

Patient Selection

- If an extreme increase in lip volume is desired

Injection Scheme and Planning (→ Technique 21 – Figs. 1, 2)

Accurate analysis and marking of the zones being treated is the prerequisite for a good treatment result. This combination of the bolus and fanning techniques can be used to produce prominent lifting of the middle part of the lip. The increase in volume depends on the amount of material delivered. The recommendation is to start with four boluses, especially if thin lips are being treated. The four boluses that are placed into the center of the lip determine the shape. The bigger these boluses, the more "bee-stung" the lips will become. In this technique, once a comprehensive analysis has been conducted (see Chap. 1.6, p. 27 ff.), it is vital to respect the underlying anatomical conditions because it is often impossible to carry out an extreme lip volumization treatment without producing a "duck's bill" effect or lines at the mouth corners. Furthermore, the boundaries of the lips' tissue structures may not admit any more volume, so that the material could migrate into other areas, producing unsightly deformities. We recommend proceeding moderately with this technique and agreeing with the patient that the treatment goal needs to be achieved in small steps. The lateral segments of the lips can be adjusted after the initial boluses are placed.

Technique: bolus and fanning technique
Direction of insertion: into the vermillion and across the course of the muscle
Layer: intramuscular
Material: class "M/L soft" product
Volume: depending on the patient's wishes, 1.0 ml to max. 1.5 ml in total
Needle: 27–29G sharp needle
Anesthesia: lidocaine cream, conduction anesthesia

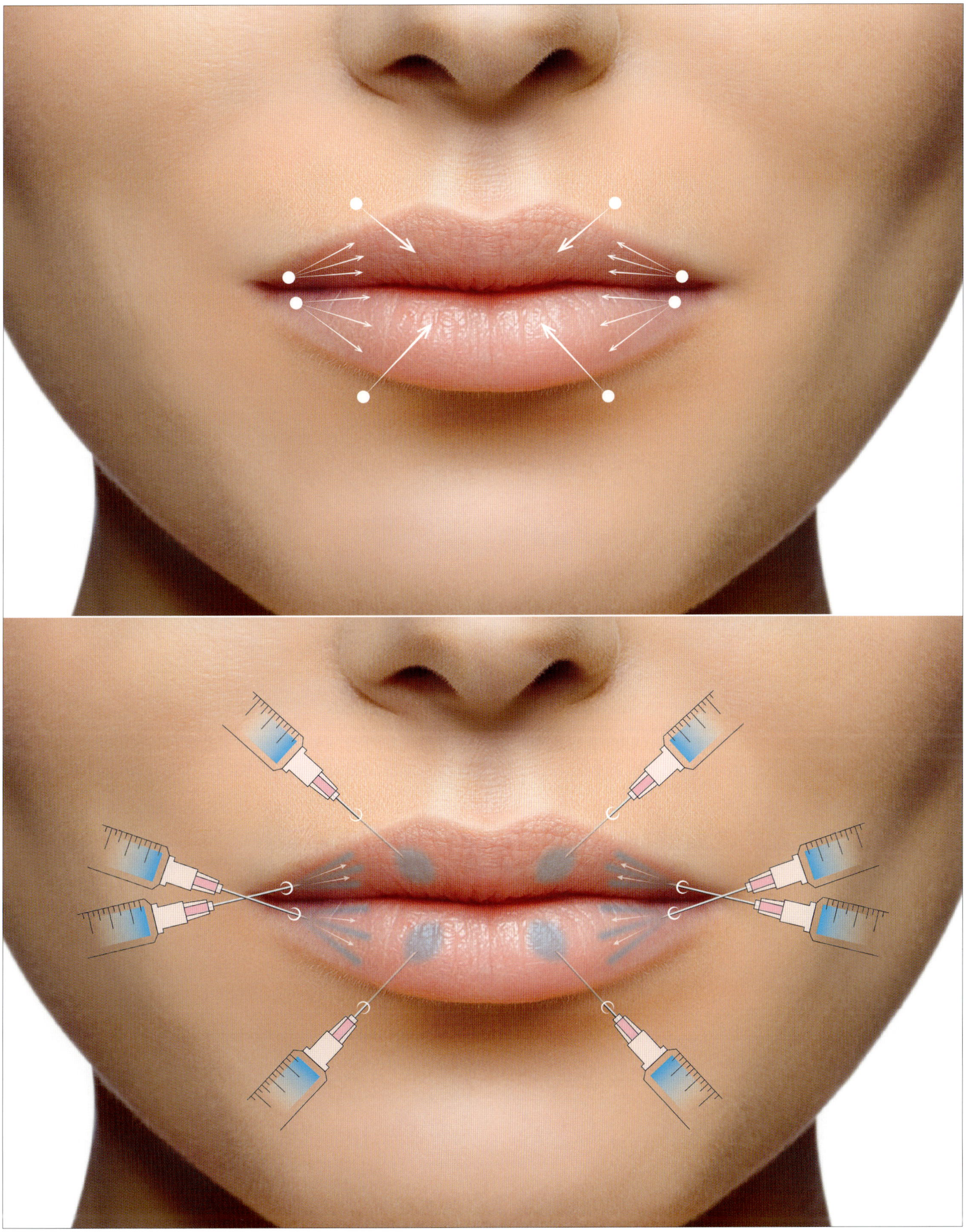

Technique 21 – Figs. 1, 2 Injection scheme and planning for extreme augmentation – bolus and fanning technique (sharp needle).

Treatment Method (→ Technique 21– Figs. 3–8)

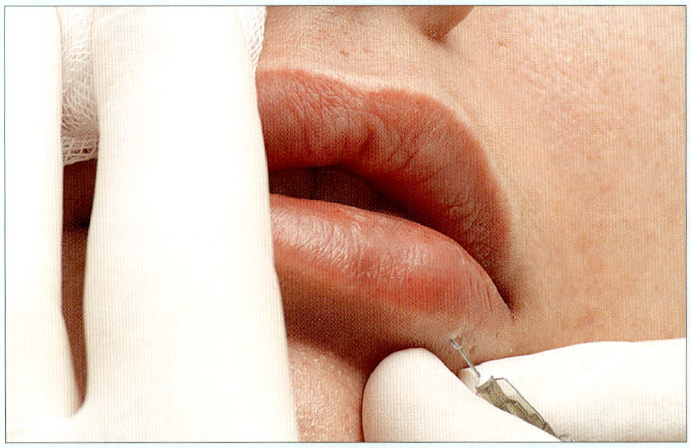

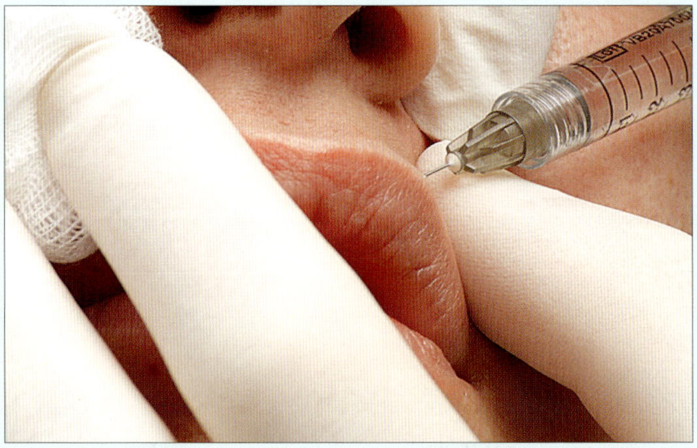

Technique 21 – Figs. 3, 4 To begin with, place one bolus per quadrant. Inject through the cutaneous part of the lip: the tip of the needle needs to be in the center of the target zone. This can be checked with a finger before delivering the material, by palpating the tip of the needle through the skin of the lip. The bolus becomes clearly visible once the material has been delivered.

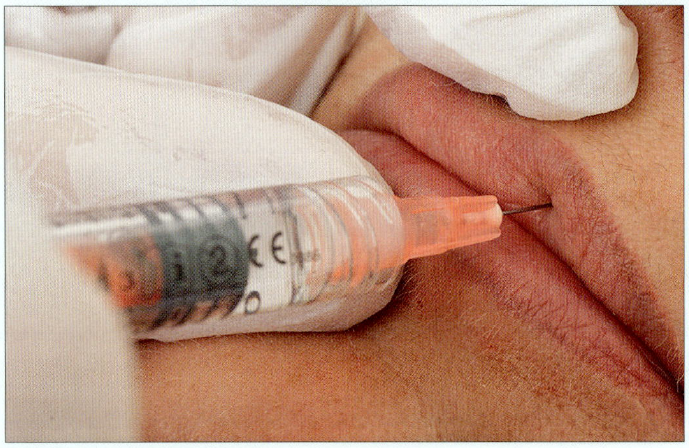

Technique 21 – Fig. 5 Alternatively, it is also possible to inject into the center of the lip directly from the front. This is easier for the therapist, but more painful for the patient.

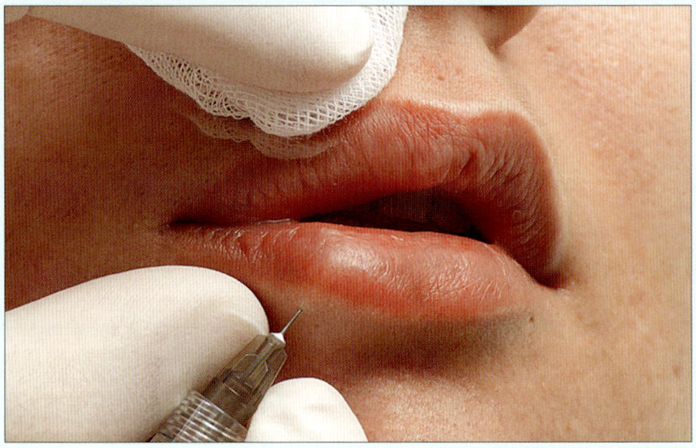

Technique 21 – Fig. 6 If a harmonious result is to be achieved, even with extreme lip volumization, care should be taken to ensure that the final treatment outcome is for the lower lip to be bigger than the upper one (see Golden Ratio, p. 32 ff.).

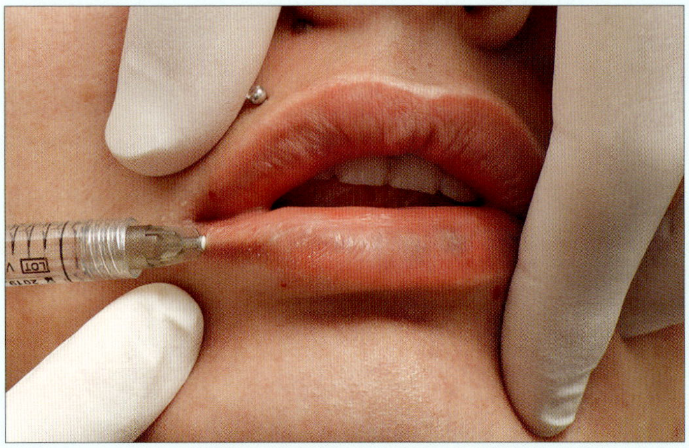

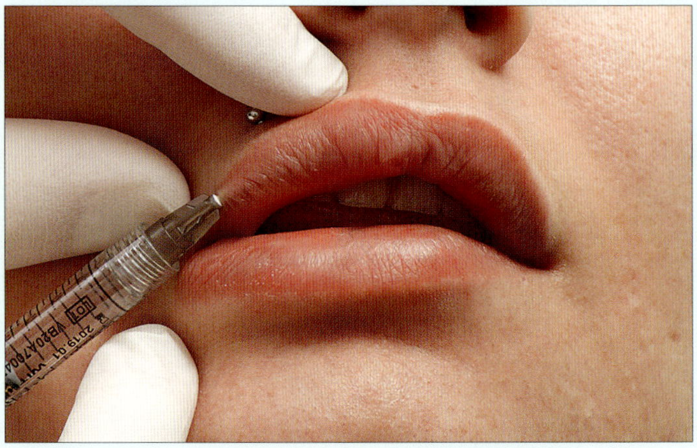

Technique 21 – Figs. 7, 8 Once the four boluses have been placed, fill the lateral segments of the lip to produce a harmonious result. The fanning technique with the sharp needle is used for this, placing 2–4 lines depending on how much volume was previously administered in bolus form. The amount of material delivered is at the discretion of the therapist and needs to be agreed with the patient. Delivering too much material can widen the mouth considerably, making it appear unnatural.

Important Notes

- The amount of material delivered is at the discretion of the therapist and needs to be agreed with the patient.
- Delivering too much material can widen the mouth considerably, distort it, and cause a "duck's bill" effect, making it appear unnatural.

Possible Side Effects

Slight reddening, rarely inflammation, commonly hematomas, more severe swellings, pain for 2–3 days

Undesirable Side Effects

Inflammation, overcorrection, and non-uniform delivery of material with resultant alteration of the shape of the lip, nodule formation, asymmetry, necrosis

Treatment Protocol at a Glance

- History, evaluation, and patient information
- Informed consent form
- Photo documentation: "before" images
- Analysis and marking of the areas to be treated
- Cleaning
- Thorough disinfection
- Local anesthesia (lidocaine cream) or conduction anesthesia if required
- Injection technique: bolus and fanning techniques
- Layer: intramuscular
- Material: class "M/L soft" product
- Volume: depending on the patient's wishes, 1.0 ml to max. 1.5 ml in total
- Needle: 27–29G sharp needle
- No massage
- Cooling if required
- Heparin cream for hematomas, ibuprofen p.o., arnica
- Photo documentation: "after" images
- Advice on dos and don'ts after the procedure
- Follow-up appointment for a check-up after 8–14 days

9.4.8 TECHNIQUE 22

Augmentation from the Dry/Wet Boundary (Sharp Needle)

This technique allows lips with a volume deficiency, i.e. thin lips, to be enlarged slightly. However, the technique has its limits if the lips are extremely thin. In general, the result is better with young, naturally thin lips than with lips that have undergone age-related atrophy and have become inverted.

Patient Selection

- For thin lips or where little of the vermillion is visible. To select suitable patients, it is necessary to distinguish between inverted lips that have undergone age-related atrophy (see Technique 23, p. 218 ff.) and lips that are merely deficient in volume.

Injection Scheme and Planning (→ Technique 22 – Figs. 1, 2 a+b)

9

The material is placed along the dry/wet boundary, with three lines each injected into the upper and lower lip. If the width of the upper lip also needs increasing, the two lines close to the mouth corners are injected with the same volume of material as the medial line. The further the line is extended toward the corner of the mouth, the more strongly the mouth will be widened. If the medial area is to be the focus of the volumization, the material should be tapered toward the sides. The upper lip is less "forgiving" than the lower lip, as its contour and shape define the expression of the mouth. If it is altered too much, the oral region will look odd.

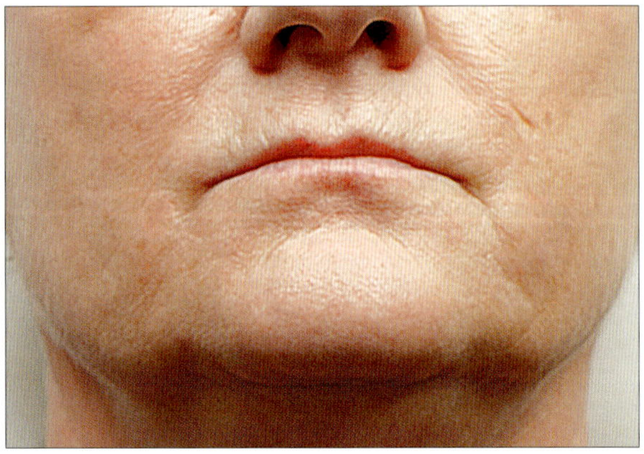

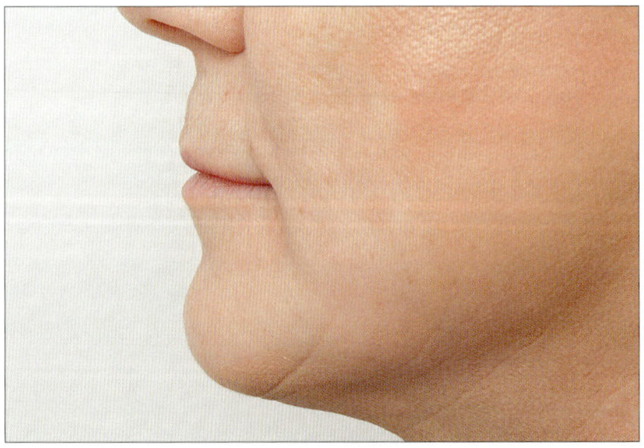

Lips that show age-related atrophy and have become inverted (left), and the thin lips of a younger patient (right).

Technique: linear technique
Direction of insertion: along the body of the muscle following the dry/wet boundary
Layer: subcutaneous in the vermillion over the orbicularis oris muscle
Material: class "M soft" product
Volume: max. 0.1 ml per line, 0.6 ml in total
Needle: 27–29G sharp needle, 20 mm
Anesthesia: lidocaine cream if required, conduction anesthesia if required

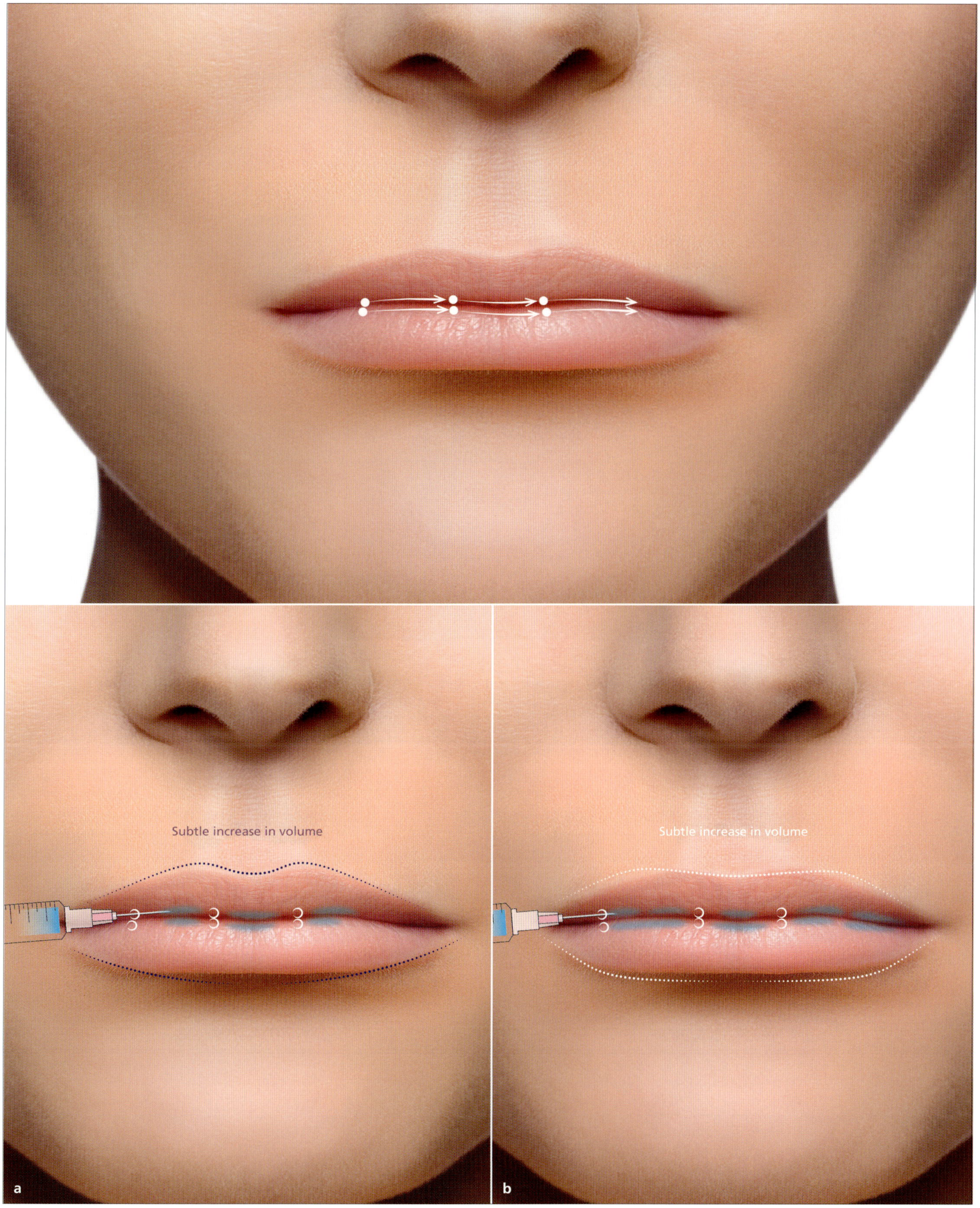

Technique 22 – Figs. 1, 2 a+b Injection scheme and planning for the augmentation of thin lips from the dry/wet boundary (sharp needle). If the lip is to be augmented in the center to increase the volume, the material should be placed into the dry/wet boundary of the center region (a). If the whole lip is to be everted slightly, it is important to inject the material over its entire length (b).

9

Treatment Method (→ Technique 22 – Figs. 3, 4)

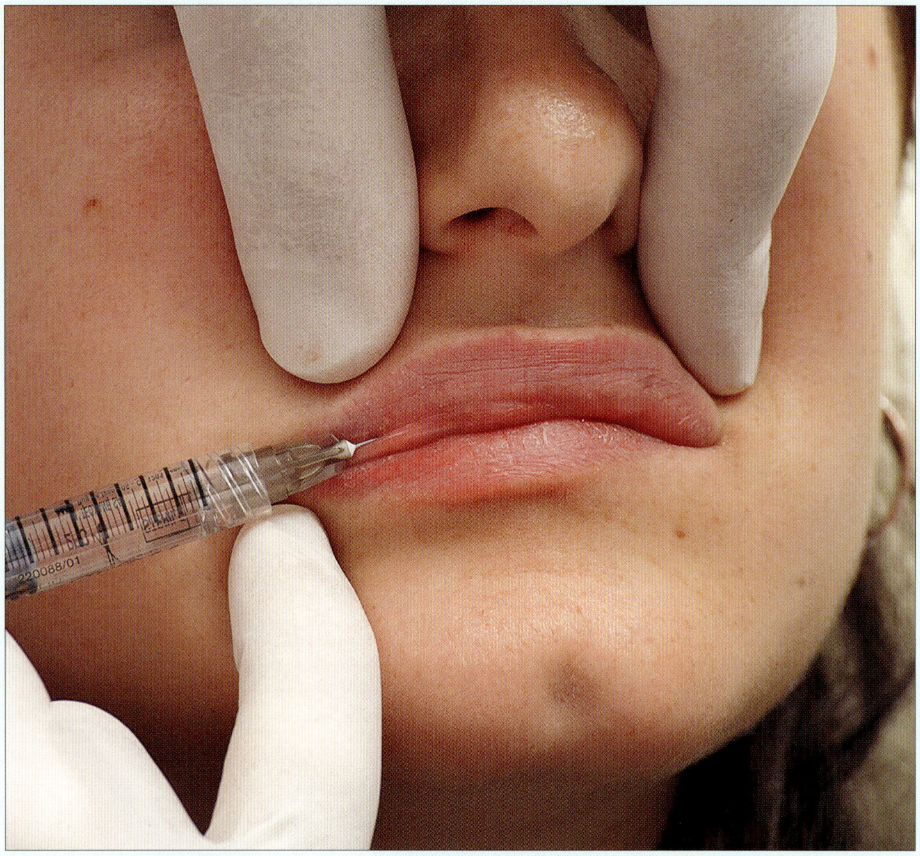

Technique 22 – Fig. 3 The more volume is introduced into the posterior region of the mucous membrane, the more the lip will protrude. The patient may be able to feel the bolus of material (which produces the lifting effect) with the tongue. Stretch the lip gently between the thumb and forefinger and roll it slightly upward until the dry/wet boundary becomes visible. Slowly inject the lip using the linear technique, with regular visual checks of the volume of material delivered.

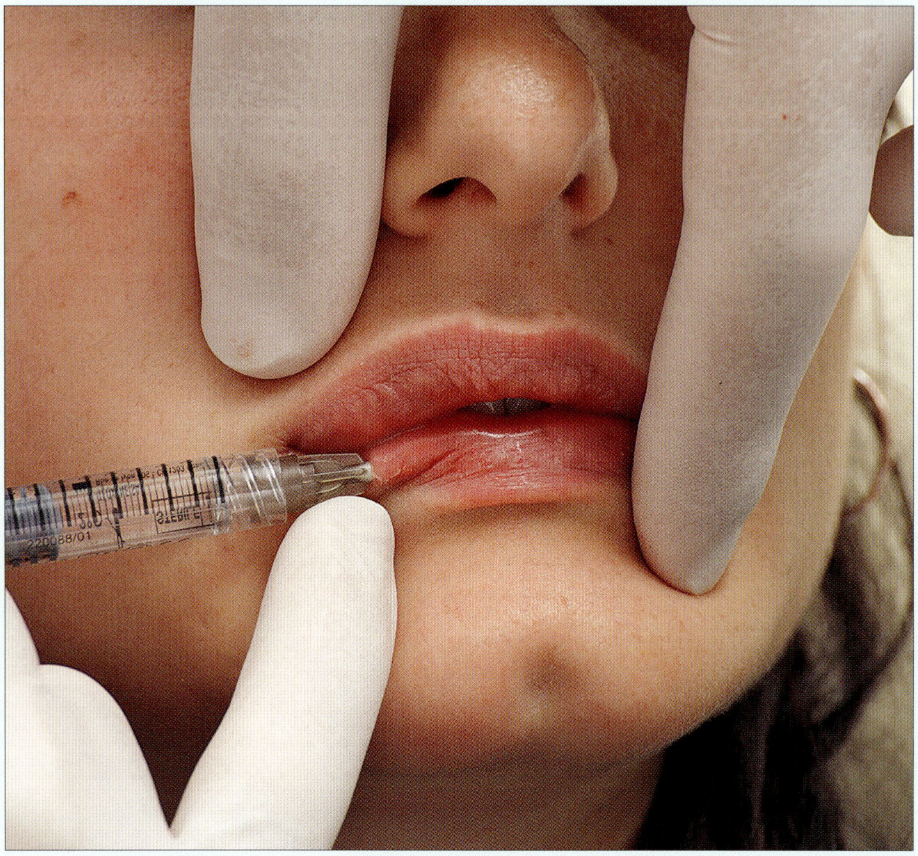

Technique 22 – Fig. 4 The lip can also be everted and then injected.

Important Notes

- After the treatment, the patient should be asked to stretch the lips and to smile. This shows up any irregularities so that they can be corrected.

Possible Side Effects

Rarely inflammation, internal hematomas, mild to more severe swellings

Undesirable Side Effects

Inflammation, overcorrection, and non-uniform delivery of material with resultant alteration of the shape of the lip, nodule formation, asymmetry

Treatment Protocol at a Glance

- History, evaluation, and patient information
- Informed consent form
- Photo documentation: "before" images
- Analysis and marking of the areas to be treated
- Cleaning
- Thorough disinfection
- Local anesthesia (lidocaine cream) or conduction anesthesia if required
- Injection technique: linear technique, 3 lines each into the upper and lower lip
- Layer: subcutaneous in the vermillion over the orbicularis oris muscle
- Material: class "M soft" product
- Volume: max. 0.1 ml per line, 0.6 ml in total
- Needle: 27–29G sharp needle, 20 mm
- Massage if required
- Cooling if required
- Heparin cream for hematomas, ibuprofen p.o., arnica
- Photo documentation: "after" images
- Advice on dos and don'ts after the procedure
- Follow-up appointment for a check-up after 8–14 days

9.4.9 TECHNIQUE 23
Augmentation from the Mucous Membrane (Sharp Needle)

The treatment goal is for thin, inverted lips to be brought forward by targeted injections. As opposed to Technique 22, the material is injected into the mucous membrane located in front of the teeth, and the teeth are used as supports.

Patient Selection

- For thin, flattened, inverted lips, with little visible vermillion or lips that show age-related atrophy
- Patients with mandibular overbite

Injection Scheme and Planning (→ Technique 23 – Figs. 1, 2)

After disinfecting the mucosa thoroughly, the boluses are injected directly into the mucous membrane close to the dry/wet boundary. As the material is placed into the mucous membrane as a bolus, and the teeth provide firm resistance, the lip is pushed forward and turned out slightly. Of course, the success of this procedure is always dependent on the position of the teeth, the substance of the jaw (see Chap. 1.6.3, p. 36 ff.), the natural vermillion of the lips, and the patient's age. Three to seven boluses of c. 0.02 ml are placed into the upper lip, depending on the underlying anatomical conditions. The recommendation for the lower lip is to inject at 3 points, to make the lower lip appear somewhat more prominent. Here, the volume delivered per point is 0.05 ml or more. This depends on the position of the teeth in the mandible.

Technique: bolus technique

Direction of insertion: from the front or from the side

Layer: supramucosal, at the boundary between the vermillion and the mucous membrane

Material: class "M soft" product

Volume: c. 0.2 ml into the upper lip and 0.3 ml into the lower one, depending on the deficit

Needle: 27G sharp needle, 20 mm

Anesthesia: lidocaine cream, conduction anesthesia if required

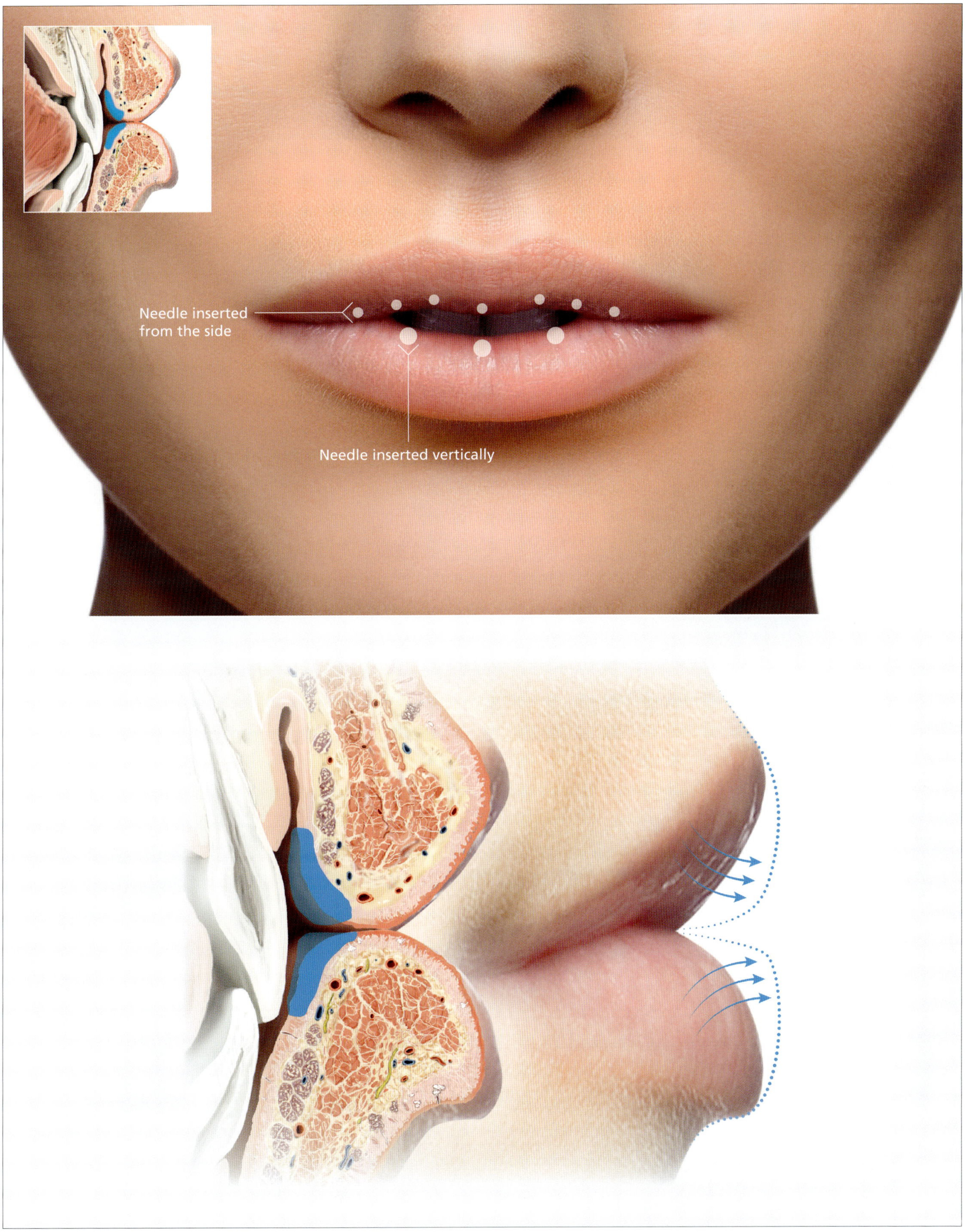

Technique 23 – Figs. 1, 2 Injection scheme and planning for the augmentation of thin lips from the mucous membrane (sharp needle).

Treatment Method (→ Technique 23 – Figs. 3–5)

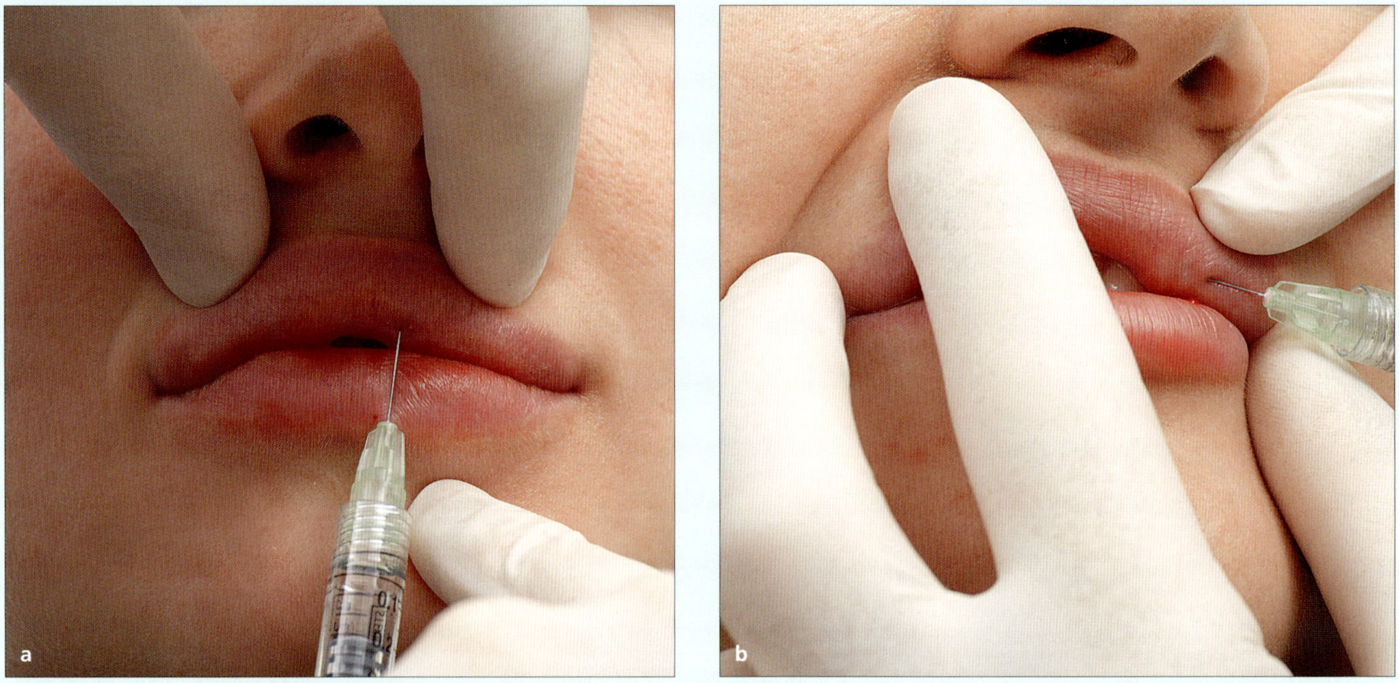

Technique 23 – Figs. 3 a+b Evert the lip with the aid of the forefinger and thumb until the mucous membrane becomes visible. This needs to be disinfected again. Then, deliver a bolus of c. 0.02 ml, as required, into the upper lip mucosa. Insert the needle either vertically (a) into the center of the target area or from the side (b), so that the needle bevel is close to the mucous membrane in the oral cavity. Having done so, assess the result and correct if required. Repeat the procedure on the other side with exactly the same amount of HA.

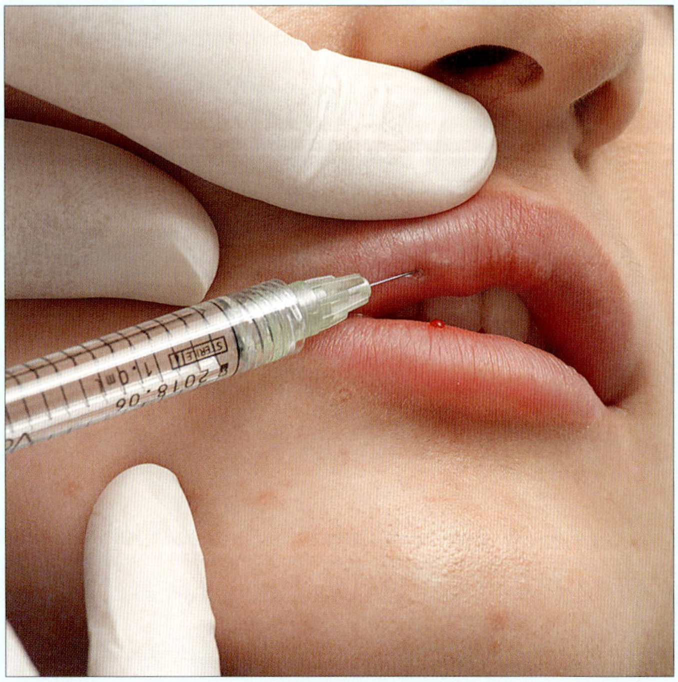

Technique 23 – Fig. 4 The image shows the bolus emerging from the needle.

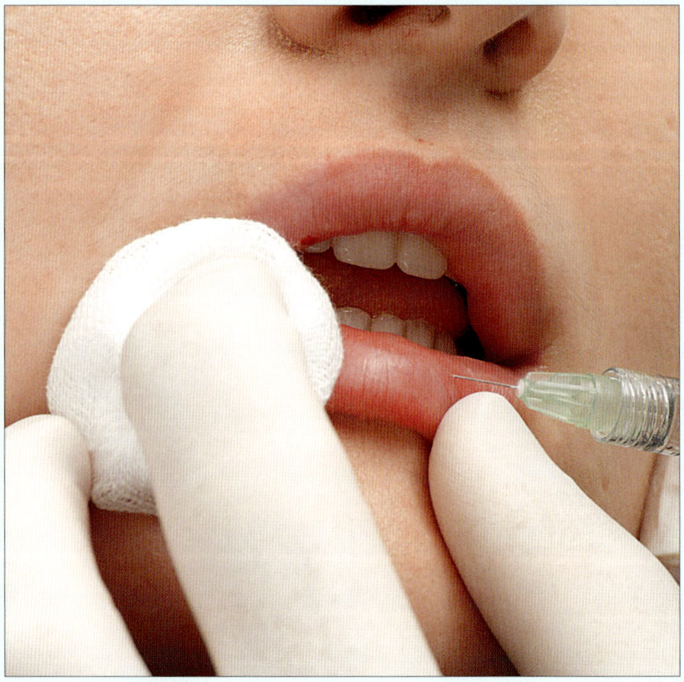

Technique 23 – Fig. 5 Injection into the lower lip mucosa at 3 points with boluses of c. 0.05 ml each, to give prominence to the lower lip.

Important Notes

- The gloves need to be dry to allow the lip to be everted properly.
- The everted lip needs to be held in place so that it does not slip back, as this would prevent the material from being injected into the desired site.

Possible Side Effects

Slight reddening, rarely inflammation, rarely hematomas, mild to more severe swellings

Undesirable Side Effects

Inflammation, overcorrection, asymmetry, nodules, necrosis

Treatment Protocol at a Glance

- History, evaluation, and patient information
- Informed consent form
- Photo documentation: "before" images
- Analysis and marking of the areas to be treated
- Cleaning
- Thorough disinfection
- Local anesthesia (lidocaine cream), conduction anesthesia if required
- Injection technique: bolus technique
- Layer: supramucosal, at the boundary between the vermillion and the mucous membrane
- Material: class "M soft" product
- Volume: c. 0.2 ml into the upper lip and 0.3 ml into the lower one, depending on the deficit
- Needle: 27G sharp needle, 20 mm
- No massage
- Cooling if required
- Heparin cream for hematomas, ibuprofen p.o., arnica
- Photo documentation: "after" images
- Advice on dos and don'ts after the procedure
- Follow-up appointment for a check-up after 8–14 days

9.4.10 TECHNIQUE 24

Volumization with or without Tubercle Accentuation (Sharp Needle)

This technique has been used ever since fillers have been in existence and is suitable for refreshing the lips by augmenting them gently (see also Technique 17, p. 194 ff.). It is easy to use as the material can be placed with great accuracy. Uniform delivery of the material is the key factor in producing a harmonious lip shape.

The technique offers a number of potential variations. It is also suitable for correcting any areas of asymmetry; this requires accurate pre-treatment planning regarding how much material to deliver.

Patient Selection

- For thinner lips, a small mouth or wrinkled lips
- If more lip volume is desired

Injection Scheme and Planning (→ Technique 24 – Figs. 1–4)

The material is injected into the selected, marked region, with frequent visual checks of the syringe plunger to monitor delivery because the lips swell quickly There are two possible variants.

Variant 1: The middle section of each lip is volumized with four or more lines (depending on needle length) without taking the shape of the lip into consideration, resulting in undifferentiated augmentation of the middle section. The tubercle is not filled because the needle does not go across it (it stops short of the center of the lip). Doing so causes a subtle realignment of the oral fissure. This method is suitable for symmetrical, shapely lips that merely require augmentation of their overall volume. Following an accurate analysis, the curvature of the lips can be perfected by observing them from the side and correcting any flattening. If the curvature does recede toward the oral fissure, the material is placed closer to the dry/wet boundary to fashion a convex shape.

Variant 2: If the tubercle needs particular accentuation, the linear technique is used so that the lines running parallel to the Cupid's bow intersect in the median tubercle. This causes marked augmentation of this central prominence and gives the lips their characteristic expression. The material is injected into the vermillion. The median tubercle of the upper lip is accentuated by placing the material into the middle of the upper lip from the side, giving the oral fissure an "M" shape.

Technique: linear technique
Direction of insertion: along the body of the muscle
Layer: subcutaneous in the vermillion over the orbicularis oris muscle
Material: class "S/M soft" product
Volume: c. 0.6 ml in total
Needle: 27G sharp needle, 20 mm
Anesthesia: lidocaine cream

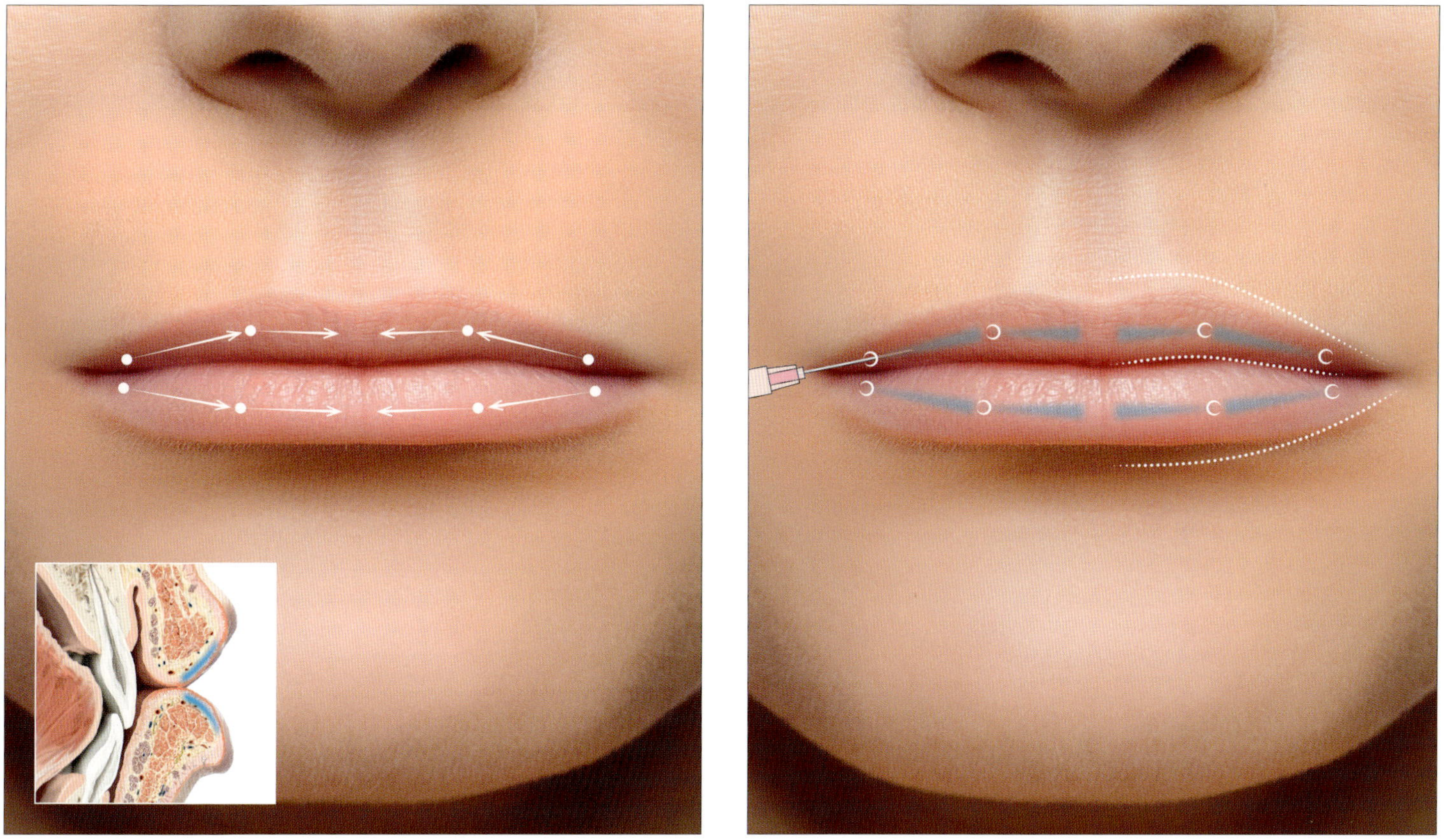

Technique 24 – Figs. 1, 2 Injection scheme and planning for undifferentiated volumization of the medial sections of the lips (sharp needle).

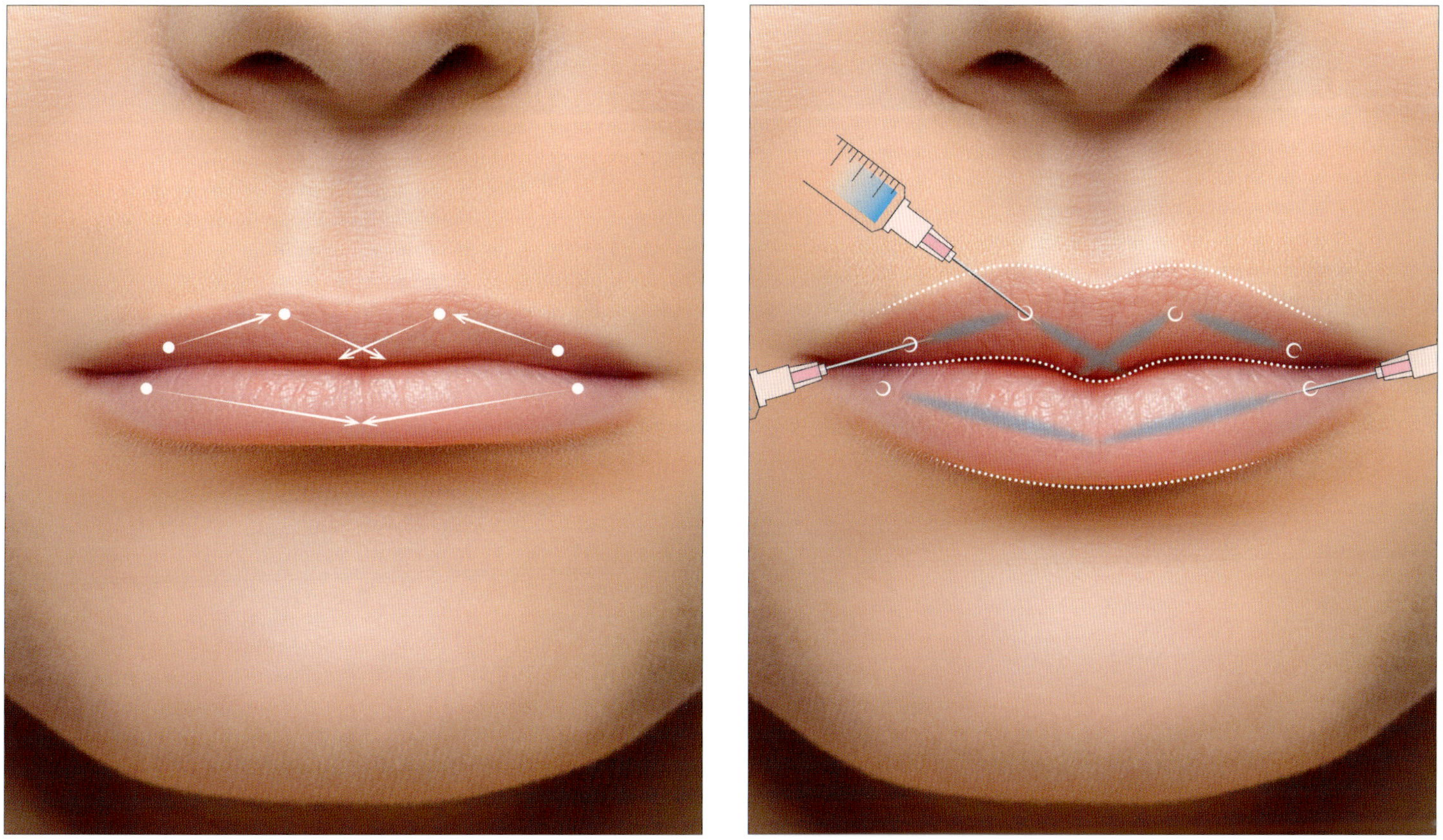

Technique 24 – Figs. 3, 4 Injection scheme and planning for volumization with tubercle accentuation (sharp needle).

Treatment Method (→ Technique 24 – Figs. 5–11)

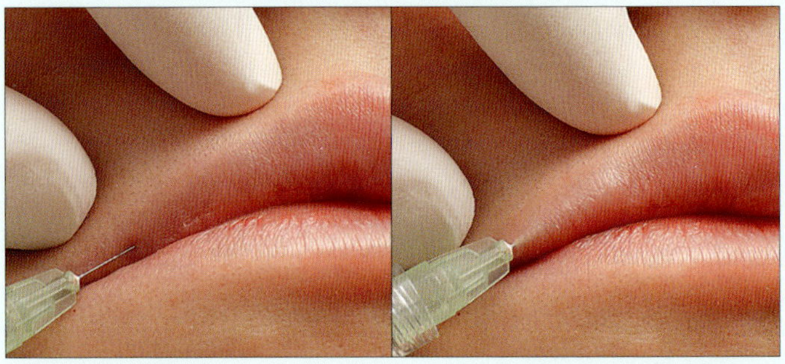

Technique 24 – Fig. 5 With the thumb and forefinger of the free hand, apply gentle pressure to the cutaneous part of the upper lip to evert and stretch the lip slightly. Insert the needle to about 2 cm in length and deliver the material uniformly by retrograde injection, tapering it off near the end. The needle should be clearly visible in the slightly everted lip.

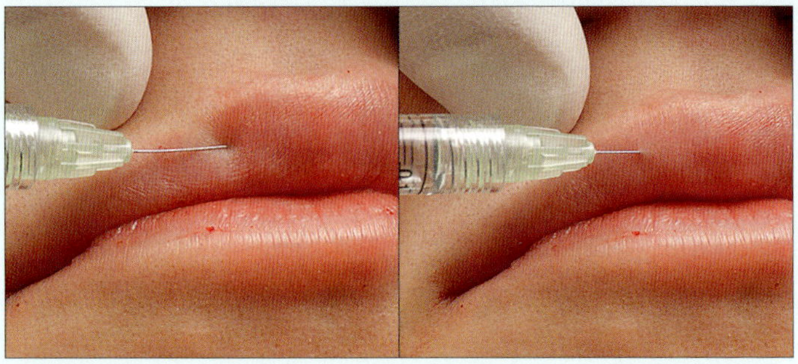

Technique 24 – Fig. 6 To accentuate the tubercle, pull the lip gently upward and outward, and inject at the level of the Cupid's bow toward the center of the tubercle. Deliver the material by retrograde injection.

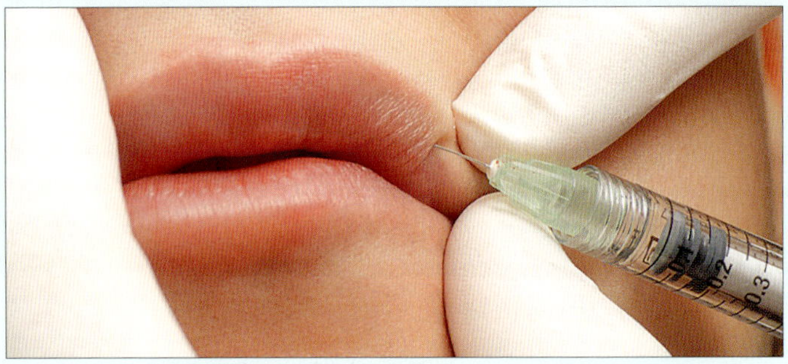

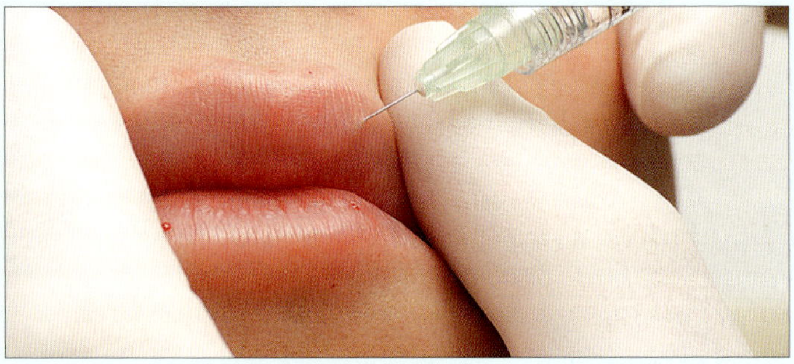

Technique 24 – Figs. 7, 8 When injecting on the other side, make sure that exactly the same amount of material is delivered. For this reason, the lips should no longer be stretched while injecting the material, so that the therapist can check that the material is being delivered symmetrically based on the outward lifting of the tissue.

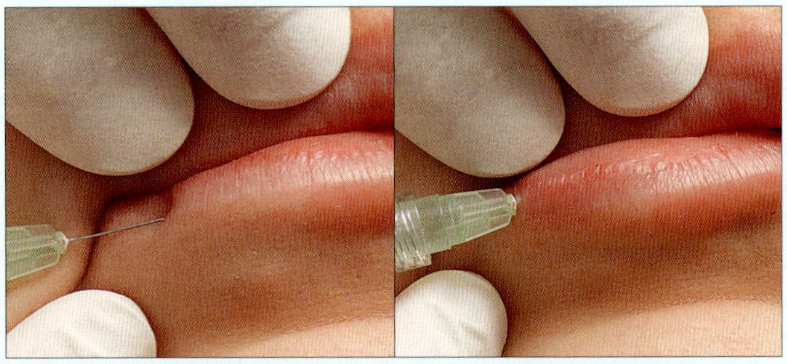

Technique 24 – Fig. 9 Using the little finger of the injecting hand or the thumb of the free hand, pull the lip gently outward and fill by linear retrograde injection in three sequences. In each case, the middle segment should be filled with slightly more volume than the two segments by the mouth corners. Monitor the syringe plunger visually to check for uniform delivery of the material.

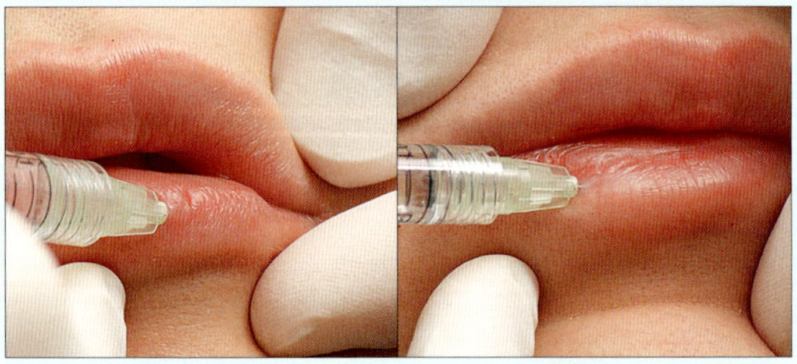

Technique 24 – Fig. 10 The therapist can inject the lower lip fully from one side. If the injection is being given from the right side, the patient only needs to rotate the head slightly from right to left.

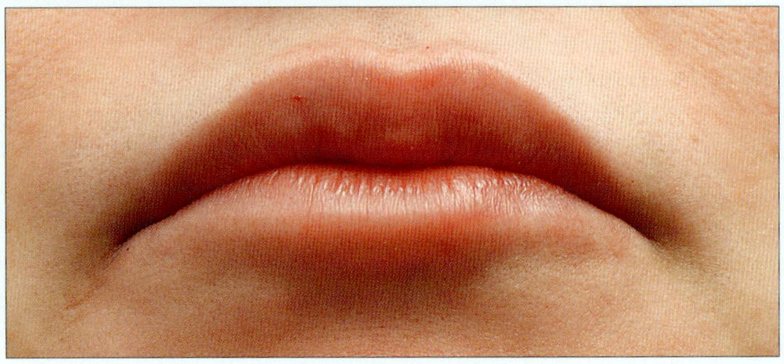

Technique 24 – Fig. 11 A final visual and palpatory check is important. There must be no areas of asymmetry.

Important Notes

- The palpatory check is important. There must be no lumps or irregularities.
- If the therapist applies some wound cream to the lips immediately after the treatment and massages the lips gently between the thumbs and forefingers of both hands, this palpation will clearly show if the material has been uniformly distributed. Any minor irregularities can also be corrected by doing this.
- The immediate result of the injection can be assessed by asking the patient to stretch the mouth into a wide smile directly after the treatment. This can also be used to check if the material has been distributed uniformly.

Possible Side Effects

Slight reddening, rarely inflammation, hematomas, mild to more severe swellings

Undesirable Side Effects

Overcorrection with resultant alteration of the shape of the lip or nodule formation, asymmetry due to non-uniform delivery of material, necrosis

Treatment Protocol at a Glance

- History, evaluation, and patient information
- Informed consent form
- Photo documentation: "before" images
- Analysis and marking of the areas to be treated
- Cleaning
- Thorough disinfection
- Local anesthesia (lidocaine cream) or conduction anesthesia if required
- Injection technique: linear technique, 4 lines into the upper lip, 3–4 lines into the lower lip
- Layer: subcutaneous in the vermillion over the orbicularis oris muscle
- Material: class "S/M soft" product
- Volume: c. 0.6 ml in total
- Needle: 27G sharp needle, 20 mm
- Massage may be applied
- Cooling if required
- Heparin cream for hematomas, ibuprofen p.o., arnica
- Photo documentation: "after" images
- Advice on dos and don'ts after the procedure
- Follow-up appointment for a check-up after 8–14 days

9.4.11 TECHNIQUE 25

Volumization – Bolus Technique (Sharp Needle)

This technique produces augmentation deep inside the lips by placing boluses of HA directly into the vermillion. The treatment is preceded by an accurate analysis of the area to be filled.

Patient Selection

- Where there is a volume deficit or if the patient wants strong lip augmentation
- Beautification
- Correcting areas of asymmetry

Injection Scheme and Planning (→ Technique 25 – Figs. 1, 2)

Boluses are placed deep into the vermillion by injecting with a sharp needle. The material is introduced from either the lateral or the medial side, or directly from the front and in the dorsal direction. The depth of insertion is determined to ensure that the needle tip is located in the center of the planned bolus, in the muscle of the lip. If the bolus is placed too superficially, it may become visible when the patient speaks or smiles, which would be undesirable. The volume of material delivered is checked visually. The hyaluronic acid should be soft, i.e. it should show a moderate degree of crosslinking and a medium calibration rate (Sattler & Sommer 2015).

Technique: bolus technique
Direction of insertion: into the body of the muscle, from the side or from the front
Layer: vermillion, intramuscular in the orbicularis oris muscle
Material: class "M/L soft" product
Volume: max. 0.25 ml per bolus in the upper lip, 0.3–0.5 ml per bolus in the lower lip, max. 1.5 ml in total
Needle: 27G sharp needle
Anesthesia: Lidocaine cream, conduction anesthesia

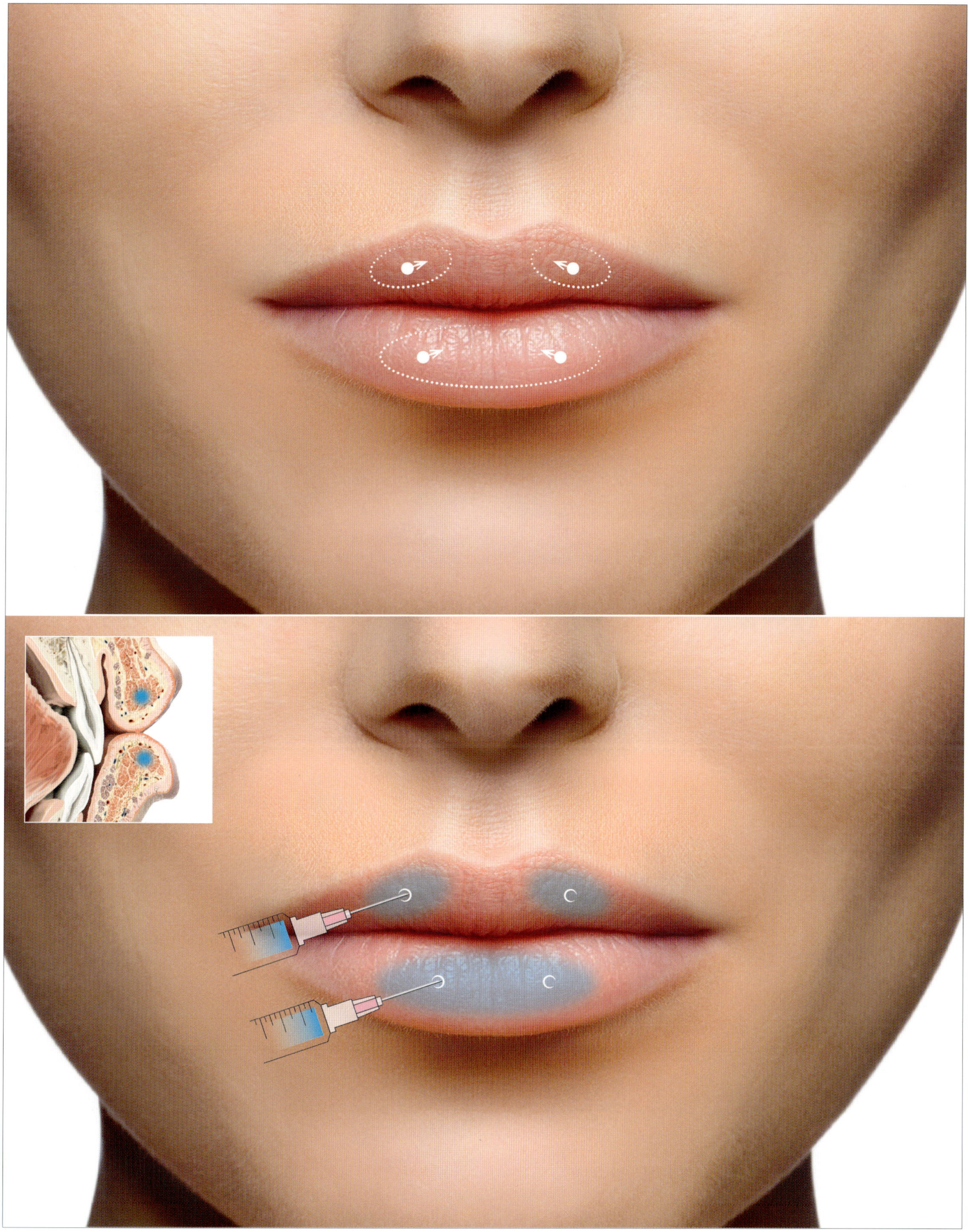

Technique 25 – Figs. 1, 2 Injection scheme and planning for volumization – bolus technique (sharp needle).

Treatment Method (→ Technique 25 – Figs. 3–6)

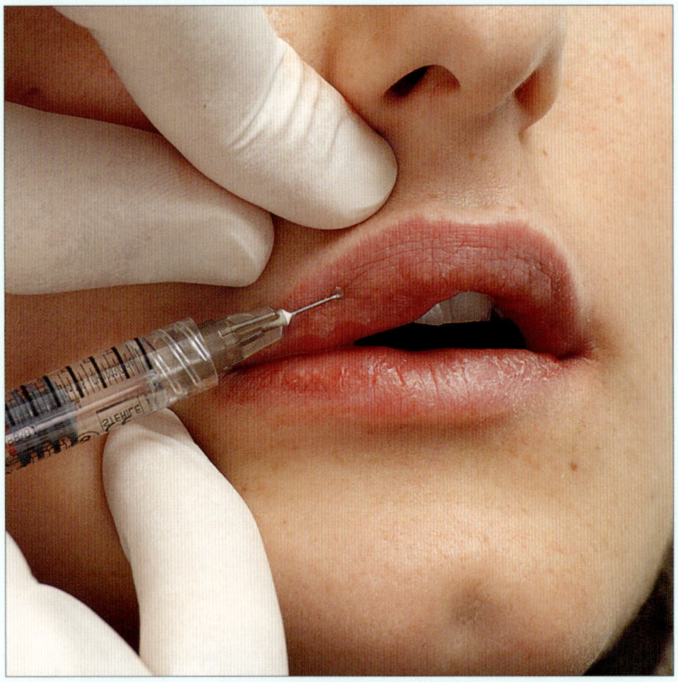

Technique 25 – Fig. 3 Place the material into areas where there is a volume deficit. Here, the needle is directed from the side toward the middle. The advantage of doing so is that the depot can be spread out slightly, making it easy to see where the material is located.

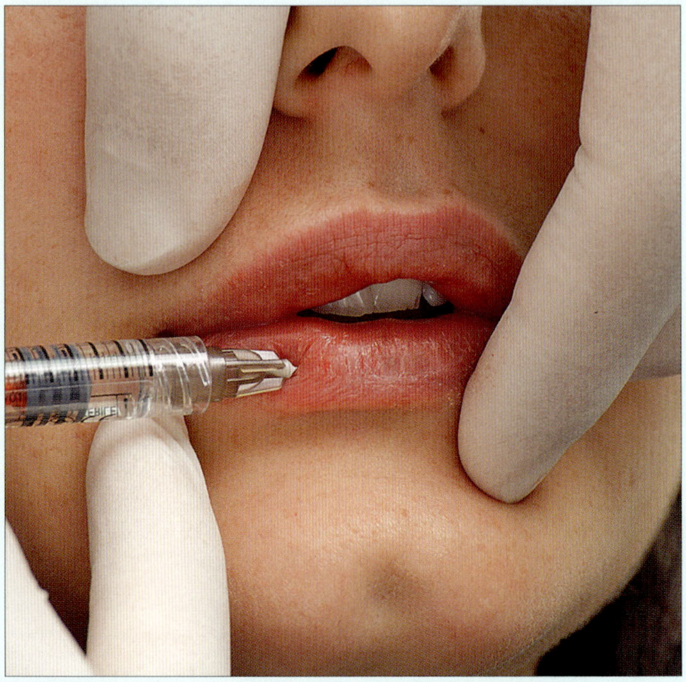

Technique 25 – Fig. 4 Place the material deep (3–5 mm, depending on the thickness of the lip) into the muscle. This makes the lip augmentation "softer" because there is sufficient tissue above the bolus at this depth.

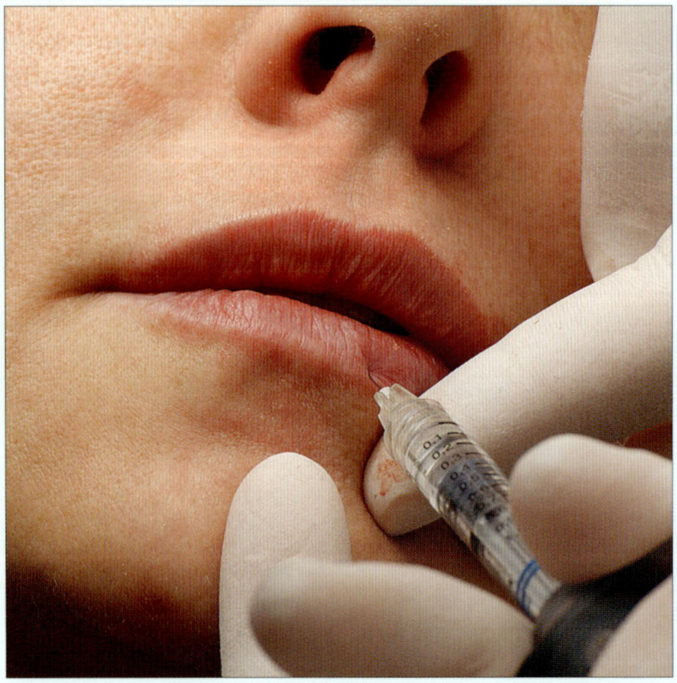

Technique 25 – Fig. 5 Alternatively, place the material as a bolus directly from the front and slightly more superficially. This fixes it into one place so that it is not distributed over the whole area, which enhances the forward curvature of the lip.

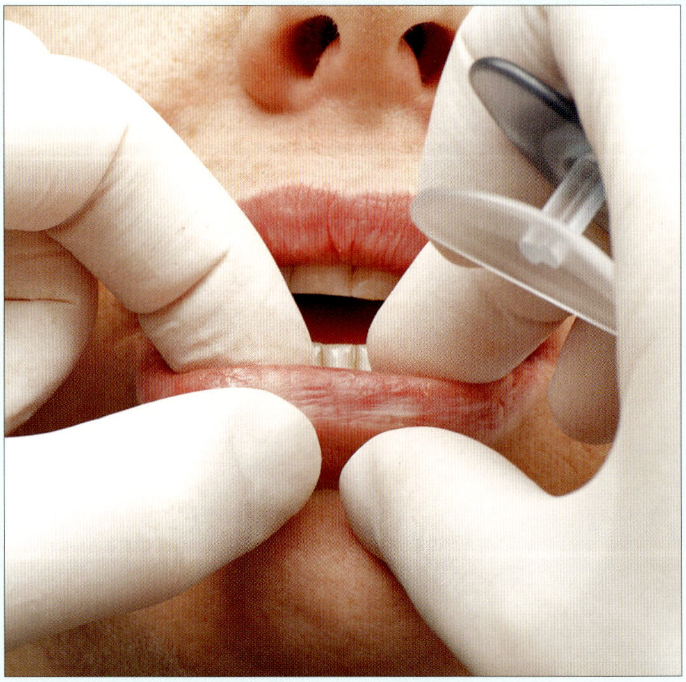

Technique 25 – Fig. 6 Massage after the treatment is recommended with the bolus technique to prevent any unevenness.

Important Notes

- If too much material is placed as a bolus, cohesion/aggregation of the HA may occur in rare cases. Therefore, smaller depots or boluses should be injected.
- Care should be taken that the lip (especially if the mouth is small) does not recede too much at its lateral ends near the mouth corners. Should this be the case, it is also advisable to place additional, smaller corrective boluses in this region.

Possible Side Effects

Slight reddening, rarely inflammation, commonly hematomas, more severe swellings, cohesive aggregation of the boluses, connective tissue encapsulation and induration

Undesirable Side Effects

Inflammation, overcorrection with resultant alteration of the shape of the lip or nodule formation, asymmetry due to non-uniform delivery of material, necrosis

Treatment Protocol at a Glance

- History, evaluation, and patient information
- Informed consent form
- Photo documentation: "before" images
- Analysis and marking of the areas to be treated
- Cleaning
- Thorough disinfection
- Local anesthesia (lidocaine cream) or conduction anesthesia if required
- Injection technique: bolus technique, 2 boluses each into the upper and lower lip
- Layer: vermillion, intramuscular into the orbicularis oris muscle
- Material: class "M/L soft" product
- Volume: max. 0.25 ml per bolus in the upper lip, 0.3–0.5 ml per bolus in the lower lip, max. < 1.5 ml in total
- Needle: 27G sharp needle
- Massage
- Cooling if required
- Heparin cream for hematomas, ibuprofen p.o., arnica
- Photo documentation: "after" images
- Advice on dos and don'ts after the procedure
- Follow-up appointment for a check-up after 8–14 days

9.4.12 TECHNIQUE 26

Volumization – Cutaneous Part of the Lip Technique (Sharp Needle)

Lip volume is increased by the specific placement of small HA boluses into the vermillion. Access is via a needle puncture into the cutaneous part of the lip. This technique is less painful than the classic injection, in which the material is injected into the vermillion directly from the front.

Patient Selection

- Where there is a volume deficit or if the patient wants gentle to moderate lip augmentation
- Beautification by building up specific lip areas
- Correcting areas of asymmetry

Injection Scheme and Planning (→ Technique 26 – Figs. 1, 2)

The areas that need filling are marked. A sharp needle is inserted into the cutaneous part of the lip and is then advanced forward through it and into the center of the vermillion. The needle insertion sites are located about 0.5–1 cm above and below the lip contours, respectively. The material is delivered with frequent visual checks, injecting it into the center of the lip as a bolus, approaching from the cutaneous part of the lips and below the contour. This produces targeted augmentation at specific points. The amount of material delivered varies as required. In general, more material is injected into the four central points of the lip than into the areas close to the mouth corners.

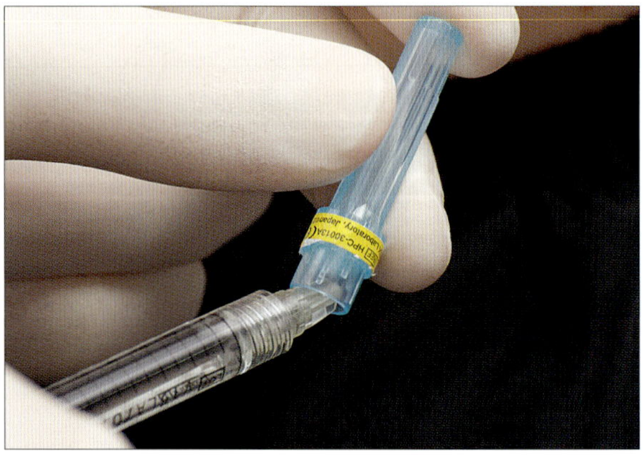

To achieve the ideal angle of insertion, the needle has been bent around 40 degrees with the bevel facing up, allowing it to reach the target area more easily.

Technique: bolus technique

Direction of insertion: starting from the cutaneous part of the lip, inject centrally into the muscle in the vermillion, LL: upward from below, OL: downward from the top

Layer: vermillion, intramuscular in the orbicularis oris muscle

Material: class "S/M soft" product

Volume: max. 0.1 ml per bolus, c. 0.5 ml in total

Needle: 27–29G sharp needle, 20 mm

Anesthesia: lidocaine cream

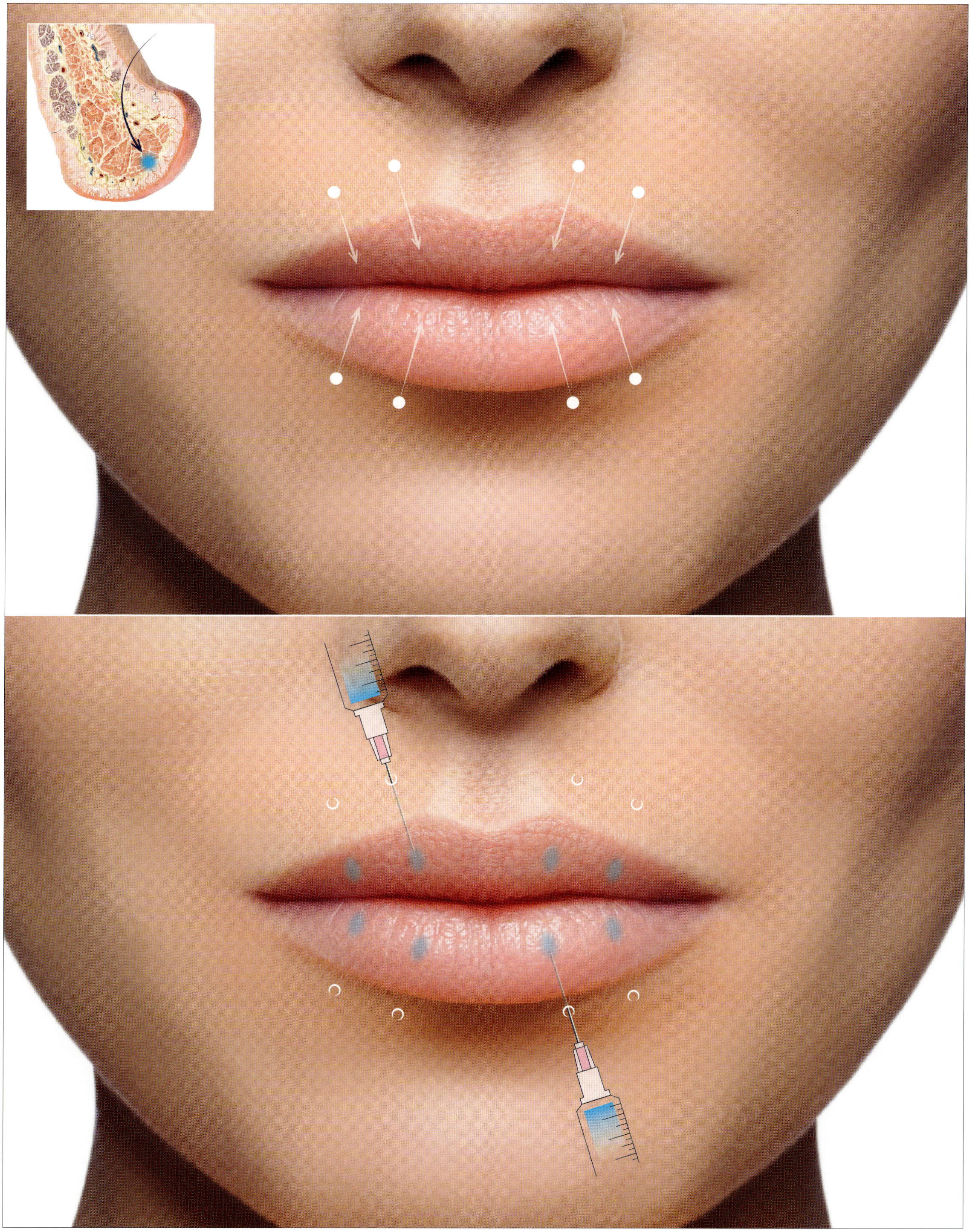

Technique 26 – Figs. 1, 2 Injection scheme and planning for volumization – cutaneous part of the lip technique (sharp needle).

Treatment Method (→ Technique 26 – Figs. 3–8)

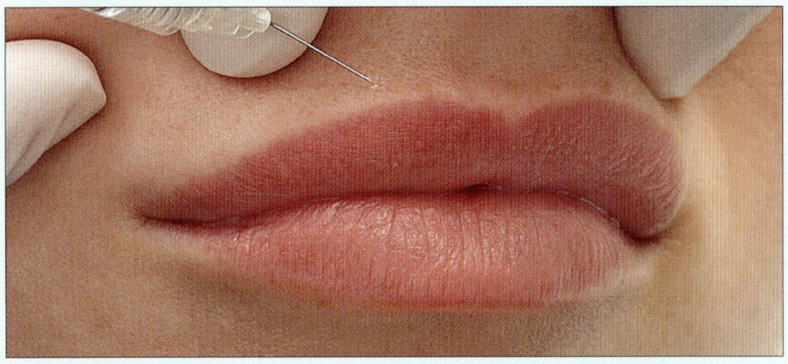

Technique 26 – Fig. 3 Stretch the lip gently when inserting the needle and advance it into the center of the vermillion in a concave arch.

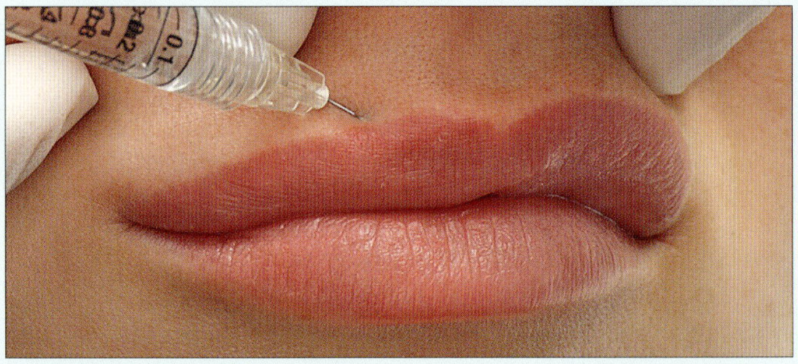

Technique 26 – Fig. 4 Deliver the material at one location as a bolus. The bigger the bolus, the more prominent the lip will become.

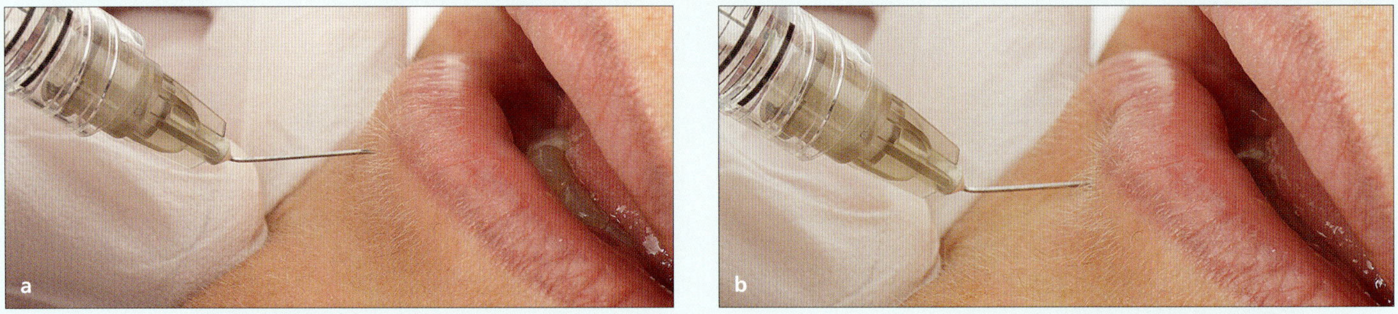

Technique 26 – Fig. 5 a+b Bend the tip of the needle slightly with the bevel facing up (a, use the open end of the safety cap for this, see video) so that it points directly at the target (b, note the angle of insertion). Introduce it into the skin very slowly, as this minimizes pain. While delivering the material, leave the skin unstretched in order to see where the material is going. Ensure uniform delivery of material by visual checks of the syringe plunger and of the treatment area.

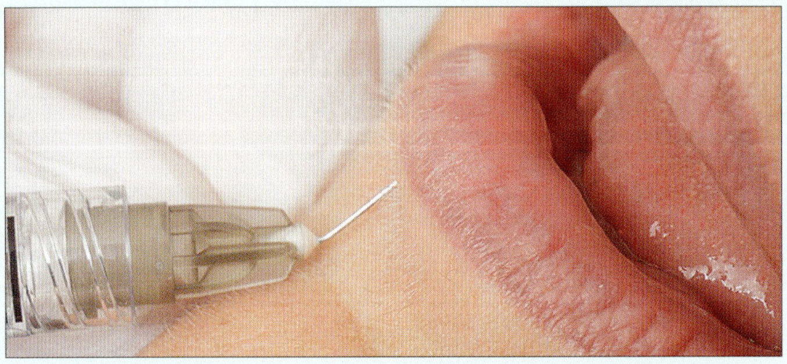

Technique 26 – Fig. 6 To reach the center of the lip muscle when approaching it from below, dip the syringe downward.

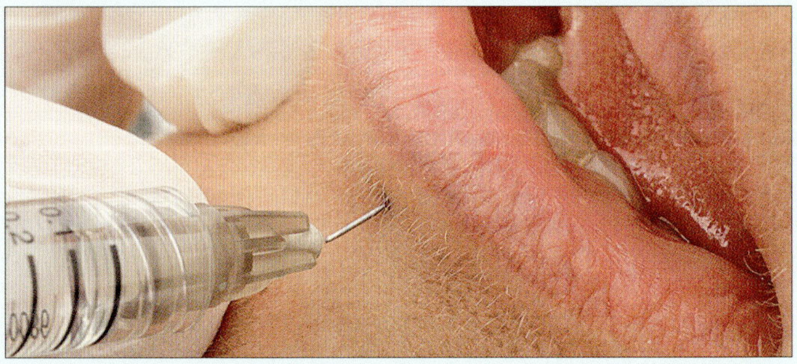

Technique 26 – Fig. 7 While the material is being delivered, the needle should be in the tissue without tearing it: the lip should be in a relaxed state with the mouth slightly open, allowing the therapist to control the augmentation of the lip by checking how much volume is being delivered. If the tip of the needle goes too far toward the mucosa of the oral cavity, the patient would be able to feel the bolus with the tongue. This can be prevented if the therapist uses a fingertip to check where the needle is located before delivering the material.

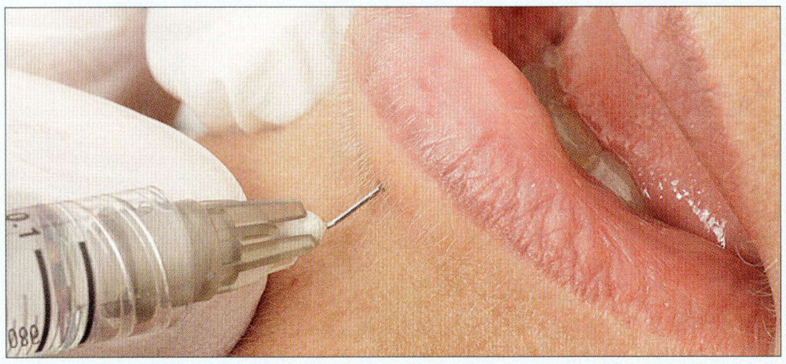

Technique 26 – Fig. 8 The material has reached the lip and has lifted it subtly. The tip of the needle should be located around 3–5 mm below the skin. If the needle tip gets too close to the surface of the skin, the injected material may protrude too much, producing an unnatural result.

Important Notes

- The immediate result of the treatment can be seen if the patient is asked to stretch the mouth into a wide smile directly after the injection. This is also used to check for a uniform injection.
- It is advisable to massage away any uneven spots.

Possible Side Effects

Slight reddening, rarely inflammation, hematomas, mild to more severe swellings

Undesirable Side Effects

Overcorrection with the resultant alteration of the shape of the lip or nodule formation, asymmetry due to non-uniform delivery of material, necrosis

Treatment Protocol at a Glance

- History, evaluation, and patient information
- Informed consent form
- Photo documentation: "before" images
- Analysis and marking of the areas to be treated
- Cleaning
- Thorough disinfection
- Local anesthesia if required (lidocaine cream), conduction anesthesia
- Injection technique: bolus technique, 4 boluses each into the upper and lower lip
- Layer: vermillion, intramuscular in the orbicularis oris muscle
- Material: class "S/M soft" product
- Volume: max. 0.1 ml per bolus, c. 0.5 ml in total
- Needle: 27–29G sharp needle, 20 mm
- Massage if required
- Cooling if required
- Heparin cream for hematomas, ibuprofen p.o., arnica
- Photo documentation: "after" images
- Advice on dos and don'ts after the procedure
- Follow-up appointment for a check-up after 8–14 days

9.4.13 TECHNIQUE 27

Extreme Volumization and Shaping – Multiple Injection Technique (Sharp Needle)

This technique not only produces very prominent lip augmentation but also enables the simple correction of deficits and areas of asymmetry with pinpoint accuracy. There is considerable latitude with regard to the type and volume of material selected as well as the number of lines injected. For this reason, the patient's wishes need to be elucidated definitively and with care. Since the material is not injected too close to the surface, the lip is given a very soft and harmonious shape.

Patient Selection

- Where there is a volume deficit or if the patient wants extreme lip augmentation
- A current beautification trend since 2018

Injection Scheme and Planning (→ Technique 27 – Figs. 1–5)

The technique is highly versatile. For extreme augmentation of the lips, the injection is given carefully and slowly with a sharp needle. The needle is inserted at the lip contour, with the bevel facing up, aiming forward into the vermillion toward the oral fissure. The material is delivered by anterograde injection into the center of the lip (into the orbicularis oris muscle) and by retrograde injection, tapering off toward the lip margin. There is a lot of scope for technical variants here. Lip shape can be influenced by how and where the material is placed.

Technique: linear technique

Direction of insertion: across the body of the muscle

Layer: vermillion, subcutaneous over the orbicularis oris muscle

Material: class "M soft" product

Volume: max. 1.0–2.0 ml in total

Needle: 27–29G sharp needle

Anesthesia: lidocaine cream, conduction anesthesia

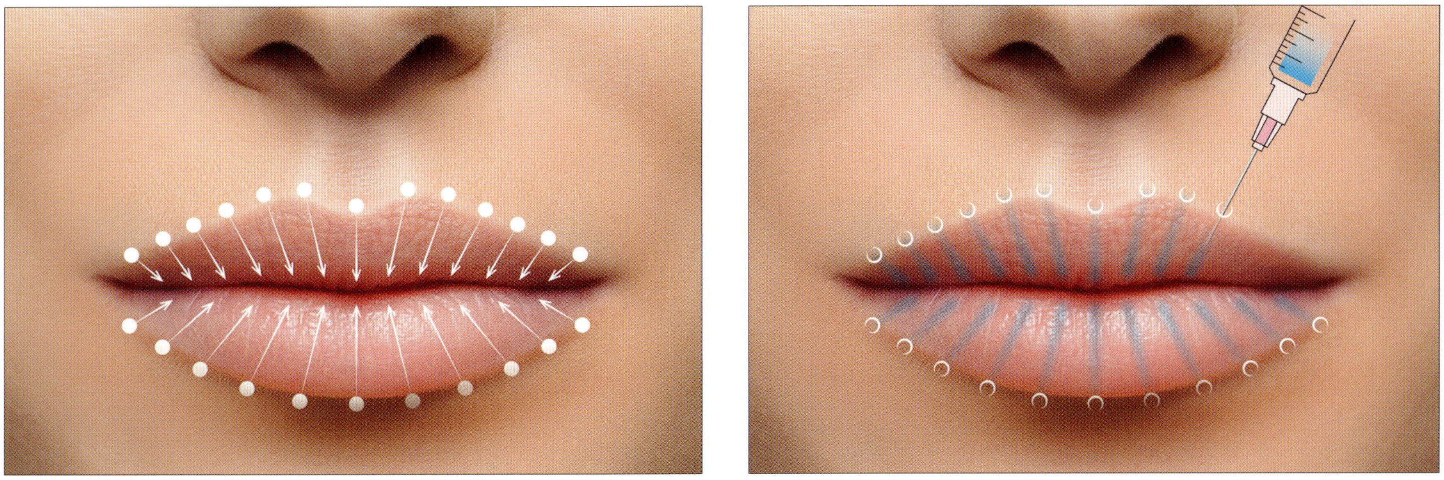

Technique 27 – Figs. 1, 2 Injection scheme and planning for extreme volumization and shaping – multiple injection technique (sharp needle).

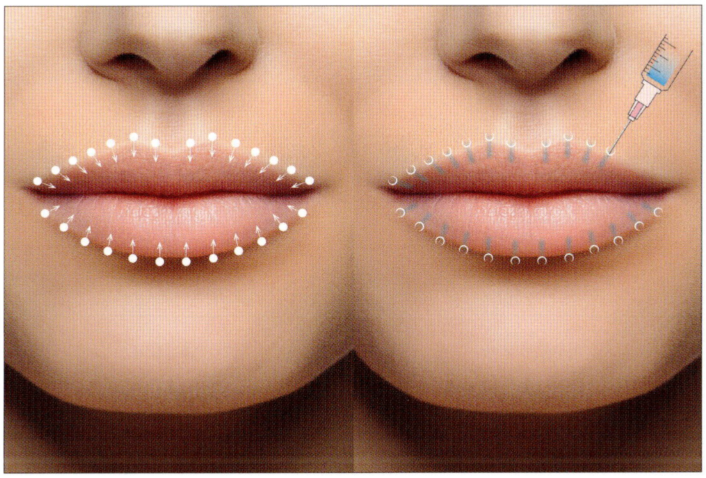

Technique 27 – Fig. 3 (Variant 1): If the needle entry points are placed closer together and the depth of insertion is reduced, the volume is placed closer to the lip margin, thus accentuating its curvature.

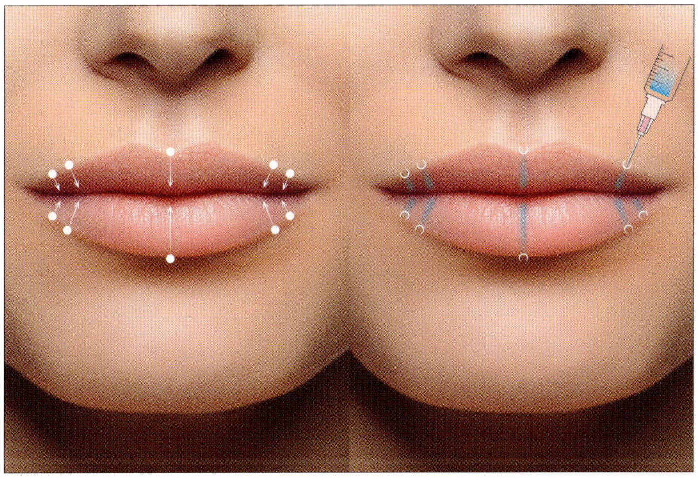

Technique 27 – Fig. 4 (Variant 2): By injecting more volume at the lateral ends and accentuating the tubercle at the center of the lip, one can highlight the "butterfly shape" of the upper lip, widen thin lips or correct the flattening of the upper lip near the mouth corners, pushing this area forward or augmenting it.

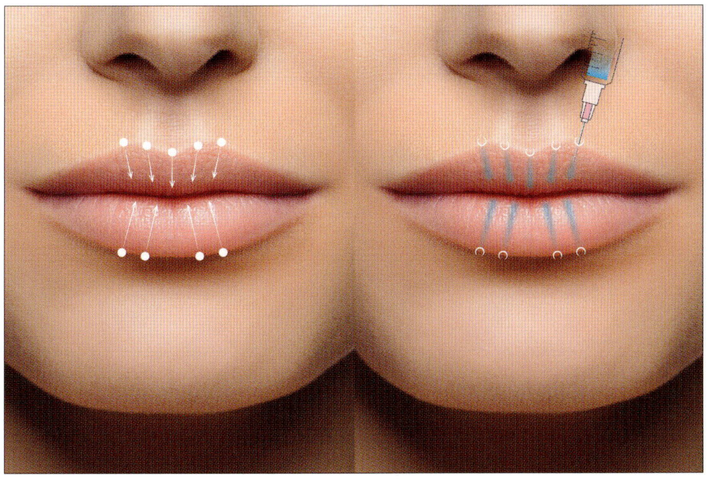

Technique 27 – Fig. 5 (Variant 3): Delivering material into the center of the lip causes targeted shaping and accentuation of the medial part of the lip if it is weakly defined or if it recedes.

Treatment Method (→ Technique 27 – Figs. 6, 7)

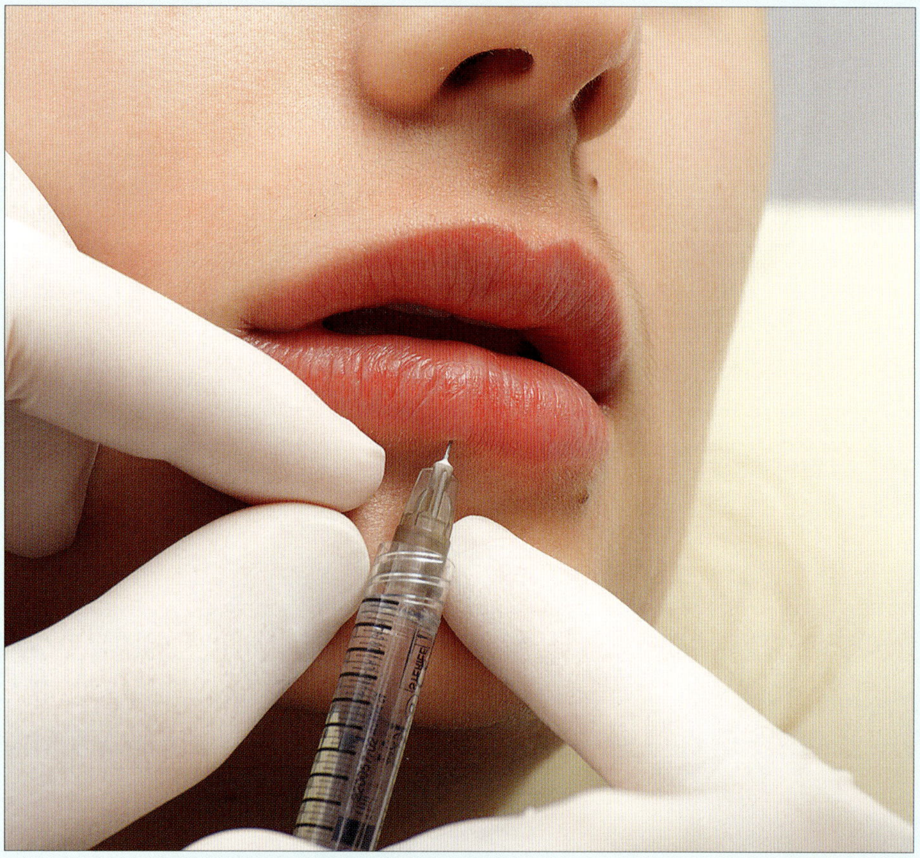

Technique 27 – Fig. 6 The lip needs to be very loose and relaxed, and the needle must not pull on the tissue; otherwise, it will not be possible to see how much material is being delivered. Volume delivery should be controlled by visual checks.

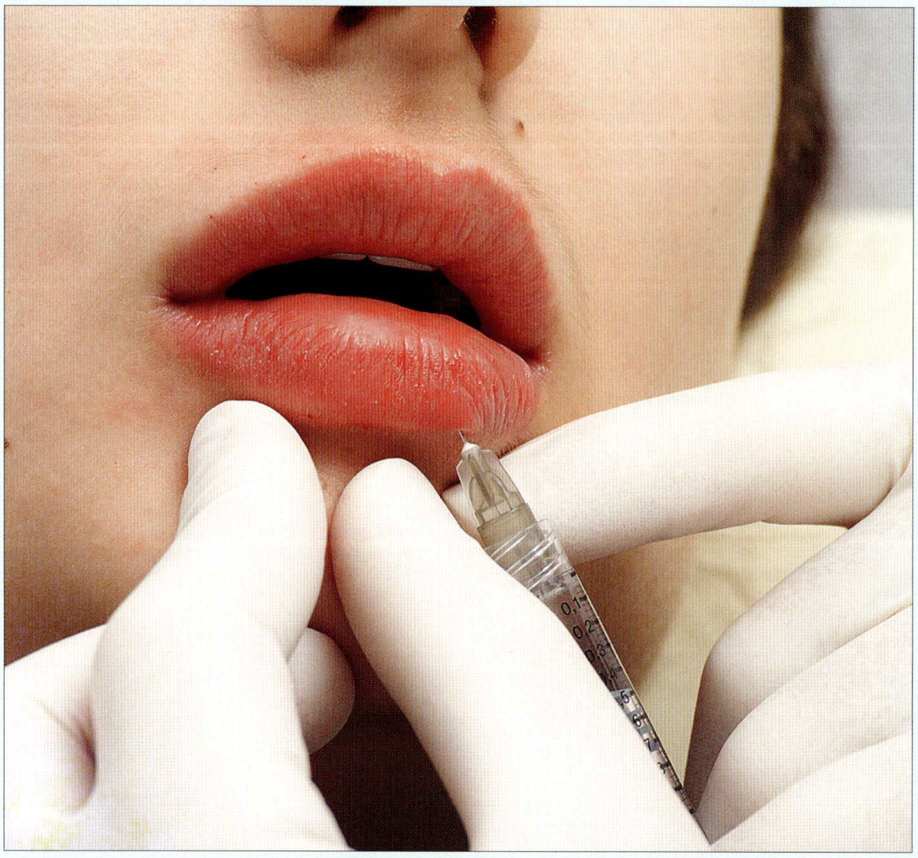

Technique 27 – Fig. 7 The therapist can check carefully with a fingertip whether the tip of the needle is in the desired location. The needle tip should not come too close to the mucous membrane of the oral cavity because a bolus may otherwise be formed, which the patient is likely to find irritating and which would call the treatment outcome into question.

Important Notes

- In the preparatory phase, it is necessary to define exactly how much material is to be delivered. The amount of material and its distribution in the lateral direction can influence the thickness and width of the mouth.
- This technique is highly traumatizing and associated with pain and swellings of the lip.
- A two-session approach is recommended to optimize the treatment result.

Possible Side Effects

Slight reddening, rarely inflammation, hematomas, mild to more severe swellings, pain for 2–4 days after the treatment

Undesirable Side Effects

Inflammation, overcorrection with resultant alteration of the shape of the lip or nodule formation, asymmetry due to non-uniform delivery of material, necrosis

Treatment Protocol at a Glance

- History, evaluation, and patient information
- Informed consent form
- Photo documentation: "before" images
- Analysis and marking of the areas to be treated
- Cleaning
- Thorough disinfection
- Local anesthesia if required (lidocaine cream), conduction anesthesia
- Injection technique: linear technique
- Layer: vermillion, subcutaneous over the orbicularis oris muscle
- Material: class "M soft" product
- Volume: max. 1.0–2.0 ml in total
- Needle: 27–29G sharp needle
- No massage
- Cooling if required
- Heparin cream for hematomas, ibuprofen p.o., arnica
- Photo documentation: "after" images
- Advice on dos and don'ts after the procedure
- Follow-up appointment for a check-up after 8–14 days

9.4.14 TECHNIQUE 28

Volumization and Shaping – "Lip Tenting Technique" according to Tom van Eijk (Sharp Needle)

The "lip tenting technique" can be used to produce a convex curvature of the upper lip (van Eijk 2014, 2017). The shape and volume of the lips are controlled by administering numerous small injections with a sharp needle to gently lift the lip roll, i.e. the paler, softer tissue directly above the vermillion (see Fig. 1.5, p. 5), optimizing the canine region of the lip arch without producing a "duck's bill" effect. The shape of the philtrum can be improved simply by treating the curvature of the lip and not injecting directly into the philtrum.

Patient Selection

- Where there is a volume deficit or if the patient wants gentle lip volume augmentation
- Correcting areas of asymmetry or to improve lip shape
- For small or narrow lips that recede at the side, with inward flattening in profile view

Injection Scheme and Planning (→ Technique 28 – Figs. 1, 2)

The "lip tenting technique" involves injecting with a sharp needle just outside the lip margin. The needle is inserted into the lip roll and guided toward the middle of the lip. When the needle is withdrawn, a small amount of HA is injected (less than 0.03 ml/injection), to add volume within the muscular part of the lip and to form columnar structures that accentuate the lip roll. The lip roll itself must not be filled so as to avoid thickening of the lip margin. It is important for the filler to be covered with sufficient lip tissue, i.e. it should not be injected too superficially in order to avoid any visible artefacts. Thanks to the multiple injections, the risk that large individual volumes of gel will lead to palpable or even visible clumps is minimal (Braun et al. 2010).

The first injection into the upper lip is given directly at the mouth corner, and the injections are then repeated every 2–3 mm in the medial direction along the upper lip, up to the philtrum. The first injection into the lower lip is placed 5–7 mm from the mouth corner, and further injections are administered at intervals of 2–3 mm until just short of the middle of the lower lip. Since the injections into the middle of the lip are diagonal, they intersect, producing a bigger volume and stabilizing the middle of the lower lip.

The technique causes bleeding and trauma. It is painful for the patient if no conduction anesthesia is administered as it involves numerous incisions with a sharp needle. It requires skill and experience because very small amounts of material need to be delivered very uniformly.

Technique: linear technique
Direction of insertion: diagonally across the body of the muscle
Layer: vermillion, intramuscular into the orbicularis oris muscle
Material: class "S/M viscous" product
Volume: c. 1.0–1.5 ml in total
Needle: 27–30G sharp needle
Anesthesia: conduction anesthesia with adrenaline

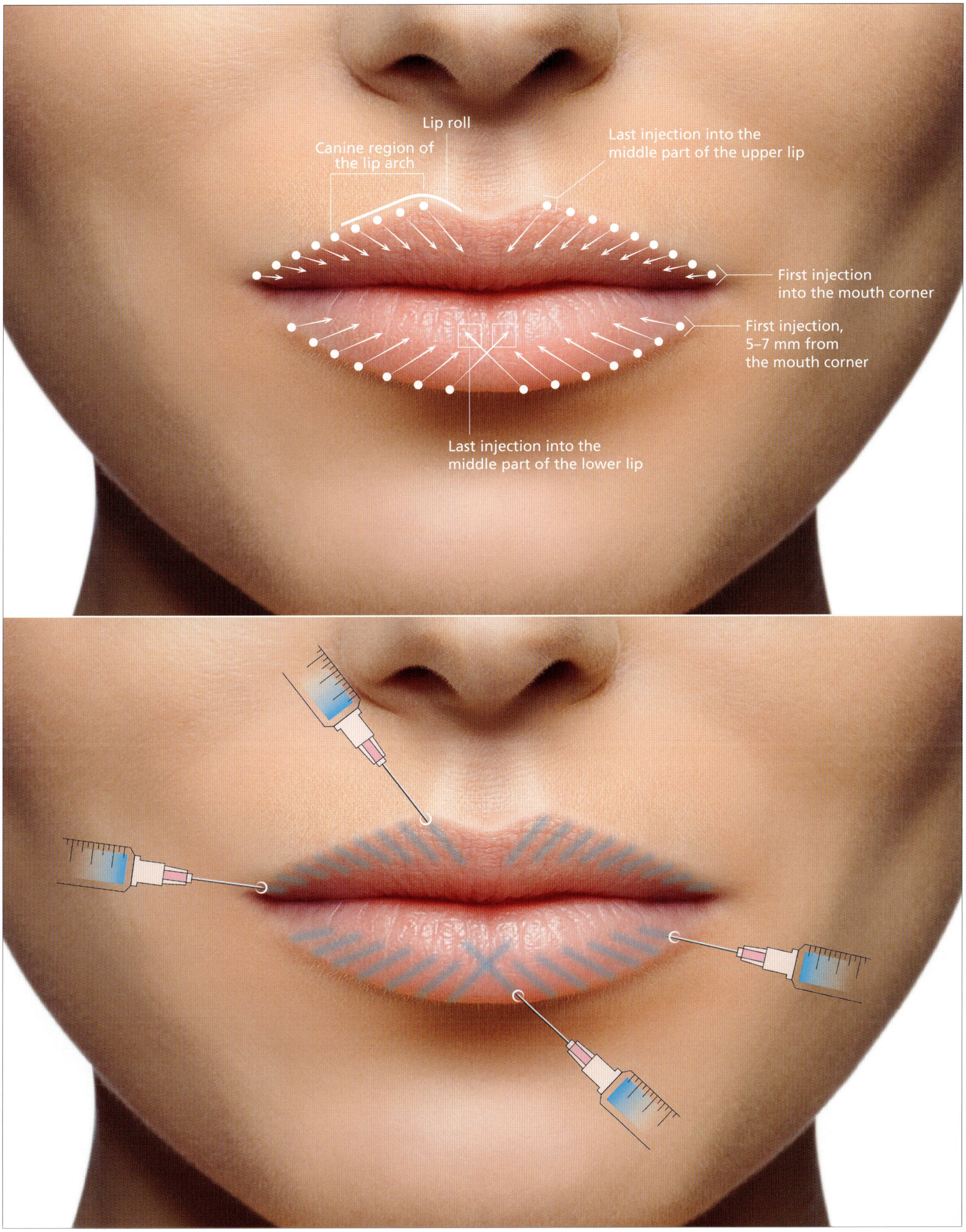

Technique 28 – Figs. 1, 2 Injection scheme and planning for volumization and shaping – "Lip Tenting Technique" according to Tom van Eijk (sharp needle).

Treatment Method (→ Technique 28 – Figs. 3–6)

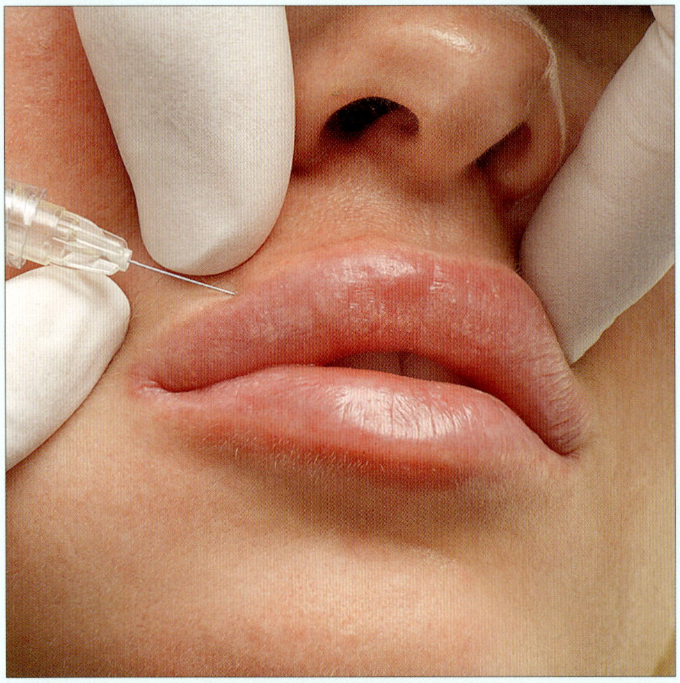

Technique 28 – Fig. 3 Stretch the lip gently between the thumb and forefinger. Insert the needle into the lip roll at the mouth corner. Advance it into the intramuscular layer of the lip tissue to about 5 mm, toward the center. Lift the tip of the needle slightly to see whether it is located at the correct depth. Deliver the material slowly by retrograde injection, applying uniform pressure.

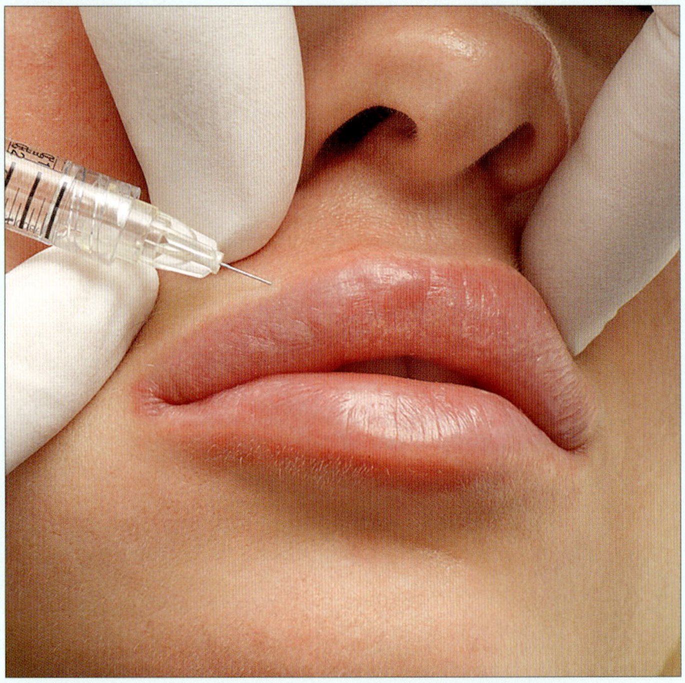

Technique 28 – Fig. 4 Starting from the mouth corner, administer additional injections at intervals of 2–3 mm up to the middle of the lip.

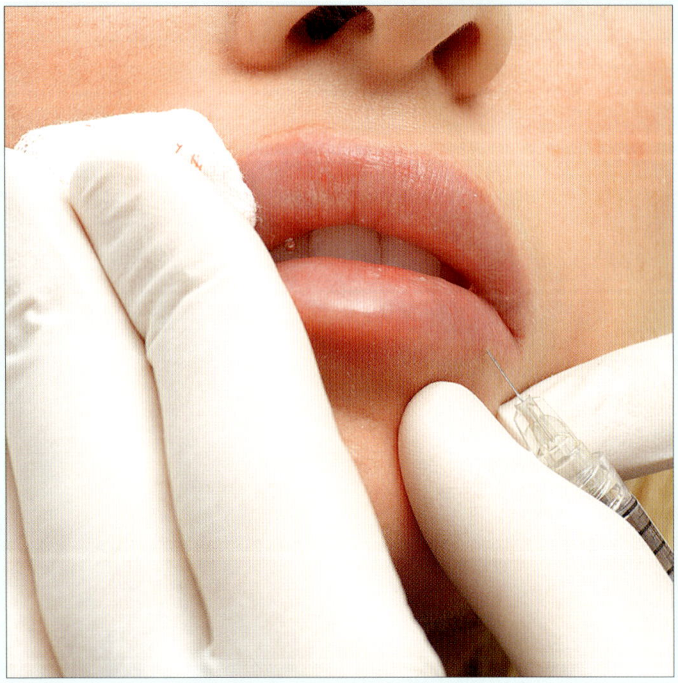

Technique 28 – Fig. 5 To achieve a natural result in the lower lip, it is advisable not to administer any injections about 5 mm from the corner of the mouth. Start with the part of the lip close to the mouth corner and inject in the medial direction.

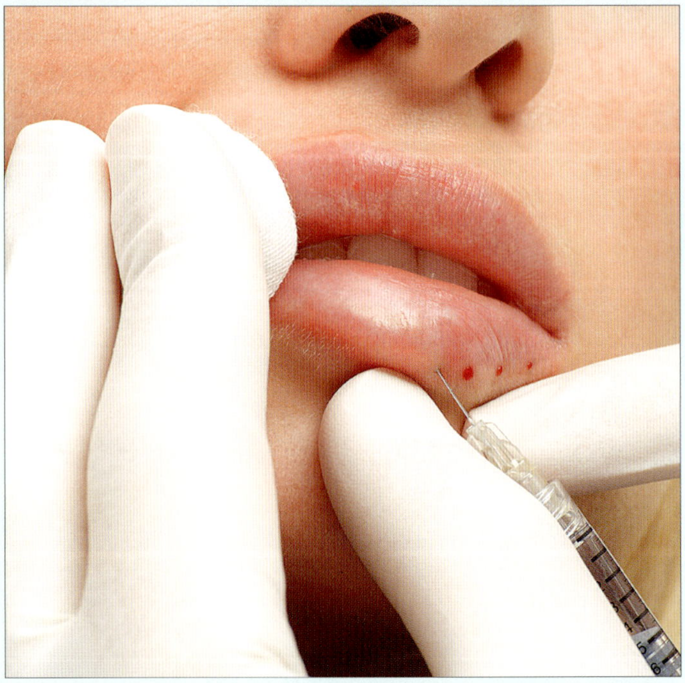

Technique 28 – Fig. 6 While doing so, evert and stretch the lip gently. The injection lines should intersect in the middle, so that the volume added here produces slight augmentation of the middle of the lower lip.

9

Important Notes

- If the lip is asymmetric, the needle can be inserted vertically at the site of the asymmetry. A tiny amount of material is then injected to remedy this.
- It is possible to restore the symmetry of the upper lip with the "lip tenting technique" by injecting a bit more filler vertically into the relevant upper lip quadrants.
- If the patient wants to have a more striking Cupid's bow, one injection should be given vertically from the lip roll at the Cupid's bow toward the dry/wet boundary, and the material delivered by retrograde injection.
- The technique is highly traumatizing and is associated with pain and swellings of the lips. It is therefore important for the patient not to have been treated with any blood-thinning drugs before the treatment.
- The therapist should change the needle frequently, as it become blunt very quickly and causes more pain when inserted.
- A two-session approach is recommended to optimize the treatment result.

Possible Side Effects

Commonly pain, reddening, more severe internal bleeding, hematomas, mild to more severe swellings, rarely inflammation

Undesirable Side Effects

Overcorrection with resultant alteration of the shape of the lip or nodule formation, asymmetry due to non-uniform delivery of material, necrosis

Treatment Protocol at a Glance

- History, evaluation, and patient information
- Informed consent form
- Photo documentation: "before" images
- Analysis and marking of the areas to be treated
- Cleaning
- Thorough disinfection
- Conduction anesthesia with adrenaline
- Injection technique: linear technique
- Layer: vermillion, intramuscular into the orbicularis oris muscle
- Material: class "S/M viscous" product
- Volume: ca. 1.0–1.5 ml in total
- Needle: 27–30G sharp needle
- No massage
- Cooling if required
- Heparin cream for hematomas, ibuprofen p.o., arnica
- Photo documentation: "after" images
- Advice on dos and don'ts after the procedure
- Follow-up appointment for a check-up after 8–14 days

9.5 Perioral Volume

Loss of volume from the fat compartments in the perioral region manifests in the form of shadows that appear at the apices of the lips during speaking, eating or whistling. In the early stage, these shadows are only apparent during any mimic activity. In the advanced stage, the loss of volume is evident without this activity and takes the form of deep lines, wrinkling, and drooping of the oral commissures and marionette lines, which is intensified by the sagging of the lax cheek tissue. The techniques in this section treat shadows and areas of unevenness caused by a lack of volume and mimic activity in the perioral region.

9.5.1 TECHNIQUE 29

Volumization – Labiomental Fold (Sharp Needle)

Treatment of the labiomental fold aims to fill the shadow between the lips and chin, visually elongating the chin so that the face appears more youthful. Two approaches are recommended for treating this area, namely the bolus and depot technique.

Patient Selection

- Where there is loss of volume or age-related or genetically determined shortening of the distance between lip and chin
- Where this distance has been shortened due to the strong contraction of the mentalis muscle, bone loss, malpositioned teeth or dental abrasion as a result of bruxism

Technique: bolus technique (1), depot technique (2)

Direction of insertion: directly from the front (1), horizontal (2)

Layer: supraperiosteal (1), subcutaneous (2)

Material: class "M/L viscous" product (1), class "M/L viscous" product for deep shadows, softer product for smaller, more superficial shadows (2)

Volume: max. 0.5 ml

Needle: 25G sharp needle

Anesthesia: lidocaine cream

Injection Scheme and Planning (→ Technique 29 – Figs. 1–4)

The **bolus technique** is suitable for large shadows or indentations. The material is placed into the deepest shadow between the lip and chin. It is often enough to place a large bolus into the center of this shadow. The needle is guided in directly from the front toward the center of the shadow, until the needle touches the periosteum. The needle is then withdrawn by 1–2 mm and the material delivered until the tissue is lifted and the shadow reduced.

If larger amounts of HA are given, these should be divided into several injections. For example, if the treatment area is so extensive that the result after delivering a bolus of c. 0.5 ml is barely visible, the additional material should be divided into 2–3 other, smaller boluses (see Figs. 1 and 2, below), since the HA can exhibit cohesive behavior and may become encapsulated in rare cases. Dividing the material into several smaller boluses greatly limits this risk.

The **depot technique** differs from the bolus technique in that several smaller boluses are placed over or beside each other in the shadow of the labiomental fold, thus forming a depot. This technique is the preferred option where the fold is very deep in order to prevent connective tissue encapsulation of the material if large amounts are placed at one location. The treatment area is marked, and the material is delivered until the tissue comes forward and the shadow is reduced. The syringe approaches from the side, and the needle is inserted horizontally, parallel to the lip. The material is injected subcutaneously and not placed onto the periosteum.

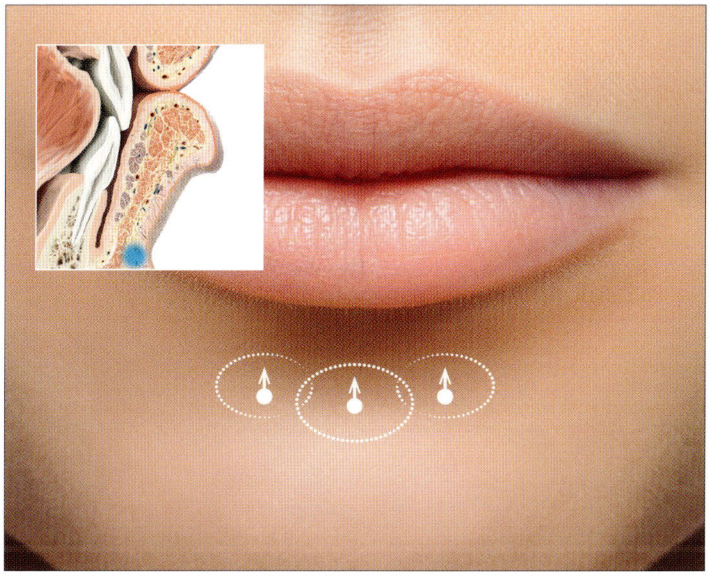

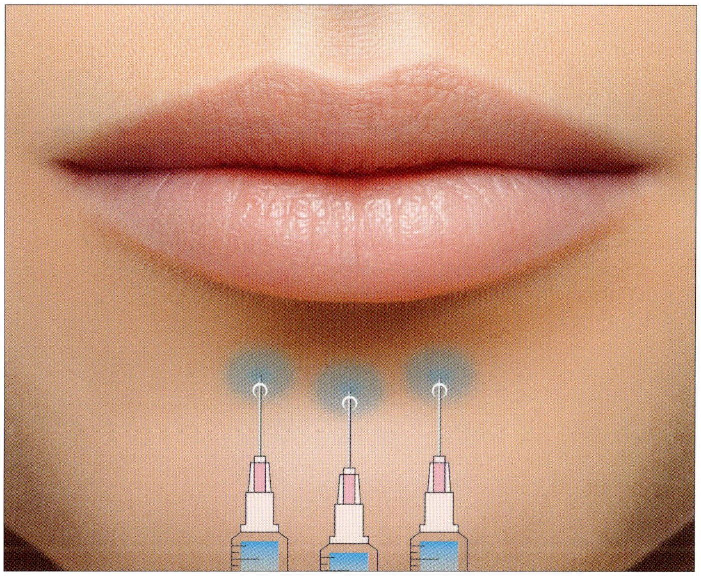

Technique 29 – Figs. 1, 2 Injection scheme and planning for **Variant 1: volumization of the labiomental fold using the bolus technique (sharp needle).**

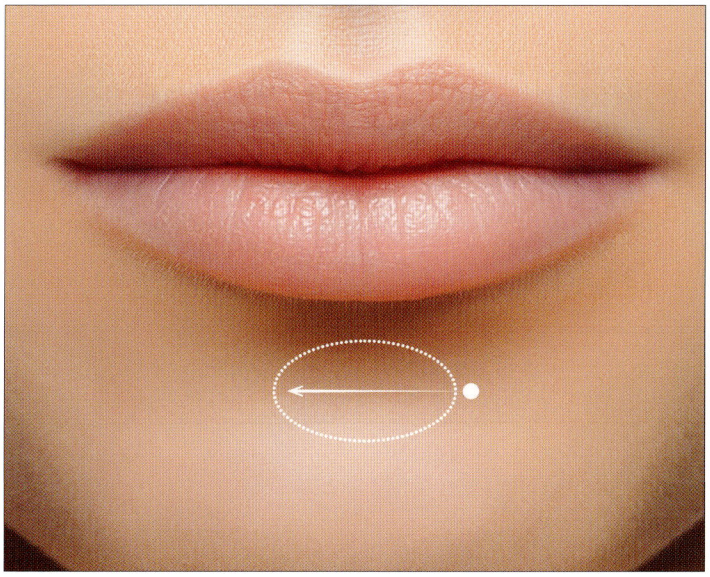

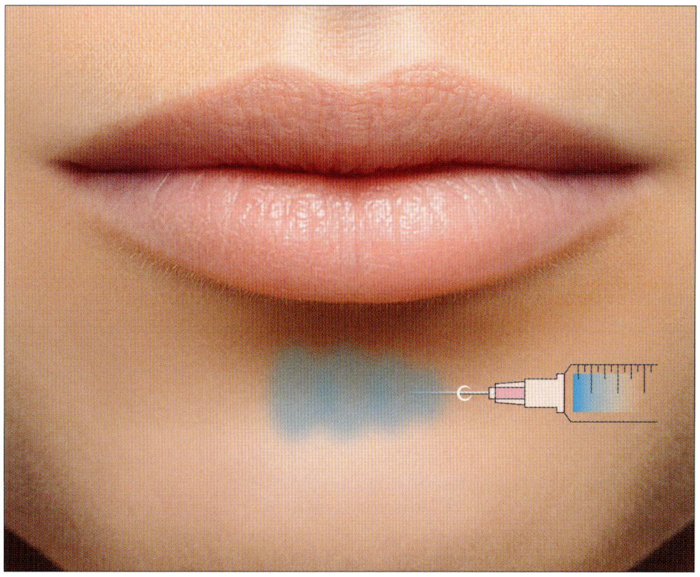

Technique 29 – Figs. 3, 4 Injection scheme and planning for **Variant 2: volumization of the labiomental fold using the depot technique (sharp needle).**

Treatment Method (→ Technique 29 – Figs. 5, 6)

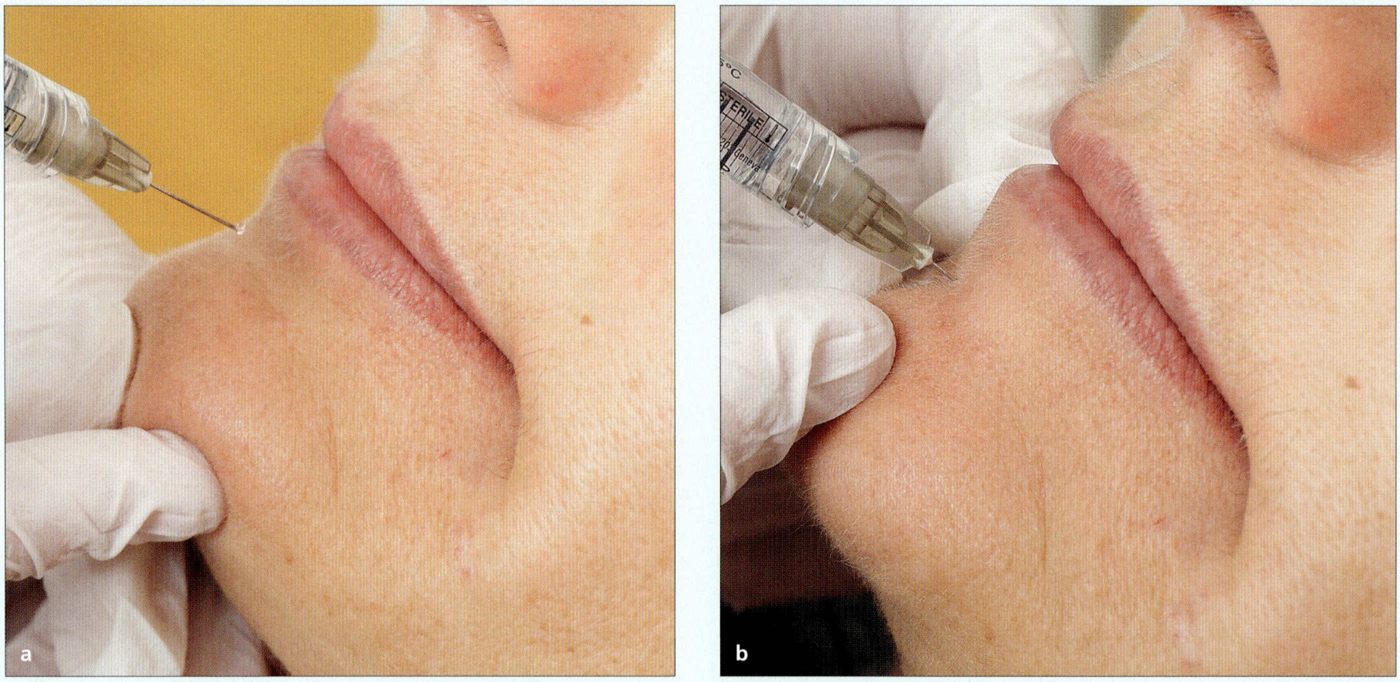

Technique 29 – Fig. 5 a+b (Variant 1, bolus technique): Using the little finger, support the injecting hand against the patient's chin (a). A steady hand is needed because the needle will touch the periosteum. The steadier the hand, the less pain the patient will experience. Once the needle has touched the periosteum, withdraw it by c. 1–2 mm and place 1–3 boluses of material, injecting vertically and directly from the front, onto the periosteum in the center of the shadow. The bone acts as a support. Placement of the material pushes the tissue forward so that the labiomental fold is already barely visible (b).

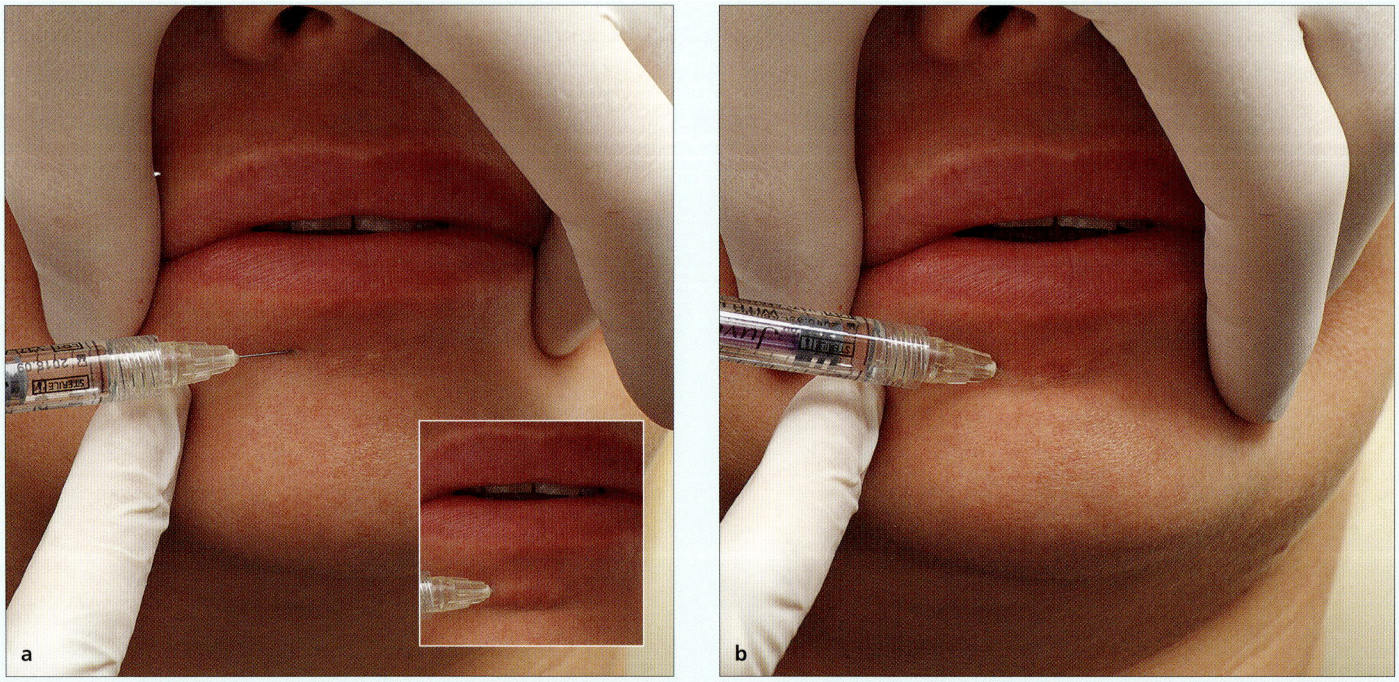

Technique 29 – Fig. 6 a+b (Variant 2, depot technique): Having marked the shadow area, stretch the skin slightly. Insert the needle into the outermost edge of this area (a). Advance the needle to the end of the marked area and deliver the material by retrograde injection. Check if the needle is in the correct skin layer by lifting it slightly (inset image). The skin bulges softly around the needle in the subcutaneous layer. Continue delivering the material until the shadow disappears and the tissue comes forward (b). Most of the volume should be placed in the deepest part of the shadow.

Important Notes

- It is advisable to aspirate first due to the risk of injecting the material into a blood vessel.
- Treatment of the labiomental fold is often performed in combination with the administration of botulinum toxin into the mentalis muscle. This relaxes the chin and counters the cobblestone effect, which encourages a deepening of the labiomental fold.
- The region can also be treated subcutaneously with a cannula.

Possible Side Effects

Slight reddening, rarely inflammation, rarely hematomas, mild swellings, slight pain up to 2 days after the treatment

Undesirable Side Effects

Inflammation, overcorrection or nodule formation, asymmetry due to non-uniform delivery of material, necrosis

Treatment Protocol at a Glance

- History, evaluation, and patient information
- Informed consent form
- Photo documentation: "before" images
- Analysis and marking of the areas to be treated
- Cleaning
- Thorough disinfection
- Local anesthesia if required (lidocaine cream)
- Injection technique: bolus technique (variant 1) or depot technique (variant 2)
- Layer: supraperiosteal and subcutaneous, respectively
- Material: class "M/L viscous" or "M/L soft" product
- Volume: max. 0.5 ml in total
- Needle: 25G sharp needle
- No massage
- Cooling if required
- Heparin cream for hematomas, ibuprofen p.o., arnica
- Photo documentation: "after" images
- Advice on dos and don's after the procedure
- Follow-up appointment for a check-up after 8–14 days

9.5.2 TECHNIQUE 30

Augmentation – Chin Region (Sharp Needle)

Augmentation of the chin can have a harmonizing effect on the overall appearance of the oral region.

Patient Selection

- For a weak or receding chin

Injection Scheme and Planning (→ Technique 30 – Figs. 1, 2)

Following an accurate analysis from the front and from the side (see Chap. 1.6, p. 27 ff.), the locations where the HA boluses will be placed are marked. The injections are given vertically from the front with a sharp needle. The material is delivered slowly until the tissue is pushed forward and the deficit is corrected. A material with a lower degree of crosslinking should be used, and not too much should be placed at a single site as it may, at worst, become encapsulated with connective tissue. For this reason, the recommended procedure here is also to divide larger volumes into several boluses or treatment sessions if necessary.

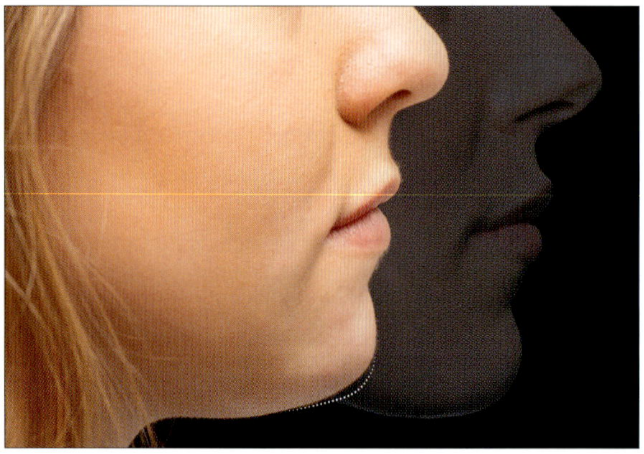

To create harmony in the oral region, the aim in this case is to augment the slightly receding chin.

Technique: bolus technique
Direction of insertion: centrally into the middle of the chin
Layer: intramuscular, supraperiosteal
Material: class "M/L viscous" product
Volume: highly dependent on the indication and should be calculated individually, generally 0.1 – < 0.2 ml per bolus
Needle: 25G sharp needle
Anesthesia: lidocaine cream

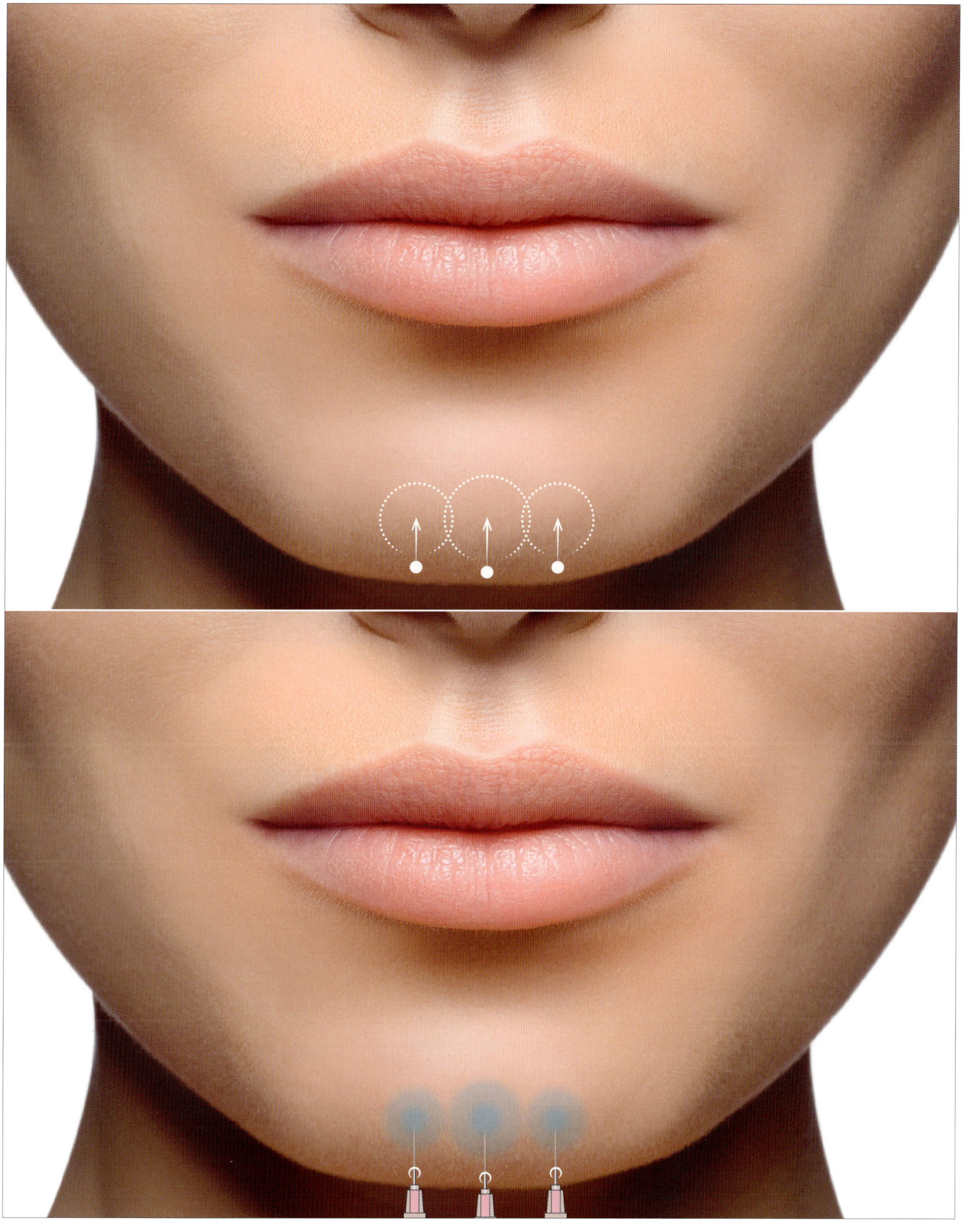

Technique 30 – Figs. 1, 2 Injection scheme and planning for augmentation – chin region (sharp needle).

Treatment Method (→ Technique 30 – Fig. 3)

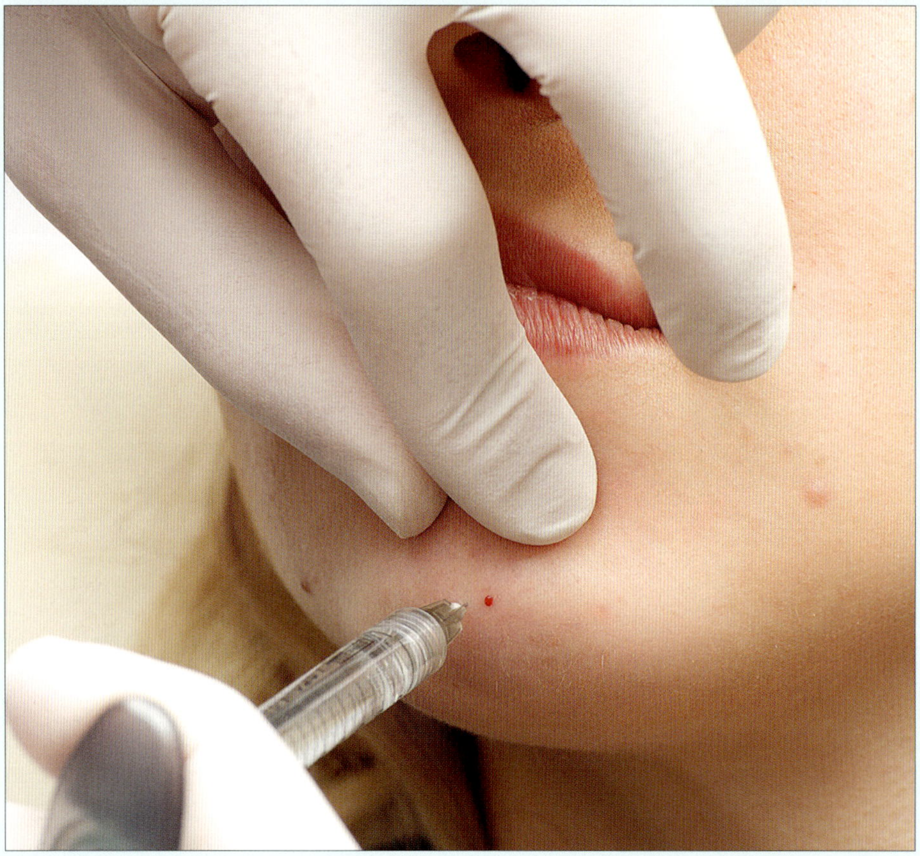

Technique 30 – Fig. 3 Insert the needle directly into the muscle, compressing the tissue to aid insertion. The periosteum acts as a support. Check that the needle tip is located in the target region. It is important to view the chin from the side after administering each bolus, to identify any spots where there is still a volume deficit; this is not always possible if viewing from the front alone.

Important Notes

- It is advisable to aspirate to prevent intravascular injection.
- Contact with the bone is very much to be desired, to avoid injecting the material into the exit point of the mental nerve.

Possible Side Effects

Slight reddening, rarely inflammation, rarely hematomas, mild swelling

Undesirable Side Effects

Inflammation, delivery of excessive material with resultant alteration of the chin or nodule formation, necrosis

Treatment Protocol at a Glance

- History, evaluation, and patient information
- Informed consent form
- Photo documentation: "before" images
- Analysis and marking of the areas to be treated
- Cleaning
- Thorough disinfection
- Local anesthesia if required (lidocaine cream)
- Injection technique: bolus technique
- Layer: intramuscular, supraperiosteal
- Material: class "M/L viscous" product
- Volume: highly dependent on the indication and should be calculated individually, generally 0.1 – < 0.2 ml per bolus
- Needle: 25G sharp needle
- No massage
- Cooling if required
- Heparin cream for hematomas, ibuprofen p.o., arnica
- Photo documentation: "after" images
- Advice on dos and don'ts after the procedure
- Follow-up appointment for a check-up after 8–14 days

9.5.3 TECHNIQUE 31
Volumization – Vertical Injection Technique (Sharp Needle)

The aim of this injection technique is to correct wrinkles, skin indentations, and shadows that are produced by muscle contractions when eating or pursing the mouth (see the image below).

Patient Selection

- In age-related loss of volume from the perioral fat compartments or a genetically determined volume deficit

Injection Scheme and Planning (→ Technique 31 – Figs. 1, 2)

The injection is given with the mouth and chin relaxed using a sharp needle inserted directly into the center of the indentation that has developed in the muscle. The material is delivered until the tissue lifts and the skin retraction disappears. The volume of material given should correlate with the size of the skin retraction. However, care should be taken to divide the material into several smaller boluses as there is a risk of connective tissue encapsulation if too much material is delivered. Once the material is injected, the movement of the muscle is blocked slightly and the area under the visible indentation is filled. The amount of material administered can vary greatly and depends on the depth of the skin retraction.

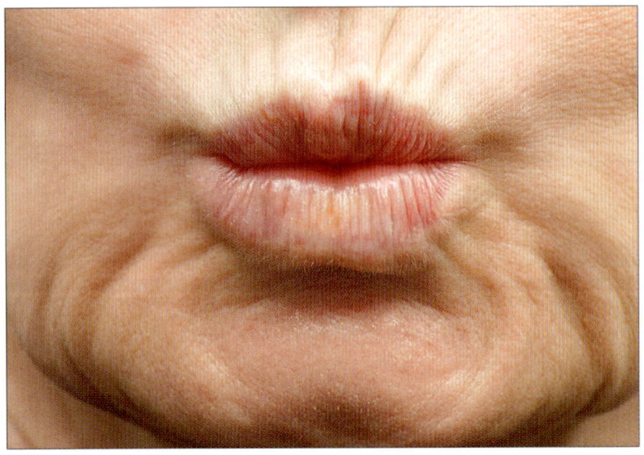

The lines are rarely visible when the mouth is in a relaxed state. Pursing the mouth or pulling up the skin immediately reveals the skin indentations.

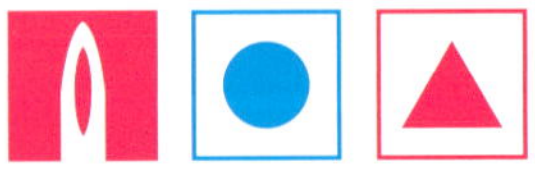

Technique: bolus technique
Direction of insertion: into the body of the muscle
Layer: intramuscular
Material: class "M/L soft" product for small indentations, "M/L viscous" for deeper indentations
Volume: dependent on the depth of the skin retraction: 0.5–1.0 ml
Needle: 25G sharp needle
Anesthesia: lidocaine cream

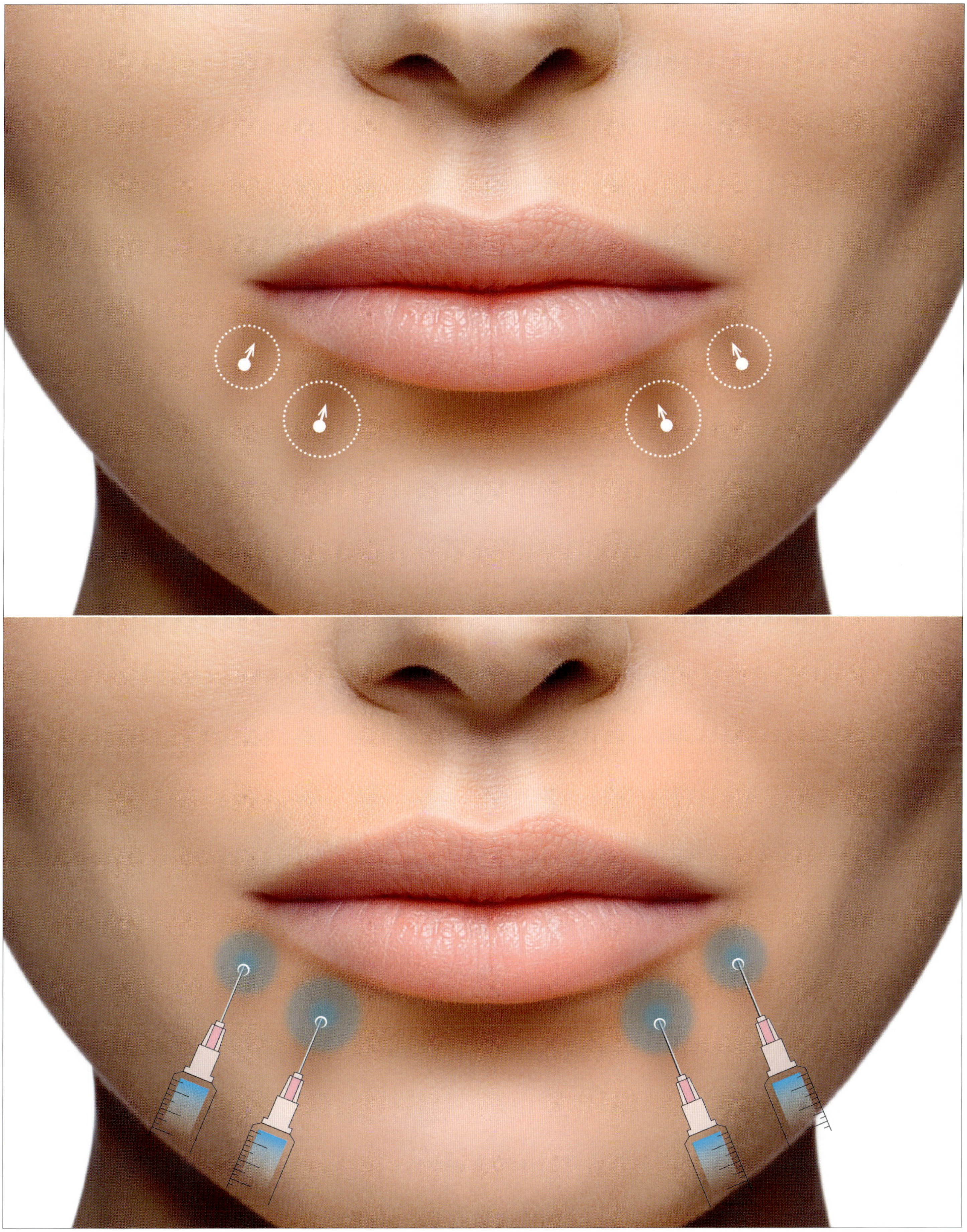

Technique 31 – Figs. 1, 2 Injection scheme and planning for volumization – vertical injection technique (sharp needle).

Treatment Method (→ Technique 31 – Figs. 3, 4)

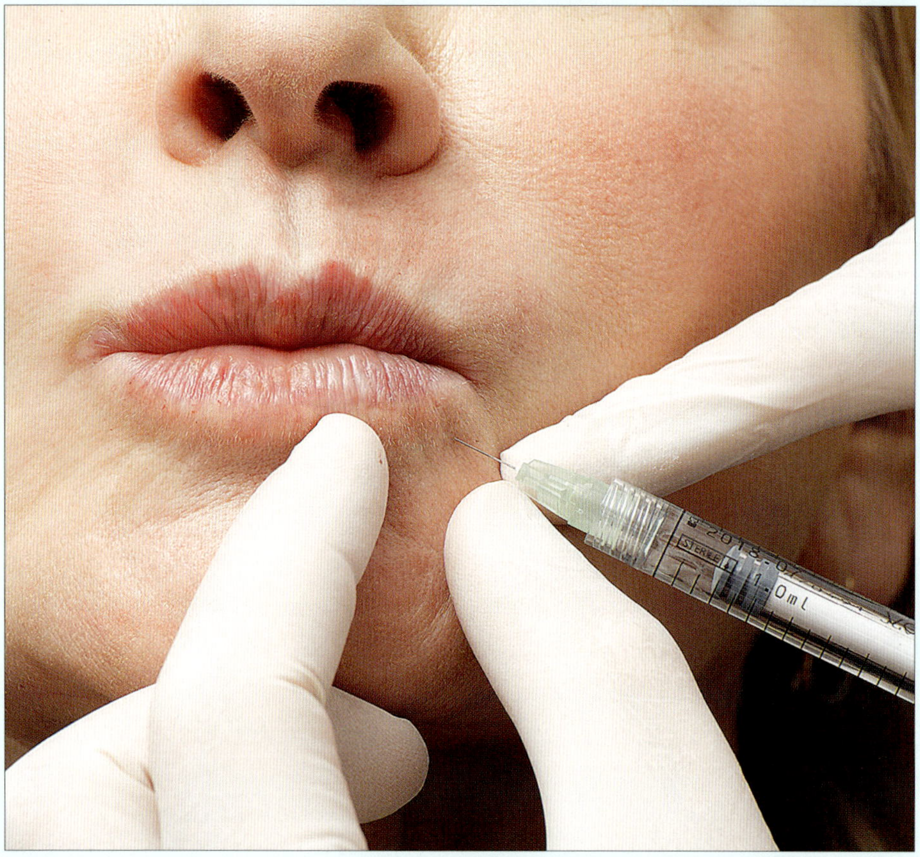

Technique 31 – Fig. 3 The procedure is not complicated. After aspirating to prevent intravascular injection, inject very slowly, directly into the center of the indentation; the mouth should be relaxed. The other side (see image) has been injected already, showing that the injected area has been lifted considerably.

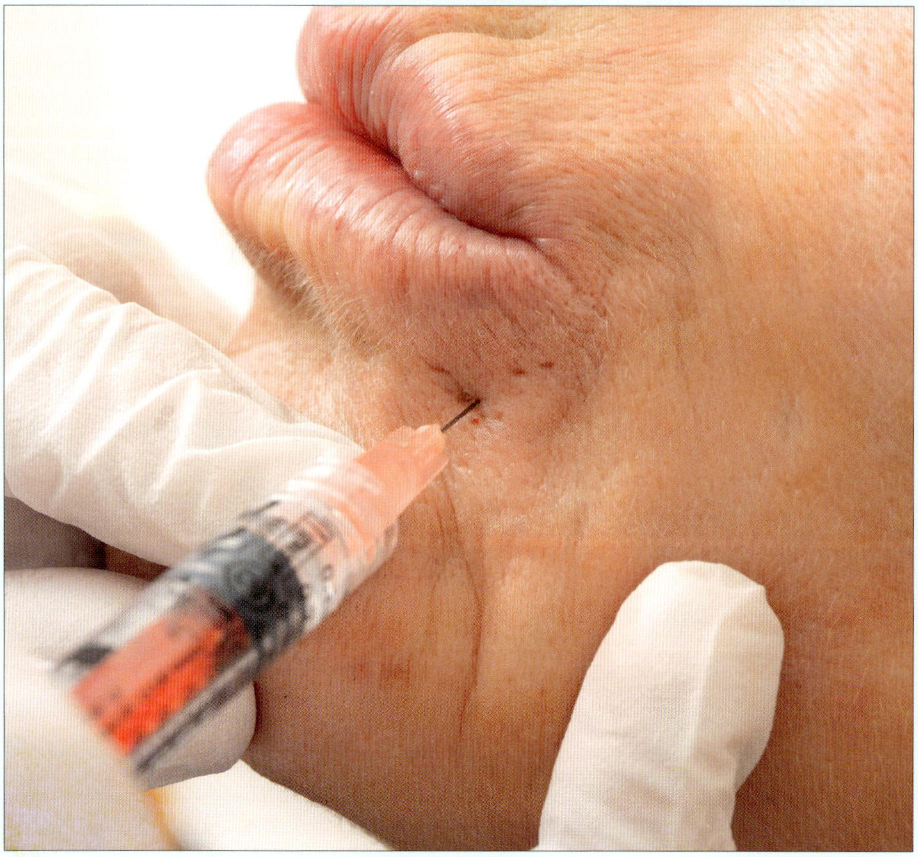

Technique 31 – Fig. 4 Insert the needle to a depth of 3 mm into the shadow while the patient keeps the mouth pursed. Deliver the material until the shadow disappears. If the shadows are as deep as shown here, up to 0.2 ml of material may be required.

Important Notes

- Prior aspiration is recommended due to the risk of injecting the material into a blood vessel.
- The material should be divided into several small boluses due to the risk of connective tissue encapsulation if too much material is delivered.

Possible Side Effects

Slight reddening, rarely inflammation, rarely hematomas, mild swellings

Undesirable Side Effects

Inflammation, overcorrection with resultant nodule formation, asymmetry due to non-uniform delivery of material

Treatment Protocol at a Glance

- History, evaluation, and patient information
- Informed consent form
- Photo documentation: "before" images
- Analysis and marking of the areas to be treated
- Cleaning
- Thorough disinfection
- Local anesthesia if required (lidocaine cream)
- Injection technique: bolus technique
- Layer: intramuscular
- Material: class "M/L soft" product for small indentations, "M/L viscous" for deeper indentations
- Volume: dependent on the depth of the skin retraction: 0.5–1.0 ml
- Needle: 25G sharp needle
- No massage
- Cooling if required
- Heparin cream for hematomas, ibuprofen p.o., arnica
- Photo documentation: "after" images
- Advice on dos and don'ts after the procedure
- Follow-up appointment for a check-up after 8–14 days

9.5.4 TECHNIQUE 32

Volumization – Fine Marionette Lines I (Sharp Needle)

The aim of this technique (and of Technique 33 that follows it) is to achieve subtle, symmetrical filling of incipient marionette lines and to reinforce the mouth corners. Reinforcing the mouth corners and reducing the lines that form beside them gives the mouth a rather more youthful and friendly appearance.

Patient Selection

- For marionette lines and mouth corner wrinkles, flattening and/or slight sagging of the mouth corners

9

Injection Scheme and Planning (→ Technique 32 – Figs. 1, 2)

The combined injection of four lines of material mitigates the marionette lines and stabilizes the mouth corners. Each corner is stabilized with two lines of material 1-cm long, injected along the mouth corner contours. Sagging of the mouth corner is prevented with two lines of material injected from below to provide support.

The first of these lines of material runs along the upper lip contour close to the mouth corner. The second line runs along the lower lip contour, again close to the mouth corner. The third line (2-cm long) runs below the mouth corner and perpendicularly to the lip margin. The fourth line (2-cm long) runs at a slightly acute angle toward the lip margin, close to the third line of material.

Technique: linear technique
Direction of insertion: along and across the lip contours at the mouth corners
Layer: subcutaneous
Material: class "M viscous" product
Volume: 0.05 ml per line, c. 0.4 ml in total
Needle: 27G sharp needle
Anesthesia: lidocaine cream

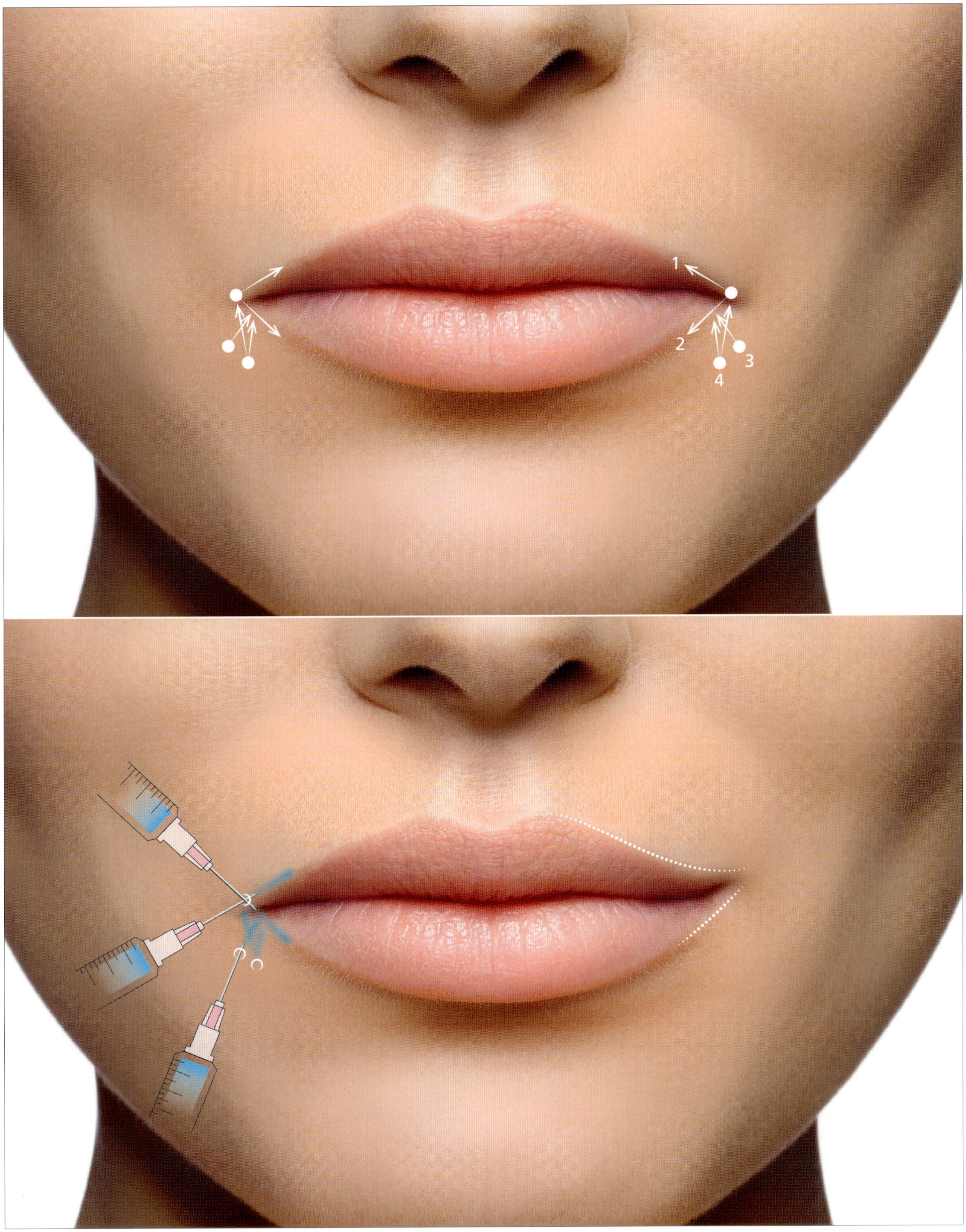

Technique 32 – Figs. 1, 2 Injection scheme and planning for the volumization of fine marionette lines using the linear technique (sharp needle).

Treatment Method (→ Technique 32 – Figs. 3–7)

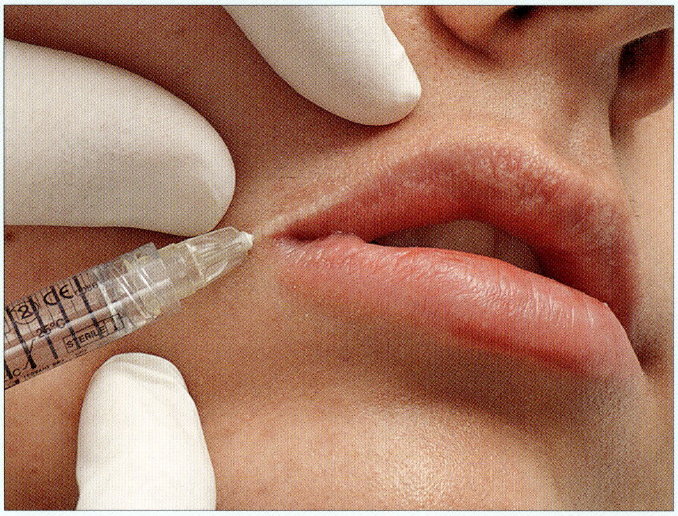

Technique 32 – Fig. 3 To reinforce the lip contour, start in the upper lip at the mouth corner.

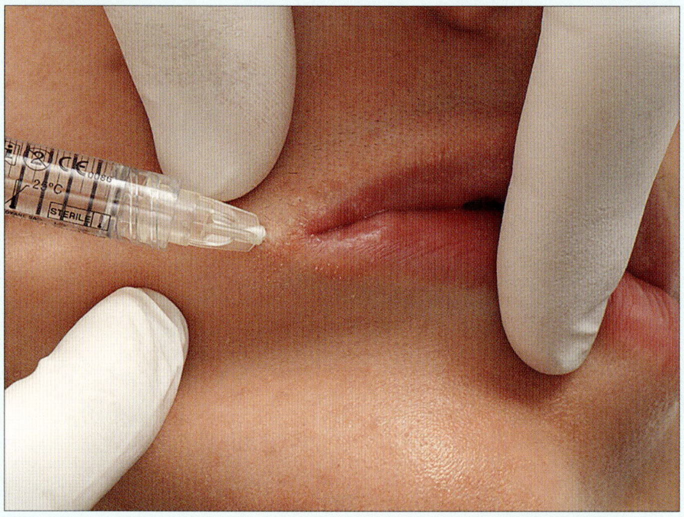

Technique 32 – Fig. 4 Repeat the procedure at the mouth corner in the lower lip.

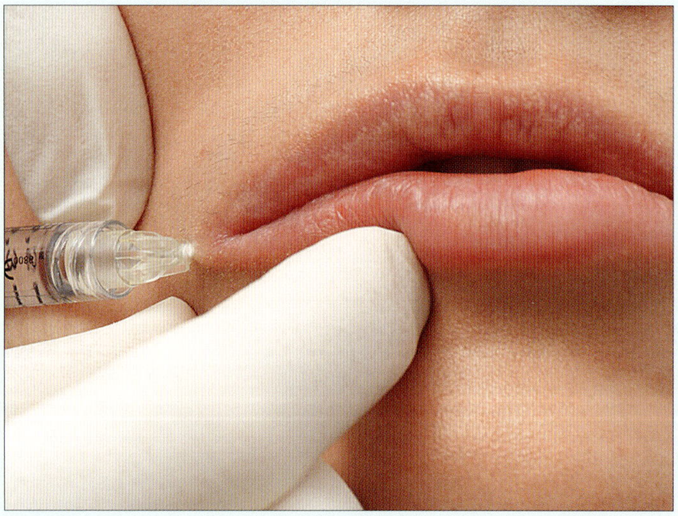

Technique 32 – Fig. 5 The upper and lower lip can also be injected from one entry point at the mouth corner, using the linear technique.

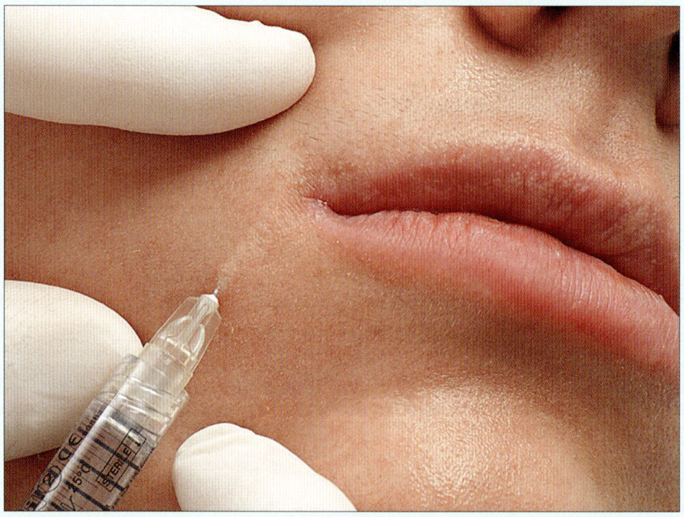

Technique 32 – Fig. 6 The mouth corner can be reinforced by using the **fanning technique**, starting from below the mouth. Inject 2–3 lines of material from the lateral side of the mouth corner, going in the medial direction.

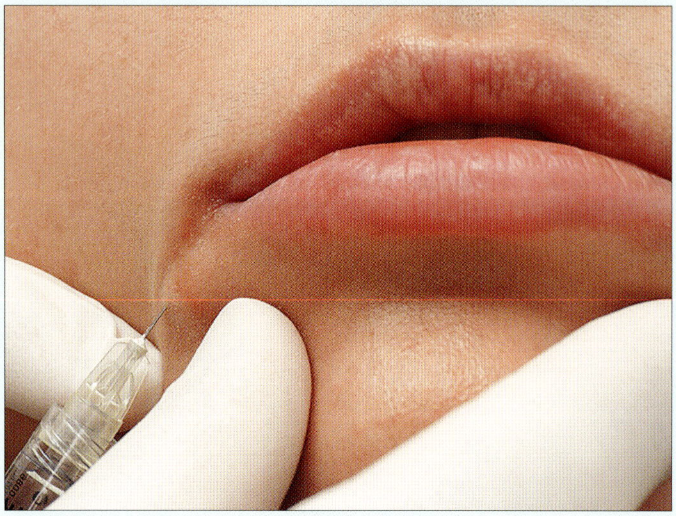

Technique 32 – Fig. 7 Should the delivered material push through the skin, producing an irregular skin surface, the area may be held flat with the thumb to cause compression.

Important Notes

- Prior aspiration is recommended due to the risk of injecting the material into a blood vessel.
- The mouth corners should not show any cracks or inflammation before the treatment as this could lead to complications that take a long time to heal.
- In general, the mouth corner treatment needs to be repeated once or twice, depending on the severity of the wrinkling or sagging. Combining the treatment with a build-up of the marionette lines is often a good option.

Possible Side Effects

Slight reddening, rarely inflammation, rarely hematomas, rarely mild swellings

Undesirable Side Effects

Inflammation, overcorrection with resultant alteration of the shape of the lip or nodule formation, asymmetry due to non-uniform delivery of material, necrosis

Treatment Protocol at a Glance

- History, evaluation, and patient information
- Informed consent form
- Photo documentation: "before" images
- Analysis and marking of the areas to be treated
- Cleaning
- Thorough disinfection
- Local anesthesia if required (lidocaine cream), conduction anesthesia
- Injection technique: linear technique
- Layer: subcutaneous
- Material: class "M viscous" product
- Volume: 0.05 ml per line, c. 0.4 ml in total
- Needle: 27G sharp needle
- No massage
- Cooling if required
- Heparin cream for hematomas, ibuprofen p.o., arnica
- Photo documentation: "after" images
- Advice on dos and don'ts after the procedure
- Follow-up appointment for a check-up after 8–14 days

9.5.5 Technique 33

Volumization – Fine Marionette Lines II (Sharp Needle)

This technique will also produce subtle, symmetrical filling of incipient marionette lines and reinforcement of the mouth corners to give the mouth a more youthful and friendly aspect.

Patient Selection

- For marionette lines and mouth corner wrinkles, flattening and slight sagging of the mouth corners

Injection Scheme and Planning (→ Technique 33 – Figs. 1, 2)

An alternative to Technique 32 in patients with incipient marionette lines is to inject the material directly into the center of the shadow or skin indentation using the bolus technique. The treatment area is marked. Injecting the bolus under compression is recommended to ensure accurate application and to avoid overcorrection. To do this, the area being treated is grasped between the thumb and forefinger, and a bolus of 0.05–0.1 ml is delivered slowly into the center. The pressure applied in this way compresses the surrounding blood vessels, limiting the risk of necrosis and preventing the material from escaping into the mouth.

Technique: bolus technique
Direction of insertion: from the front going diagonally upward
Layer: subcutaneous, intramuscular (depending on the thickness of the tissue)
Material: class "M viscous" product
Volume: 0.05–0.1 ml per bolus, c. 0.2 ml in total
Needle: 25–27G sharp needle
Anesthesia: lidocaine cream

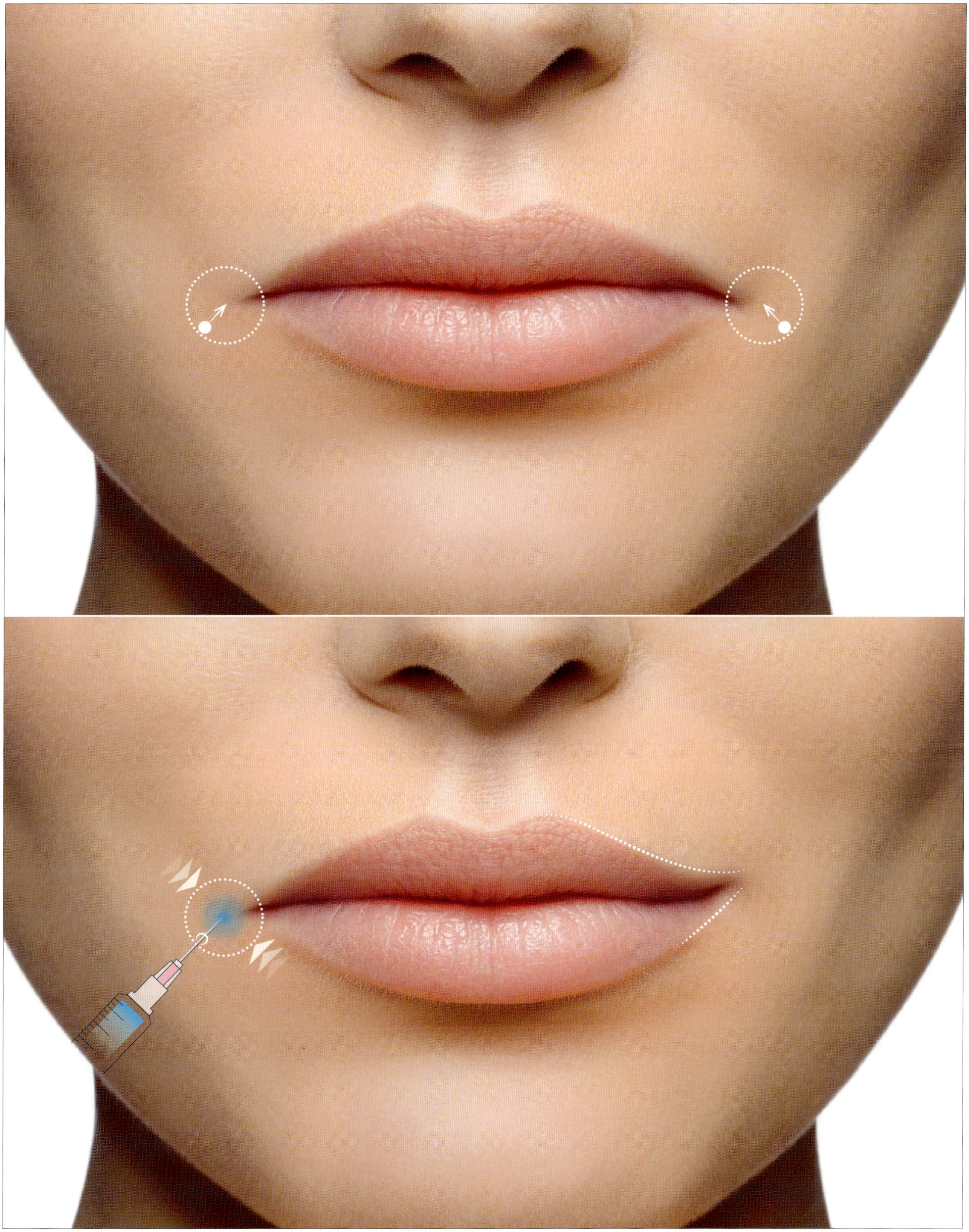

Technique 33 – Figs. 1, 2 Injection scheme and planning for the volumization of fine marionette lines using the bolus technique (sharp needle).

Treatment Method (→ Technique 33 – Figs. 3, 4)

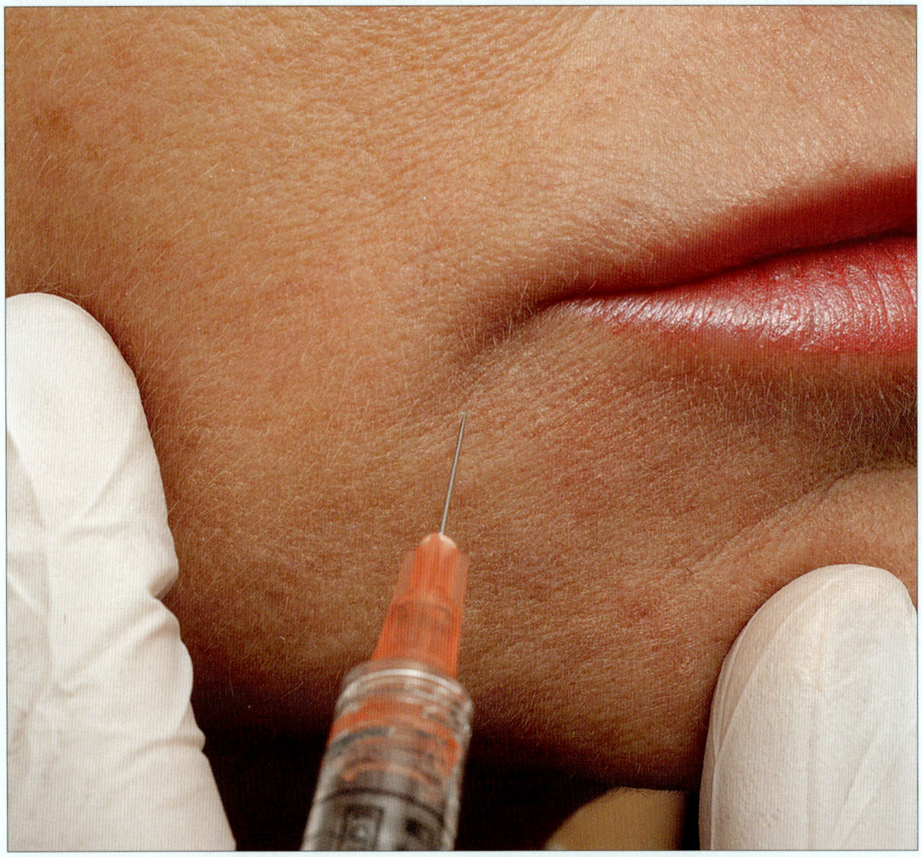

Technique 33 – Fig. 3 Deliver the bolus directly into the center of the shadow. Keep injecting the material until the tissue lifts and the shadow disappears.

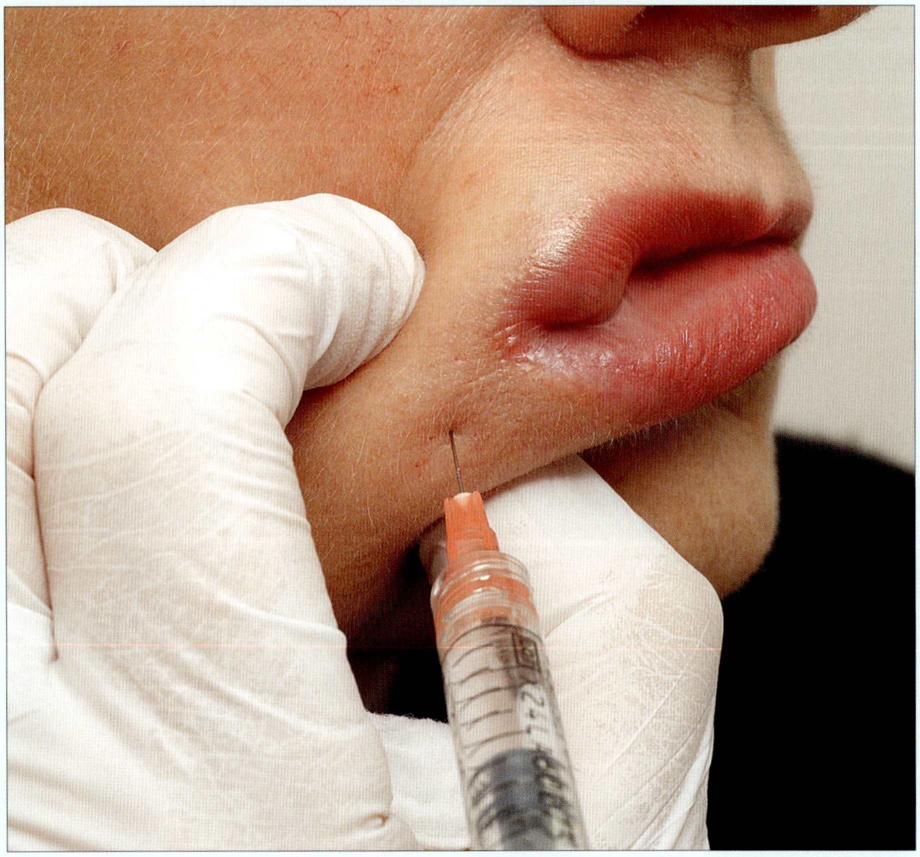

Technique 33 – Fig. 4 As an alternative, grasp the tissue between the thumb and forefinger so that it bulges outward. The pressure exerted with this hold forces the material into the target area. This procedure is recommended where there is septal damage in the tissue, which makes it more difficult to place the material at a specific location. Plunge the needle into the tissue to a depth of 1–3 mm and deliver the material slowly.

Important Notes

- Prior aspiration is recommended due to the risk of injecting the material into a blood vessel.
- The mouth corners should not show any cracks or inflammation before the treatment as this could lead to complications that take a long time to heal.
- In general, the mouth corner treatment needs to be repeated once or twice, depending on the severity of the wrinkling or sagging. Combining the treatment with filling of the marionette lines is often a good option.
- HA fillers with different degrees of crosslinking can be superimposed to improve the result even further.

Possible Side Effects

Slight reddening, rarely inflammation, rarely hematomas, rarely mild swellings

Undesirable Side Effects

Inflammation, overcorrection with resultant alteration of the shape of the lip or nodule formation, asymmetry due to non-uniform delivery of material, necrosis

Treatment Protocol at a Glance

- History, evaluation, and patient information
- Informed consent form
- Photo documentation: "before" images
- Analysis and marking of the areas to be treated
- Cleaning
- Thorough disinfection
- Local anesthesia if required (lidocaine cream), conduction anesthesia
- Injection technique: bolus technique
- Layer: subcutaneous, intramuscular
- Material: class "M viscous" product
- Volume: 0.05–0.1 ml per bolus, c. 0.2 ml in total
- Needle: 25–27G sharp needle
- No massage
- Cooling if required
- Heparin cream for hematomas, ibuprofen p.o., arnica
- Photo documentation: "after" images
- Advice on dos and don'ts after the procedure
- Follow-up appointment for a check-up after 8–14 days

9.5.6 Technique 34

Augmentation – Marionette Lines (Sharp Needle)

The treatment goal is to achieve harmonious correction of marionette lines. This involves subtle, symmetrical reinforcement of the oral commissure area by filling the region between the mouth corner and the end of the mentalis muscle. There are four different approaches for marionette line treatment, which can also be performed using a cannula (see Technique 35, p. 266 ff.).

Patient Selection

- In age-related loss of volume or thinning of the mouth corners
- Patients with sagging mouth corners and shadows due to their facial type
- In patients with genetically determined, hypertrophic extensions of the nasolabial folds

Injection Scheme and Planning (→ Technique 34 – Figs. 1–8)

Volume replacement in the cutaneous part of the lower lip reinforces this region, thereby supporting the mouth corners. The corner area also loses its perioral shadows, which has a rejuvenating effect. The technique involves gentle filling of the marionette lines using the fanning technique, causing mobilization of the attached muscles.

Technique: fanning technique, criss-cross technique
Direction of insertion: see Technique 34, Figs 1–8
Layer: subdermal, subcutaneous
Material: class "M viscous" or "M soft" product, depending on indication
Volume: 0.05–0.1 ml per line
Needle: 27G sharp needle
Anesthesia: lidocaine cream

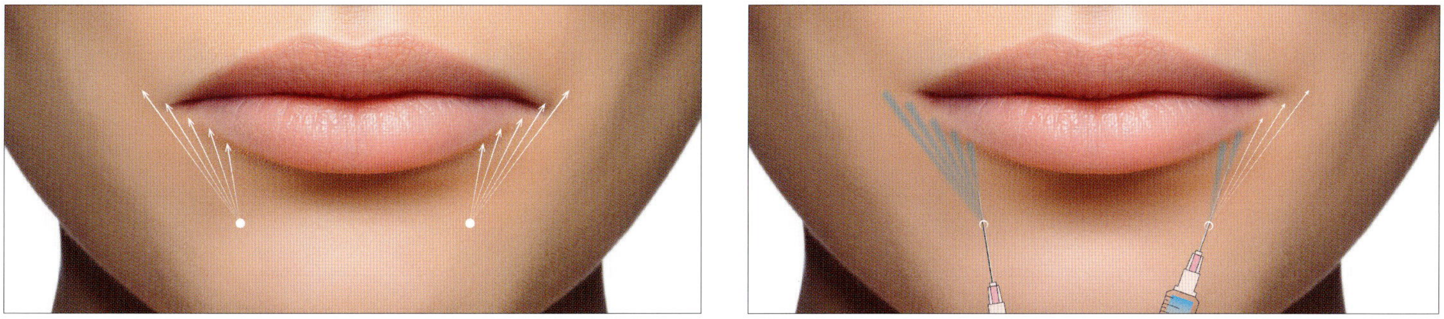

Technique 34 – Figs. 1, 2 Injection scheme and planning for **Variant 1: augmentation – marionette lines (sharp needle).** The material is injected into the target areas in a fan shape from the single needle entry point (the tip of the "fan") located on each side. By directing the needle upward, more volume can be placed at the mouth corners and at the end of the lip. This reinforces the supportive effect. The material is injected toward the mouth and the mouth corners using the linear technique.

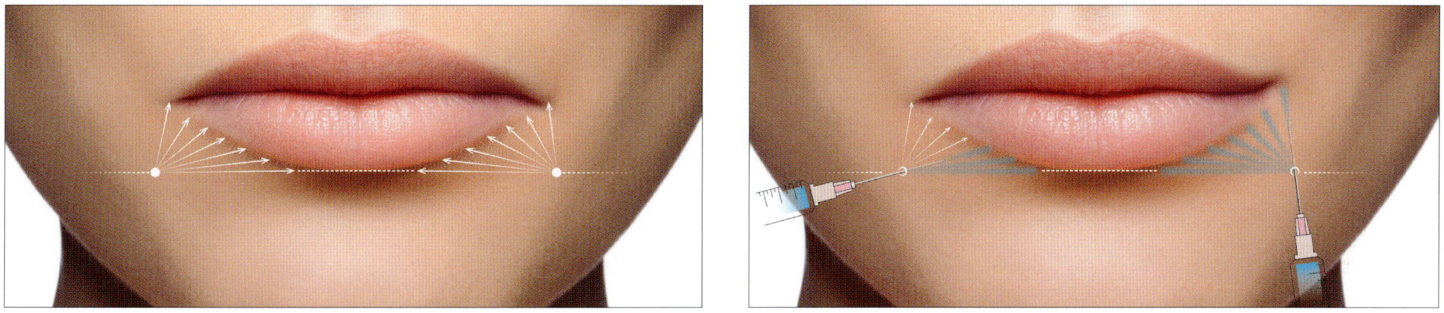

Technique 34 – Figs. 3, 4 Injection scheme and planning for **Variant 2: Augmentation – marionette lines (sharp needle).** If there is a lateral volume deficit below the lip, the needle insertion point is marked along the imaginary line running through the lowest point of the lower lip (dashed line); from there, several lines of material are injected up to the lip margin. By injecting numerous adjacent lines, the therapist can define the material placement very accurately and correct even the finest areas of asymmetry.

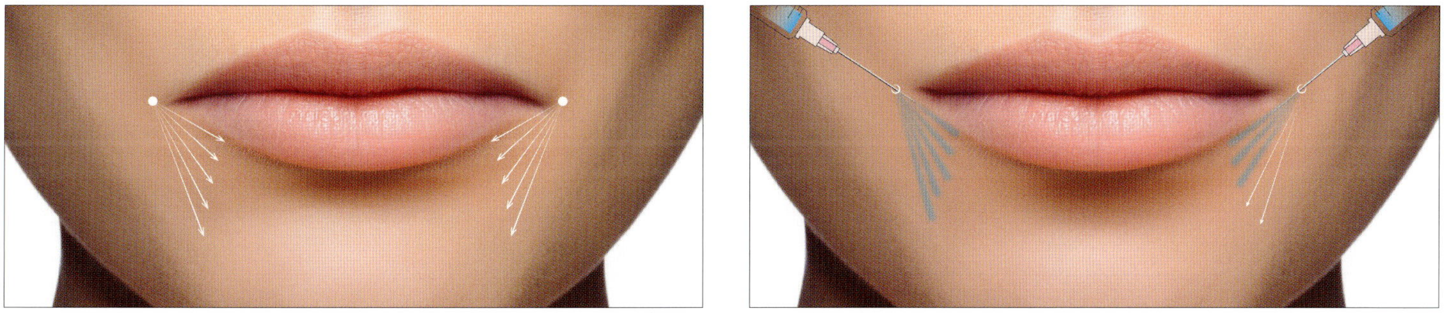

Technique 34 – Figs. 5, 6 Injection scheme and planning for **Variant 3: Augmentation – marionette lines (sharp needle).** Here, the needle insertion point is directly at the mouth corner. This approach is the preferred option if the lip contours are to be integrated into the treatment. Only one entry point is needed per side, from which several lines of material are injected toward the middle of the chin, using the fanning technique.

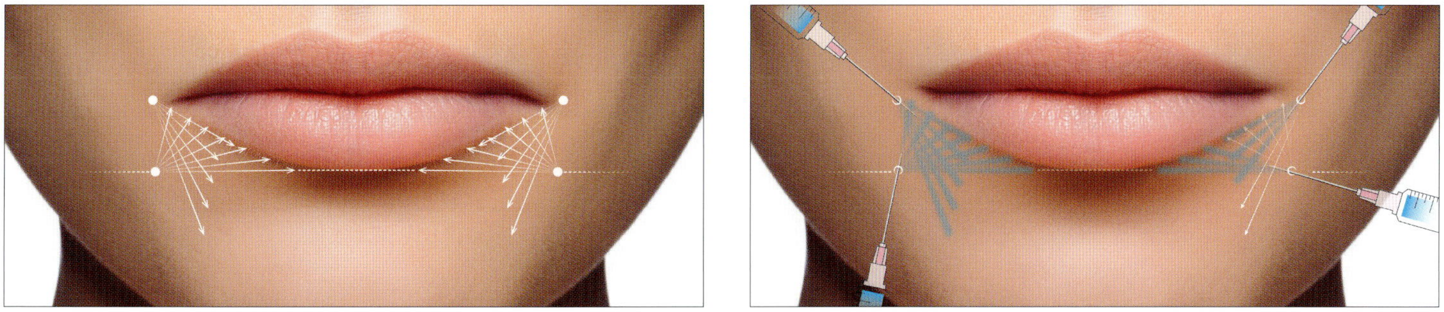

Technique 34 – Figs. 7, 8 Injection scheme and planning for **Variant 4: Augmentation – marionette lines (sharp needle).** The sandwich technique is recommended for extremely pronounced marionette lines. It combines filling of the lost fat compartments with support of the mouth corners. The volume deficit is first filled by deep subcutaneous injection toward the middle of the chin using the fanning technique; a second fan is then superimposed over this (criss-cross technique), with the material injected more superficially into the subcutaneous layer in the direction of the lower lip contour. This procedure stabilizes the area, which also counteracts mimic wrinkles.

Treatment Method (→ Technique 34 – Figs. 9–12)

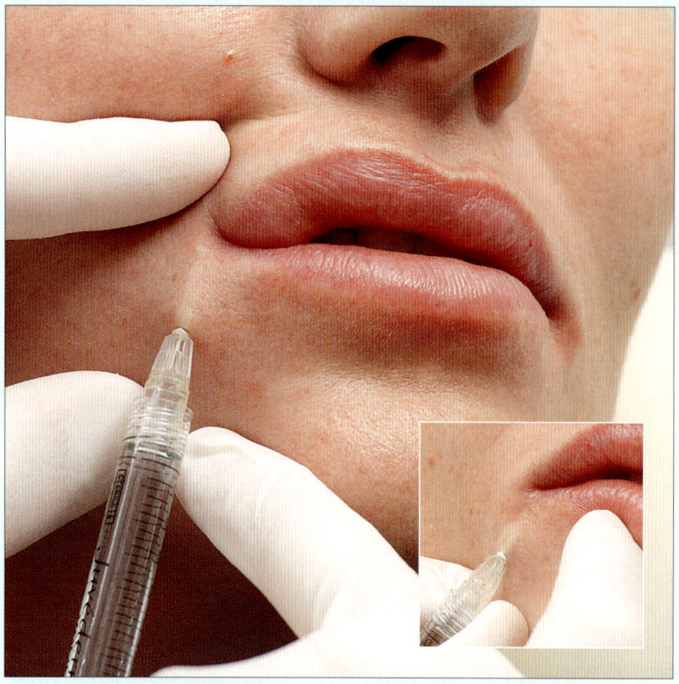

Technique 34 – Fig. 9 (Variant 1): The mouth corner is first reinforced from below. From a needle insertion point 1 cm below the mouth corner, inject several lines at the mouth corner using the fanning technique, advancing in the medial direction and ending at the lip margin. Areas of different size may be treated, depending on the needle length used.

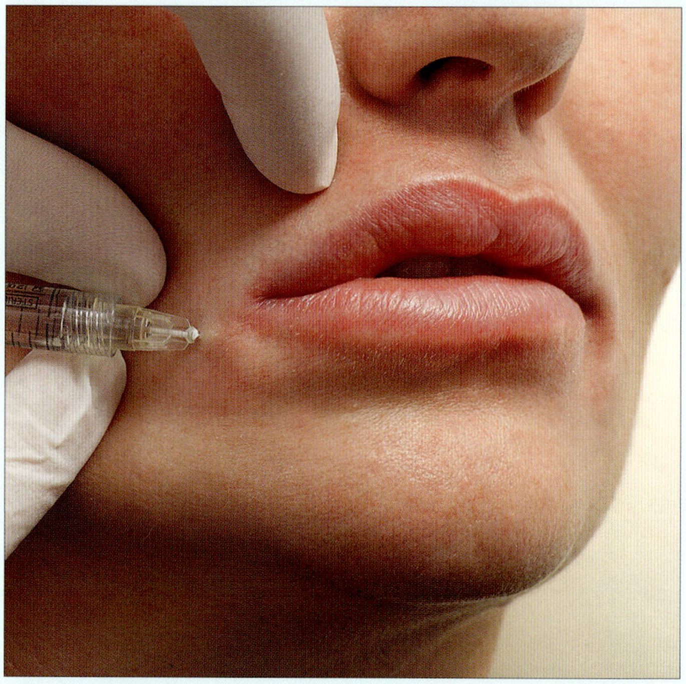

Technique 34 – Fig. 10 (Variant 2): Approaching from the lateral side, inject several lines of material below the lip contour from one entry point, using the fanning technique. If the material forms a somewhat irregular bulge, as shown in this image, it is advisable to reach into the oral cavity with the forefinger and squeeze the material between the thumb and forefinger until the irregularities disappear.

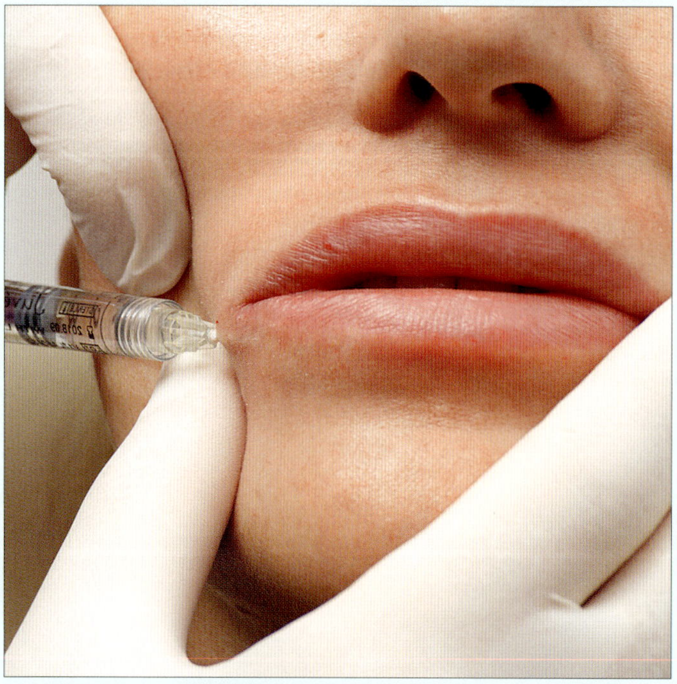

Technique 34 – Fig. 11 (Variant 3): It is easier to treat the oral commissure if the entire lower lip region is stretched.

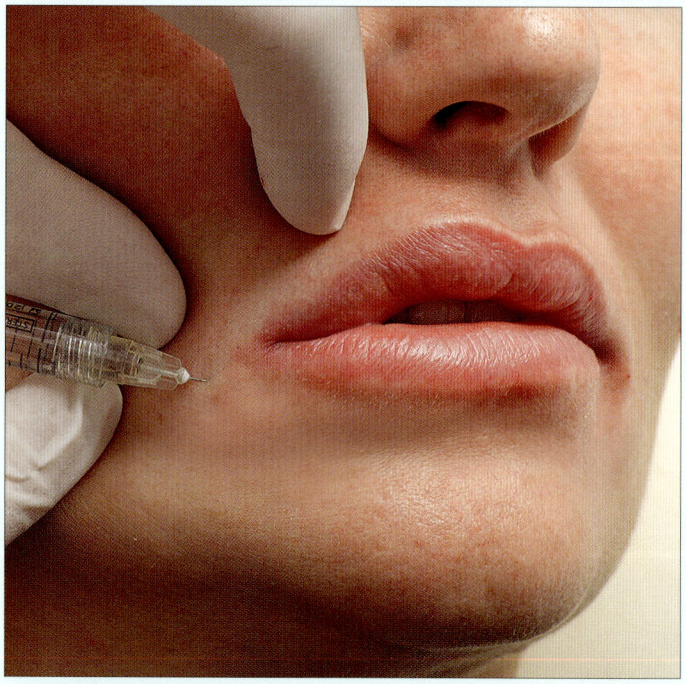

Technique 34 – Fig. 12 (Variant 4): Superimposing the layers can lead to slightly uneven areas. These can generally be corrected by massage.

Important Notes

- As a general rule, the mouth corner treatment needs to be repeated 1–2 times, depending on the extent of the wrinkling or sagging. For this reason, it is very useful to combine the treatment with filling of the marionette lines, as this gives added support to the tissue.

Possible Side Effects

Slight reddening, rarely inflammation, commonly hematomas, mild swellings

Undesirable Side Effects

Inflammation, overcorrection, nodule formation, asymmetry due to non-uniform delivery of material, necrosis

Treatment Protocol at a Glance

- History, evaluation, and patient information
- Informed consent form
- Photo documentation: "before" images
- Analysis and marking of the areas to be treated
- Cleaning
- Thorough disinfection
- Local anesthesia if required (lidocaine cream)
- Injection technique: fanning technique, criss-cross technique
- Layer: subdermal, subcutaneous, depending on the depth of lines and shadows
- Material: class "M viscous" or "M soft" product, depending on indication
- Volume: 0.05–0.1 ml per line
- Needle: 27G sharp needle
- Gentle massage
- Cooling if required
- Heparin cream for hematomas, ibuprofen p.o., arnica
- Photo documentation: "after" images
- Advice on dos and don'ts after the procedure
- Follow-up appointment for a check-up after 8–14 days

9.5.7 Technique 35

Augmentation – Marionette Lines (Blunt Cannula)

The treatment goal is to achieve harmonious correction of marionette lines. This involves symmetrical reinforcement of the oral commissure area by filling the region between the mouth corner and the end of the mentalis muscle using a cannula. A large area can be filled subcutaneously in this way. The advantage of the cannula technique is that fewer blood vessels are damaged, resulting in fewer hematomas and swellings, and patients experience less pain after the treatment. However, when using the cannula technique, it is more difficult to superimpose different layers or to guide the cannula itself in a controlled manner.

Patient Selection

- In age-related loss of volume or thinning of the mouth corners
- Patients with sagging mouth corners and shadows due to their facial type
- In patients with genetically determined, hypertrophic extensions of the nasolabial folds

Injection Scheme and Planning (→ Technique 35 – Figs. 1–6)

Volume replacement in the cutaneous part of the lower lip reinforces this region, thus supporting the mouth corners. The corner area also loses its perioral shadows, which has a rejuvenating effect. The technique involves filling of the marionette lines using the fanning technique, causing mobilization of the attached muscles. The material is injected into the target areas in a fan shape from the single needle entry point (the tip of the "fan") located on each side. Placement of the tip of the fan may vary according to the treatment goal and depends on the indication. The entry point for the cannula is prepared with a Nokor needle. The length of the cannula used depends on the treatment area. Before delivering the material, the tissue layers in the region being treated are teased apart to allow the material to distribute itself over a wide area. Any irregularities can be readily massaged away after the treatment. We present three variants here, which differ slightly in terms of their mode of action.

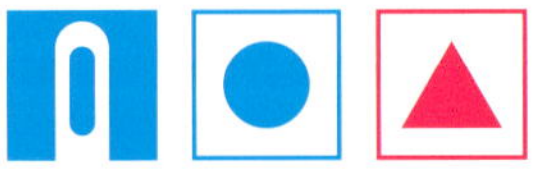

Technique: fanning technique

Direction of insertion: see Technique 35, Figs. 1–6

Layer: subcutaneous

Material: class "M viscous" or "M soft" product, according to indication

Volume: 0.05–0.1 ml per line

Needle: 27G blunt cannula

Anesthesia: lidocaine (skin wheal technique)

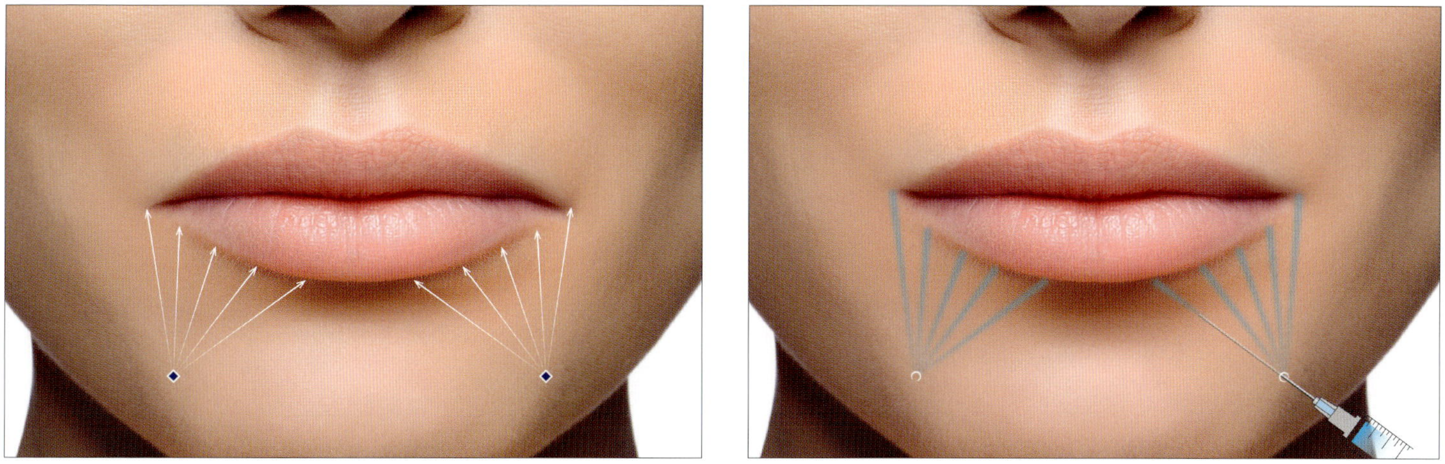

Technique 35 – Figs. 1, 2 Injection scheme and planning for **Variant 1: Augmentation – marionette lines (blunt cannula).** This technique is often used when the marionette lines – caused by sagging or volume loss – involve deep mimic lines or pronounced shadows, and when the reduced fat compartments need replacing. Starting from a needle insertion point around 2 cm below the mouth corner, several lines of material are injected at the mouth corner and toward the lower lip margin, using the fanning technique. By directing the needle upward, more volume can be placed at the mouth corners and at the edge of the lip. This reinforces the supportive effect. The cannula is advanced toward the lip gently and without using force, taking care that the tip of the cannula does not penetrate into the lip itself. Areas of different sizes may be treated, depending on the needle length used.

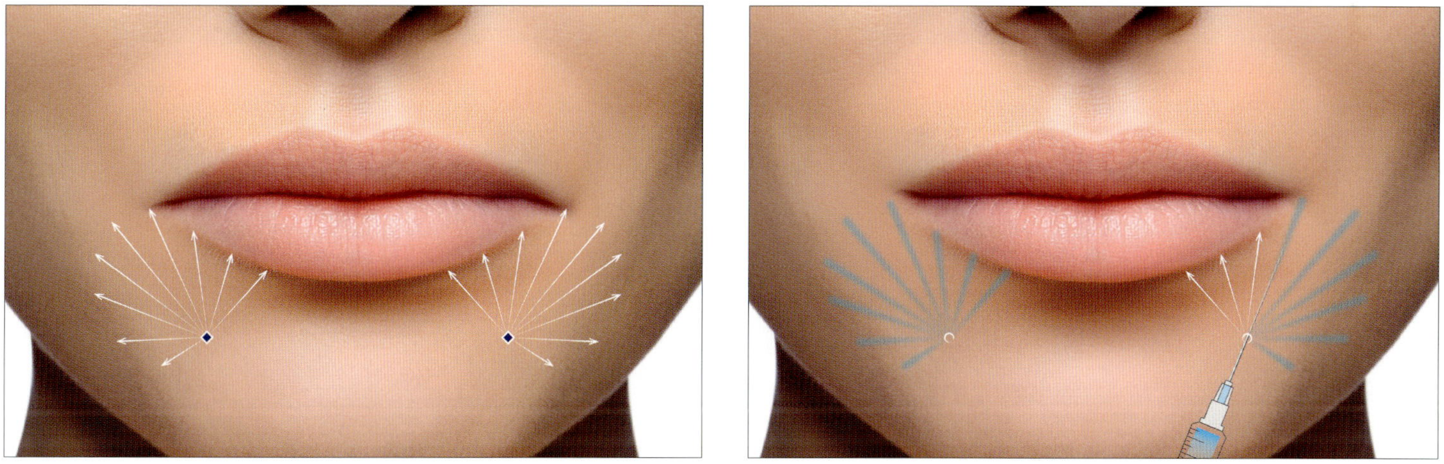

Technique 35 – Figs. 3, 4 Injection scheme and planning for **Variant 2: augmentation – marionette lines (blunt cannula).** In this technique variant, the needle insertion point below the mouth corners is located further in the medial direction, toward the center of the chin. It is suitable for the eradication of deep marionette lines with concomitant lifting of the lateral lip region.

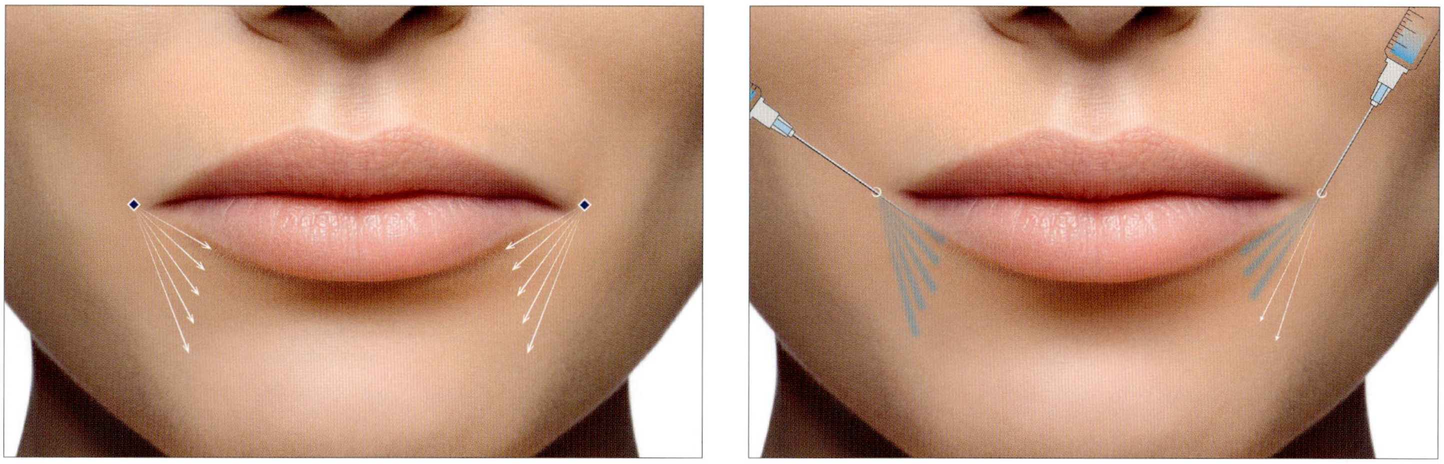

Technique 35 – Figs. 5, 6 Injection scheme and planning for **Variant 3: augmentation – marionette lines (blunt cannula).** This most commonly used variant of the cannula method not only stabilizes the mouth corners, but also firms up the lower lip contour and treats the marionette lines. The needle insertion point is located 2–3 mm from the mouth corner. Only one entry point is needed per side, from which several lines of material are injected toward the middle of the chin using the fanning technique.

Treatment Method (→ Technique 35 – Figs. 7, 8)

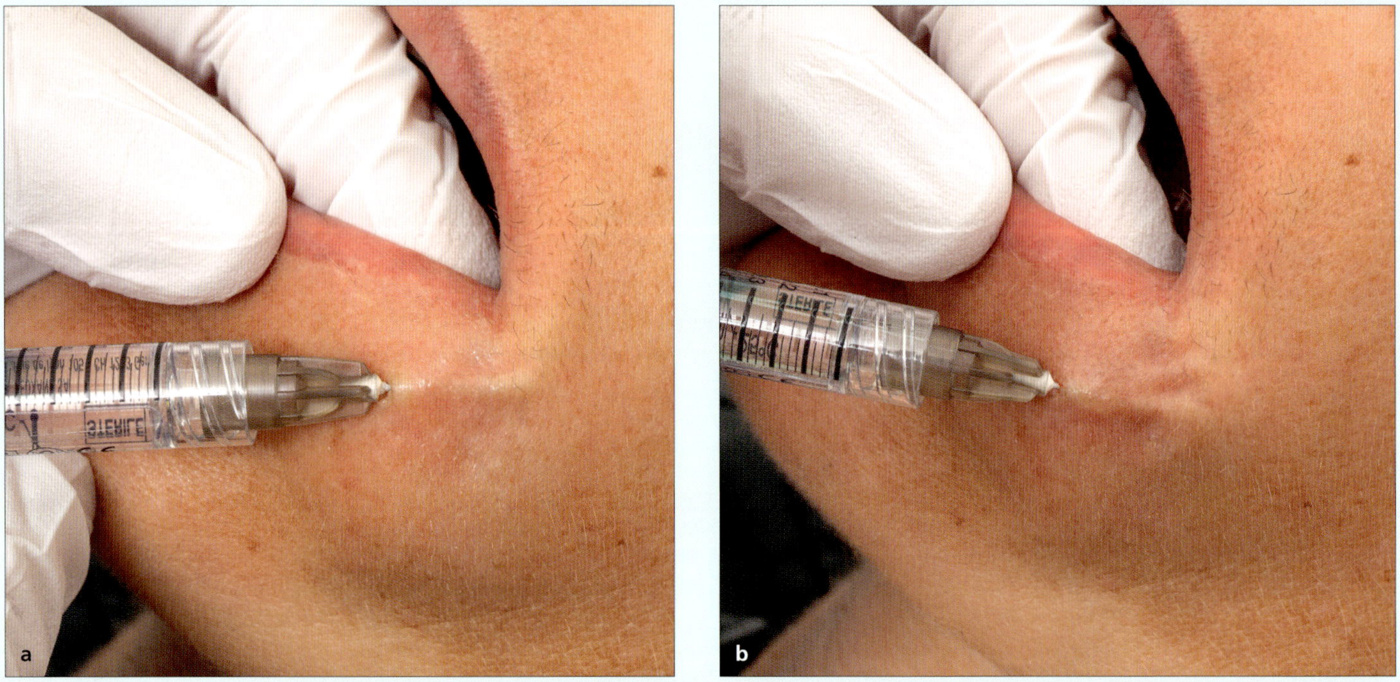

Technique 35 – Fig. 7 a+b (Variant 2): When using the fanning technique with a cannula, a triangular area is injected, the shadow filled, and the tissue stabilized at the same time. A short cannula (25 mm) was used here.

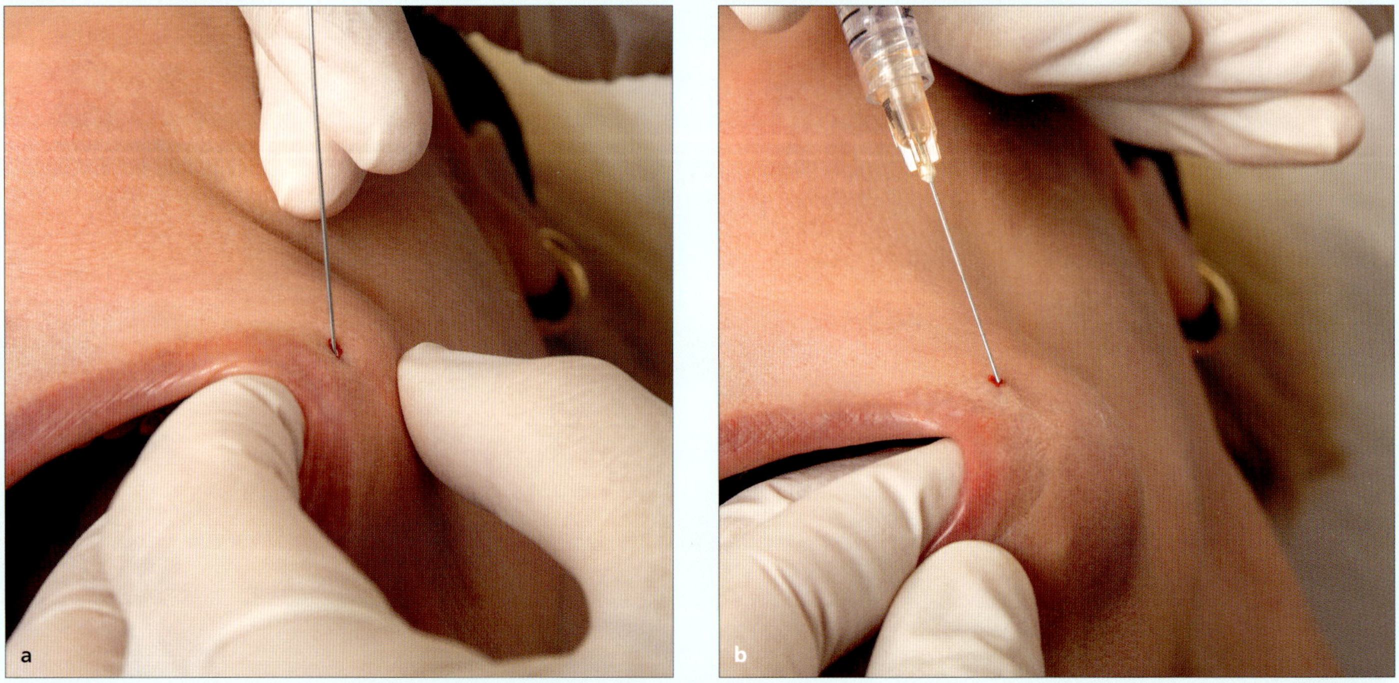

Technique 35 – Fig. 8 a+b (Variant 3): Use of a longer cannula (38–50 mm) is recommended when injecting downward in the medial direction from the mouth corner. Pulling the cheek forward between thumb and forefinger allows the long cannula to be guided more easily and to overcome any resistance in the tissue. Holding the tissue in place with the thumb and forefinger makes it easier for the tissue layers to be teased apart, and also allows the therapist to see where the cannula is located.

Important Notes

- The technique is easier to implement if the treatment chair is tilted backward at an angle of 30–45 degrees, and if the therapist can stand side on to the patient.
- The therapist does not see the treatment area from the front; during the preliminary analysis, it is therefore necessary to note exactly how much material needs to be introduced into which zone. During the injection, the amount of material being delivered needs to be closely monitored by watching the syringe plunger.
- The treatment should start with small amounts of HA, and the patient brought back into the vertical position between injections to check the interim result.
- The viscosity of the HA should be selected according to skin thickness and wrinkle depth. More viscous materials should be used where the tissue needs to provide greater support, while thin, delicate skin needs a soft, less viscous HA filler.

Possible Side Effects

Slight reddening, rarely inflammation, hematomas possible due to pre-pricking with the Nokor needle, mild swellings

Undesirable Side Effects

Inflammation, overcorrection, nodule formation, asymmetry due to non-uniform delivery of material, necrosis

Treatment Protocol at a Glance

- History, evaluation, and patient information
- Informed consent form
- Photo documentation: "before" images
- Analysis and marking of the areas to be treated
- Cleaning
- Thorough disinfection
- Local anesthesia if required (lidocaine cream)
- Injection technique: fanning technique
- Layer: subcutaneous
- Material: class "M viscous" or "M soft" product, according to indication
- Volume: 0.05–0.1 ml per line
- Needle: 27G blunt cannula
- Gentle massage
- Cooling if required
- Heparin cream for hematomas, ibuprofen p.o., arnica
- Photo documentation: "after" images
- Advice on dos and don'ts after the procedure
- Follow-up appointment for a check-up after 8–14 days

9.5.8 Technique 36

Augmentation – Windmill Technique: Marionette Lines, Lips, Perioral Region (Blunt Cannula)

This technique allows the entire oral region to be augmented without leaving the entry point on either side or changing the cannula. With a bit of skill, it is even possible to use different materials for the whole area with one and the same cannula. Of course, the radius can be increased as well.

Patient Selection

- Patients who want to correct age-related or genetically determined volume loss and wrinkles in the perioral region and lips as well as marionette lines

Injection Scheme and Planning (→ Technique 36 – Figs. 1, 2)

If the needle insertion point is placed 3–5 mm laterally of the mouth corner, the skin will need to be pre-pricked in the various different directions with a Nokor needle.

First, the blunt cannula is used to fill the tissue in the subcutaneous layer toward the middle of the chin using the fanning technique. After this, individual lines of material are injected in the direction of the lower lip contour and center, the dry/wet boundary of the lower and upper lip, the upper lip center and contour, and into the perioral upper lip region up to the nasolabial fold. However, it is also possible to work in reverse order, starting with the upper lip.

The material may be changed according to indication and treatment goal: a more viscous HA is used for stabilizing treatment of the lower lip area, which also counteracts mimic wrinkles, while a softer HA is used for lip volumization, and a soft, small-particle HA is used for upper lip revitalization. It is advisable to withdraw the cannula fully, change the cannula and material, and then inject into the next region through the same entry point. When changing the material, it is also possible to unscrew the syringe while leaving the cannula in the tissue.

Technique: fanning technique
Direction of insertion: over a radius of c. 160 degrees in the medial direction
Layer: subcutaneous
Material: class "S/M viscous" or "S/M soft" product, depending on region and indication
Volume: 0.05–0.1 ml per line
Needle: 27G blunt cannula
Anesthesia: lidocaine (skin wheal technique)

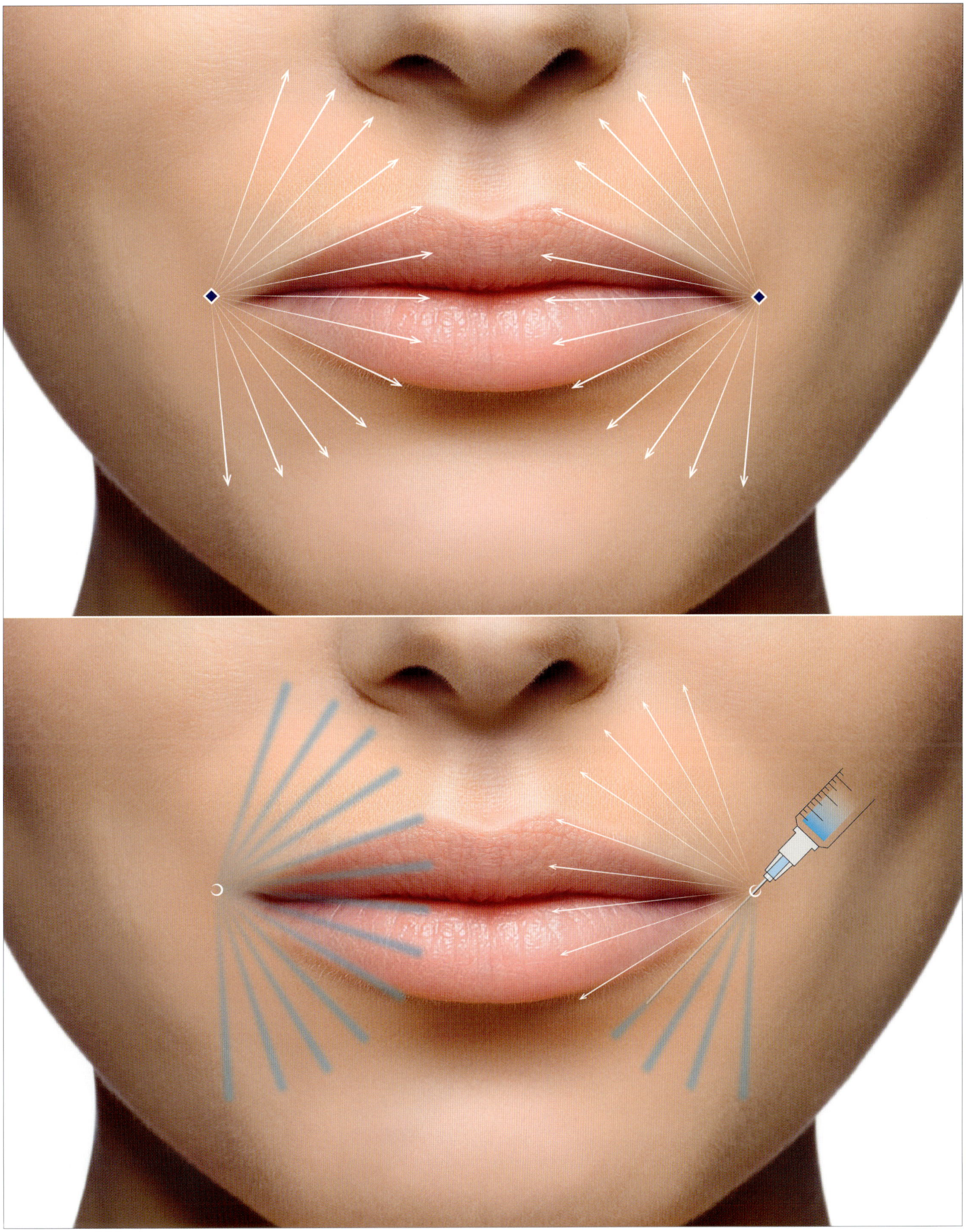

Technique 36 – Figs. 1, 2 Injection scheme and planning for augmentation – windmill technique: marionette lines, lips, perioral region (blunt cannula).

Treatment Method (→ Technique 36 – Figs. 3–5)

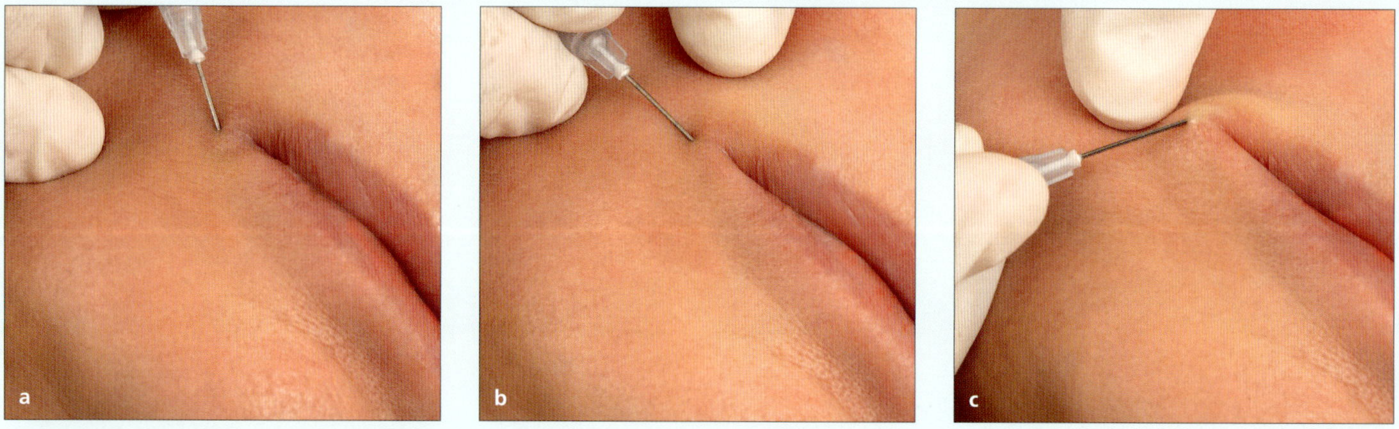

Technique 36 – Fig. 3 a–c To make it possible to inject with the cannula in all directions, pre-prick with the Nokor needle in the three directions into which the cannula needs to be introduced: downward (a), in the medial direction (b), upward (c). This facilitates the insertion of the cannula.

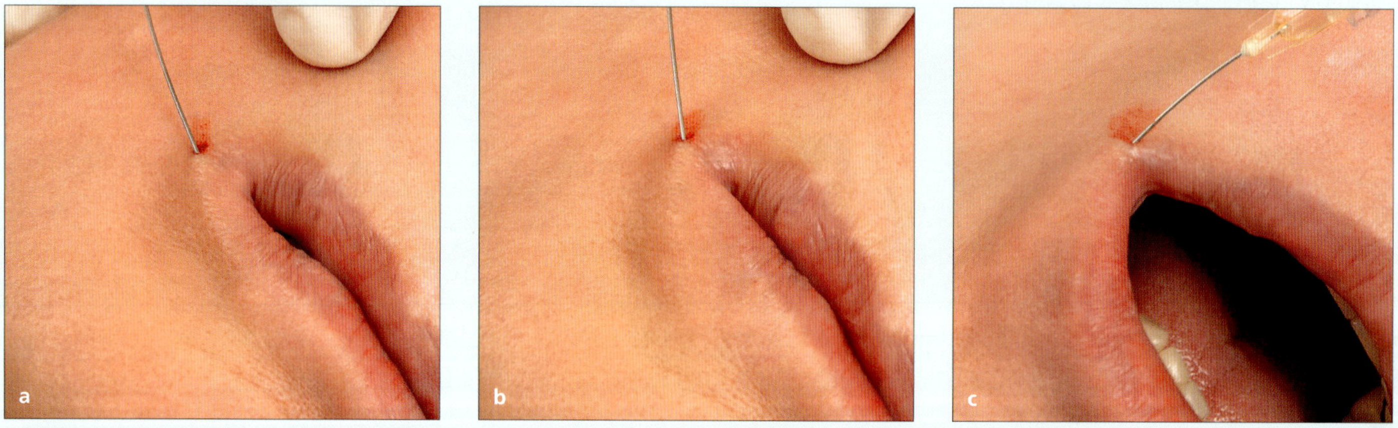

Technique 36 – Fig. 4 a–c Treatment of the lower lip region: lifting the cannula shows in which tissue layer it is located; in this case, in the subcutis (a). Using the fanning technique, place the different lines of material next to each other, working downward. Stretching the skin of the cheek makes is easier to move the cannula gently through the tissue toward the chin fold (b). Where the cannula needs to be guided vertically downward (c) on the patient's right side, it is more convenient for a right-handed therapist to be positioned slightly further behind the patient's head, with the treatment chair lowered.

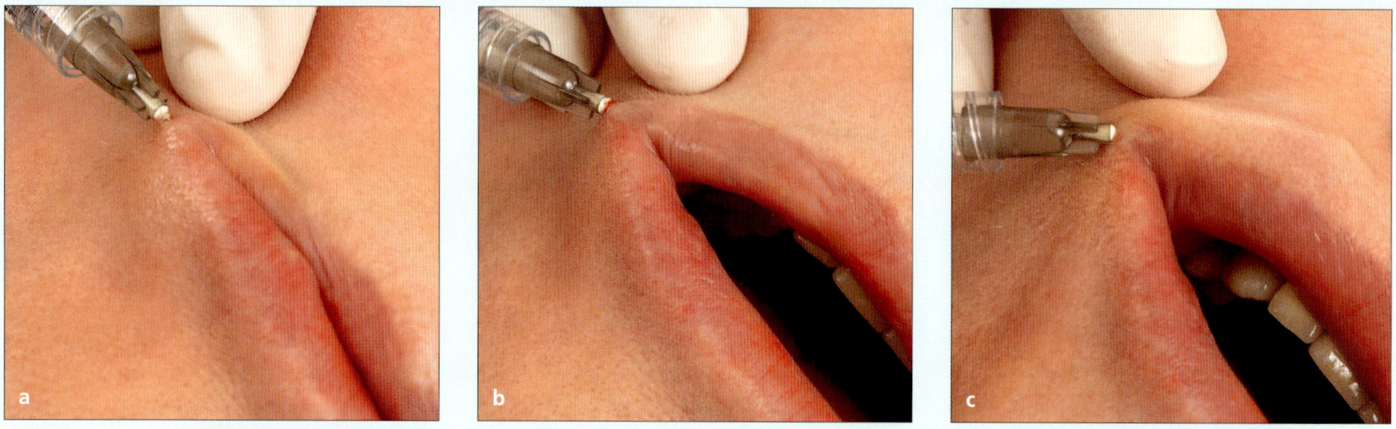

Technique 36 – Fig. 5 a–c Treatment of the upper lip: inject the required number of lines, depending on the treatment goal, through the same entry point (a). In this slightly older patient, the upper lip was injected with only one line at the dry/wet boundary (b), to prevent the "duck's bill" effect while still introducing some volume. The cutaneous part of the upper lip was hydrated with a skin booster (c).

Important Notes

- It is possible to use the same cannula all the time if it is left in the skin while the syringe containing the HA filler is unscrewed and changed. This allows different materials to be introduced into different regions of the lip.
- Insertion and withdrawal of the cannula carries an infection risk. Therefore, the cannula should be changed if it is withdrawn.
- It is essential to ensure that the cannula does not come into contact with anything non-sterile outside the region being injected.
- If the tissue layers in the treatment area are teased apart, the material is distributed more evenly and produces fewer uneven areas.

Possible Side Effects

Slight reddening, rarely inflammation, hematomas possible due to pre-pricking with the Nokor needle, mild swellings

Undesirable Side Effects

Inflammation, overcorrection, nodule formation, asymmetry due to non-uniform delivery of material, necrosis

Treatment Protocol at a Glance

- History, evaluation, and patient information
- Informed consent form
- Photo documentation: "before" images
- Analysis and marking of the areas to be treated
- Cleaning
- Thorough disinfection
- Local anesthesia if required (lidocaine cream)
- Injection technique: fanning technique
- Layer: subcutaneous
- Material: class "S/M viscous" or "S/M soft" product, depending on region and indication
- Volume: 0.05–0.1 ml per line
- Needle: 27G blunt cannula
- Gentle massage
- Cooling if required
- Heparin cream for hematomas, ibuprofen p.o., arnica
- Photo documentation: "after" images
- Advice on dos and don'ts after the procedure
- Follow-up appointment for a check-up after 8–14 days

9.6 Shaping, Beautification

The techniques presented in this section involve making changes or improvements in lip shape where there are areas of asymmetry, previous treatments or genetically determined deficits. Fashion, along with trends attributed to the zeitgeist and to beauty ideals in general, also play a role in prompting a desire to alter the shape and expression of the lips. This also involves changes and improvements to young, intact lips, which is referred to as "beautification." Examples include accentuation of the Cupid's bow or tubercles, lifting the mouth corners, creating the stomion, etc. In this section, we have concentrated on the most common indications and have ignored the extremes.

9.6.1 Technique 37

Subtle Mouth Corner Lift (Sharp Needle)

The mouth corners are lifted by injecting the contours of the lateral lower lip. This results in a more cheerful facial expression. The materials used and the volume of material delivered are the defining factors. This technique is suitable for minimal support or accentuation to stabilize the mouth corners.

Patient Selection

- For still young and intact lips where a minimal lift is required

Injection Scheme and Planning (→ Technique 37 – Figs. 1, 2)

This minimal injection treatment gives some support to the mouth corners and refreshes them. The material is injected subdermally at the vermillion border, starting from the mouth corner and into the last 0.5–1 cm of the upper lip. The needle is inserted into the mouth corner. Caution: do not inject into the upper lip corner, to allow the treated segment of the lower lip to curve upward gently and lift the mouth corner.

Technique: linear technique
Direction of insertion: starting from the mouth corner and ending max. 1 cm toward the middle of the lip
Layer: subdermal
Material: class "S/M viscous" product
Volume: 0.05–0.1 ml per line
Needle: 27–29G sharp needle
Anesthesia: lidocaine cream

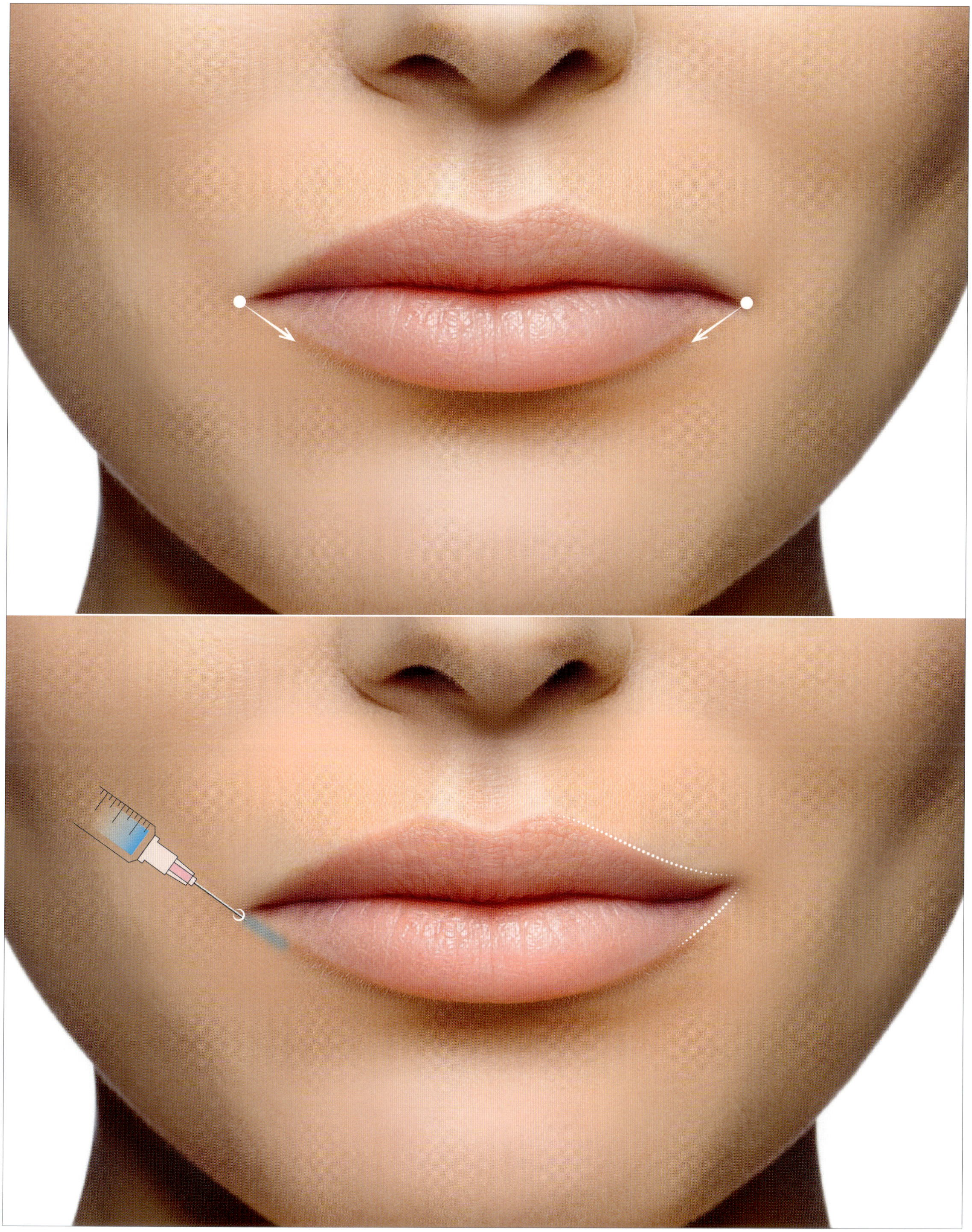

Technique 37 – Figs. 1, 2 Injection scheme and planning for the subtle mouth corner lift (sharp needle).

9

Treatment Method (→ Technique 37 – Figs. 3, 4)

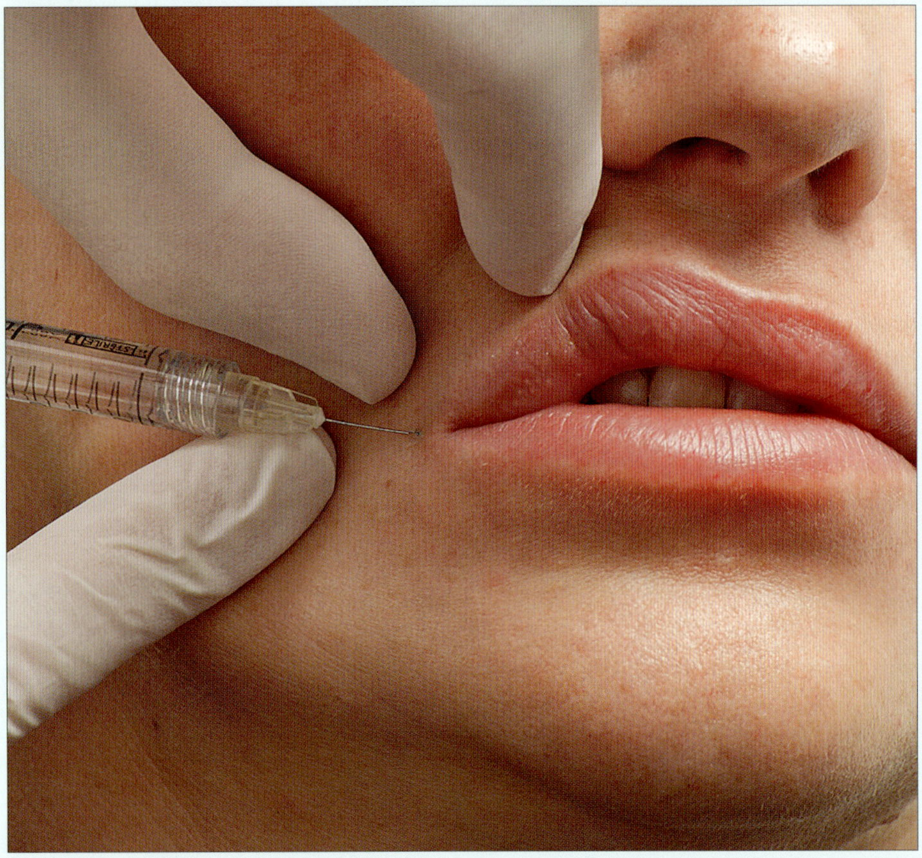

Technique 37 – Fig. 3 Pull this lip area apart slightly so that the mouth corner is clearly visible. Insert the needle precisely into the lower lip part of the mouth corner.

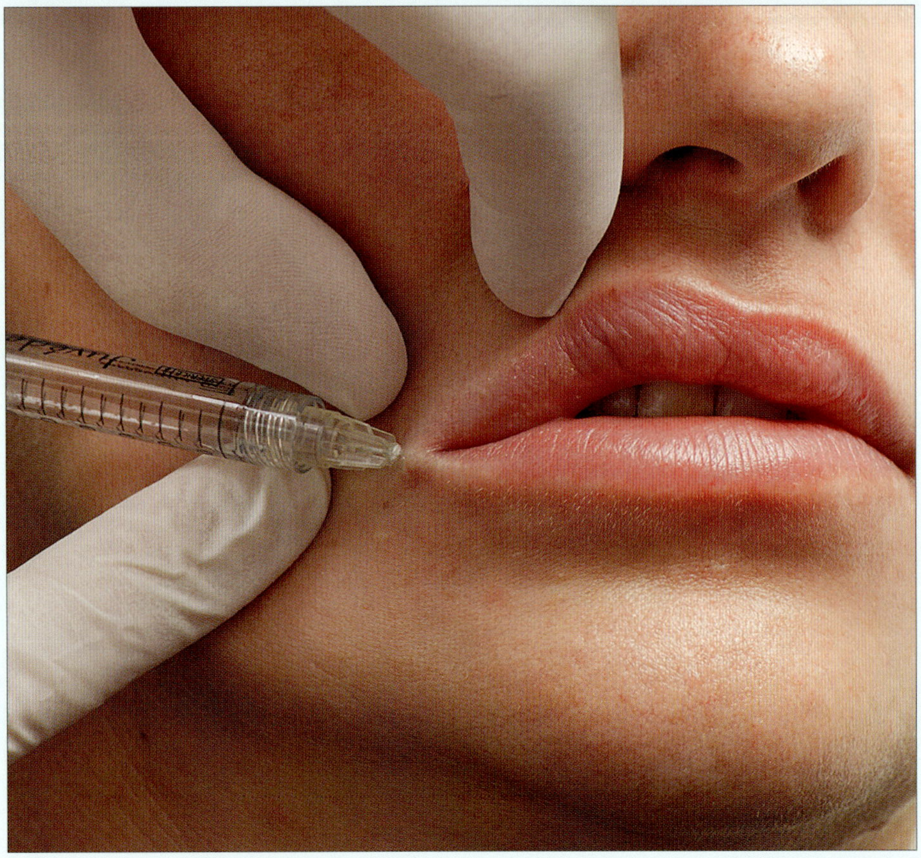

Technique 37 – Fig. 4 Administer c. 0.05–0.1 ml into the contour of the lower lip. Advance the needle tip c. 0.5 cm in the medial direction within the lip contour. Deliver the material by retrograde injection toward the mouth corner.

Important Notes

- If the skin is older and already damaged or if the mouth corners have been pulled down by gravity, use the next technique (Technique 38) to achieve a satisfactory result.
- If there is pronounced sagging of the mouth corners, the marionette lines will need to be treated as well.

Possible Side Effects

Slight reddening, rarely inflammation, rarely hematomas, rarely mild swellings

Undesirable Side Effects

Asymmetry due to non-uniform delivery of material or nodule formation, Tyndall effect if the injection is too superficial, necrosis

Treatment Protocol at a Glance

- History, evaluation, and patient information
- Informed consent form
- Photo documentation: "before" images
- Analysis and marking of the areas to be treated
- Cleaning
- Thorough disinfection
- Local anesthesia if required (lidocaine cream)
- Injection technique: linear technique
- Layer: subdermal
- Material: class "S/M viscous" product
- Volume: 0.05–0.1 ml per line
- Needle: 27–29G sharp needle
- Gentle massage
- Cooling if required
- Heparin cream for hematomas, ibuprofen p.o., arnica
- Photo documentation: "after" images
- Advice on dos and don'ts after the procedure
- Follow-up appointment for a check-up after 8–14 days

9.6.2 Technique 38

Classic Mouth Corner Lift (Sharp Needle)

The mouth corners are lifted by injecting the contours of the lateral lower lip and – if a higher degree of correction is required – of the upper lip. This results in a more cheerful facial expression. Depending on the degree of sagging at the mouth corners, it is not always possible to lift them so that they are pulled above the horizontal line. However, bringing the mouth corners into the horizontal can already produce a very positive change in facial expression.

Two approaches, which show only minor differences and are dependent on the indication, are presented here. The materials used and the volume of material delivered are the defining factors. Either the first or the second variant should be considered, depending on the extent of the mouth corner sagging.

Patient Selection

- For sagging of the mouth corners of varying extent

Injection Scheme and Planning (→ Technique 38 – Figs. 1–6)

If the mouth corners are only slightly downturned, the material is injected subcutaneously at the vermillion border of the lower lip, along an imaginary line that extends beyond the lip up to the risorius muscle (see image on the right). The needle is inserted into the lower lip c. 0.5 cm from the mouth corner and directed toward it. Injecting into the upper lip is not advisable as the lifting effect will be lost otherwise.

If the mouth corners are very downturned, more material (a double line) is placed at the mouth corners and the upper lip is included in the treatment plan. The first puncture is made on the lower lip contour c. 1 cm short of the mouth corner, and the needle is advanced up to the risorius muscle. The mouth corner region is given added support and reinforcement with a second line of material coming from below and directed toward the mouth corner. In addition, 1–2 lines are injected into the upper lip, close to the mouth corner. To ensure that the lifting effect is not countered by delivering material into the upper lip, and that no counterpressure is built up from above, it is important not to inject any material into the first 1–3 mm of the lip margin at the mouth corners.

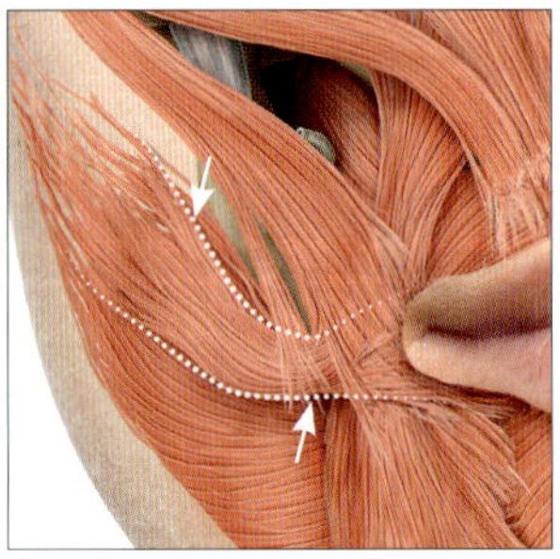

Musculature of the oral region with the risorius muscle.

Technique: linear technique

Direction of insertion: c. 1.0 cm short of the mouth corner toward the risorius muscle; upper lip: ca. 0.5 cm from the mouth corner toward the middle of the lip

Layer: subcutaneous

Material: class "S/M viscous" product

Volume: max. 0.1 ml per line, c. 0.4 ml in total

Needle: 27–29G sharp needle

Anesthesia: lidocaine cream

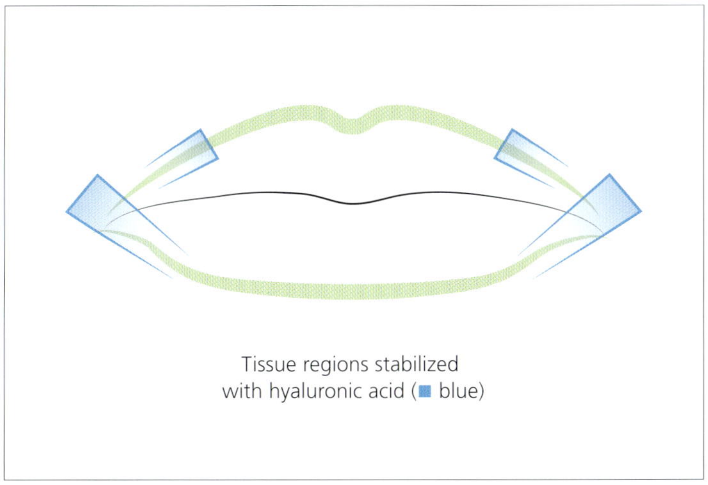

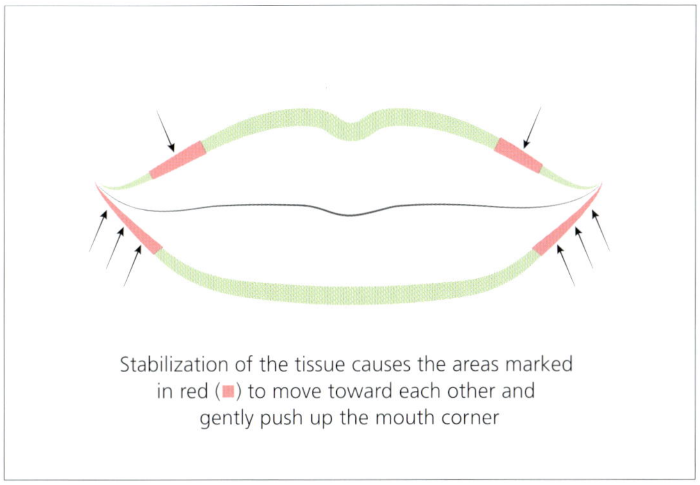

Technique 38 – Figs. 1, 2 The added reinforcement of the upper lip region produced by administering a line of material into the upper lip, starting c. 0.5 cm away from the mouth corner on the medial side, gently pushes this section downward. Leaving the segment of the upper lip close to the mouth corner untreated causes this area to be pushed up by the pressure from the lower lip: this lifts the mouth corners slightly and gives the mouth a smiling, positive expression. To achieve this, it is necessary to ensure that no material is injected into the first 1–2 mm at the lip margin of the upper part of the mouth corner.

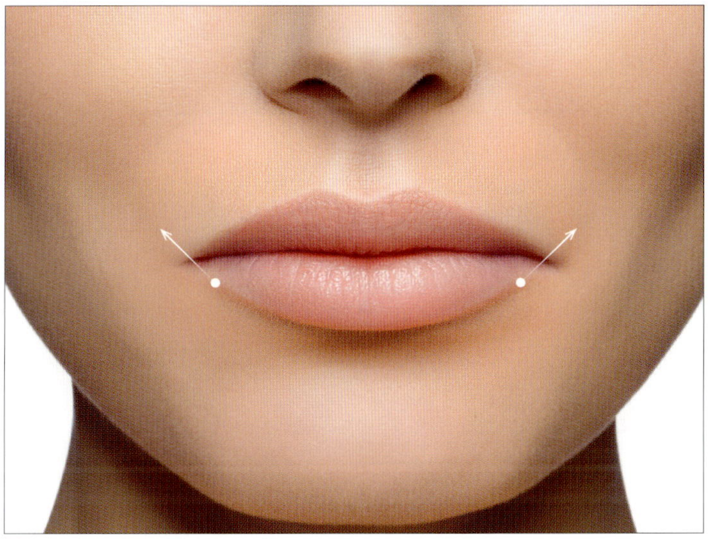

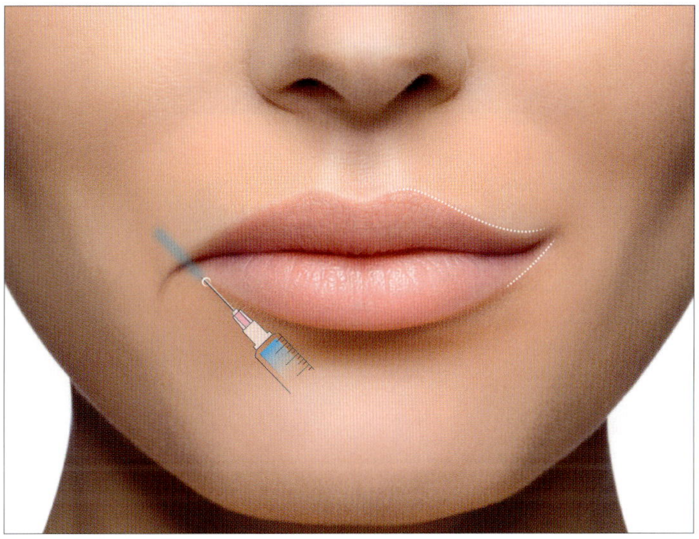

Technique 38 – Figs. 3, 4 Injection scheme and planning for **Variant 1: classic lift by injecting at the mouth corners (sharp needle).**

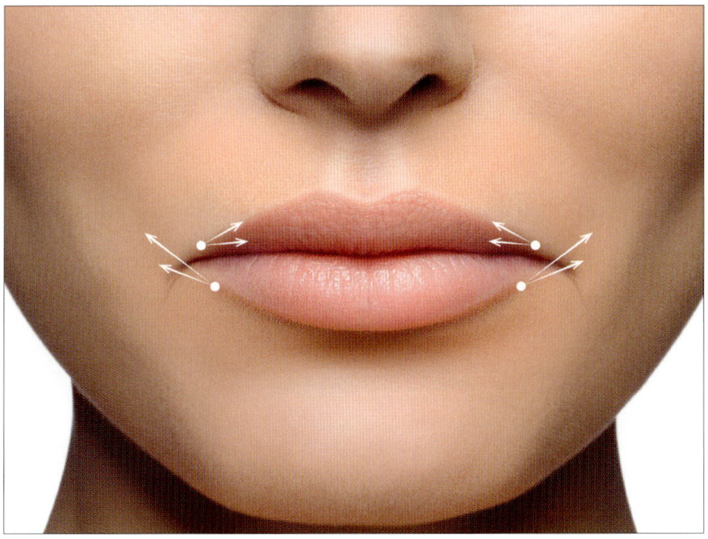

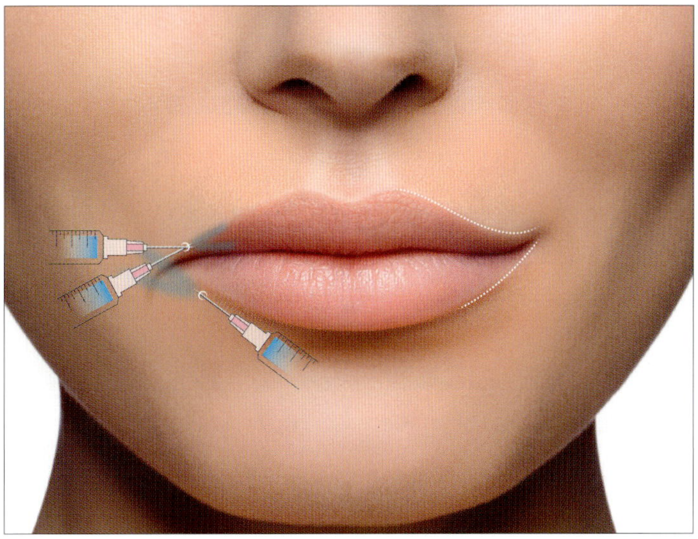

Technique 38 – Figs. 5, 6 Injection scheme and planning for **Variant 2: classic mouth corner lift by injecting into the lower and upper lips (sharp needle).**

9

Treatment Method (→ Technique 38 – Figs. 7–10)

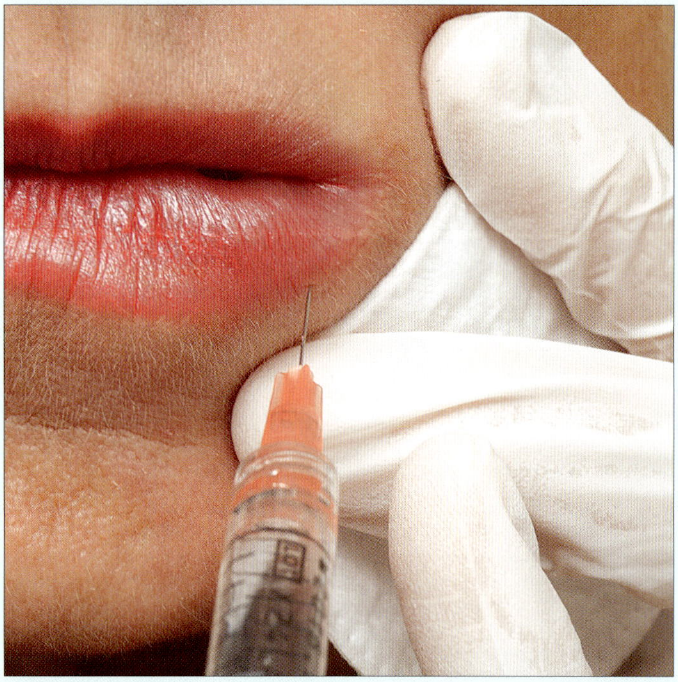

Technique 38 – Fig. 7 (Variant 1+2): Insert the needle 0.5–1 cm short of the mouth corner. Evert the lip slightly to ensure that the needle is accurately directed.

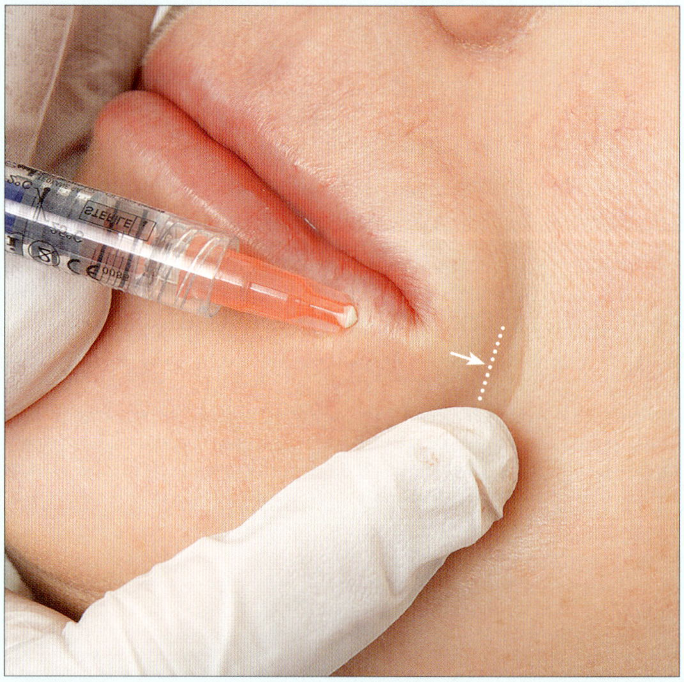

Technique 38 – Fig. 8 (Variant 1): Inject only 1 line of material beyond the mouth corner and up to the risorius muscle.

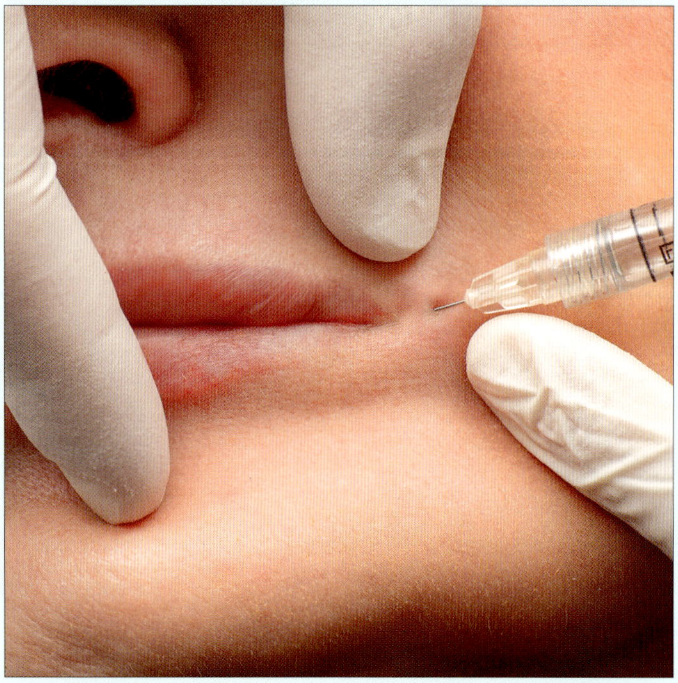

Technique 38 – Fig. 9 (Variant 1+2): Another option is to approach from the lateral side of mouth corner. It is important to ensure that the material is injected 0.5–1.0 cm beyond the mouth corner.

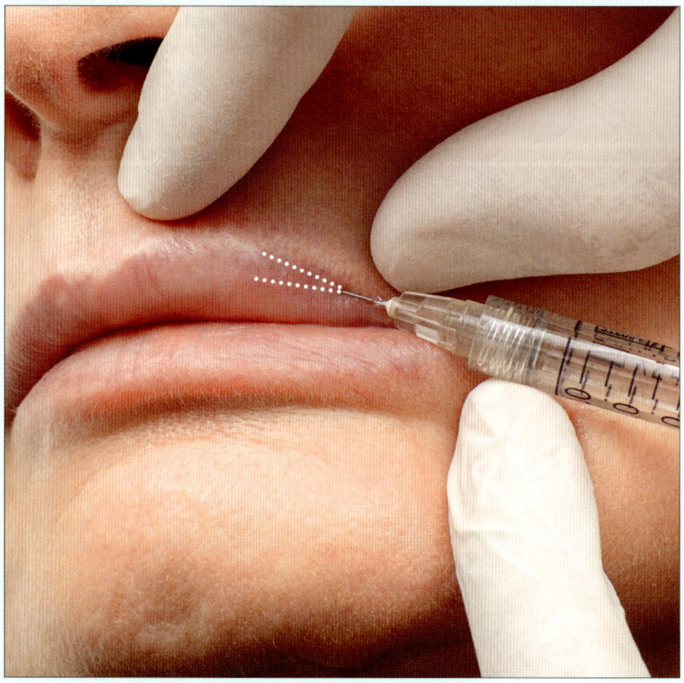

Technique 38 – Fig. 10 (Variant 2): Deliver 1–2 lines of material c. 0.7-cm long into the upper lip by retrograde injection using the fanning technique, injecting c. 3–5 mm away from the mouth corner. This strengthens the effect of the mouth corner lift. During the injection, stretch the lip gently with the opposite hand.

Important Notes

- If there is pronounced sagging of the mouth corners, the marionette lines will need to be treated as well.

Possible Side Effects

Slight reddening, rarely inflammation, rarely hematomas, rarely mild swellings

Undesirable Side Effects

Asymmetry due to non-uniform delivery of material or nodule formation, Tyndall effect if the injection is too superficial, necrosis

Treatment Protocol at a Glance

- History, evaluation, and patient information
- Informed consent form
- Photo documentation: "before" images
- Analysis and marking of the areas to be treated
- Cleaning
- Thorough disinfection
- Local anesthesia if required (lidocaine cream)
- Injection technique: linear technique
- Layer: subcutaneous
- Material: class "S/M viscous" product
- Volume: max. 0.1 ml per line, c. 0.4 ml in total
- Needle: 27–29G sharp needle
- Gentle massage
- Cooling if required
- Heparin cream for hematomas, ibuprofen p.o., arnica
- Photo documentation: "after" images
- Advice on dos and don'ts after the procedure
- Follow-up appointment for a check-up after 8–14 days

9.6.3 Technique 39

Subtle Volumization – Tubercle Definition (Sharp Needle)

This technique produces subtle lip tubercle accentuation. This is regarded as a beauty feature in Asia, in particular, as the heart shape of the lip is accentuated.

Patient Selection

- Patients who have tubercles and a uniform lip shape and want to freshen up these features
- Patients who desire tubercle accentuation

Injection Scheme and Planning (→ Technique 39 – Figs. 1, 2)

A prominent medial tubercle produces a downward turn in the upper lip line at the oral commissure, giving the mouth a heart shape. The technique is very simple. The material is injected into the center of the selected point. The classic points for the freshening-up injection as shown here may be varied as required. When treating the upper lip, care must be taken to ensure that the material is placed at the correct point. If the injection is given further down at the dry/wet boundary, the lip is everted more prominently and thus slightly enlarged.

Technique: linear technique
Direction of insertion: from the front into the center of the marked point
Layer: 3–5 mm deep into the vermillion, from the front
Material: class "S/M soft" product
Volume: max. 0.2 ml per line
Needle: 27–29G sharp needle
Anesthesia: lidocaine cream

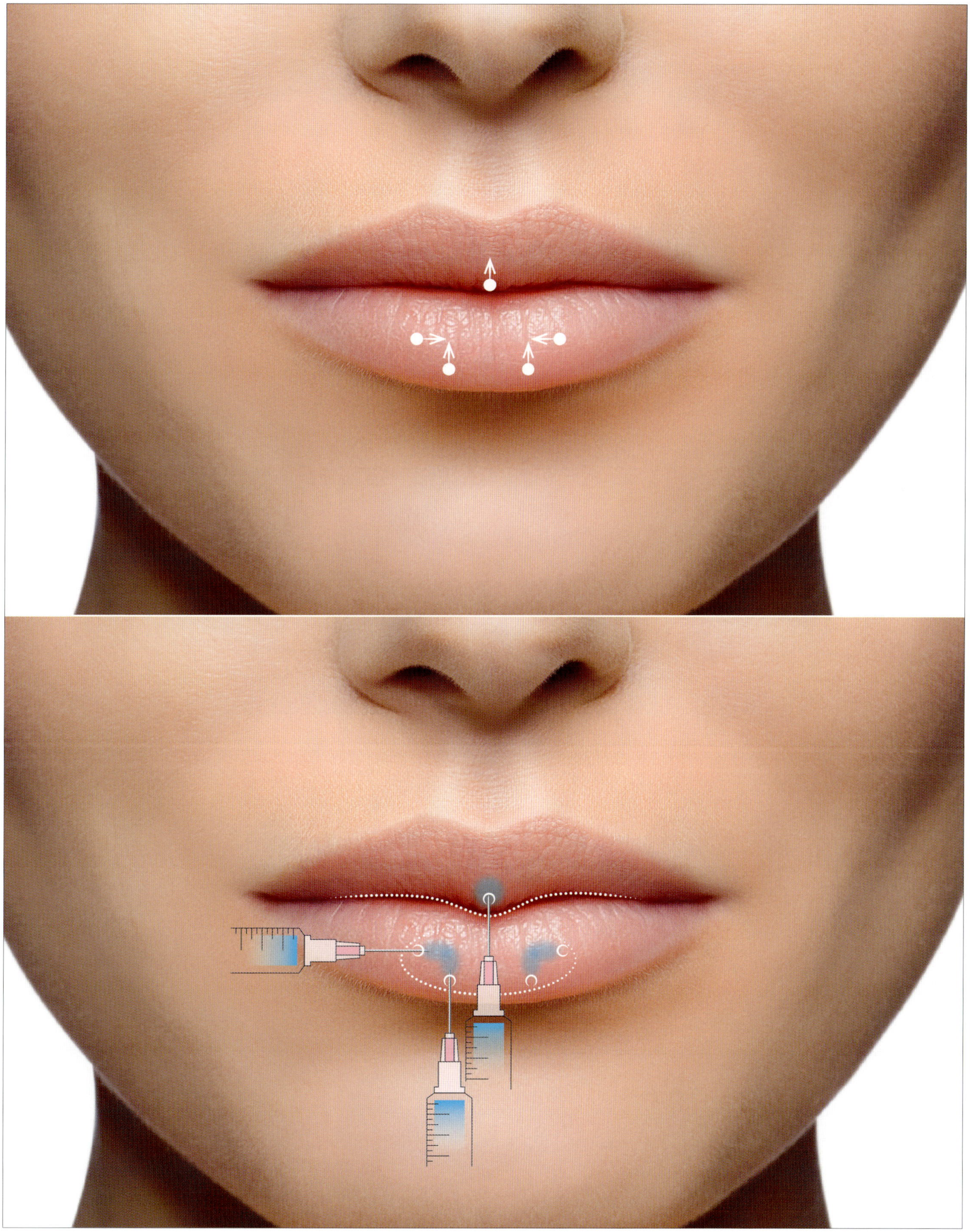

Technique 39 – Figs. 1, 2 Injection scheme and planning for subtle volumization – tubercle definition (sharp needle).

Treatment Method (→ Technique 39 – Figs. 3–5)

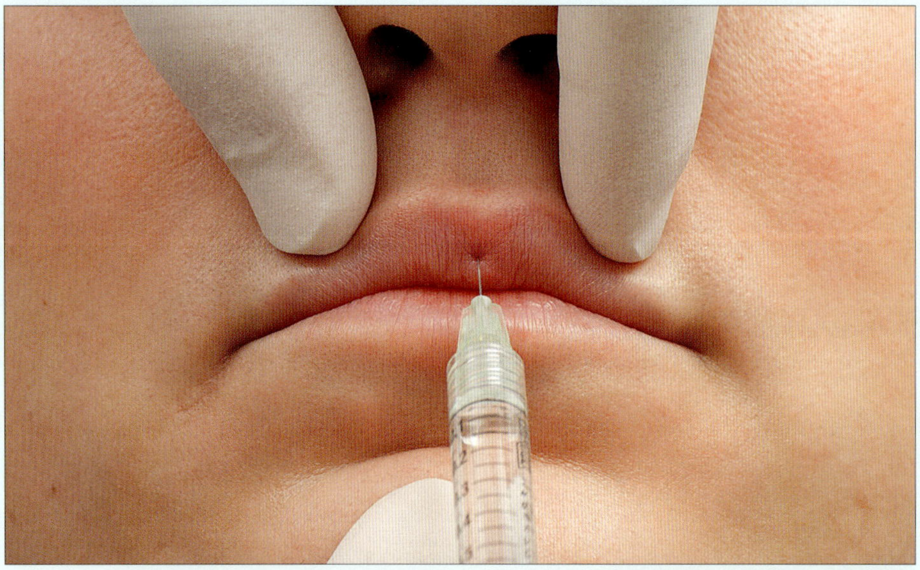

Technique 39 – Fig. 3 Slightly evert the upper lip with the forefinger and hold in place gently between the thumb and forefinger. Insert the needle at the marked point on the vermillion to a depth of c. 2–3 mm. Deliver the material with frequent checks of the syringe plunger. The material should not be placed too close to the oral mucosa because the patient will then be able to feel it with the tongue as an irritating lump.

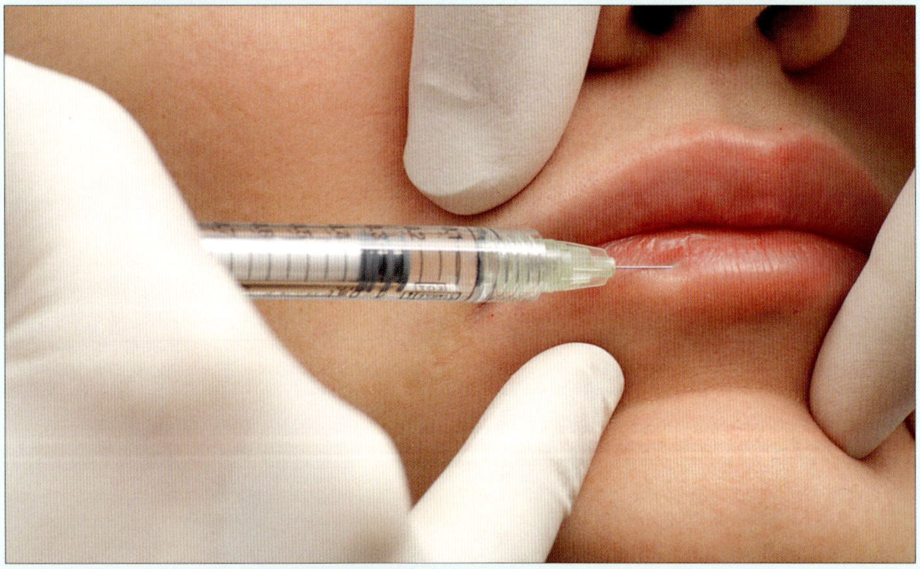

Technique 39 – Fig. 4 If the bolus needs to be distributed slightly more softly over the whole area, deliver the material into the target area from the side when injecting the lower lip tubercles.

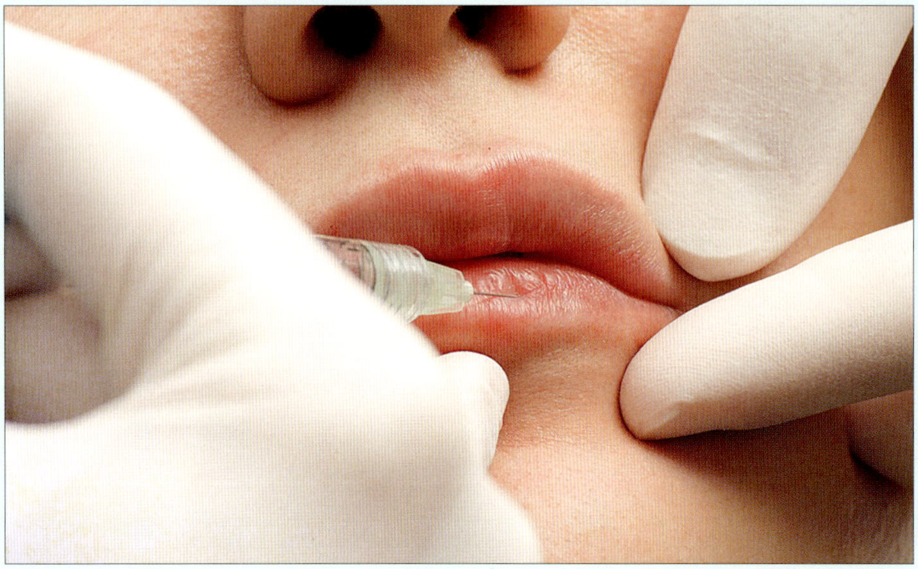

Technique 39 – Fig. 5 If the curvature of the lower lip tubercle needs to be accentuated more strongly, inject the material into the center of the target area from the front.

9

Important Notes

- This technique can cause internal bleeding due to blood vessel injuries.
- It is important not to inject too much material at each site as it may very occasionally become encapsulated.
- If harder, more highly crosslinked products than recommended are used, they may become visible as nodules when the patient smiles.
- Even if small amounts of material are delivered, swellings may occur in the first 2–4 days, obscuring the true results of the treatment.
- The immediate result of the injection can be assessed by asking the patient to stretch the mouth into a wide smile directly after the treatment. This can also be used to check if the material has been distributed uniformly.
- It is advisable to use HA products with lower crosslinking: if these do produce palpable or visible nodules, they can be massaged away more easily if required.

Possible Side Effects

Slight reddening, rarely inflammation, hematomas, commonly swellings

Undesirable Side Effects

Overcorrection with resultant alteration of the shape of the lip or nodule formation, visible bumps if the injection is too superficial, nodules that can be felt with the tongue if injecting up to the mucous membrane border, necrosis

Treatment Protocol at a Glance

- History, evaluation, and patient information
- Informed consent form
- Photo documentation: "before" images
- Analysis and marking of the areas to be treated
- Cleaning
- Thorough disinfection
- Local anesthesia if required (lidocaine cream), conduction anesthesia
- Injection technique: linear technique
- Layer: 3–5 mm deep into the vermillion, from the front
- Material: class "S/M soft" product
- Volume: max. 0.2 ml per line
- Needle: 27–29G sharp needle
- No massage, possibly gentle shaping
- Cooling if required
- Heparin cream for hematomas, ibuprofen p.o., arnica
- Photo documentation: "after" images
- Advice on dos and don'ts after the procedure
- Follow-up appointment for a check-up after 8–14 days

9.6.4 Technique 40

Contouring of the Perioral Line according to Phillip Chang (Sharp Needle)

The aim of the treatment is to lift the upper lip slightly without creating a "duck's bill" effect. The effect of the technique comprises the production of a subtle increase in substance in the cutaneous part of the upper lip. The material is distributed over a larger area, which causes a soft rounding of the entire region. A reduction of the fine perioral lines is a positive side effect (see "Lip Augmentation Technique Virginia" video by Phillip Chang, MD).

Patient Selection

- In mild, age-related lip atrophy and elongation of the cutaneous part of the lip
- For lips that recede naturally at the front and thus appear less voluminous

Injection Scheme and Planning (→ Technique 40 – Figs. 1, 2)

The injection is given into the cutaneous part of the upper lip parallel to its contour and into the vermillion of the lower lip. This causes the lip to protrude upward and outward slightly, making it appear more voluminous.

The contour is injected in a single pass with a sharp needle (27G, 38 mm) inserted into the vermillion border; the material, 0.15 ml per line, is delivered uniformly by retrograde injection. The second line is injected around 5 mm above the first line; this is also injected subcutaneously in a single pass, delivering 0.15 ml of material. In the lower lip contour, the material is injected within the vermillion (see also Technique 6, p 148 ff.). A total of 0.4 ml HA is injected into the entire lower lip contour. Conduction anesthesia is recommended.

Technique: linear technique
Direction of insertion: along the contour, parallel to the contour
Layer: subcutaneous in the vermillion/cutaneous part of the lip and above the upper lip contour in the cutaneous part
Material: class "M viscous" product
Volume: max. 1.0–1.2 ml in total
Needle: 27G sharp needle, 38 mm
Anesthesia: lidocaine cream, conduction anesthesia

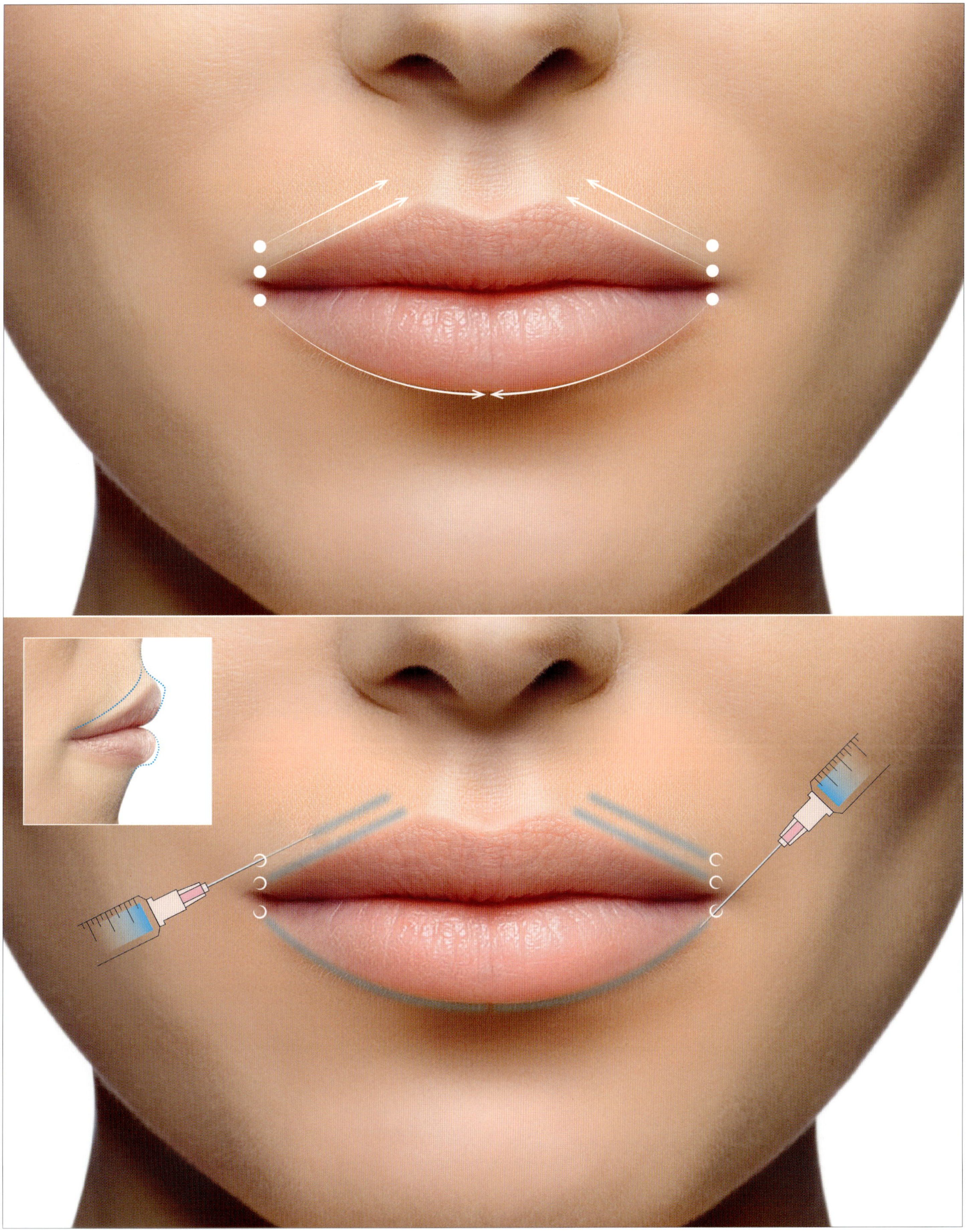

Technique 40 – Figs. 1, 2 Injection scheme and planning for contouring of the perioral line according to Phillip Chang (sharp needle).

Treatment Method (→ Technique 40 – Figs. 3, 4)

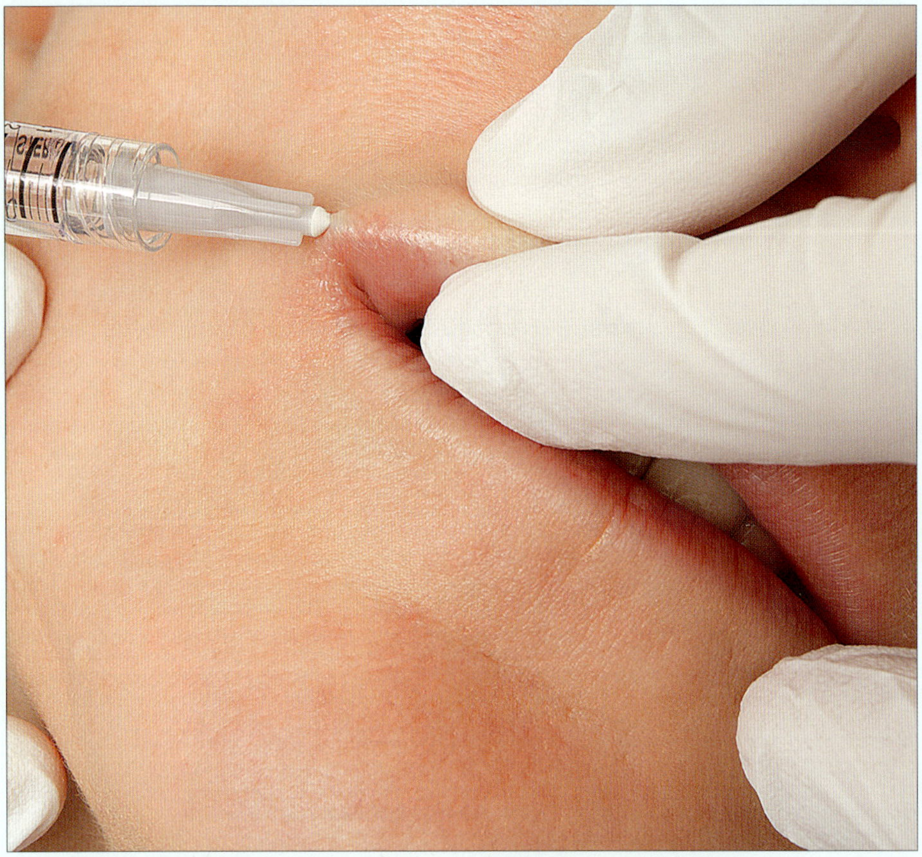

Technique 40 – Fig. 3 To place the first injection accurately into the upper lip contour, grasp the lip between the thumb and forefinger. Once in the contour, advance the needle up to the philtrum. Deliver the material by retrograde injection.

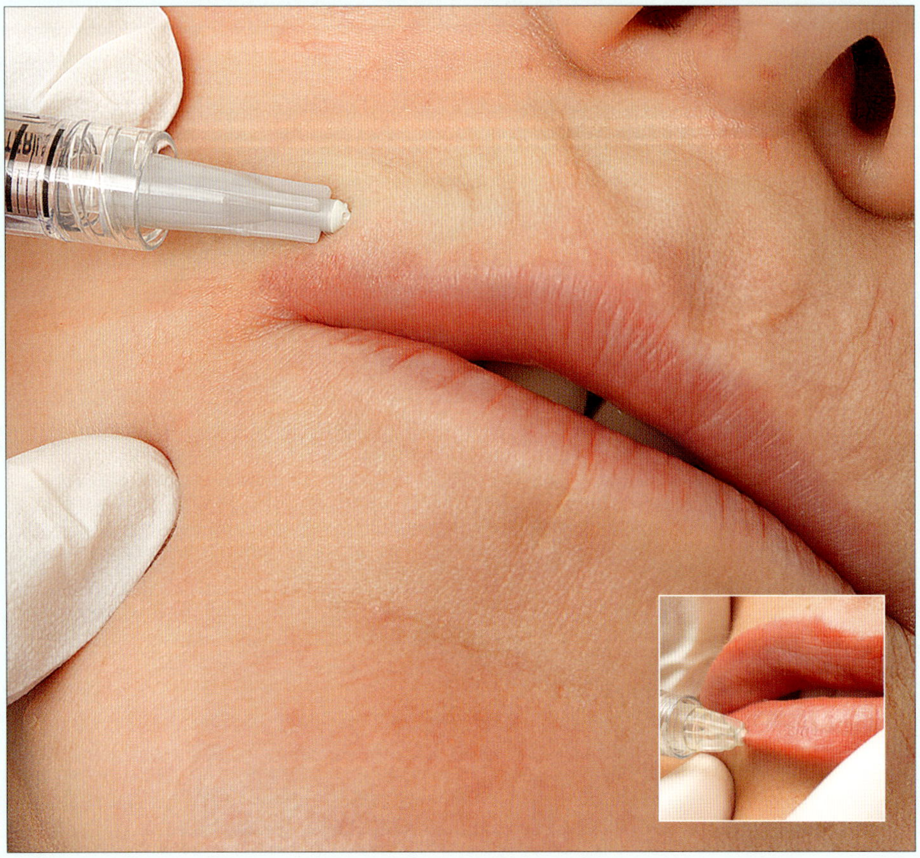

Technique 40 – Fig. 4 Administer the second injection subcutaneously 5 mm above the contour. Advance the needle up to the philtral peak. Raise the needle tip to check if it is located in the correct layer. Deliver the material by retrograde injection. Inject the lower lip contour (inset image) using the classic method described in Technique 6 (p. 148 ff.).

Important Notes

Possible Side Effects

Slight reddening, rarely inflammation, hematomas, swellings

Undesirable Side Effects

Inflammation, overcorrection with resultant alteration of the shape of the lip or nodule formation, asymmetry due to non-uniform delivery of material, necrosis

Treatment Protocol at a Glance

- History, evaluation, and patient information
- Informed consent form
- Photo documentation: "before" images
- Analysis and marking of the areas to be treated
- Cleaning
- Thorough disinfection
- Local anesthesia if required (lidocaine cream), conduction anesthesia
- Injection technique: linear technique
- Layer: subcutaneous in the vermillion/cutaneous part of the lip, and above the upper lip contour in the cutaneous part
- Material: class "M viscous" product
- Volume: max. 1.0–1.2 ml in total
- Needle: 27G sharp needle, 38 mm
- No massage
- Cooling if required
- Heparin cream for hematomas, ibuprofen p.o., arnica
- Photo documentation: "after" images
- Advice on dos and don'ts after the procedure
- Follow-up appointment for a check-up after 8–14 days

9.6.5 Technique 41

Indentation in the Center of the Lip (Sharp Needle)

A length of dental floss in combination with the bolus technique is used to create a central indentation in the lower lip, and also in the upper lip if desired, to give the lips a sensual expression.

Patient Selection

- If the patient wants to change the appearance of the lips in this way
- If the natural indentation in the center of the lip has been reduced by aging processes and the patient wishes to restore it
- Where there is a difference in volume between the upper and lower lip and/or between the right and left side of the lip

Injection Scheme and Planning (→ Technique 41 – Figs. 1, 2)

This thread treatment is used primarily in the lower lip. However, the upper lip can also be treated in this way to make the central groove more pronounced. Following an accurate analysis, the lower and upper lips are marked to divide them into four quadrants. A piece of dental floss 15-cm long is knotted at one end and threaded through the two mandibular anterior teeth so that the knot catches between the teeth at the back and can be pulled tight. The thread is now pulled over the marked point on the upper lip and toward the chin, dividing the lip in two. The same defined volume of HA is placed into the orbicularis oris muscle on either side of the taut thread, on the left and right beside the notch, thus producing an artificial groove that creates the desired visual effect.

If desired, this procedure can be repeated on the upper lip. The result depends on its volume: if the upper lip is very voluminous in the middle or if the tubercle is too prominent, the lip may become misshapen, producing an unnatural treatment result.

Technique: bolus technique
Direction of insertion: into the body of the muscle
Layer: vermillion, into the orbicularis oris muscle
Material: class "M soft" product
Volume: max. 0.15 ml per bolus, 0.6–1 ml in total
Needle: 27–29G sharp needle
Anesthesia: lidocaine cream, conduction anesthesia

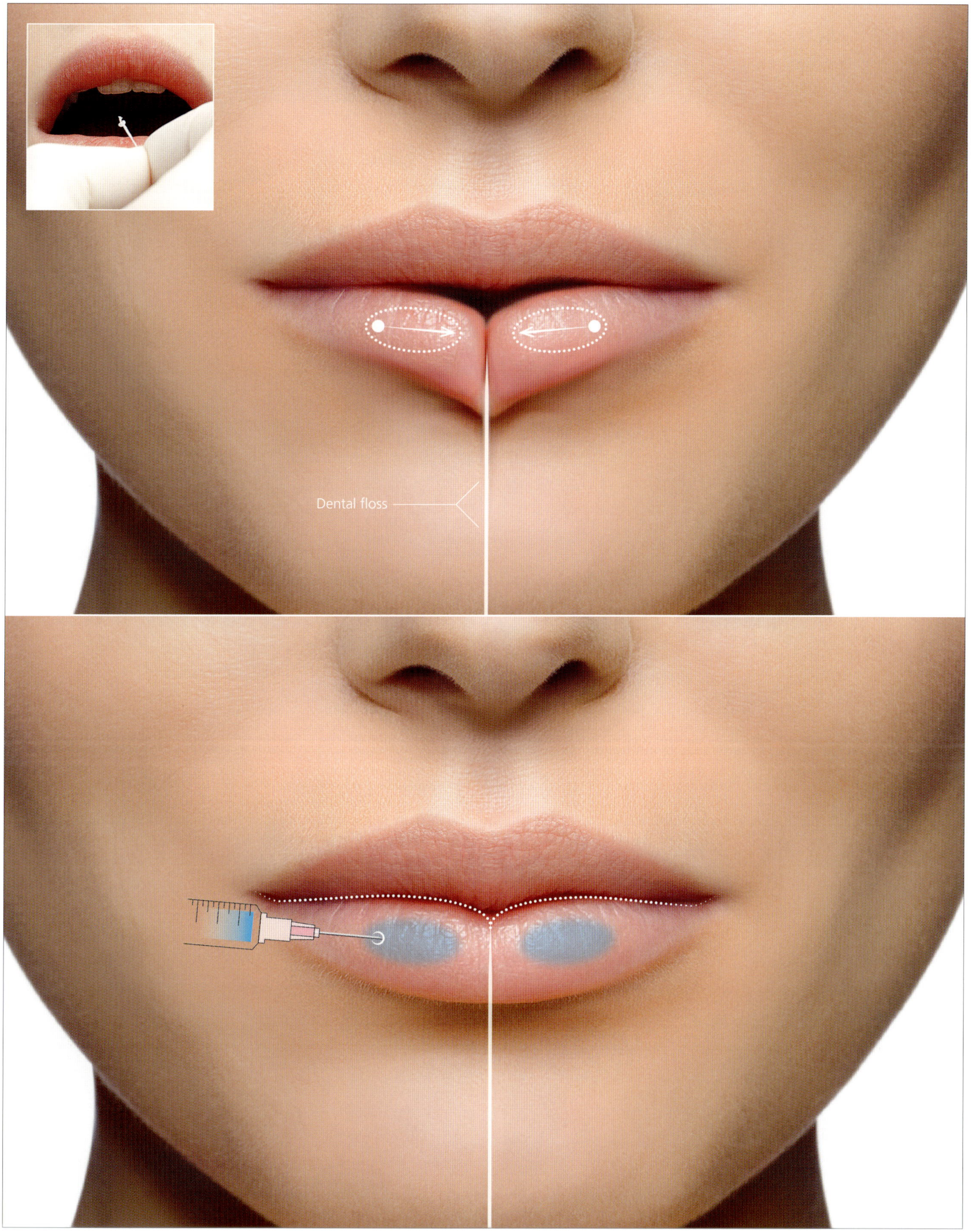

Technique 41 – Figs. 1, 2 Injection scheme and planning for an indentation in the center of the lip (sharp needle).

Treatment Method (→ Technique 41 – Figs. 3–8)

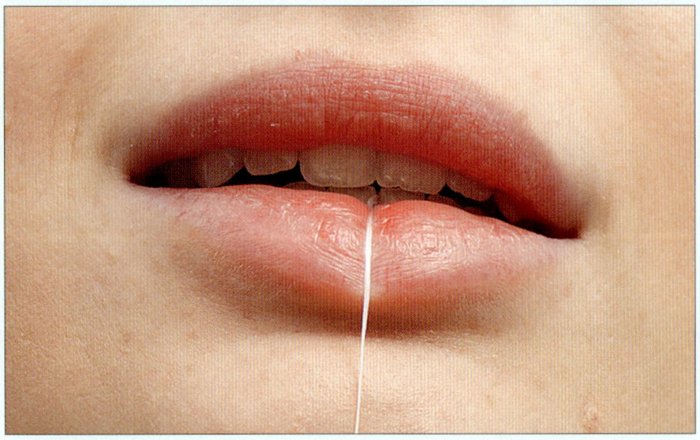

Technique 41 – Fig. 3 Knot one end of the length of floss and thread it between the two mandibular central incisors so that it lies exactly in the middle. An assistant, the therapist or the patient needs to hold the thread firmly during the treatment, maintaining the same degree of tension.

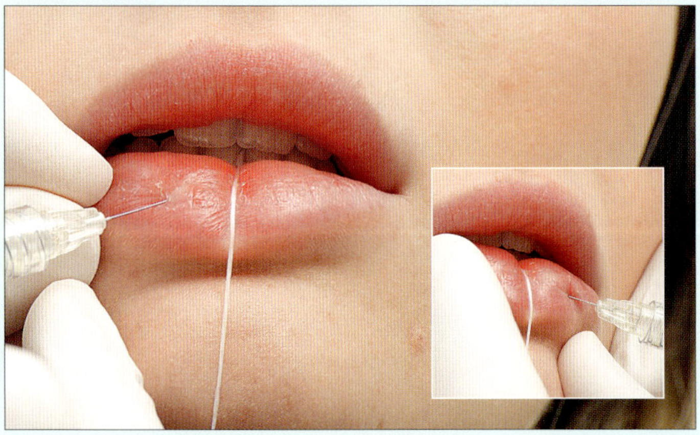

Technique 41 – Fig. 4 The first dose of material into the upper lip should always be given while keeping a close eye on the syringe to check the delivered volume. The bulge in the tissue produced by the injected bolus is clearly visible. Inject exactly the same amount of HA into the other half of the lower lip.

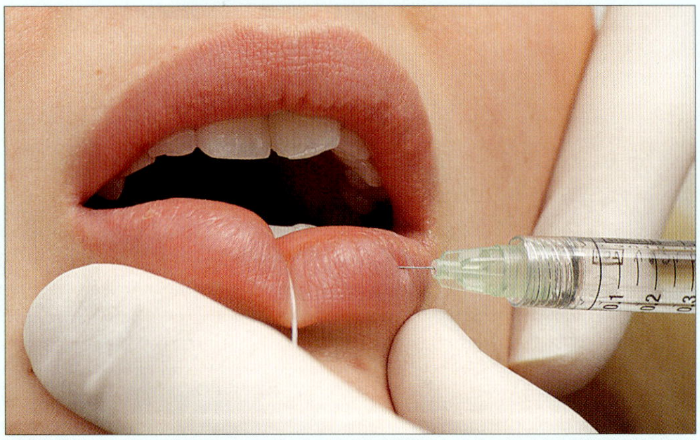

Technique 41 – Fig. 5 The closer the material is placed to the thread, the sharper the groove will be. Conversely, the further away from the thread the material is placed, the softer the indentation in the center of the lip will appear.

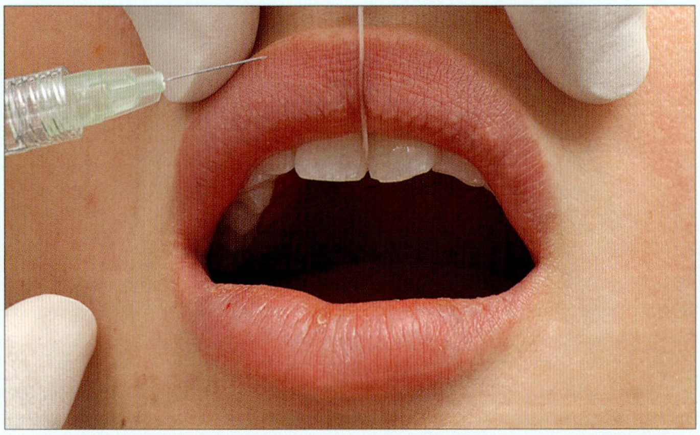

Technique 41 – Fig. 6 This procedure may be repeated a bit more moderately on the upper lip. Knot the thread and fix it into place between the two maxillary central incisors with the knot at the back, then pull upward toward the nose. If no assistant is available, pull the thread upward with the free hand, keeping the hand steady with the thumb and forefinger on the patient's upper lip.

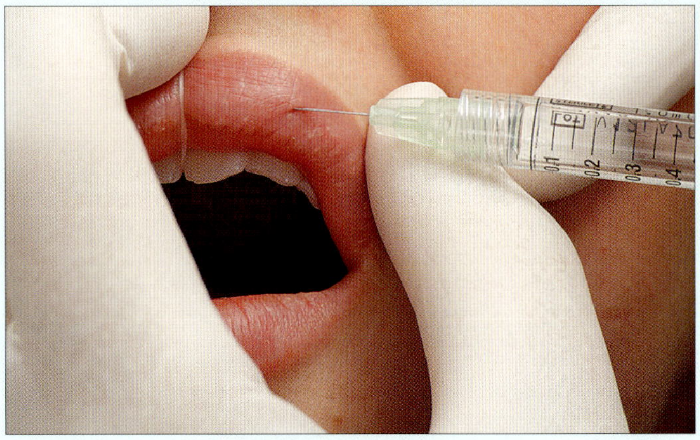

Technique 41 – Fig. 7 Alternatively, the thread may be held in place on the lip with one finger. Insert the needle from the side to inject the bolus. Repeat on the other side of the upper lip.

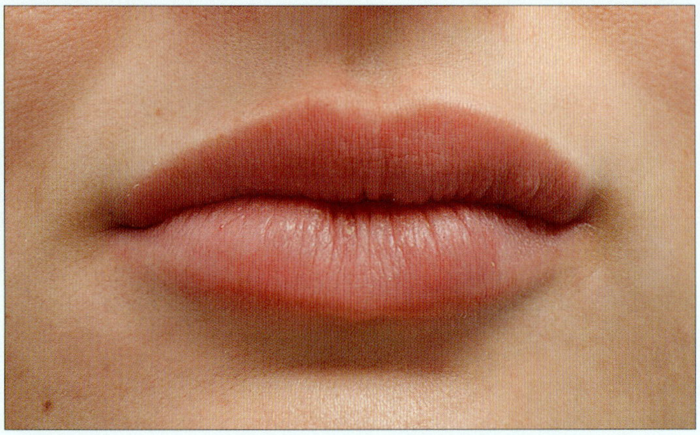

Technique 41 – Fig. 8 The desired indentation in the center of the lip can also be massaged into shape slightly.

Important Notes

- If a lip is inherently asymmetric, the therapist will need to balance this out by delivering different amounts of material on each side. For this reason, the pre-treatment analysis is very important.
- The technique is not feasible if the patient has a bridge or too little space between the central incisors. If the space is very wide, a plastic bead or a small piece of wood 1-cm long (e.g. broken off a toothpick) can be tied to the end of the thread in order to hold it in place against the teeth inside the oral cavity.

Possible Side Effects

Slight reddening, rarely inflammation, hematomas, mild to more severe swellings

Undesirable Side Effects

Inflammation, overcorrection with resultant alteration of the shape of the lip or nodule formation, asymmetry due to non-uniform delivery of material, necrosis

Treatment Protocol at a Glance

- History, evaluation, and patient information
- Informed consent form
- Photo documentation: "before" images
- Analysis and marking of the areas to be treated
- Cleaning
- Thorough disinfection
- Local anesthesia if required (lidocaine cream), conduction anesthesia
- Injection technique: bolus technique, 2 boluses each into the lower and upper lip
- Layer: vermillion, into the orbicularis oris muscle
- Material: class "M soft" product
- Volume: max. 0.15 ml per bolus, 0.6–1 ml in total
- Needle: 27–29G sharp needle
- No massage, possibly gentle shaping
- Cooling if required
- Heparin cream for hematomas, ibuprofen p.o., arnica
- Photo documentation: "after" images
- Advice on dos and don'ts after the procedure
- Follow-up appointment for a check-up after 8–14 days

9.6.6 Technique 42

Widening the Arch of the Lower Lip (Sharp Needle)

The aim here is to use HA injections to achieve a subtle, symmetrical realignment of the arch of the lower lip in the lateral direction in order to make the lower lip appear fuller and wider.

Patient Selection

- If the Cupid's bow is too spread out or the lower lip is too small
- If the patient desires a modeling and beautification treatment

Injection Scheme and Planning (→ Technique 42 – Figs. 1, 2)

The points on the lower lip opposite the Cupid's bow are subtly accentuated. As the distance between the injection points increases, the lateral realignment of the lower lip becomes more pronounced. The injection is given with a sharp needle using the linear technique. The needle is inserted 1 cm below the lower lip contour, at points located below each Cupid's bow peak, and no more than one third of the entire width of the lip from the mouth corner toward the center (see Fig. 2, left). The material is injected along a line that runs from the chin toward the vermillion, with the needle going upward. The material is delivered only once the needle is in the vermillion itself. The volume of material placed into the vermillion depends on how much the edge of the lip is to be accentuated. The material is delivered by retrograde injection. If the aim is to widen the lower lip visually, the distance to the mouth corner is reduced (see Fig. 2, right).

Optional: To further realign and stabilize the lip contour between the two points, an additional line may be injected into the contour between the first two points. To define this line clearly, it is helpful to use the thumb and forefinger to exert pressure against the material while it is being injected.

Technique: linear technique
Direction of insertion: upward from below
Layer: subcutaneous
Material: class "M viscous" product
Volume: c. 0.1 ml per line/bolus, c. 0.2 ml in total
Needle: 27G sharp needle
Anesthesia: lidocaine cream

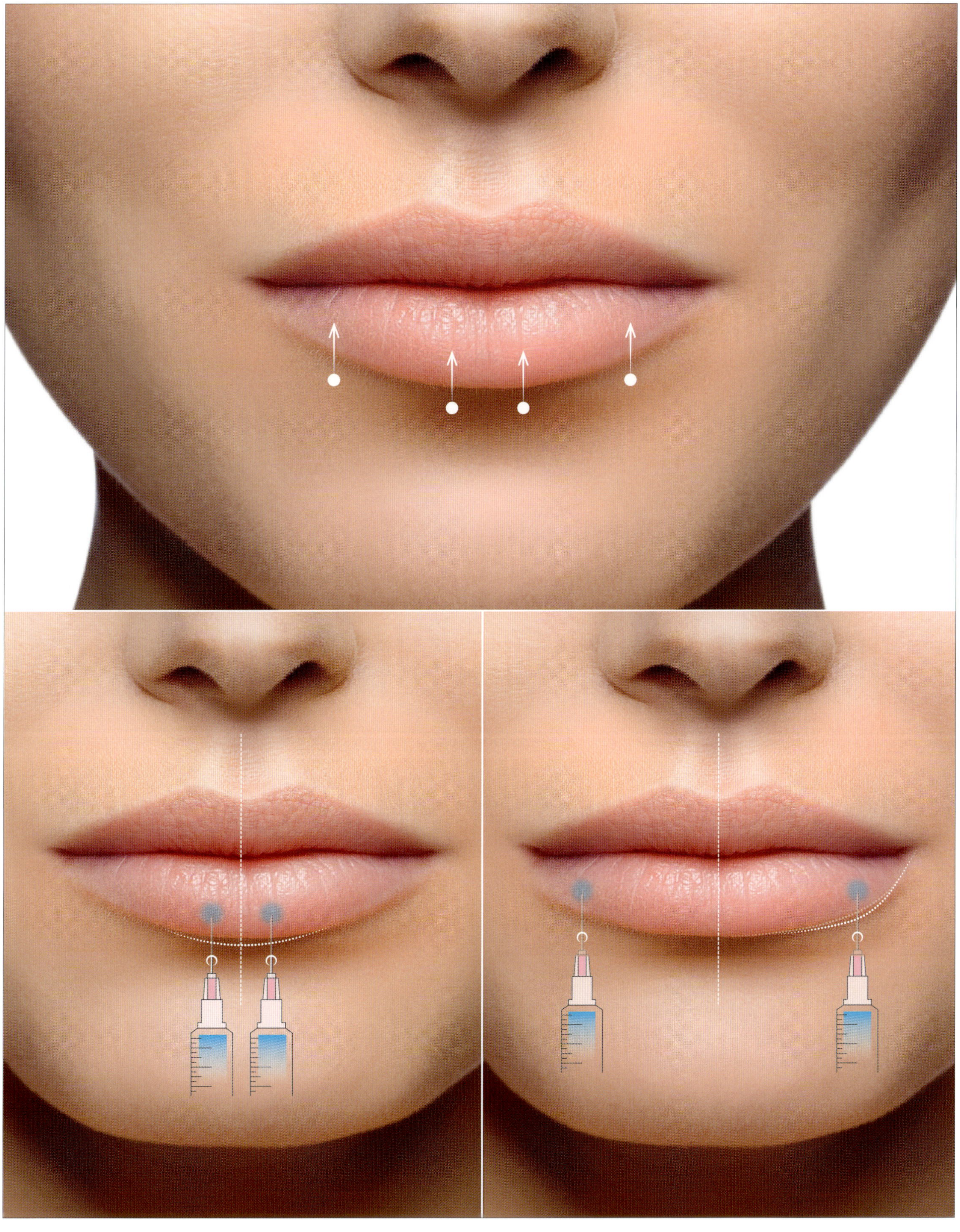

Technique 42 – Figs. 1, 2 Injection scheme and planning for widening the arch of the lower lip (sharp needle).

Treatment Method (→ Technique 42 – Figs. 3, 4)

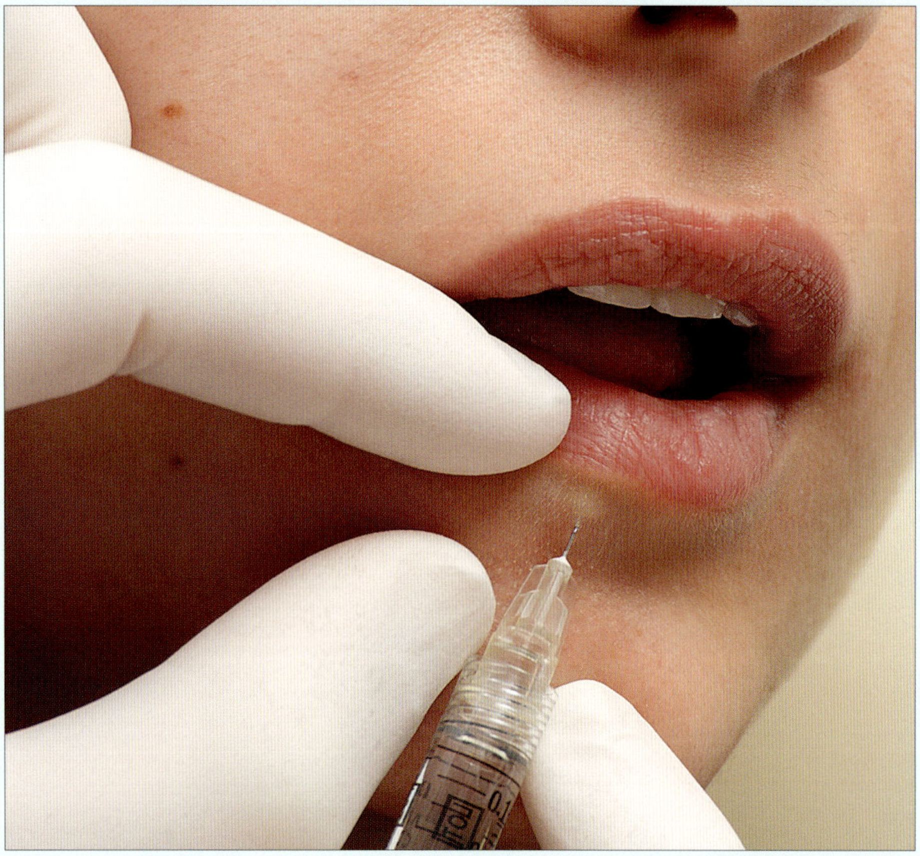

Technique 42 – Fig. 3 Mark the zones to be treated before the injection. Pull the lip up gently and hold it in place so that the needle can be placed accurately. Deliver the material as a bolus that tapers off toward the end in order to create the desired edge.

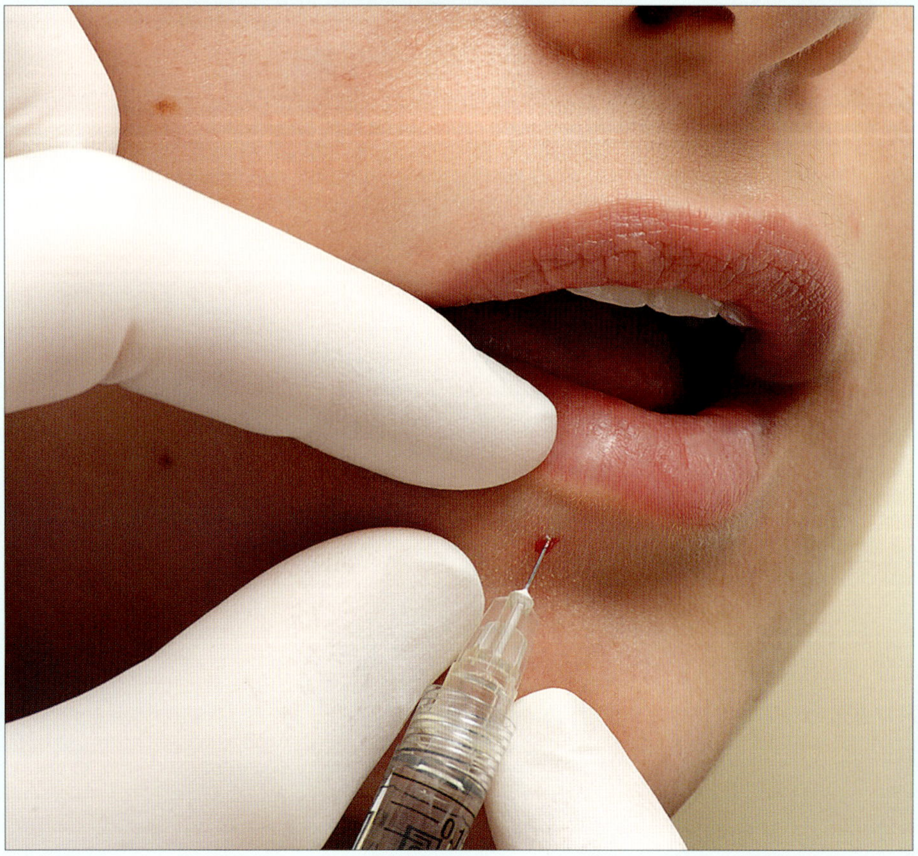

Technique 42 – Fig. 4 The material shows up as a small bulge close to the lip contour.

9

Important Notes

- The material should not be placed too superficially. The injection starts when the needle is located within the vermillion.
- To make the edge of the lip more prominent, it may be shaped slightly with the thumb and forefinger.

Possible Side Effects

Slight reddening, rarely inflammation, rarely hematomas, rarely swellings

Undesirable Side Effects

Inflammation, overcorrection with resultant alteration of the shape of the lip or nodule formation, asymmetry due to non-uniform delivery of material, necrosis

Treatment Protocol at a Glance

- History, evaluation, and patient information
- Informed consent form
- Photo documentation: "before" images
- Analysis and marking of the areas to be treated
- Cleaning
- Thorough disinfection
- Local anesthesia if required (lidocaine cream)
- Injection technique: linear technique
- Layer: subcutaneous
- Material: class "M viscous" product
- Volume: c. 0.1 ml per line/bolus, c. 0.2 ml in total
- Needle: 27G sharp needle
- No massage, possibly gentle shaping
- Cooling if required
- Heparin cream for hematomas, ibuprofen p.o., arnica
- Photo documentation: "after" images
- Advice on dos and don'ts after the procedure
- Follow-up appointment for a check-up after 8–14 days

9.6.7 Technique 43

Correcting a Previously Treated Lip (Sharp Needle)

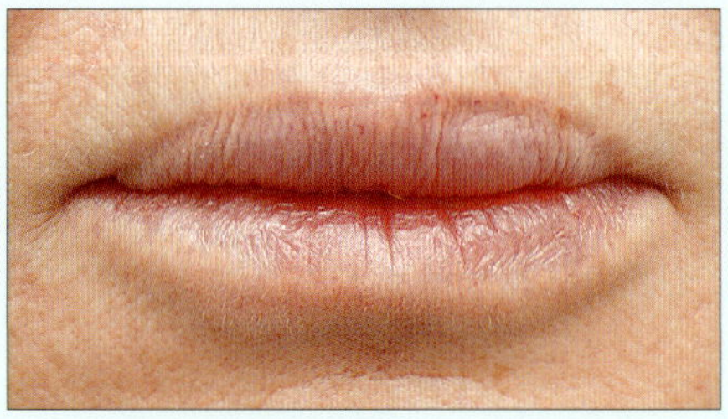

When patients present to the practice with previously treated lips that need correction, their lips show irregularities, nodules, and areas of asymmetry that can be perceived visually or by touch (see image on the right). The causes include encapsulated HA boluses or excess HA placed as a depot in one place, non-uniform injections or even scarring due to frequent injections. The treatment goal is to correct these deformities – either by breaking up or dissolving the nodules (see Chap. 6.4.1, p. 87) or, as shown here, by correcting the irregularities with the administration of HA.

One common and undesirable side effect of filler treatments is that injected HA is encapsulated with connective tissue at certain points and cannot be absorbed if the material was delivered irregularly or in excessive amounts. If the therapist is unable to dissolve or break up these pockets of material, the surrounding tissue can be carefully filled with a soft HA to even out the irregularities.

In addition, if frequent bolus injections are given into the lip, the hollows created in the tissue once these boluses have been absorbed may remain in place. If the material "slips" into a tissue pocket of this type during an injection and fails to distribute uniformly through the tissue, this can also cause irregularities. Where this is the case, it is advisable to inject less or to perform the treatment in two sessions.

Patient Selection

- If there are palpable or visible irregularities in the lip following a filler treatment

Injection Scheme and Planning (→ Technique 43 – Figs. 1–6)

Correction of previously treated lips is a challenge for every therapist. First, it will be necessary to determine which product was injected and when. Then, the therapist needs to decide whether to inject the previously treated lips with HA to even out the irregularities or to correct them in some other way. Depending on the indication, the corrective treatment requires the use of the linear, point, and/or bolus technique.

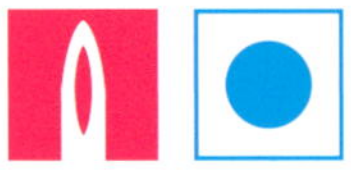

Technique: linear, point and/or bolus technique, depending on how much material needs to be injected in which layer
Material: class "S/M soft" product
Volume: depending on requirement
Needle: 27–30G sharp needle
Anesthesia: lidocaine cream, conduction anesthesia

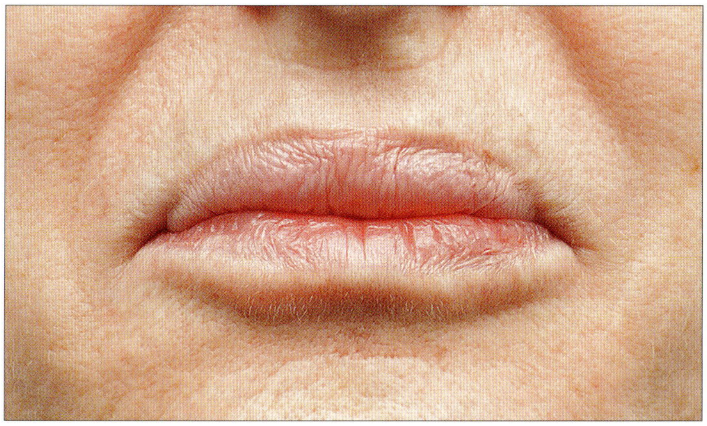

Technique 43 – Fig. 1 If the patient presses the lips together tightly, this action clearly reveals where the unwanted material is located.

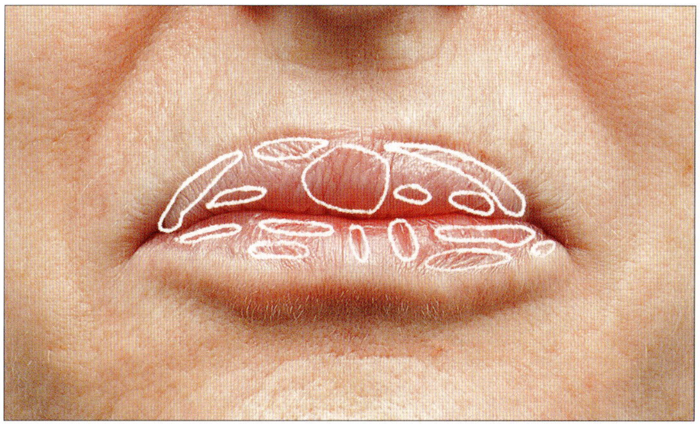

Technique 43 – Fig. 2 Precise mapping of the irregularities with the aid of a marker is essential when drawing up a treatment plan and is a prerequisite for a good treatment result. The markings show up the irregularities created by the previous treatment, defining areas that need to be injected to even out the texture of the lips.

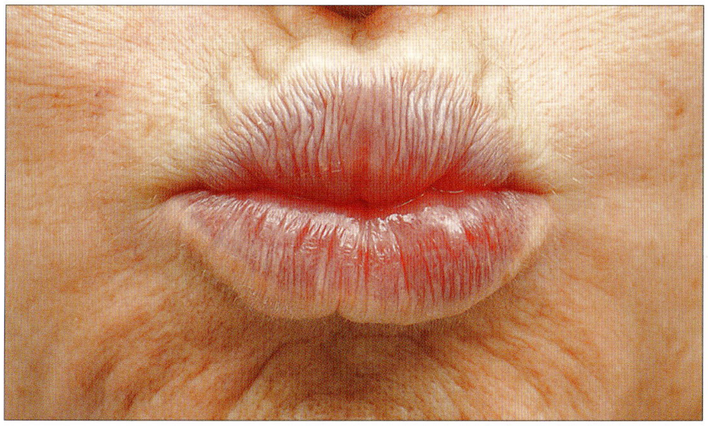

Technique 43 – Fig. 3 For a comprehensive analysis of the treatment requirements, the lips should be observed when moving ...

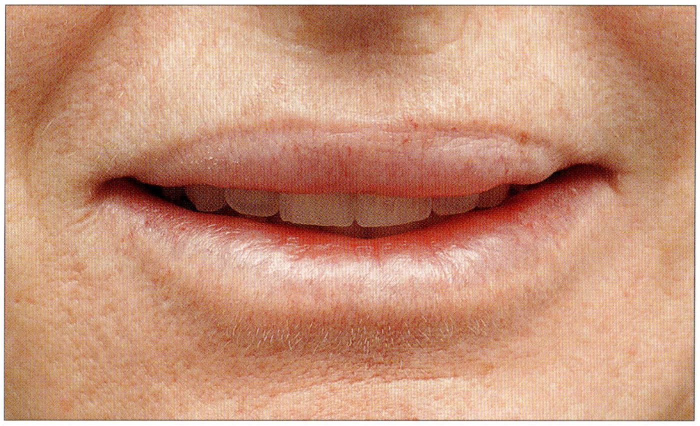

Technique 43 – Fig. 4 ... and when they are in a relaxed state.

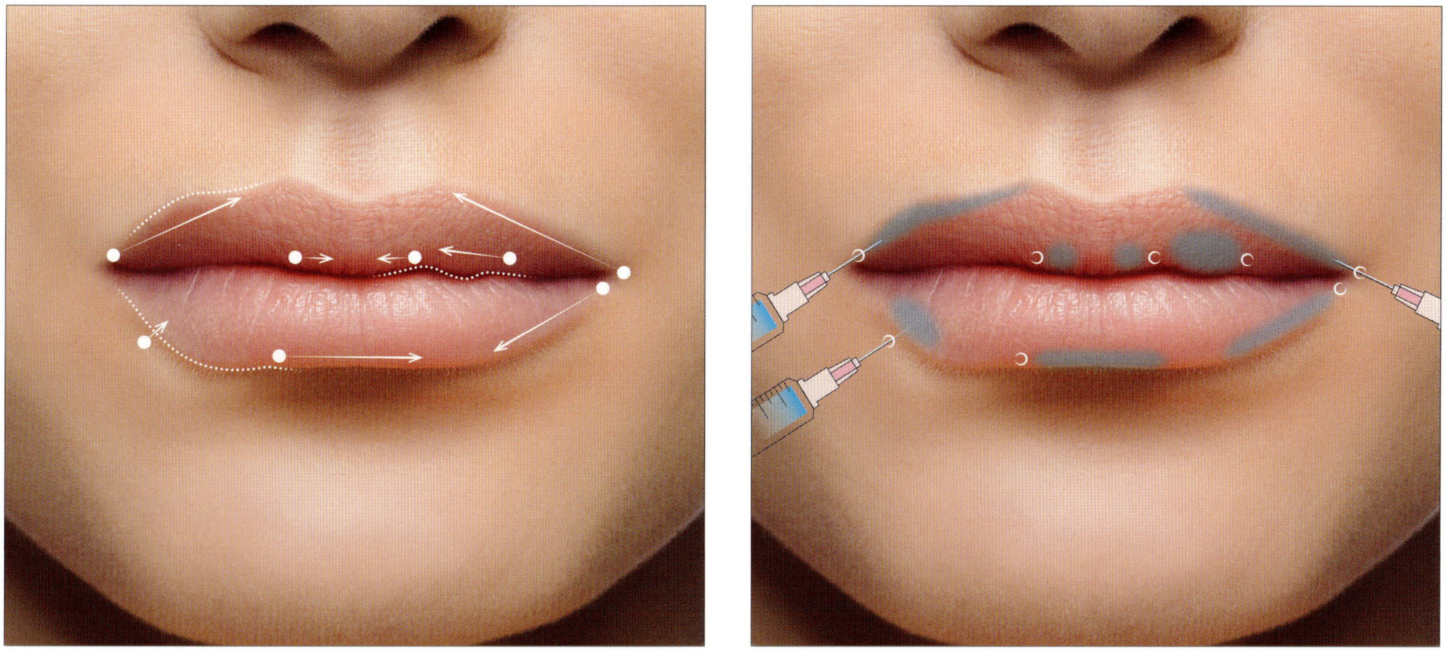

Technique 43 – Figs. 5, 6 Injection scheme and planning for correcting a previously treated lip (sharp needle).

Treatment Method (→ Technique 43 – Figs. 7–10)

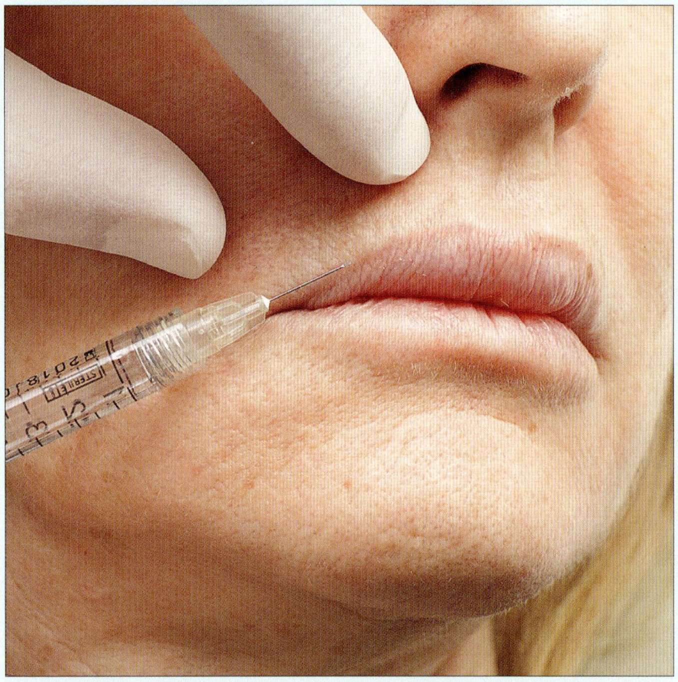

Technique 43 – Fig. 7 Stretch the skin area gently with the thumb and forefinger to reduce pain. First insert the sharp needle into the vermillion along the shadow below the contour, directing the needle toward the philtrum.

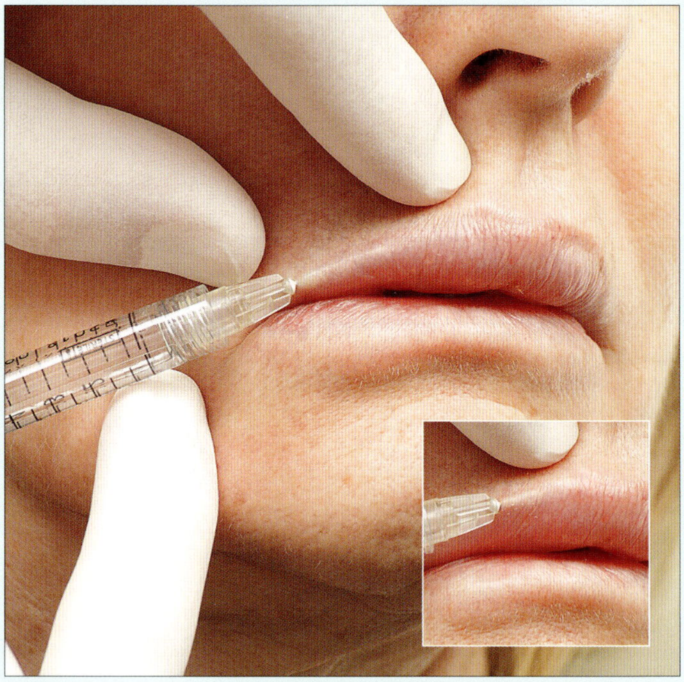

Technique 43 – Fig. 8 While the material is being delivered, the lips need to be relaxed so that the therapist can see where the material is going in.

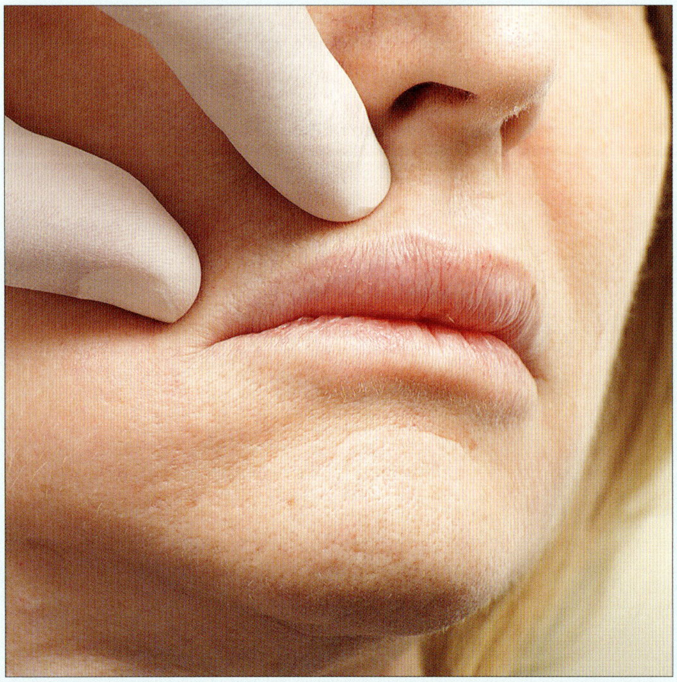

Technique 43 – Fig. 9 Visual check: result after the correction of irregularities caused by injections into the right upper lip, in comparison with the left side.

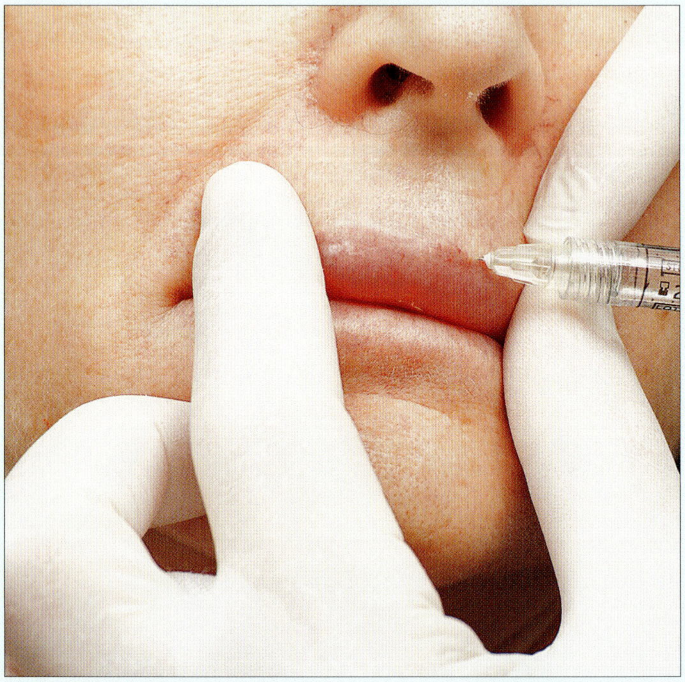

Technique 43 – Fig. 10 The visible boluses remaining after the previous treatment need to be evened out from all sides by injecting HA. Hold the tissue in place without stretching it. Any overcorrection must be avoided.

Important Notes

- It is often a challenge to correct large nodules uniformly.

Possible Side Effects

Slight reddening, rarely inflammation, commonly hematomas, more severe swellings, pain for 2–3 days

Undesirable Side Effects

Inflammation, overcorrection with resultant alteration of the shape of the lip or nodule formation, asymmetry due to non-uniform delivery of material, necrosis

Treatment Protocol at a Glance

- History, evaluation, and patient information
- Informed consent form
- Photo documentation: "before" images
- Analysis and marking of the areas to be treated
- Cleaning
- Thorough disinfection
- Local anesthesia (lidocaine cream) or conduction anesthesia if required
- Injection technique: linear, point, and/or bolus technique
- Layer: according to indication
- Material: class "S/M soft" product
- Volume: as required
- Needle: 27–30G sharp needle
- No massage
- Cooling if required
- Heparin cream for hematomas, ibuprofen p.o., arnica
- Photo documentation: "after" images
- Advice on dos and don'ts after the procedure
- Follow-up appointment for a check-up after 8–14 days

9.6.8 Technique 44

Correcting Areas of Asymmetry (Sharp Needle/Blunt Cannula)

In most cases, any asymmetry of the lips – regardless of whether it was caused by an injury, whether it is a side effect of injection treatments or whether it is genetically determined – can only be corrected to a limited extent.

Patient Selection

- For asymmetrically shaped lips

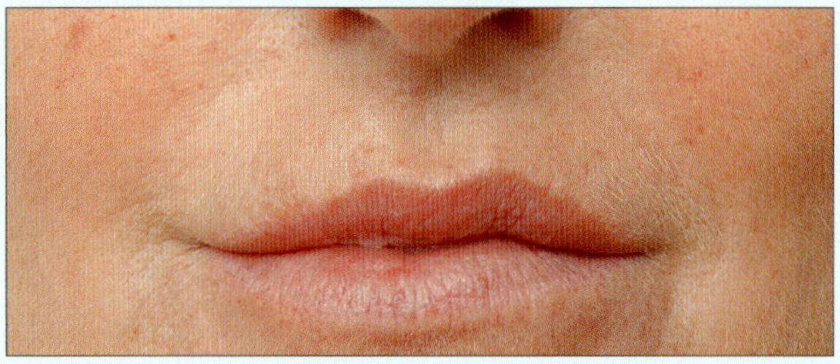

Asymmetries of the upper and lower lip that need correcting.

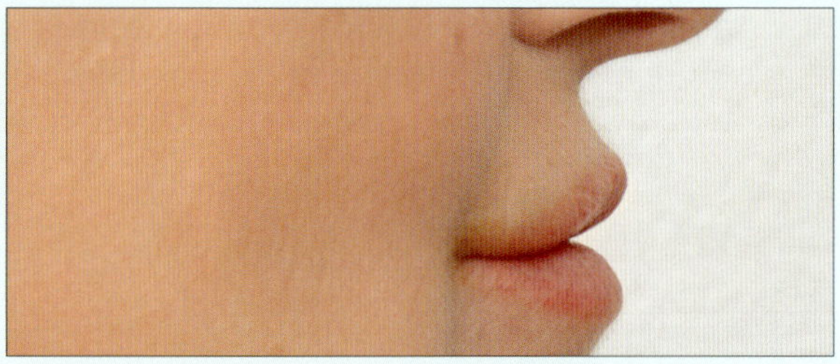

Side view of the inwardly folded right upper lip.

9

Injection Scheme and Planning (→ Technique 44 – Figs. 1, 2)

Correction of an asymmetric lip is a challenge for every therapist, as the limits are often set by the anatomical conditions. Once the reasons for the asymmetry have been determined, the lips are subjected to a detailed analysis and the zones that need treatment are marked, as in the following examples:

1. The lower lip lacks pigmentation on the left side. This cannot always be balanced out with an HA injection. The volume deficit, which causes additional narrowing of the left lower lip, can be built up by the targeted delivery of small boluses (see Techniques 25 or 26, pp. 226 ff. and 230 ff., respectively).

2. The upper part of the right upper lip is flattened. Here, the therapist can attempt to balance out the volume either with the cannula technique or with a sharp needle.

3. The upper lip is inverted on the right side between the mouth corner and the Cupid's bow. HA injection into the dry/wet boundary using the pillar technique (see Technique 45, p. 306 ff.) may be used in an attempt to evert it slightly and bring it forward, making the vermillion more visible.

4. The right philtrum is flattened, and the right Cupid's bow peak is lower than the left one. This can be adjusted with Techniques 9 and 10 (see pp. 160 ff. and 164 ff., respectively).

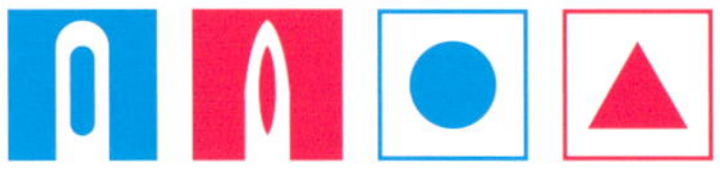

Technique: linear, point, and/or bolus technique, depending on how much material needs to be injected into which layer
Material: class "S/M soft" and/or "S/M viscous" product, according to indication
Volume: depending on requirement
Needle: 27–29G sharp needle, 27G blunt cannula
Anesthesia: lidocaine cream, conduction anesthesia

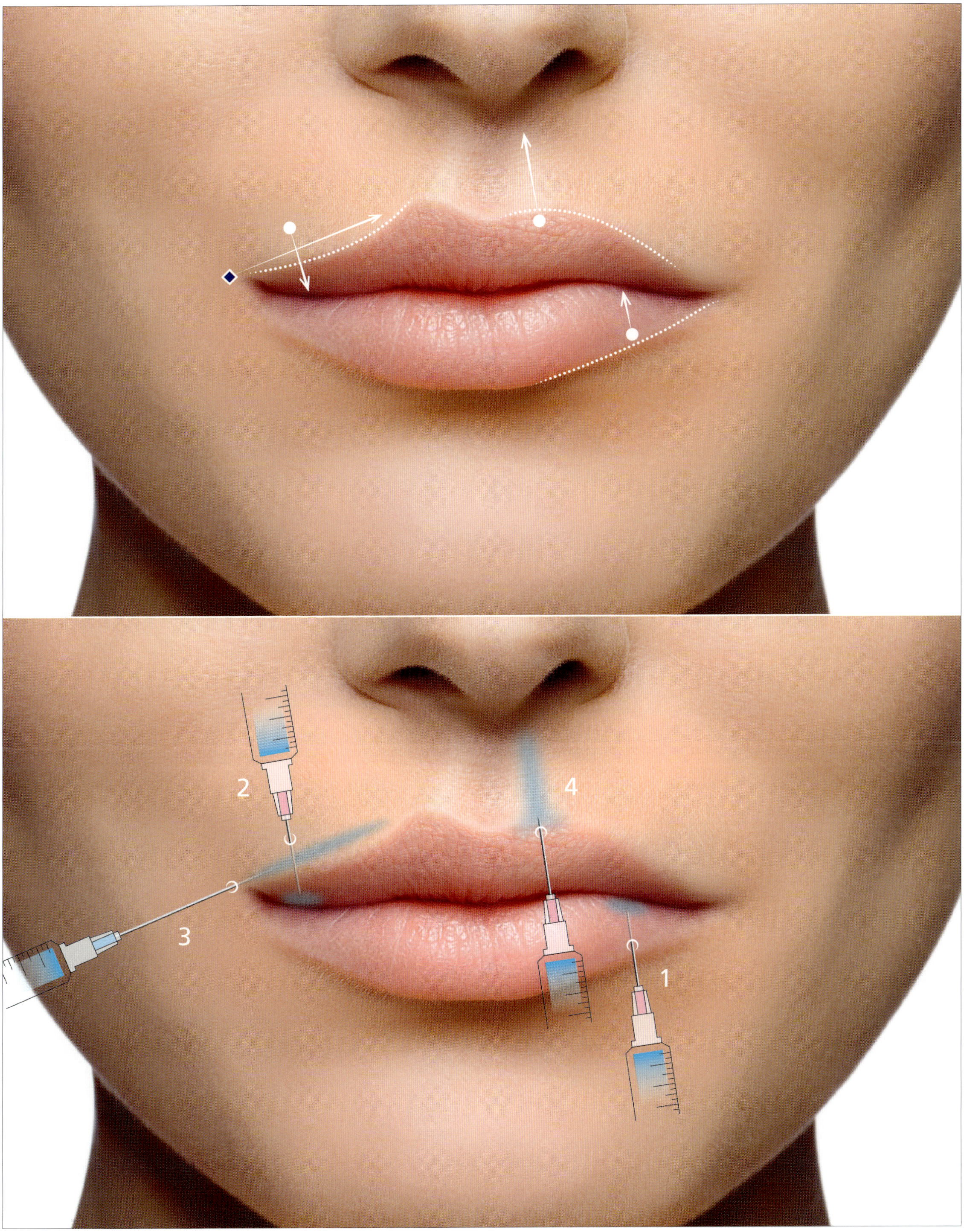

Technique 44 – Figs. 1, 2 Injection scheme and planning for correcting areas of asymmetry (sharp needle/blunt cannula).

Treatment Method (→ Technique 44 – Figs. 3–8)

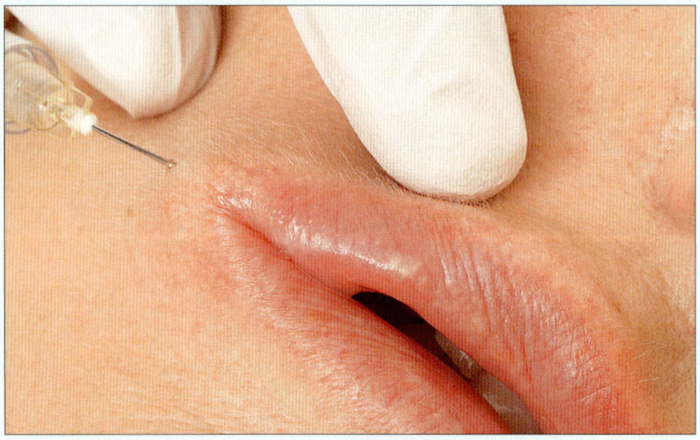

Technique 44 – Fig. 3 Using the linear technique with a cannula, inject the HA into the lower part of the right upper lip across the dry/wet boundary.

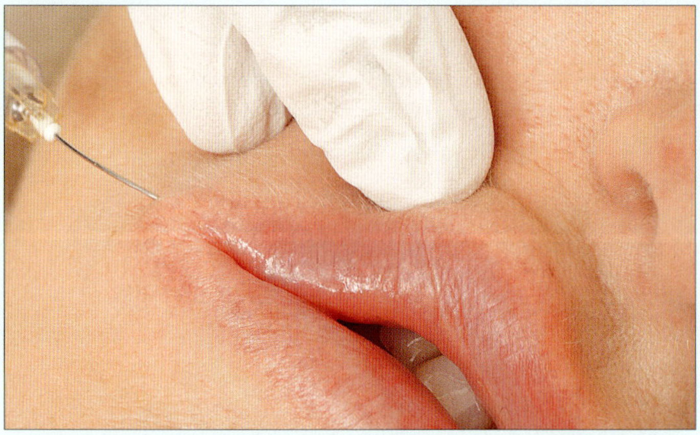

Technique 44 – Fig. 4 Pull the lip upward with the opposite hand so that the dry/wet boundary becomes visible. Negotiate the cannula into the wet zone, teasing apart the tissue, and bring the right upper lip forward more prominently by delivering one or two parallel lines of HA. Add a bit of volume to the lower lip as well (not shown).

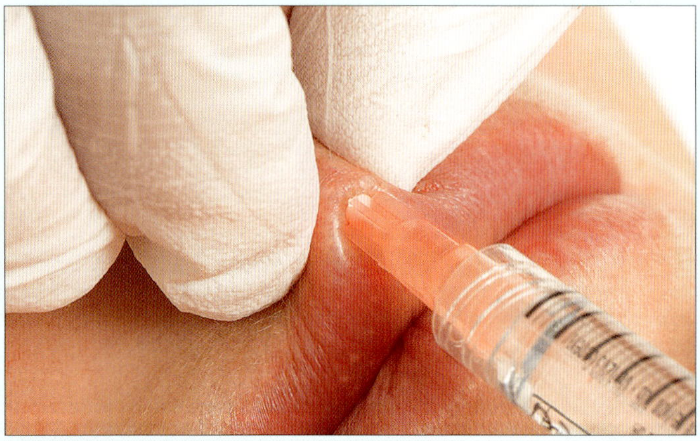

Technique 44 – Fig. 5 The Cupid's bow can be pulled upward slightly by reconstructing the right philtrum.

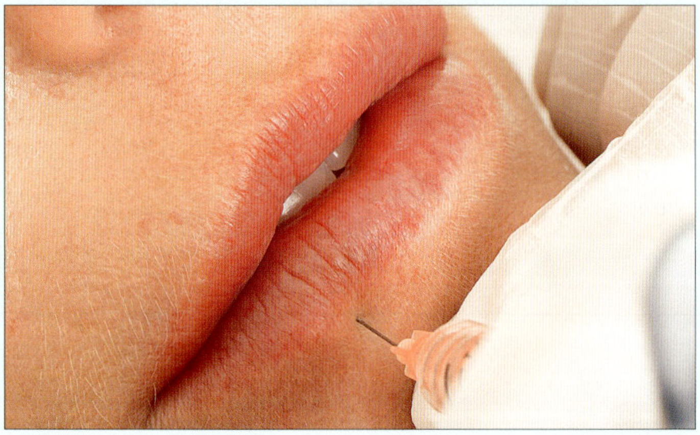

Technique 44 – Fig. 6 Use the bolus technique through the cutaneous part of the lip (Technique 24) if specific points of the lip need to be brought forward.

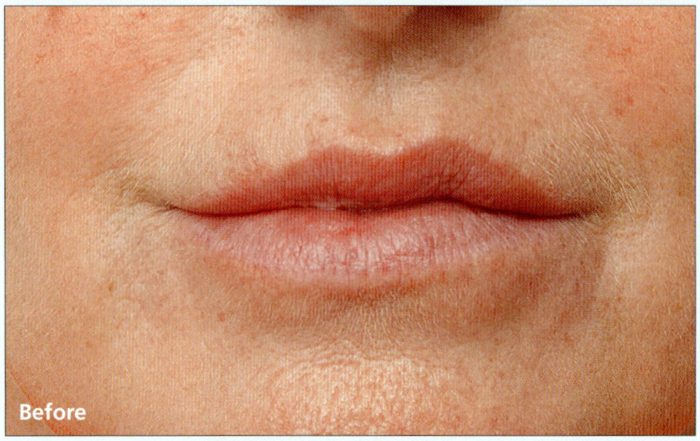

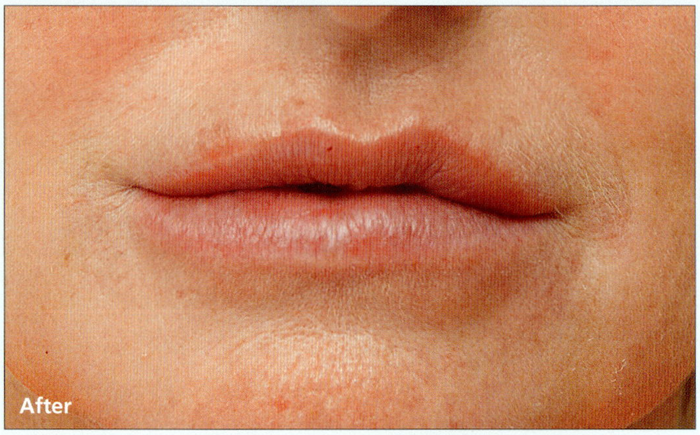

Technique 44 – Figs. 7, 8 Before/after comparison: the result in the upper lip shows only a slight improvement in the asymmetry, and the lower lip needs to be drawn in with permanent makeup to optimize the result.

Important Notes

- Where any asymmetry is present, the limits of what it feasible are often tight. Genetically determined asymmetric lip shapes can only be corrected to a limited extent, and the same applies to any asymmetry of motor origin.
- During the treatment, the patient should be observed from the front in a relaxed state after each HA injection, to see if the shape has been balanced out.
- Once the treatment has been completed, the patient should be asked to say "cheese," to purse the lips, to open them slightly, to close them without tension, and to smile. This mobilization of the lips makes it possible to see if the HA has been uniformly distributed.

Possible Side Effects

Slight reddening, rarely inflammation, commonly hematomas, more severe swellings, pain for 2–3 days

Undesirable Side Effects

Inflammation, overcorrection with resultant alteration of the shape of the lip or nodule formation, asymmetry due to non-uniform delivery of material, necrosis

Treatment Protocol at a Glance

- History, evaluation, and patient information
- Informed consent form
- Photo documentation: "before" images
- Analysis and marking of the areas to be treated
- Cleaning
- Thorough disinfection
- Local anesthesia (lidocaine cream) or conduction anesthesia if required
- Injection technique: linear, point and bolus technique
- Layer: according to indication
- Material: class "S/M soft" and/or "S/M viscous" product, according to indication
- Volume: depending on requirement
- Needle: 27–29G sharp needle, 27G blunt cannula
- No massage
- Cooling if required
- Heparin cream for hematomas, ibuprofen p.o., arnica
- Photo documentation: "after" images
- Advice on dos and don'ts after the procedure
- Follow-up appointment for a check-up after 8–14 days

9.6.9 Technique 45
Augmentation of the Upper Lip – "Pillar Technique" according to Anil Rajani (Sharp Needle)

This technique (Rajani 2019) can be used to bring an upper lip slightly forward where the flat segments of the lip have become so inverted that the vermillion is no longer visible. The first thing to analyze is whether the lip is folded inward or if it shows too little volume. This technique has its limitations if the lips are extremely thin and have little volume.

Patient Selection

- If the lateral parts of the upper lip are very thin and inverted
- Where the vermillion is barely visible while the middle lip segment is normal

Injection Scheme and Planning (→ Technique 45 – Figs. 1, 2)

The technique involves placing 5–6 depots per upper lip half at the dry/wet boundary: each time, the needle is inserted at the lip contour and advanced from the contour through the vermillion, through the orbicularis oris muscle and up to the oral fissure, at the dry/wet boundary. The material is delivered in small boluses as required, by retrograde injection, tapering it off right up to the contour. To ensure that the needle reaches the dry/wet boundary in a straight line, the lip needs to be everted slightly and consistently during the injection. The material is delivered with stringent visual monitoring.

Technique: linear/bolus combination technique
Direction of insertion: starting from the vermillion border and toward the dry/wet boundary
Layer: into the vermillion through the orbicularis oris muscle up to the dry/wet boundary
Material: class "M soft" or "M viscous" product
Volume: max. 0.05 ml per line/bolus, max. 0.5 ml in total
Needle: 27G sharp needle
Anesthesia: lidocaine cream, conduction anesthesia if required

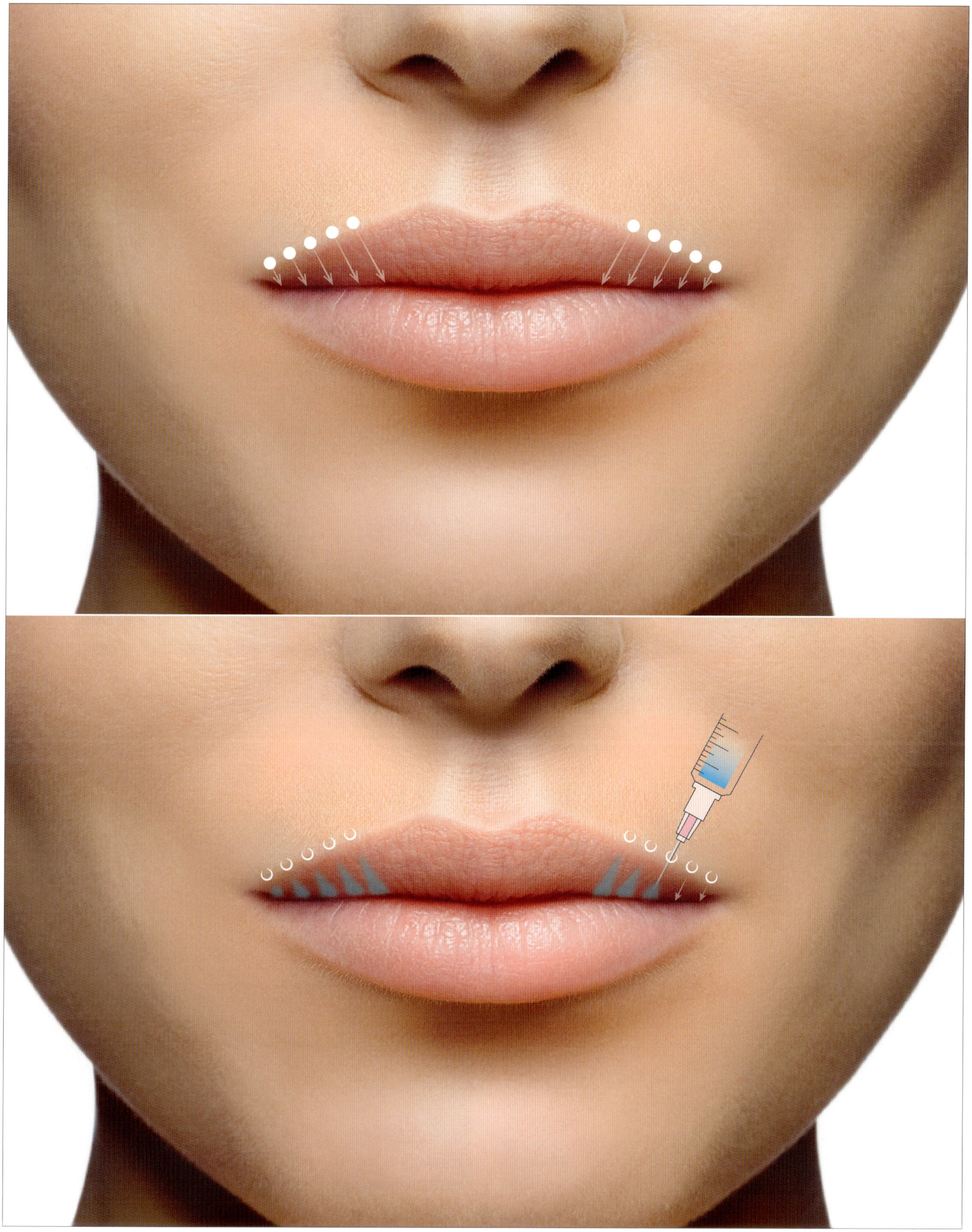

Technique 45 – Figs. 1, 2 Injection scheme and planning: augmentation of the upper lip – "Pillar Technique" according to Anil Rajani (sharp needle).

Treatment Method (→ Technique 45 – Figs. 3, 4)

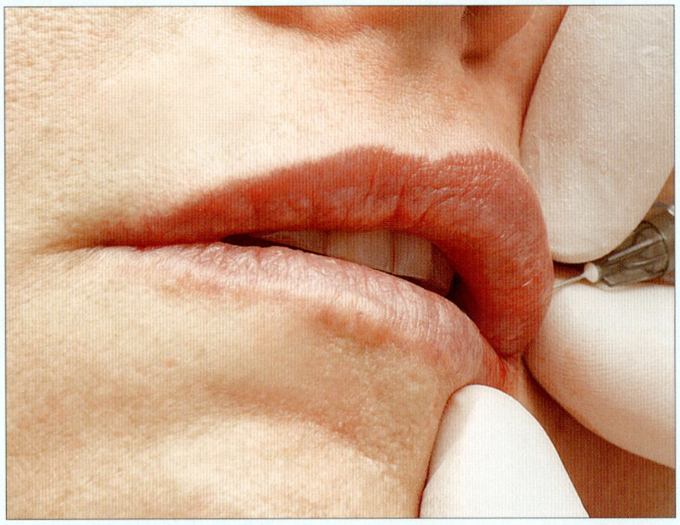

Technique 45 – Fig. 3 Inject the material into the dry/wet boundary of the upper lip. Evert the lip slightly with the opposite hand until the dry/wet boundary becomes visible. Starting at the contour, insert the sharp needle directly through the muscle and up to the dry/wet boundary, without perforating the skin there. Deliver the material in small, droplet-like boluses. Repeat this procedure, starting from the mouth corner up to the center of the lip, depending on the volume deficit.

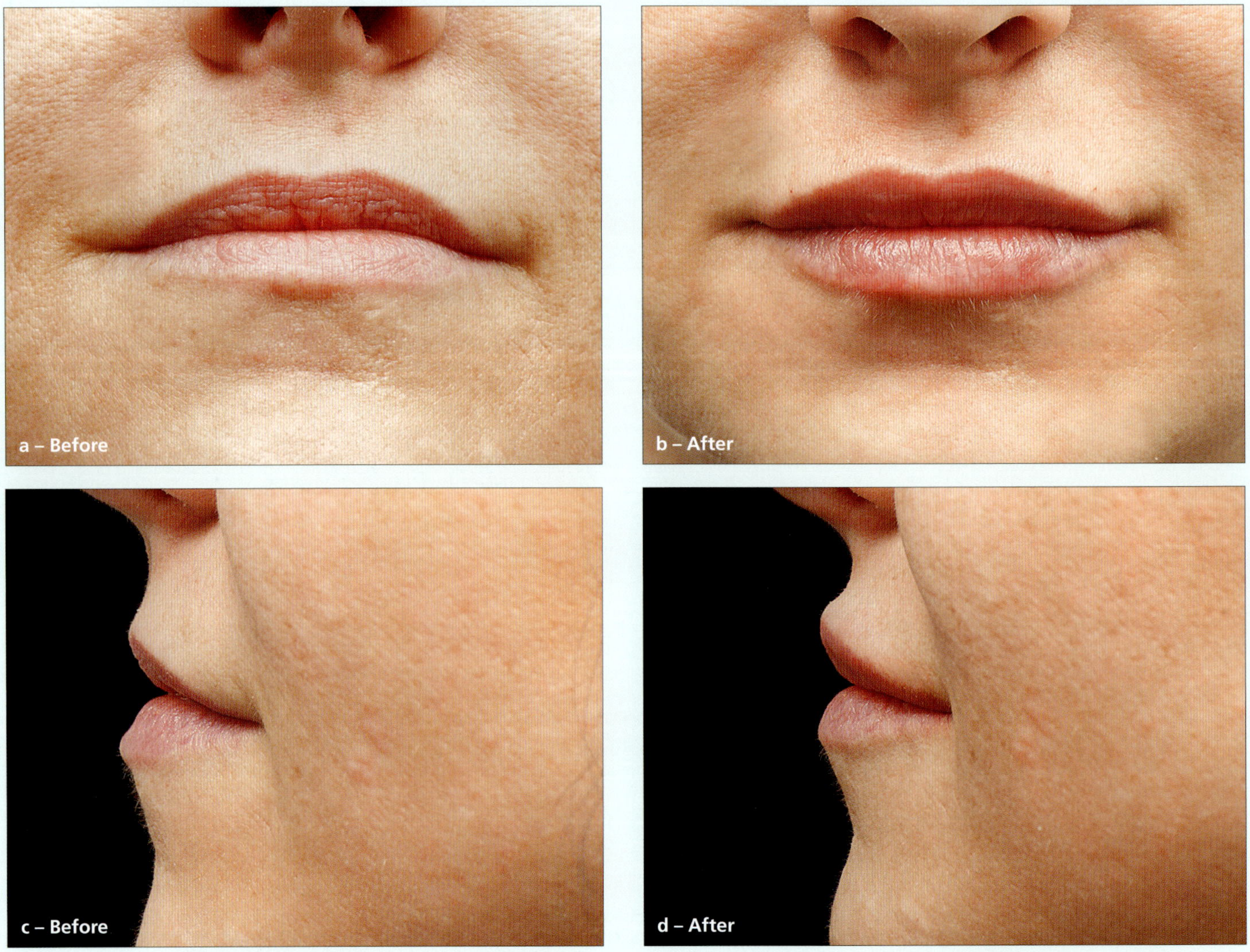

Technique 45 – Fig. 4 a–d Before/after comparison: the improvement is clearly visible in both the front and side views.

Important Notes

- Optimal improvements are not to be expected if the lips are extremely narrow and have little volume.
- After the treatment, the patient should be asked to stretch the lips and smile to reveal any irregularities, so that these can then be corrected.

Possible Side Effects

Rarely inflammation, internal hematomas, mild to more severe swellings

Undesirable Side Effects

Nodule formation or asymmetry due to non-uniform delivery of material

Treatment Protocol at a Glance

- History, evaluation, and patient information
- Informed consent form
- Photo documentation: "before" images
- Analysis and marking of the areas to be treated
- Cleaning
- Thorough disinfection
- Local anesthesia (lidocaine cream), conduction anesthesia if required
- Injection technique: linear/bolus combination technique
- Layer: into the vermillion through the orbicularis oris muscle up to the dry/wet boundary
- Material: class "M" product
- Volume: max. 0.05 ml per line/bolus, max. 0.5 ml in total
- Needle: 27G sharp needle
- No massage
- Cooling if required
- Heparin cream for hematomas, ibuprofen p.o., arnica
- Photo documentation: "after" images
- Advice on dos and don'ts after the procedure
- Follow-up appointment for a check-up after 8–14 days

10 The 45 Lip Treatment Techniques: An Overview

10 The 45 Lip Treatment Techniques: An Overview

The table in this chapter lists the 45 lip treatment techniques and their key features, providing the therapist with an at-a-glance guide to the relevant aspects of the treatment for each indication. The techniques selected for each treatment goal are at the discretion of – and depend on the skill of – the therapist. Our recommendation for difficult indications, in particular, is to undergo training in the use of various techniques to extend your experience.

- **HYDRATION, REVITALIZATION:** Techniques T1–T4 involve the superficial skin layers. Neocollagenesis is stimulated by perforating the tissue in the cutaneous part of the lip with numerous needle punctures. The tissue is hydrated as a result of the water-binding capacity of certain types of hyaluronic acid (HA).
- **ACCENTS:** In techniques T5–T10, minimal accents are placed in the lip region, without significantly changing the appearance of the lips.
- **PERIORAL LINES:** Techniques T11–T14 aim to treat radial, mimic, and smoker's lines; it should be noted that the demarcations between these three wrinkle types are fluid.
- **LIP VOLUME:** Techniques T15–T28 use various methods to fill the lips to differing degrees.
- **PERIORAL VOLUME:** Techniques T29–T36 treat shadows and areas of unevenness caused by lack of volume and mimic activity in the perioral region.
- **SHAPING, BEAUTIFICATION:** Techniques T37–T45 involve making changes to the shape of the lips to address congenital asymmetries, as yet uncorrected effects of previous treatments, and genetically determined imperfections. They are also used in response to patients' desires to alter the shape, contour or expression of their lips. This also involves changes and improvements to young, intact lips, which is referred to as "beautification." Such changes are frequently motivated by beauty ideals influenced by fashion and trends.

No.	Lip Treatment Technique	Category	Degree of Difficulty	Indication
T1	**Hydration and revitalization – cutaneous part of the lip (sharp needle)**	Hydration, revitalization	💉	Dry skin, actinic skin damage, very fine lines
T2	**Hydration – cutaneous part of the lip (blunt cannula)**	Hydration, revitalization	💉💉	Dry skin, actinic skin damage, very fine lines
T3	**Hydration – vermillion (blunt cannula)**	Hydration, revitalization	💉💉	Dry lips
T4	**Revitalization – vermillion (according to Patrick Trevidic, sharp needle)**	Hydration, revitalization	💉💉	Dry lips
T5	**Fresh up (sharp needle)**	Accents	💉	Flat lips, aging lips, patients who want minimal lip augmentation
T6	**Contouring and enhancement (sharp needle)**	Accents	💉	Irregular or flattened contour, radial lines
T7	**Contouring (blunt cannula)**	Accents	💉💉	Irregular or flattened contour, radial lines, patients who want a prominent contour
T8	**Contouring/reshaping of the Cupid's bow (sharp needle)**	Accents	💉	Poorly defined Cupid's bow
T9	**Contouring of the philtrum (sharp needle)**	Accents	💉	Inherent or age-related flattening of the philtrum
T10	**Modeling of the philtrum and Cupid's bow (sharp needle)**	Accents	💉💉	Inherent or age-related flattening of the Cupid's bow and philtrum, patients who want a heart-shaped upper lip

Table 10.1 The 45 lip treatment techniques with HA fillers: an overview (continued on pp. 314–317)

Abbreviations and Symbols in the Table "The 45 lip treatment techniques with HA fillers: an overview"

No. **Lip treatment technique number**

Degree of difficulty of the lip treatment technique: Level 1

Degree of difficulty of the lip treatment technique: Level 2

SN **Sharp needle**

BC **Blunt cannula**

XS **HA particle size** (stands for a thin material with no lifting capacity, suitable for revitalization and hydration of the skin)

S **HA particle size** (stands for a material with very small particles, suitable for the finest lines and wrinkles)

M **HA particle size** (stands for a material of medium thickness with lifting capacity, suitable for lines of medium depth)

L **HA particle size** (stands for a thicker material with lifting capacity, suitable for deep lines)

● **Soft HA consistency** (low-crosslinked gel)

▲ **Viscous HA consistency** (high-crosslinked gel)

ml **Milliliter**

Treatment Goal	Needle/ Cannula	Material	HA Consistency	Injection Technique	Needle Size (Gauge)	Total Volume of HA (c.)
Rejuvenation	SN	XS	●	Point technique	30–33	0.01 ml/point, < 1.0 ml in total
Rejuvenation	BC	XS	●	Fanning technique	27–30	1.0 ml–1.5 ml
Rejuvenation	BC	XS/S	●	Linear technique	27–30	1.0 ml
Rejuvenation	SN	XS	●	Fanning technique	27	1.0 ml
Rejuvenation	SN	S/M	▲	Point technique	27–30	0.03 ml/point
Rejuvenation	SN	S/M	▲	Linear technique	27–30	0.5 ml
Rejuvenation	BC	S/M	▲	Linear technique	27–30	0.5 ml
Rejuvenation/Beautification	SN	S/M	▲	Linear technique	27–30	0.2 ml
Rejuvenation/Beautification	SN	M	▲	Linear technique	27	0.2 ml
Rejuvenation/Beautification	SN	S/M	▲	Linear technique	27–30	0.4 ml

Table 10.1 (continued)

No.	Lip Treatment Technique	Category	Degree of Difficulty	Indication
T11	**Linear and fishbone technique for perioral lines (sharp needle)**	Perioral lines	💉	Melomental folds, deeper radial lines
T12	**Perioral point technique, modification by stretching or compression (sharp needle)**	Perioral lines	💉	Melomental folds, deeper radial lines
T13	**Perioral blanching technique (sharp needle)**	Perioral lines	💉💉	Melomental folds, superficial radial lines
T14	**"Fern pattern technique" according to Tom van Eijk (sharp needle)**	Perioral lines	💉💉	Moderate to deeply indented radial lines
T15	**Minimal four-point volume replacement (sharp needle)**	Lip volume S (minimal)	💉	Patients who want very subtle lip augmentation
T16	**Subtle volume replacement (sharp needle)**	Lip volume S (minimal)	💉	Volume deficit, thin lips, older lips
T17	**Subtle lip augmentation (sharp needle)**	Lip volume M (moderate)	💉	Volume deficit, thin lips, older lips
T18	**Classic augmentation (sharp needle)**	Lip volume L (strong)	💉💉	Volume deficit, thin lips
T19	**Moderate augmentation (blunt cannula)**	Lip volume M (moderate)	💉💉	Volume deficit, thin lips, older lips
T20	**Classic to strong augmentation (blunt cannula)**	Lip volume L (strong)	💉💉	Patients who want strong lip augmentation
T21	**Extreme augmentation – bolus and fanning technique (sharp needle)**	Lip volume L (strong)	💉💉	Patients who want strong lip augmentation
T22	**Augmentation from the dry/wet boundary (sharp needle)**	Lip volume S (minimal)	💉💉	Very thin lips
T23	**Augmentation from the mucous membrane (sharp needle)**	Lip volume S (minimal)	💉💉	Very thin, inverted lips, also in cases of malpositioned teeth
T24	**Volumization with or without tubercle accentuation (sharp needle)**	Lip volume M (moderate)	💉💉	Thin lips, flattened tubercles, older lips, patients who want shaping and beautification
T25	**Volumization – bolus technique (sharp needle)**	Lip volume L (strong)	💉	Thin lips, patients who want more volume, lips showing age-related atrophy
T26	**Volumization – cutaneous part of the lip technique (sharp needle)**	Lip volume M (moderate)	💉💉	Volumization, correcting areas of asymmetry, shaping
T27	**Extreme volumization and shaping – multiple injection technique (sharp needle)**	Lip volume L (strong)	💉💉	Patients who want strong augmentation and lip shape definition
T28	**Volumization and shaping – "Lip tenting technique" according to Tom van Eijk (sharp needle)**	Lip volume M (moderate)	💉💉	Patients who want more volume, augmentation, refreshing, shaping

Treatment Goal	Needle/ Cannula	Material	HA Consistency	Injection Technique	Needle Size (Gauge)	Total Volume of HA (c.)
Rejuvenation	SN	XS/S	●	Linear, fishbone technique	27–30	< 0.5 ml
Rejuvenation	SN	XS/S	●	Point technique, also linear technique	27–30	< 0.5 ml
Rejuvenation	SN	XS/S	●	Point blanching technique	27–33	0.01–0.02 ml/ point, < 0.5 ml in total
Rejuvenation	SN	S	▲	Short linear technique	27–30	0.02 ml/line
Rejuvenation/Beautification	SN	M	●	Point technique	27	0.2 ml
Rejuvenation/Beautification	SN	S/M	●	Linear technique	27	0.3 ml
Rejuvenation/Beautification	SN	S/M	●	Linear technique	27	< 0.4 ml
Beautification	SN	M/L	●	Fanning technique	27	1.0 ml
Rejuvenation/Beautification	BC	S/M	●	Linear technique	27	0.5 ml–1.0 ml
Beautification	BC	M/L	●	Fanning technique	27	1.0–1.2 ml
Beautification	SN	M/L	●	Bolus/fanning technique	27–29	1.0–1.5 ml
Rejuvenation/Beautification	SN	M	●	Linear technique	27–29	0.6 ml
Beautification	SN	M	●	Bolus technique	27	0.5–1.0 ml
Rejuvenation/Beautification	SN	S/M	●	Bolus technique	27–29	0.6 ml
Rejuvenation/Beautification	SN	M/L	●	Bolus technique	27	1.0 ml < 1.5 ml
Rejuvenation/Beautification	SN	S/M	●	Bolus technique	27–29	0.5 ml
Beautification	SN	M	●	Linear technique	27–29	1.0–2.0 ml
Rejuvenation/Beautification	SN	S/M	▲	Linear technique	27–30	1.0–1.5 ml

Table 10.1 (continued)

No.	Lip Treatment Technique	Category	Degree of Difficulty	Indication
T29	**Volumization – labiomental fold (sharp needle)**	Perioral volume	💉	Lengthening the lower part of the lip in age-related shortening of the distance between lip and chin
T30	**Augmentation – chin region (sharp needle)**	Perioral volume	💉	Harmonization of the chin
T31	**Volumization – vertical injection technique (sharp needle)**	Perioral volume	💉	Perioral shadows formed by mimic activity
T32	**Volumization – fine marionette lines I (sharp needle)**	Perioral volume	💉	Sagging mouth corners, wrinkling, mouth corner lines
T33	**Volumization – fine marionette lines II (sharp needle)**	Perioral volume	💉💉	Sagging mouth corners, wrinkling, mouth corner lines
T34	**Augmentation – marionette lines (sharp needle)**	Perioral volume	💉💉	Marionette lines, shadows
T35	**Augmentation – marionette lines (blunt cannula)**	Perioral volume	💉💉	Marionette lines, shadows
T36	**Augmentation – windmill technique: marionette lines, lips, perioral region (blunt cannula)**	Perioral volume	💉💉	Marionette lines, shadows
T37	**Subtle mouth corner lift (sharp needle)**	Shaping, beautification	💉💉	Downturned mouth corners
T38	**Classic mouth corner lift (sharp needle)**	Shaping, beautification	💉💉	Downturned mouth corners
T39	**Subtle volumization – tubercle definition (sharp needle)**	Shaping, beautification	💉💉	Lip tubercle definition or shaping
T40	**Contouring of the perioral line according to Phillip Chang (sharp needle)**	Shaping, beautification	💉💉	Raising of the upper lip
T41	**Indentation in the center of the lip (sharp needle)**	Shaping, beautification	💉💉	Definition of the lip center
T42	**Widening the arch of the lower lip (sharp needle)**	Shaping, beautification	💉💉	Improving lip shape if the lower lip is too small
T43	**Correcting a previously treated lip (sharp needle)**	Shaping, beautification	💉💉	Correction of deficits
T44	**Correcting areas of asymmetry (sharp needle/blunt cannula)**	Shaping, beautification	💉💉	Harmonization
T45	**Augmentation of the upper lip – "Pillar Technique" according to Anil Rajani (Sharp Needle)**	Shaping, beautification	💉💉	Harmonization and shaping of the upper lip

Treatment Goal	Needle/Cannula	Material	HA Consistency	Injection Technique	Needle Size (Gauge)	Total Volume of HA (ca.)
Rejuvenation/Beautification	SN	M/L	● ▲	Bolus, depot technique	25	0.5 ml
Beautification	SN	M/L	▲	Bolus technique	25	< 0.2 ml/bolus
Rejuvenation	SN	M/L	● ▲	Bolus technique	25	0.5–1.0 ml
Rejuvenation	SN	M	▲	Linear technique	27	0.4 ml
Rejuvenation	SN	M	▲	Bolus technique	25–27	0.2 ml
Rejuvenation	SN	M	● ▲	Fanning/criss-cross technique	27	0.5–1.0 ml
Rejuvenation	BC	M	● ▲	Fanning technique	27	0.5–1.0 ml
Rejuvenation	BC	M	● ▲	Fanning technique	27	0.5–1.0 ml
Beautification	SN	S/M	▲	Linear technique	27–29	0.05–1.0 ml/line
Beautification	SN	S/M	▲	Linear technique	27–29	0.4 ml
Beautification	SN	S/M	●	Linear technique	27–29	0.2 ml
Rejuvenation/Beautification	SN	M	▲	Linear technique	27; 38 mm	1.0–1.2 ml
Beautification	SN	M	●	Bolus technique	27–29	0.6–1.0 ml
Beautification	SN	M	▲	Linear technique	27	0.2 ml
Beautification	SN	S/M	●	Linear, point, bolus technique	27–30	As required
Beautification	SN/BC	S/M	● ▲	Linear, point, bolus technique	SN: 27–29; BC: 27	As required
Beautification	SN	M	● ▲	Linear/bolus combination technique	27	Max. 0.5 ml

11 Case Examples

11 Case Examples

The following examples include certain tricky indications that are often encountered in routine practice such as "older lips," "thin mouth" or "previously treated lips." When it comes to older lips, the indications are often similar, and the patient's desire for a treatment is the defining factor. The technique the therapist chooses to use depends on the indication, the therapist's experience, and the patient's budget. For each of the cases presented in this chapter, we recommend a selection of techniques divided into two levels of difficulty, allowing the therapist to choose whether to concentrate on basic techniques or whether to embark on more complex challenges:

TECHNIQUE – LEVEL 1

TECHNIQUE – LEVEL 2

Some techniques are used in almost all of the cases, since older lips are generally characterized by loss of moisture, contour, and volume. In our examples, we have indicated all the potential treatments that could be implemented; in reality, this is not always possible due to the restrictions of budget. However, having a broad palette of options allows the therapist to present the patient with a detailed offer and the optimum treatment during the pre-treatment consultation.

The selection of techniques presented in this chapter may be used according to the therapist's preferences and are based on the treatment goal. Thus, for example, several types of contouring may be recommended, while only one technique would actually be used.

Moreover, revitalization with low-crosslinked products is possible, and frequently advisable, in almost every patient, extending the scope of the treatment. Since the recommended techniques have been divided into two levels of difficulty, inexperienced therapists can focus on the basic techniques, while experienced therapists can extend their range to include the more challenging methods (see also Chap. 10, p. 312 ff. with regard to the classification of techniques into degrees of difficulty).

The color scheme used to mark the treatment areas provides the therapist with an indication of the heading that the respective treatment technique falls under (see also Chap. 10, p. 312 ff.), namely:

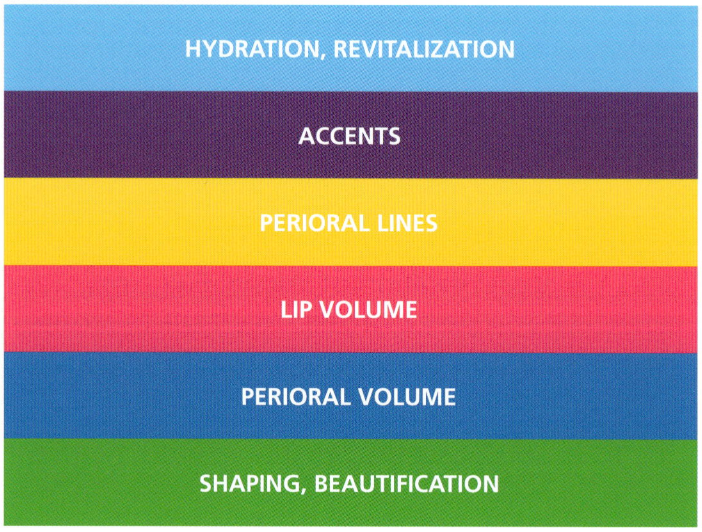

11.1 Perioral Lines, Atrophied Mouth

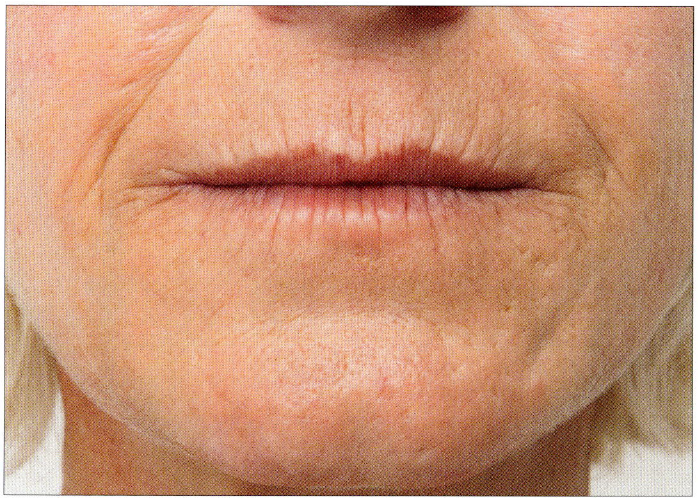

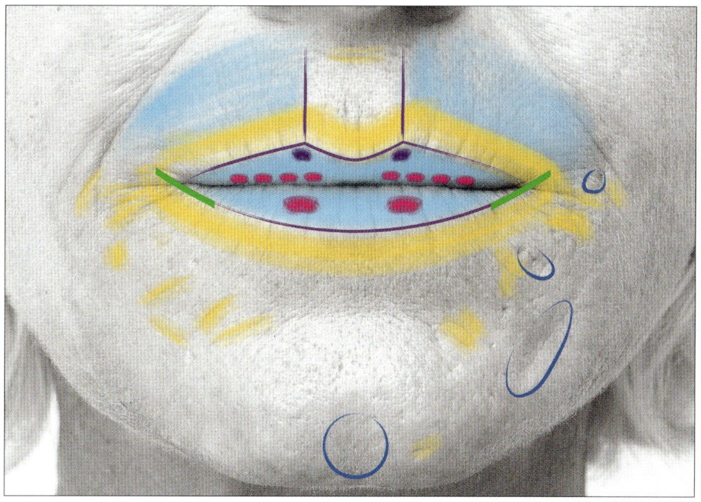

Status: 50-year-old woman, smoker, menopausal, actinic skin damage, slightly atrophied and very wrinkled, dry lips

Treatment Planning with Injection Volumes

Perioral hydration: 0.5 ml
Hydration of the lips: 0.5 ml

Enhance contours: 0.5 ml
Accentuate philtrum: 0.3 ml
Fresh up: 0.2 ml

Smooth out perioral lines: 0.5 ml

Fill lower lip: 0.3 ml
Fill and evert upper lip: 0.3 ml

Correct lines/shadows
(vertical injection technique): 0.4 ml

Lift mouth corners: 0.3 ml

Caution

- The treatment requires meticulous planning and should be agreed with the patient because its success, especially when treating radial lines, depends on having several treatments sessions (2–3 at intervals of 2–3 weeks).
- The procedure should be guided by the patient's wishes and budget.
- There are various options for building up lip volume (see below).
- Once the lip volume has been filled to the required level, wait 2–3 weeks before hydrating the vermillion.

Potential lip treatment techniques to be used according to the therapist's preference and experience

Level 1		Level 2	
T1	Hydration ●	**T3**	Hydration (vermillion) ●
T5	Fresh up ▲	**T4**	Revitalization (vermillion) according to Patrick Trevidic ●
T6	Contouring ▲	**T7**	Lip contouring ▲
T8	Contouring (Cupid's bow) ▲	**T13**	Perioral lines (blanching technique) ●
T9	Contouring (philtrum) ▲	**T14**	Smoothing perioral lines (fern pattern technique) ▲
T12	Smoothing (radial lines) ●	**T23**	Volumization (mucous membrane) ●
T15	Four-point volume replacement ●	**T38**	Mouth corner lift ▲
T16	Lip volumization (subtle) ●		
T30	Augmentation (chin region) ▲		
T31	Volumization (vertical injection technique) ▲		

11.2 Older Mouth with Thin Lips

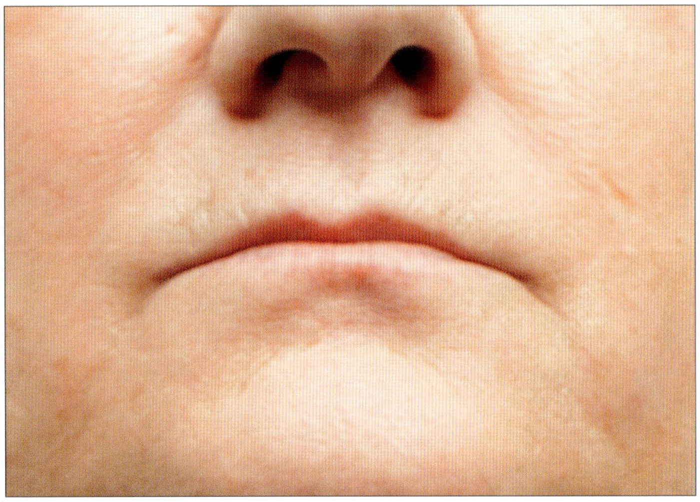

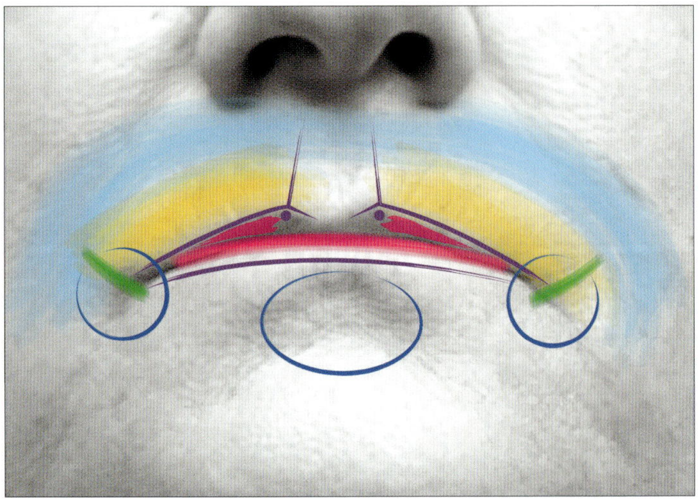

Status: 55-year-old woman, thin lips atrophied by aging, perioral lines over the upper lip, oral commissure lines, downturned mouth corners, flattened philtrum, large-pored skin texture, blurred contours, deep labiomental fold

Treatment Planning with Injection Volumes

- (light blue) Perioral revitalization: 1.0 ml
- (purple) Contouring: 0.5 ml
  Contour the philtrum and Cupid's bow peaks: 0.3 ml
  Upper lip fresh up: 0.1 ml
- (yellow) Smooth out perioral lines: 0.2 ml
- (pink) Subtle upper and lower lip filling: 0.5 ml
- (blue) Volumization of the marionette lines: 0.4 ml
  Lift the labiomental fold: 0.3 ml
- (green) Lift mouth corners: 0.1 ml

Caution

- The volume build-up should take place in small steps to allow any irregularities to be corrected properly.
- Treating older lips is a challenge because the anatomical changes that occur throughout the oral region impose their own limits on the extent to which lip shape can be influenced (see Chap. 1.4.7, p. 22 f.). The top priority here should be to refresh the lips gently, revitalize the perioral region, and mitigate the marionette lines. Lip augmentation would produce an unnatural result.

Potential lip treatment techniques to be used according to the therapist's preference and experience			
Level 1		**Level 2**	
T1	Hydration ●	**T7**	Lip contouring ▲
T5	Fresh up ▲	**T19**	Augmentation (moderate) ●
T6	Contouring ▲	**T22**	Volumization (dry/wet boundary) ●
T8	Contouring (Cupid's bow) ▲	**T24**	Volumization (vermillion with tubercle accentuation) ●
T9	Contouring (philtrum) ▲	**T26**	Volumization (cutaneous part of the lip) ●
T12	Smoothing (radial lines) ●	**T35**	Augmentation (marionette lines) ● ▲
T29	Volumization (labiomental fold) ▲	**T38**	Mouth corner lift (strong) ▲

11.3 Previously Treated Lips

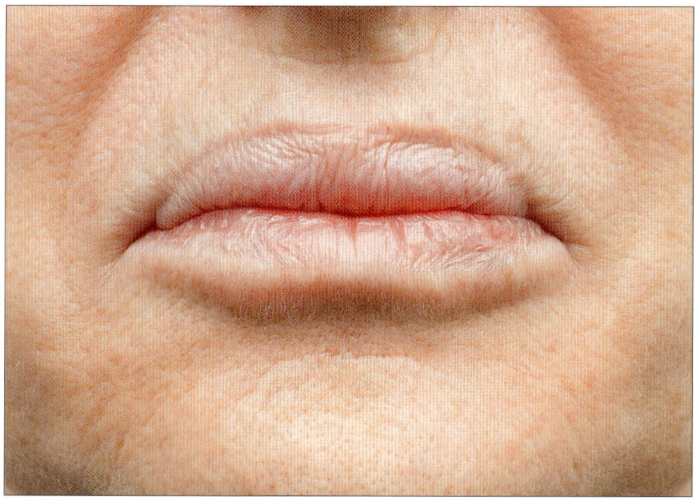

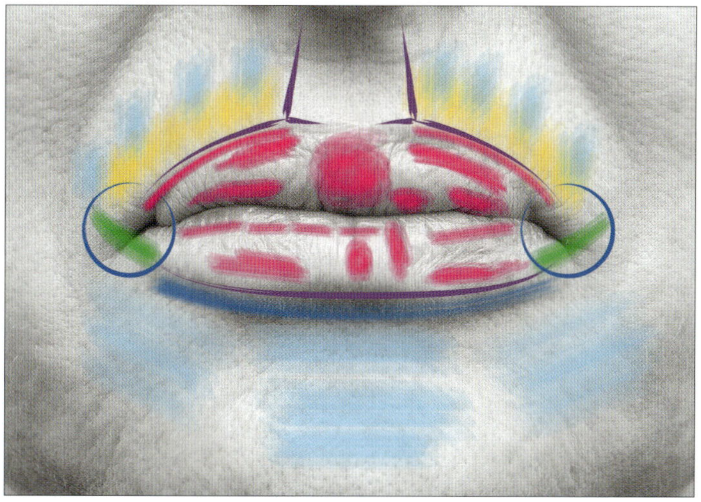

Status: 38-year-old woman, previously treated lips (with autologous fat tissue), areas of soft, irregular thickening, has not had any further treatments for the past two years

Treatment Planning with Injection Volumes

- Perioral hydration: 0.5 ml
- Contour the philtrum and Cupid's bow: 0.2 ml
  Upper and lower lip contouring: 0.5 ml
- Smooth out perioral lines: 0.3 ml
- Correct deficits: 0.5 ml
- Correct shadows under the lower lip: 0.3 ml
  Volumization of the marionette lines: 0.4 ml
- Lift mouth corners: 0.4 ml

Caution

- The challenge lies in uniform adjustment of the lips by filling and shaping.
- Assessing the specific treatment needs is not easy and requires a good eye.
- The first and most important step is to clarify the history: What product was used for the previous treatment? What was done to even out any irregularities?
- A low-crosslinked, small-particle product should be used as the material for correcting the volume deficits in order to ensure that the various transitional zones are smoothed out uniformly.

Potential lip treatment techniques to be used according to the therapist's preference and experience

Level 1		**Level 2**	
T1	Hydration ●	**T7**	Lip contouring ▲
T6	Contouring ▲	**T26**	Volumization (cutaneous part of the lip) ●
T9	Contouring (philtrum) ▲	**T35**	Augmentation (marionette lines, shadows below the lower lip contour) ●
T12	Smoothing (radial lines) ●	**T37**	Mouth corner lift (subtle) ●
T15	Four-point volume replacement ●	**T38**	Mouth corner lift (strong) ▲
		T43	Correcting a previously treated lip ●

11.4 Oral Commissure Lines, Thin Lower Lip, Minor Asymmetries, Dry Upper Lip

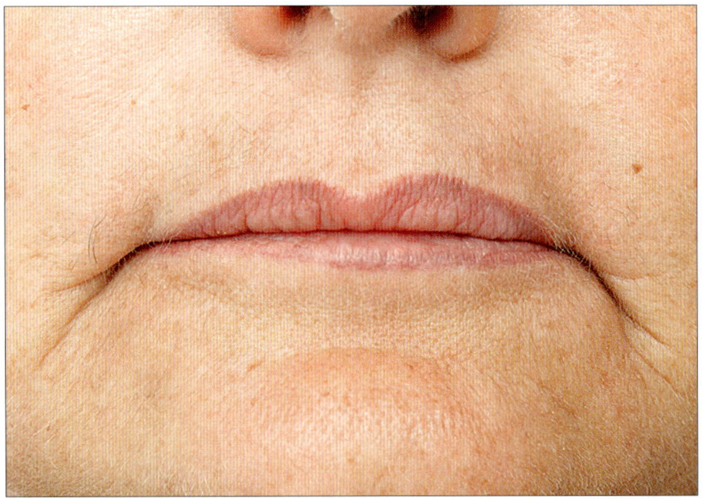

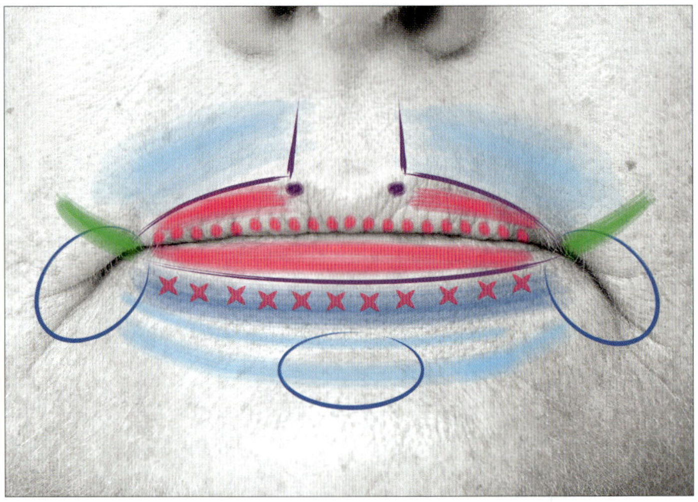

Status: 45-year-old woman, very pronounced marionette lines, extremely thin lower lip that tapers off on the right side, upper lip tapering off slightly on the right side, extremely dry lines in the vermillion, large-pored perioral skin

Treatment Planning with Injection Volumes

Perioral revitalization: 1.0 ml

Fresh up: 0.2 ml
Contour lower and upper lip: 0.5 ml
Contour philtrum: 0.3 ml

Lower lip volumization: 0.5 ml
Upper lip volumization (subtle): 0.2 ml
Correct areas of asymmetry: 0.2 ml

Smooth out oral commissure lines: 0.7 ml
Correct shadows under the lower lip and the labiomental fold: 0.3 ml

Lift mouth corners: 0.4 ml

Caution

- The pronounced marionette lines are very difficult to treat.
- Only slight improvements are to be expected.
- Another 1–2 treatment sessions will be needed.

Potential lip treatment techniques to be used according to the therapist's preference and experience			
Level 1		**Level 2**	
T1	Revitalization ●	**T7**	Lip contouring ▲
T5	Fresh up ▲	**T22**	Augmentation from the dry/wet boundary ●
T6	Contouring ▲	**T26**	Volumization (cutaneous part of the lip) ●
T9	Contouring (philtrum) ▲	**T28**	Lip tenting technique according to Tom van Eijk ▲
T15	Four-point volume replacement ●	**T33**	Volumization (marionette lines) ▲
T16	Lip volumization (subtle) ●	**T34**	Volumization (marionette lines) ▲
T29	Volumization (labiomental fold) ▲	**T38**	Mouth corner lift ▲

11.5 Perioral Shadows and Areas of Asymmetry

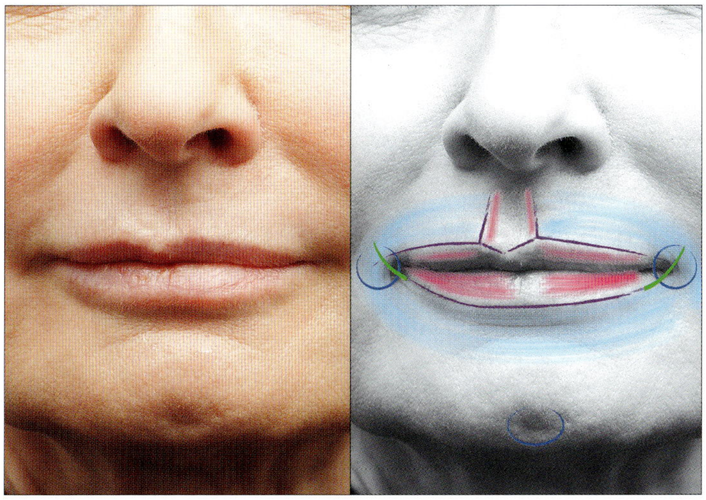

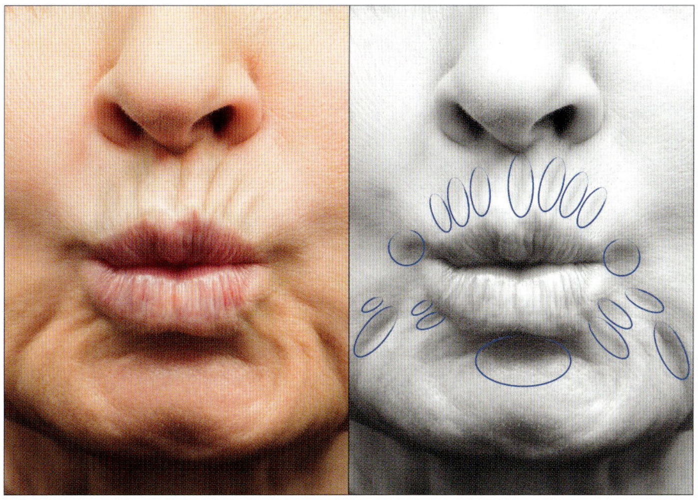

Status: 60-year-old woman, very pronounced perioral shadows during mimic activity, sagging of the perioral zone, dry skin, areas of asymmetry in the lips, irregular contours

Treatment Planning with Injection Volumes

- Perioral hydration: 1.0 ml (light blue)
- Contour lower and upper lip: 0.6 ml; Contour philtrum Cupid's bow: 0.2 ml (purple)
- Volumize lips and correct slight asymmetries: 0.7 ml (pink)
- Correct perioral shadows: 1.5 ml; Correct labiomental fold: 0.5 ml (blue)
- Reinforce mouth corners: 0.2 ml (green)

> **Caution**
>
> - The perioral shadows should be injected with the patient's mouth pursed, inserting the needle directly into the shadow.
> - Any palpable uneven areas can be smoothed out by gentle massage.

Potential lip treatment techniques to be used according to the therapist's preference and experience			
Level 1		**Level 2**	
T1	Hydration ●	**T3**	Hydration (vermillion) ●
T6	Contouring ▲	**T7**	Lip contouring ▲
T8	Contouring (Cupid's bow) ▲	**T26**	Volumization (cutaneous part of the lip) ●
T9	Contouring (philtrum) ▲	**T28**	Lip tenting technique according to Tom van Eijk ▲
T12	Smoothing (radial lines) ●	**T37**	Mouth corner lift (subtle) ▲
T17	Lip augmentation (subtle) ●	**T40**	Contouring according to Phillip Chang ▲
T29	Volumization (labiomental fold) ▲	**T44**	Correcting areas of asymmetry ●
T31	Volumization (vertical injection technique) ●		

11.6 Asymmetric Mouth

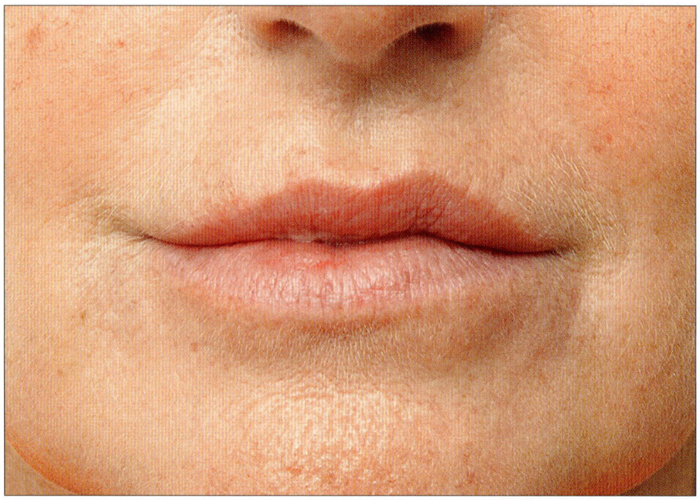

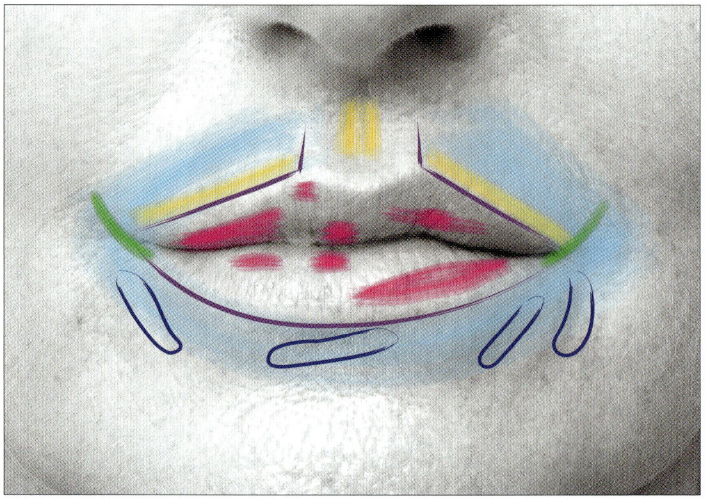

Status: 38-year-old woman, asymmetric lips, dry lips, very fine perioral lines, lip contour absent in places, perioral shadows

11

Treatment Planning with Injection Volumes

- (light blue) Revitalization of the lips and perioral zone: 1.0 ml
- (purple) Adjust Cupid's bow peaks and contours: 0.7 ml
Accentuate philtrum slightly: 0.1 ml
- (yellow) Smooth out perioral lines: 0.2 ml
- (pink) Fill various lip areas: 0.6 ml
- (blue) Correct shadows under the lower lip: 0.5 ml

Caution

- Correcting areas of asymmetry is not a simple task. Accurate analysis and meticulous planning are important here, as this helps the less well-trained eye to identify asymmetries.
- The procedure used to correct areas of asymmetry may vary. Techniques may be combined: the pillar technique to lift the sunken lateral section, filling with the cannula techniques, and correction using Technique 24, with constant visual checks.
- For the tapering right upper lip, the contour should be drawn in the cutaneous part of the lip; for the left upper lip, this should be done in the vermillion.

Potential lip treatment techniques to be used according to the therapist's preference and experience			
Level 1		**Level 2**	
T1	Hydration ●	**T2**	Hydration (cutaneous part of the lip) ●
T6	Contouring ▲	**T7**	Lip contouring ▲
T9	Contouring (philtrum) ▲	**T19**	Augmentation (moderate) ●
T12	Smoothing (radial lines) ●	**T22**	Augmentation from the dry/wet boundary ●
T31	Volumization (vertical injection technique) ●	**T24**	Volumization (vermillion with tubercle accentuation) ●
		T26	Volumization (cutaneous part of the lip) ●
		T35	Augmentation (marionette lines) ●
		T44	Correcting areas of asymmetry ●
		T45	Augmentation of the upper lip – Pillar Technique according to Anil Rajani ▲

11.7 Beautification of Young, Full Lips

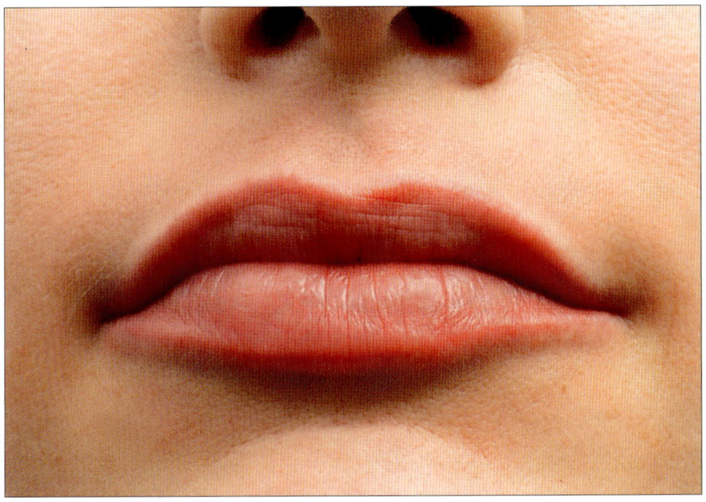

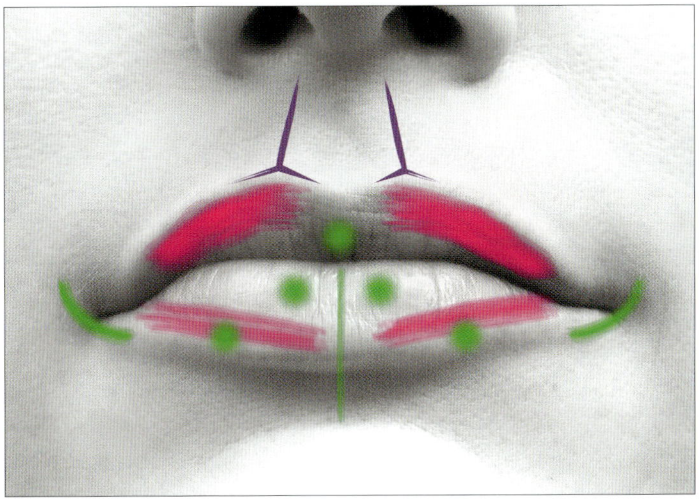

Status: 25-year-old woman, full and attractive mouth, wants augmentation of the lips to enhance their sensual effect

Treatment Planning with Injection Volumes

Purple:
Accentuate Cupid's bow and peaks: 0.05 ml
Accentuate philtrum slightly: 0.1 ml

Pink:
Subtly fill upper and lower lip: 0.6 ml

Green:
Lift mouth corners: 0.1 ml
Accentuate stomion: 0.1 ml
Accentuate tubercles: 0.05 ml
Widening the arch of the lower lip: 0.1 ml

Caution

- This treatment falls under the category "Beautification," and the patient's wishes are often driven by a fashion trend.
- If the patient requests a treatment to fit in with a fashion trend, this needs to be elicited in detail during the consultation and then discussed with the patient with regard to feasibility in order to avoid unrealistic expectations of what is possible.

Potential lip treatment techniques to be used according to the therapist's preference and experience

Level 1		Level 2	
T16	Lip volumization (subtle) ●	**T10**	Modeling of the philtrum and Cupid's bow ▲
T25	Volumization (bolus technique) ●	**T18**	Volumization (classic) ●
		T19	Augmentation (moderate) ●
		T24	Volumization (vermillion with tubercle accentuation) ●
		T26	Volumization (cutaneous part of the lip) ●
		T27	Volumization (extreme, multiple injection technique) ●
		T37	Mouth corner lift (subtle) ▲
		T39	Volumization (subtle) with tubercle definition ●
		T41	Indentation in the center of the lip ●
		T42	Widening the arch of the lower lip ▲

11.8 Thin Lips with Poorly Defined Contours

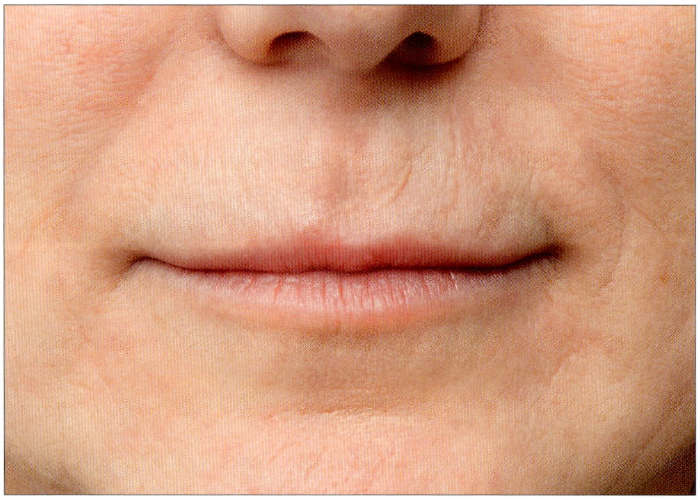

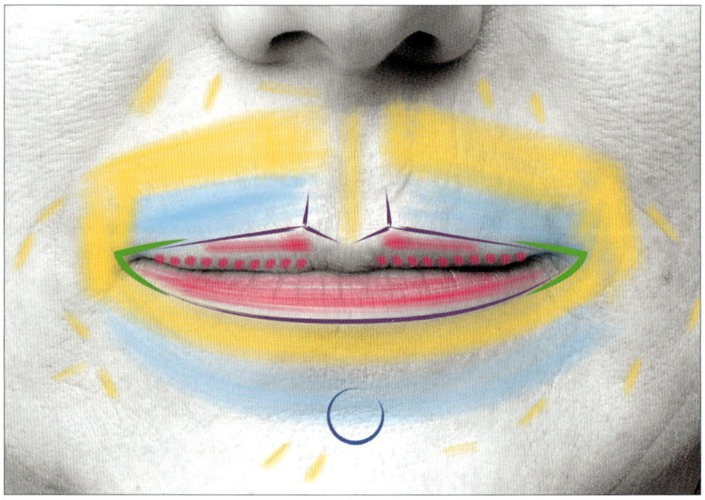

Status: 32-year-old woman, no defined contours, thin and inverted lips, skin drawn through by fine melomental folds, slight drooping of the oral commissures, small scars

Treatment Planning with Injection Volumes

- Hydration possible: 0.3–0.5 ml
- Contour philtrum: 0.2 ml
  Accentuate Cupid's bow: 0.1 ml
  Contouring: 0.5 ml
- Smooth out perioral skin texture and scars: 1.0 ml
  Smooth out melomental folds: 0.3 ml
- Subtle to moderate lower lip filling: c. 0.4 ml
  Fill upper lip subtly and in the dry/wet boundary: c. 0.2 ml
- Lift labiomental fold: 0.3 ml
- Reinforce mouth corners: 0.2 ml

Caution

- Since both the upper and lower lip are thin, the contouring material may be injected into the lip roll, causing the lip to curve upwards very gently, with soft augmentation.
- Important note: the underlying anatomical conditions must be respected here. The dental substance and jaw alignment are defining factors for the procedure.
- Delivering too much volume risks producing a "duck's bill" effect.

Potential lip treatment techniques to be used according to the therapist's preference and experience

Level 1		Level 2	
T6	Contouring ▲	T3	Hydration (vermillion) ●
T9	Contouring (philtrum) ▲	T4	Revitalization (vermillion) according to Patrick Trevidic ●
T15	Four-point volume replacement ●	T7	Lip contouring ▲
T29	Volumization (labiomental fold) ●	T10	Modeling (philtrum and Cupid's bow) ▲
		T14	Perioral lines (fern pattern technique) ▲
		T19	Augmentation (moderate) ●
		T22	Volumization (dry/wet boundary) ●
		T24	Volumization (vermillion with tubercle accentuation) ●
		T27	Volumization (extreme, multiple injection technique) ●
		T28	Lip tenting technique according to Tom van Eijk ▲
		T37	Mouth corner lift (subtle) ▲
		T45	Augmentation of the upper lip – Pillar Technique according to Anil Rajani ●

11.9 Small Mouth with a Prominent Medial Tubercle

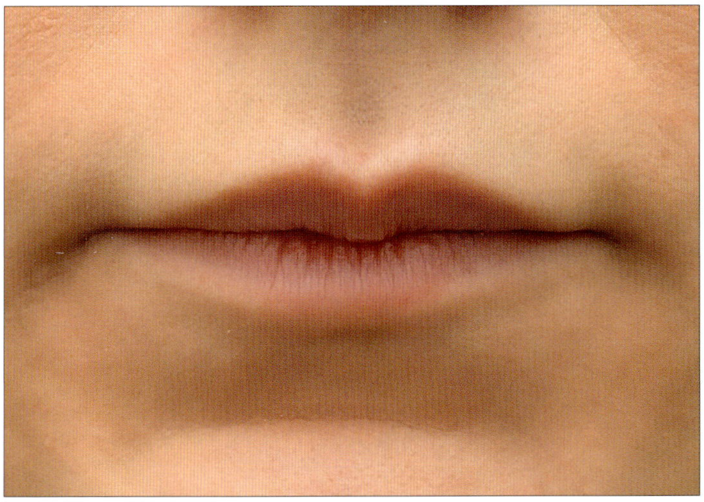

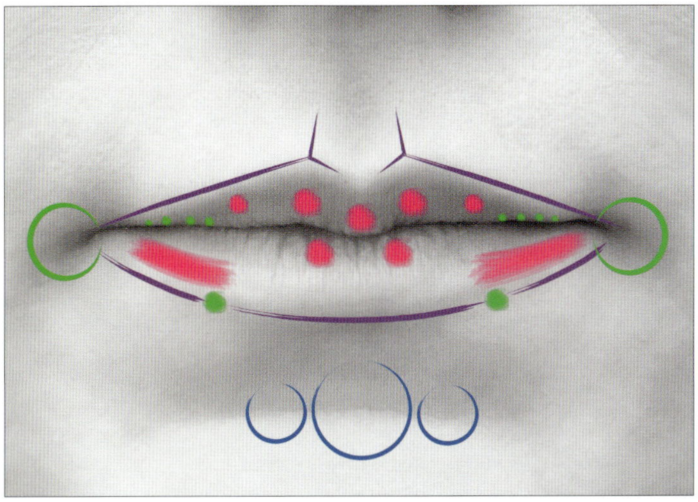

Status: 25-year-old woman, small mouth with a thin, slightly asymmetric lower lip

Treatment Planning with Injection Volumes

- (purple) Contouring (subtle): 0.3 ml
- (pink) Subtle lower lip filling: 0.4 ml
  Subtle upper lip filling: 0.1 ml
  Correct asymmetry (lower lip): 0.05 ml
- (blue) Lift labiomental fold: 0.3 ml
- (green) Reinforce mouth corners: 0.2 ml
  Widening the arch of the lower lip: 0.2 ml
  Raise the upper lip segments close to the mouth corners: 0.2 ml

Caution

- This treatment falls under the category "Beautification" because the lips are still young.
- All that needs to be done is for the volume deficit to be corrected and the shape defined more clearly.

Potential lip treatment techniques to be used according to the therapist's preference and experience			
Level 1		**Level 2**	
T6	Contouring ▲	**T7**	Lip contouring ▲
T25	Volumization (bolus technique) ●	**T19**	Augmentation (moderate) ●
T29	Volumization (labiomental fold) ●	**T23**	Augmentation from the mucous membrane ●
		T24	Volumization (vermillion with tubercle accentuation) ●
		T26	Volumization (cutaneous part of the lip) ●
		T37	Mouth corner lift (subtle) ▲
		T42	Widening the arch of the lower lip ▲
		T45	Augmentation of the upper lip – Pillar Technique according to Anil Rajani ▲

11.10 Sad, Young Mouth

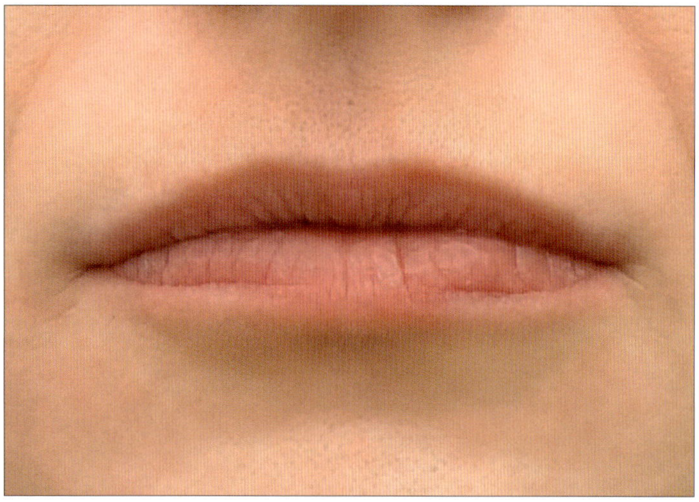

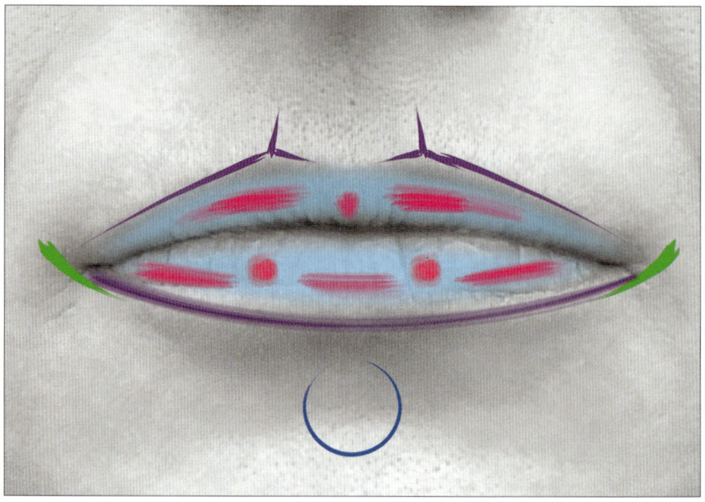

Status: 35-year-old woman, sad mouth with dry lip skin texture, irregular retractions at the lower lip margin and downturned mouth corners, poorly defined contours, philtrum, and Cupid's bow

Treatment Planning with Injection Volumes

- (light blue) Hydration (vermillion) possible: 0.4 ml
- (purple) Minimal contouring of the philtrum: 0.05 ml
  Minimal contouring of the Cupid's bow peaks: 0.05 ml
  Contouring: 0.5 ml
- (pink) Moderate lower lip filling: 0.4 ml
  Subtle upper lip filling: 0.2 ml
- (blue) Lift labiomental fold: 0.3 ml
- (green) Strongly lift mouth corners: 0.2 ml

Caution

- The retractions at the lower lip margin can be stubborn. If so, they will need to be loosened with the cannula (by teasing apart the tissue layers), and gently filled. Take care not to overcorrect!

Potential lip treatment techniques to be used according to the therapist's preference and experience

Level 1		Level 2	
T6	Contouring ▲	**T3**	Hydration (vermillion) ●
T15	Four-point volume replacement ●	**T7**	Lip contouring ▲
T25	Volumization (bolus technique) ●	**T10**	Modeling (philtrum and Cupid's bow) ▲
T29	Volumization (labiomental fold) ▲	**T19**	Augmentation (moderate) ●
		T26	Volumization (cutaneous part of the lip) ●
		T34	Augmentation (marionette lines) ▲
		T38	Mouth corner lift (strong) ▲

11.11 Dry Lips

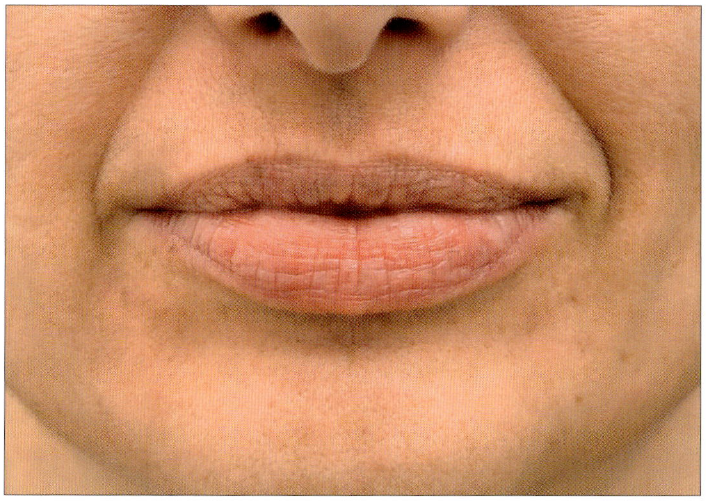

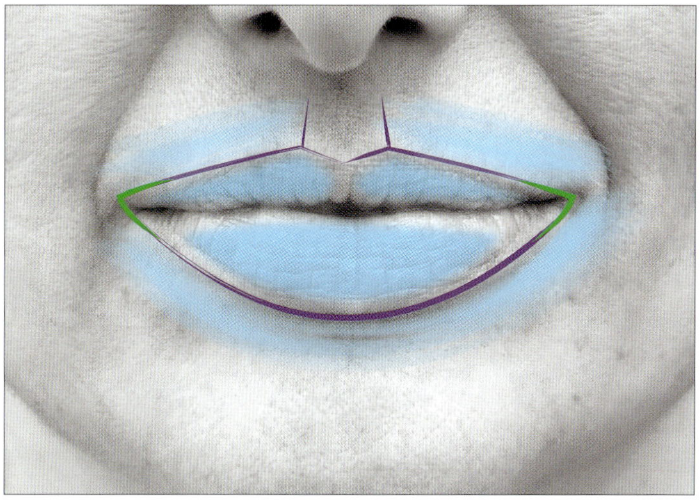

Status: 45-year-old woman, extremely dry lips with a full shape, perioral lines due to extremely dry skin, poorly defined philtrum and Cupid's bow contours, slight labiomental fold

Treatment Planning with Injection Volumes

- Perioral hydration: 1.0 ml
  Hydration of the lips with low-crosslinked gel: 1.0 ml
- Contour philtrum: 0.1 ml
  Contour Cupid's bow peaks: 0.1 ml
  Contouring: 0.5 ml
- Reinforce mouth corners: 0.1 ml

Caution

- This treatment is highly traumatizing due to the multiple injections with a sharp needle and is associated with severe swellings.
- The long-term effect is very good.

Potential lip treatment techniques to be used according to the therapist's preference and experience			
Level 1		**Level 2**	
T1	Hydration ●	**T2**	Hydration (cutaneous part of the lip) ●
T6	Contouring ▲	**T3**	Hydration (vermillion) ●
T9	Contouring (philtrum) ▲	**T4**	Revitalization (vermillion) according to Patrick Trevidic ●
T29	Volumization (labiomental fold) ●	**T7**	Lip contouring ▲
		T37	Mouth corner lift (subtle) ▲

Illustrated Guide "The Lips"

12 Appendix

References

André P, Azib N, Berros P, et al. (2012): Anatomy and Volumising Injections. Master Collection 2. Paris: E2e Medical Publishing.

Azib N (2011): Anaesthesia of the Lips prior to Filler Injection. In: Azib N, Charrier JP, Cornette de Saint Cyr B, et al.: Anatomy & Lip Enhancement. Master Collection 4. Paris: E2e Medical Publishing.

Becker-Wegerich PM (2011): Sexy Lippen. Lippenmodellierung mit der Becker-Wegerich-Technik – die sanfte Perfektionierung der individuellen Natur. Annabelle Issue 15/11:122.

Becker-Wegerich PM (2016a): Filler – Grundlagen: Lippen und Umgebung. Anatomie, Rheologie und Tipps zur Therapievorbereitung. Dermatologie Praxis 26(3):21–25.

Becker-Wegerich PM (2016b): Filler – Praxis: Lippen und Umgebung. Lippeninjektionstechniken und zu berücksichtigende unerwünschte Wirkungen. Dermatologie Praxis 26(4):26–30.

Benedetto AV (ed) (2018): Botulinum Toxins in Clinical Aesthetic Practice. 2 volumes. 3rd ed. Boca Raton: CRC Press.

Braun M, Braun S, van Eijk T (2010): Lip tenting: a simple technique for better lip enhancement. J Drugs Dermatol 9:559–560.

Brusco D (2019): Dentoskelettale Einflüsse auf die Ästhetik der Lippen. Unpublished manuscript.

Brusco D, Triaca A (2013): Skelettale und dentoalveoläre Maßnahmen zur Profiloptimierung. J Ästhet Chir 6:21–25.

Bunte.de Redaktion (2018): Geheimnis gelüftet – Das verrät deine Lippenform über deinen Charakter! https://www. bunte.de/beauty/geheimnis-gelueftet-das-verraet-deinelippenform-ueber-deinen-charakter.html (last accessed 15.12.2019).

Chang P (2014): Lip Augmentation Technique Virginia: Phillip Chang, MD. https://www.youtube.com/watch?v=93dQNCWjbWc (last accessed 09.08.2020).

Charrier JB (2011): Bone Support of the Lips: how adult orthognathic surgery can enhance the smile. In: Azib N, Charrier JP, Cornette de Saint Cyr B, et al.: Anatomy & Lip Enhancement. Master Collection 4. Paris: E2e Medical Publishing.

Cotofana S, Pretterklieber B, Lucius R, et al. (2017): Distribution Pattern of the Superior and Inferior Labial Arteries: Impact for Safe Upper and Lower Lip Augmentation Procedures. Plast Reconstr Surg 139:1075–1082.

Criollo-Lamilla G, DeLorenzi C, Karpova E, et al. (2017): Anatomy & Filler Complications. Master Collection 5. Paris: E2e Medical Publishing.

Criollo-Lamilla G, Garcia P, Trévidic P (2011): Lips and Botulinum Toxin. In: Azib N, Charrier JP, Cornette de Saint Cyr B, et al.: Anatomy & Lip Enhancement. Master Collection 4. Paris: E2e Medical Publishing.

DeLorenzi C (2014): Complications of injectable fillers, part 2: vascular complications. Aesthet Surg J 34:584–600.

DeLorenzi C (2017): New High Dose Pulsed Hyaluronidase Protocol for Hyaluronic Acid Filler Vascular Adverse Events. Aesthet Surg J 37:814–825.

Dmitrieva I (2011): Lip Enhancement: Modern Injection Products. In: Azib N, Charrier JP, Cornette de Saint Cyr B, et al.: Anatomy & Lip Enhancement. Master Collection 4. Paris: E2e Medical Publishing.

DocCheck Flexikon: Lippe. https://flexikon.doccheck.com/de/Lippe (last accessed 13.12.2019).

dpa-Meldung (2016): Wenn Schönheit zur Sucht wird. Zeit Online. https://www.zeit.de/news/2016-03/09/gesellschaft-wenn-schoenheit-zur-sucht-wird-09104802 (last accessed 13.12.2019).

Galderma (Ed.) (no date): Die Gesichtsanatomie. Information leaflet, 80 pp.

Goisis M, Guareschi M (2017): Anatomy and Proportions in Asian Patients. Paris: E2e Medical Publishing.

Gout U (2011): History of Lip Treatment. In: Azib N, Charrier JP, Cornette de Saint Cyr B, et al.: Anatomy & Lip Enhancement. Master Collection 4. Paris: E2e Medical Publishing.

Hesse Z (2016): Handbuch Faltenunterspritzung mit Hyaluronsäure. Datteln: MediNostik-Verlag.

Ibhler N, Penna V, Stark GB (2011): Ageing of the Lips: Photomorphometry, Magnetic Resonance Imaging and Histology. In: Azib N, Charrier JP, Cornette de Saint Cyr B, et al.: Anatomy & Lip Enhancement. Master Collection 4. Paris: E2e Medical Publishing.

Karam AM, Goldman MP (2014): Rejuvenation of the Aging Face. A Comprehensive Approach to Treatment. London: JP Medical Ltd.

Kechichian E, El Khoury R, Helou J (2017): Less Pain, More Gain: Lip Augmentation with Insulin Syringes. Dermatol Surg 43:979–981.

Kerscher M, Bayrhammer J, Reuther T (2008): Rejuvenating influence of a stabilized hyaluronic acid-based gel of nonanimal origin on facial skin aging. Dermatol Surg 34:720–726.

Kim H-J, Seo KK, Lee H-K, Kim J (2016): Clinical Anatomy of the Face for Filler and Botulinum Toxin Injection. Singapore: Springer Science+Business Media.

Lemaire T, Garcia P (2011): Anatomy of Lips. In: Azib N, Charrier JP, Cornette de Saint Cyr B, et al.: Anatomy & Lip Enhancement. Master Collection 4. Paris: E2e Medical Publishing.

Noël X (2011): Ageing of Upper Lips: Clinical Analysis. In: Azib N, Charrier JP, Cornette de Saint Cyr B, et al.: Anatomy & Lip Enhancement. Master Collection 4. Paris: E2e Medical Publishing.

Oberhofer E (2015): "Passen diese Lippe zu Ihnen?". Interview mit Dr. P Becker-Wegerich. Der Deutsche Dermatologe 63:51.

Padey H (2011): Male Lip Enhancement Guidelines. In: Azib N, Charrier JP, Cornette de Saint Cyr B, et al.: Anatomy & Lip Enhancement. Master Collection 4. Paris: E2e Medical Publishing.

Pavicic T (2011): Complications of Lip Treatments. In: Azib N, Charrier JP, Cornette de Saint Cyr B, et al.: Anatomy & Lip Enhancement. Master Collection 4. Paris: E2e Medical Publishing.

Penna V, Stark GB, Voigt M, Mehlhorn A, Iblher N (2015): Classification of the Aging Lips: A Foundation for an Integrated Approach to Perioral Rejuvenation. Aesthetic Plast Surg 39:1–7.

Radlanski RJ, Wesker KH (2012): Das Gesicht. Bildatlas klinische Anatomie. Berlin: KVM – Der Medizinverlag.

Rajani A (2019): Watch Lip Filler Pillar Technique with Before and After-Portland Oregon. https://youtu.be/pojaM40u2pU (last accessed 13.12.2019).

Rejuvent, Medical Spa & Surgery (2017): The Secret to Natural and Beautiful Lips – with Dr. Bouzoukis. https://www.youtube.com/watch?v=3SRk7ZZ2RlE (last accessed 15.12.2019).

Sattler G, Sommer B (2015): Bildatlas der ästhetischen Augmentationsverfahren mit Fillern. Dosierung, Lokalisation, Anwendung. 2nd Ed. Berlin: KVM – Der Medizinverlag.

Snozzi P, Van Loghem J (2018): Complication Management Following Rejuvenation Procedures with Hyaluronic Acid Fillers—an Algorithm-based Approach. Plast Reconstr Surg Glob Open 6(12):e2061.

Swift A (2017): Defining Facemaps. https://www.youtube.com/watch?v=1glLW6DCjeQ (last accessed 09.08.2020).

Swift A, Remington K (2011): BeautiPHIcation™: a global approach to facial beauty. Clin Plast Surg 38:347–377.

Thess K (2010): Körperdysmorphe Störung oder die Angst hässlich zu sein. PDP – Psychodynamische Psychotherapie 9:235–248.

Tonnard PL, Verpaele AM, Bension RH (2018): Centrofacial Rejuvenation. New York: Thieme.

van Eijk T (2007): The Fern Pattern Technique using Restylane. https://tomvaneijkkliniek.nl/fern-pattern-technique-english/ (last accessed 10.02.2020).

van Eijk T (2014): Lip Tenting Technique, Restylane Refyne. https://www.youtube.com/watch?v=uIZ0Y1yo-mA/ (last accessed 10.02.2020).

van Eijk T (2017): Lip Augmentation: Lip Tenting Technique. CosMedicList. https://www.cosmediclist.com/lip-augmentation-lip-tenting/ (last accessed 10.02.2020).

van Eijk T (2017): Lip lines injections, Fern Pattern technique. Tom van Eijk Academy. https://youtu.be/UXaMjLufB0o (last accessed 10.02.2020).

van Eijk T, Braun M (2007): A novel method to inject hyaluronic acid: the Fern Pattern Technique. J Drugs Dermatol 6:805–808.

Verner I (2011): Lip Augmentation Techniques. In: Azib N, Charrier JP, Cornette de Saint Cyr B, et al.: Anatomy & Lip Enhancement. Master Collection 4. Paris: E2e Medical Publishing.

Video Register

Name of Video Clip	Page	QR Code	URL
Technique 1	128		http://media.kvm-verlag.de/DIE_LIPPE/T01.mp4
Technique 2	132		http://media.kvm-verlag.de/DIE_LIPPE/T02.mp4
Technique 3	136		http://media.kvm-verlag.de/DIE_LIPPE/T03.mp4
Technique 5	144		http://media.kvm-verlag.de/DIE_LIPPE/T05.mp4
Technique 6	148		http://media.kvm-verlag.de/DIE_LIPPE/T06.mp4
Technique 7	152		http://media.kvm-verlag.de/DIE_LIPPE/T07.mp4
Technique 8	156		http://media.kvm-verlag.de/DIE_LIPPE/T08.mp4
Technique 9	160		http://media.kvm-verlag.de/DIE_LIPPE/T09.mp4
Technique 10	164		http://media.kvm-verlag.de/DIE_LIPPE/T10.mp4
Technique 11	168		http://media.kvm-verlag.de/DIE_LIPPE/T11.mp4
Technique 12 – Variant 1	174		http://media.kvm-verlag.de/DIE_LIPPE/T12a_Punkt-technik.mp4
Technique 12 – Variant 2	175		http://media.kvm-verlag.de/DIE_LIPPE/T12b_Deh-nungstechnik.mp4
Technique 12 – Variant 3	176		http://media.kvm-verlag.de/DIE_LIPPE/T12c_Kompres-sionstechnik.mp4
Technique 13	178		http://media.kvm-verlag.de/DIE_LIPPE/T13.mp4

Name of Video Clip	Page	QR Code	URL
Technique 14	182		http://media.kvm-verlag.de/DIE_LIPPE/T14.mp4
Technique 15	186		http://media.kvm-verlag.de/DIE_LIPPE/T15.mp4
Technique 16	190		http://media.kvm-verlag.de/DIE_LIPPE/T16.mp4
Technique 17	194		http://media.kvm-verlag.de/DIE_LIPPE/T17.mp4
Technique 18	198		http://media.kvm-verlag.de/DIE_LIPPE/T18.mp4
Technique 19	202		http://media.kvm-verlag.de/DIE_LIPPE/T19.mp4
Technique 21	210		http://media.kvm-verlag.de/DIE_LIPPE/T21.mp4
Technique 22	214		http://media.kvm-verlag.de/DIE_LIPPE/T22.mp4
Technique 23	218		http://media.kvm-verlag.de/DIE_LIPPE/T23.mp4
Technique 24	222		http://media.kvm-verlag.de/DIE_LIPPE/T24.mp4
Technique 25	226		http://media.kvm-verlag.de/DIE_LIPPE/T25.mp4
Technique 26	230		http://media.kvm-verlag.de/DIE_LIPPE/T26.mp4
Technique 27	234		http://media.kvm-verlag.de/DIE_LIPPE/T27.mp4
Technique 28	238		https://www.youtube.com/watch?v=uIZ0Y1yo-mA&feature=youtu.be

Video Register (continued)

Name of Video Clip	Page	QR Code	URL
Technique 29	242		http://media.kvm-verlag.de/DIE_LIPPE/T29.mp4
Technique 30	246		http://media.kvm-verlag.de/DIE_LIPPE/T30.mp4
Technique 31	250		http://media.kvm-verlag.de/DIE_LIPPE/T31.mp4
Technique 32	254		http://media.kvm-verlag.de/DIE_LIPPE/T32.mp4
Technique 34	262		http://media.kvm-verlag.de/DIE_LIPPE/T34.mp4
Technique 37	274		http://media.kvm-verlag.de/DIE_LIPPE/T37.mp4
Technique 38	278		http://media.kvm-verlag.de/DIE_LIPPE/T38.mp4
Technique 39	282		http://media.kvm-verlag.de/DIE_LIPPE/T39.mp4
Technique 40	286		https://www.youtube.com/watch?v=93dQNCWjbWc
Technique 41	290		http://media.kvm-verlag.de/DIE_LIPPE/T41.mp4
Technique 42	294		http://media.kvm-verlag.de/DIE_LIPPE/T42.mp4
Technique 43	298		http://media.kvm-verlag.de/DIE_LIPPE/T43.mp4
Technique 45	306		https://www.youtube.com/watch?v=pojaM40u2pU&feature=youtu.be
Wheal	80		http://media.kvm-verlag.de/DIE_LIPPE/Clip_Lidocain_Quaddel.mp4

Name of File	Page	QR Code	URL
Informed Consent Form	60		http://media.kvm-verlag.de/THE_LIPS/Informed_Consent_Form.pdf
Patient Documentation Form	60		http://media.kvm-verlag.de/THE_LIPS/TEOXANE_INFORMATION_SHEET.pdf
Checklist – Equipment	97		http://media.kvm-verlag.de/THE_LIPS/Checklist_Equipment.pdf
Checklist – Treatment Course	105		http://media.kvm-verlag.de/THE_LIPS/Checklist_Treatment_Course.pdf

Web Links

CANNULAS

TSK Laboratory Europe B.V.
www.tsklab.com

Thiébaud S.A.S.
(Thiébaud Biomedical Devices)
www.thiebaud-surgical.com

Soft Medical Aesthetics
www.sonewa.com

Needle Concept
www.needleconcept.fr

HYPODERMIC NEEDLES

www.bbraun.com
www.bd.com/en-eu/
www.micro-tech-europe.com

FILLER PRODUCTS

Allergan GmbH
www.allergan.com
www.juvederm.com

Croma-Pharma GmbH
https://at.croma.at/home-en/

Galderma
www.galderma.com
www.restylane.com

Merz Pharmaceuticals GmbH
www.belotero.com
www.merz-aesthetics.com
www.merz.com

Teoxane SA
https://www.teoxane.com/en

Image Sources

Main image, front cover
© Svetography, www.shutterstock.com

Pages 41– 43, 1.7 – Merz Scales
© Merz Pharmaceuticals GmbH
www.merz.com

Page 49, Fig. 2.2 – "Bee-stung lips"
© Volodymyr TVERDOKHLIB
www.shutterstock.com

Page 49, Fig. 2.3 – "Heart-shaped lips"
© www.doctorappleclinic.com

Page 94, Fig. 7.16 – Hyaluronidase
© RIEMSER Pharma GmbH
www.riemser.com

Page 119, Fig. 8.22, 8.23 – Cannulas
© TSK Laboratory Europe B.V.
www.tsklab.com

Index

10

10

10

T